AMINO ACIDS
Metabolism and Medical Applications

Edited by

George L. Blackburn, MD, PhD
Associate Professor of Surgery
Harvard Medical School
Director, Nutritional Support Service
New England Deaconess Hospital
Boston, Massachusetts

John P. Grant, MD
Assistant Professor of Surgery
Duke University Medical Center
Durham, North Carolina

Vernon R. Young, PhD
Professor of Nutritional Biochemistry
Massachusetts Institute of Technology
Department of Nutrition and Food Science
Cambridge, Massachusetts

John Wright • PSG Inc
Boston Bristol London
1983

Library of Congress Cataloging in Publication Data
Main entry under title:

Amino acids.

Based on a conference held Mar. 31–Apr. 2, 1982, in Raleigh, N.C.
Includes bibliographies and index.
1. Amino acids—Metabolism—Congresses. 2. Amino acids in human nutrition—Congresses. 3. Amino acids—Therapeutic use—Congresses. I. Blackburn, George L. II. Grant, John Palmer, 1942– . III. Young, Vernon R. (Vernon Robert), 1937– . [DNLM: 1. Amino acids—Congresses. QU 60 A5167 1982]
QP561.A47 1983 612′.01575 82-17328
ISBN 0-7236-7061-7

Published simultaneously by:
John Wright • PSG Inc, 545 Great Road, Littleton, Massachusetts 01460, U.S.A.
John Wright & Sons Ltd, 823–825 Bath Road
Briston BS4 5NU, England

First Printing 1983
Second Printing 1984

Printed in the United States of America.

International Standard Book Number: 07236-7061-7

Library of Congress Catalog Card Number: 82-17328

CONTRIBUTORS

Naji N. Abumrad, MD
Department of Surgery
School of Medicine
Vanderbilt University
Nashville, Tennessee

Siamak A. Adibi, MD, PhD
Clinical Nutrition Center
University of Pittsburgh School of Medicine and Department of Medicine of Montefiore Hospital
Pittsburgh, Pennsylvania

Dean W. Andersen, BS
Department of Pediatrics
College of Medicine
University of Iowa
Iowa City, Iowa

G. Harvey Anderson, PhD
Professor and Chairman
Department of Nutritional Sciences
University of Toronto
Toronto
CANADA

Samuel D. Ang, MD
Department of Surgery
The Graduate Hospital and University of Pennsylvania
Philadelphia, Pennsylvania

Thomas T. Aoki, MD
Associate Professor of Medicine
Harvard Medical School and
Senior Investigator
Joslin Diabetes Foundation
Boston, Massachusetts

Gregory J. Bagby, PhD
Associate Professor of Physiology
Louisiana State University
New Orleans, Louisiana

Edward F. Bell, MD
Department of Pediatrics
College of Medicine
University of Iowa
Iowa City, Iowa

Julien F. Biebuyck, MD, PhD
Department of Anesthesia
Milton S. Hershey Medical Center
Hershey, Pennsylvania

Dennis M. Bier, MD
Professor of Pediatrics
St. Louis Children's Hospital
St. Louis, Missouri

Bruce R. Bistrian, MD, PhD
Assistant Professor of Medicine
Assistant Director
Nutritional Support Service
Harvard Medical School
Boston, Massachusetts

George L. Blackburn, MD, PhD
Associate Professor of Surgery
Chief, Nutrition/Metabolism Laboratory
Cancer Research Institute
Harvard Medical School
Boston, Massachusetts

Julie C. Bleier, MNS, RD
Research Dietician
Emory University
Atlanta, Georgia

Murray F. Brennan, MD
Chief, Gastric and Mixed Tumor Service
Memorial Sloan-Kettering Cancer Center
New York, New York

David C. Brooks, MD
Department of Surgery
Brigham and Women's Hospital
Boston, Massachusetts

David L. Bunner, MD
United States Army Medical Research Institute of Infectious Diseases
Fort Detrick
Frederick, Maryland

John F. Burke, MD
Department of Surgery
Harvard Medical School
Massachusetts General Hospital
Boston, Massachusetts

Michael E. Burt, MD, PhD
Resident in Surgery
New York Hospital
New York, New York

Chun-Rong Chang, PhD
Department of Clinical Nutrition
Division of Surgery
City of Hope National Medical Center
Duarte, California

Rajender K. Chawla, PhD
Associate Professor of Medicine
Emory University
Atlanta, Georgia

Alan D. Cherrington, PhD
Department of Physiology
School of Medicine
Vanderbilt University
Nashville, Tennessee

Tahia T. Daabees, PhD
Department of Pediatrics
College of Medicine
University of Iowa
Iowa City, Iowa

Daniel Debonis, MD
Department of Clinical Nutrition
Division of Surgery
City of Hope National Medical Center
Duarte, California

Ralph B. Dell, MD
Professor of Pediatrics
Columbia University
New York, New York

Jaque Denis
Hopital Ste. Antoine
Paris
FRANCE

Philippe Desurmont
Hopital Regional
Lille
FRANCE

Anna Mae Diehl, MD
Fellow
Johns Hopkins University
Baltimore, Maryland

Richard E. Dinterman, BS
United States Army Medical Research Institute of Infectious Diseases
Fort Detrick
Frederick, Maryland

Lars Ekman, MD
Department of Surgery
Sahlgren's Hospital
University of Gothenburg
Gothenburg
SWEDEN

David H. Elwyn, PhD
Senior Research Associate in Biochemistry (in Surgery)
College of Physicians and Surgeons
Columbia University
New York, New York

Ljusk-Siw Eriksson
Karolinska Institute
Huddinge University Hospital
Huddinge
SWEDEN

Jean-Marc Escoffier
Hopital Ste. Marguerite
Marseille
FRANCE

Jacob J. Faintuch, MD
Assistant Professor
Department of Medicine
Hospital das Clinicas
Sao Paulo
BRAZIL

Joel Faintuch, MD
Assistant Professor of Surgery
Sao Paulo University Medical School
Sao Paulo
BRAZIL

Edward B. Fern, PhD
Clinical Nutrition and Metabolism Unit
Addenbrook Hospital
London
ENGLAND

Lloyd J. Filer, Jr, MD, PhD
Department of Pediatrics
College of Medicine
University of Iowa
Iowa City, Iowa

Kathryn Erskine Flaim, PhD
College of Medicine
Pennsylvania State University
Milton S. Hershey Medical Center
Hershey, Pennsylvania

Yoshiaki Fujita, PhD
Chief of Division of Nutrition
Tokyo Metropolitan Institute of Gerontology
Tokyo
JAPAN

Peter J. Garlick, PhD
Clinical Nutrition and Metabolism Unit
Addenbrook Hospital
London
ENGLAND

A.P. Gauthier
Hopital Ste. Marguerite
Marseille
FRANCE

N. Theresa Glanville
Department of Nutritional Sciences
University of Toronto
Toronto
CANADA

Alfred L. Goldberg, PhD
Department of Physiology and Biophysics
Harvard Medical School
Boston, Massachusetts

Richard D. Goodenough, MD
Massachusetts General Hospital
Shriners Burns Institute
Boston, Massachusetts

John P. Grant, MD
Assistant Professor of Surgery
Duke University Medical Center
Durham, North Carolina

Lars Hagenfeldt
Karolinska Institute
Huddinge University Hospital
Huddinge
SWEDEN

Alfred E. Harper, PhD
Departments of Nutritional Sciences and Biochemistry
University of Wisconsin
Madison, Wisconsin

Richard A. Hawkins, PhD
Professor of Physiology
Chief, Division of Research
Department of Anesthesia
Hershey Medical Center
The Pennsylvania State University
Hershey, Pennsylvania

Morey W. Haymond, MD
Associate Professor of Medicine
Department of Pediatrics and Medicine
Endocrine Research Unit
Mayo Clinic and Foundation
Rochester, Minnesota

William C. Heird, MD
Associate Professor of Pediatrics
Columbia University
New York, New York

H. Franklin Herlong, MD
Assistant Professor of Medicine
Johns Hopkins University
Baltimore, Maryland

L. Robert Hill, MS
Department of Clinical Nutrition
Division of Surgery
City of Hope National Medical Center
Duarte, California

Leonard J. Hoffer, MD, PhD
Fellow, Clinical Nutrition
New England Deaconess Hospital
Boston, Massachusetts

Goro Inoue, MD
Department of Nutrition
School of Medicine
University of Tokushima
Tokushima
JAPAN

Khursheed N. Jeejeebhoy, MD
Professor of Medicine
University of Toronto and
Director, Division of Gastroenterology
Toronto General Hospital
Toronto
CANADA

Leonard S. Jefferson, PhD
College of Medicine
Pennsylvania State University
Hershey Medical Center
Hershey, Pennsylvania

Siroj Kanjanapanjapol, MD
Lecturer
Department of Surgery
Ramathibodi Hospital
Bangkok
THAILAND

Auchai Kanjanapitak, MD
Associate Professor of Surgery
Department of Surgery
Ramathibodi Hospital
Bangkok
THAILAND

Irene E. Karl, PhD
Research Professor of Medicine
Department of Medicine
Washington University School of Medicine
St. Louis, Missouri

G. Raja Kapadia, MD
Department of Surgery
Brigham and Women's Hospital
Boston, Massachusetts

Isao Kawamura, PhD
Research Fellow in Surgery
Harvard Medical School
Boston, Massachusetts

John M. Kinney, MD
Professor of Surgery
Director of Surgical Metabolism Program
College of Physicians and Surgeons
Columbia University
New York, New York

Kyoichi Kishi, MD
Associate Professor
Department of Nutrition
School of Medicine
University of Tokushima
Tokushima
JAPAN

Tatsushi Komatsu, PhD
Instructor
Department of Nutrition
School of Medicine
University of Tokushima
Tokushima
JAPAN

Joel D. Kopple, MD
Division of Nephrology and Hypertension
Harbor—UCLA Medical Center
Torrance, California

William W. Lacy, MD
Department of Medicine
School of Medicine
Vanderbilt University
Nashville, Tennessee

Aurora Landel, PhD
Department of Clinical Nutrition
Division of Surgery
City of Hope National Medical Center
Duarte, California

Charles H. Lang, PhD
Post-Doctoral Fellow in Physiology
Louisiana State University
New Orleans, Louisiana

Edmund T.S. Li
Department of Nutritional Sciences
University of Toronto
Toronto
CANADA

Chun-Chih Lo, MS
Department of Clinical Nutrition
Division of Surgery
City of Hope National Medical Center
Duarte, California

Calvin L. Long, PhD
Professor of Surgery and
Biochemistry
Medical College of Ohio
Toledo, Ohio

Kent G. Lundholm, MD, PhD
Department of Surgery
Sahlgren's Hospital
University of Gothenburg
Gothenburg
SWEDEN

Marcel C.C. Machado, MD
Associate Professor of Surgery
Sao Paulo University Medical School
Sao Paulo
BRAZIL

Anke M. Mans, PhD
Department of Anesthesia
Milton S. Hershey Medical Center
Hershey, Pennsylvania

Dwight E. Matthews, PhD
Research Assistant Professor of Internal Medicine
Department of Medicine
Washington University School of Medicine
St. Louis, Missouri

Owen P. McGuinness, BS
Fellow in Physiology
Louisiana State University
New Orleans, Louisiana

George A. McNamee, Jr, VC
United States Army Medical Research Institute of Infectious Diseases
Fort Detrick
Frederick, Maryland

Margaret A. McNurlan, PhD
Department of Biochemistry
School of Medicine
St. George's Hospital
London
ENGLAND

Michael M. Meguid, MD, PhD
Department of Clinical Nutrition
Division of Surgery
City of Hope National Medical Center
Duarte, California

Carol Meredith, PhD
Laboratory of Human Nutrition
Department of Nutrition and Food Science
Massachusetts Institute of Technology
Cambridge, Massachusetts

Henri Michel
Hopital Saint-Eloi
Montpellier
FRANCE

William E. Mitch, MD
Associate Professor of Medicine
Harvard Medical School
Brigham and Women's Hospital
Boston, Massachusetts

Lyle L. Moldawer
Research Associate
Nutrition/Metabolism Laboratory
Cancer Research Institute
Harvard Medical School
Boston, Massachusetts

Kathleen J. Motil, MD, PhD
Assistant Professor of Pediatrics
Baylor University Medical School
Houston, Texas

Ferdinand Muhlbacher, MD
Surgical Staff Consultant
University of Vienna
Vienna
AUSTRIA

Hamish N. Munro, MB, DSc
Director
USDA Human Nutrition Research Center
Tufts University
Boston, Massachusetts

Stephen Nissen, DVM, PhD
Department of Pediatrics
Endocrine Research Unit
Mayo Clinic and Medical School
Rochester, Minnesota

Richard Odessey, PhD
Department of Physiology
Louisiana State University Medical Center
New Orleans, Louisiana

Ikuo Ohara
Ajinomoto Life Science Laboratory
Tokyo
JAPAN

Hiroyuki Ohashi
Ajinomoto Life Science Laboratory
Tokyo
JAPAN

Mei Ohno, PhD
Managing Director
Ajinomoto Company, Inc.
Tokyo
JAPAN

Pierre Opolon
Hopital Ste. Antoine
Paris
FRANCE

J.C. Paris
Hopital Regional
Lille
FRANCE

Harbhajan S. Paul, PhD
Assistant Professor of Medicine and Biochemistry
Montefiore Hospital
University of Pittsburgh School of Medicine
Pittsburgh, Pennsylvania

Stephen D. Phinney, MD, PhD
Research Assistant Professor of Medicine
University of Vermont
Burlington, Vermont

Arrigo A. Raia, MD
Professor of Surgery
Sao Paulo University Medical School
Sao Paulo
BRAZIL

Daniel Rudman, MD
Professor of Medicine
Director, Clinical Research Facility
Emory University
Atlanta, Georgia

Hanspeter Schwarz, MD
Research Instructor
Department of Medicine
Washington University School of Medicine
St. Louis, Missouri

Robert Smith, MD
Assistant Professor of Medicine
Harvard Medical School, and
Senior Investigator
Joslin Diabetes Foundation
Boston, Massachusetts

John J. Spitzer, MD
Professor and Head, Department of Physiology
Louisiana State University
New Orleans, Louisiana

William P. Steffee, MD, PhD
Director
Department of Medicine
St. Vincent Charity Hospital and Health Center
Cleveland, Ohio

Lewis D. Stegink, PhD
Departments of Pediatrics and Biochemistry
College of Medicine
University of Iowa
Iowa City, Iowa

T. Peter Stein, PhD
Department of Surgery
The Graduate Hospital and University of Pennsylvania
Philadelphia, Pennsylvania

Kurt E. Steiner, PhD
Department of Physiology
School of Medicine
Vanderbilt University
Nashville, Tennessee

John A. Sturman, PhD
Institute for Basic Research in Developmental Disabilities
Staten Island, New York

Toru Takami, PhD
Ajinomoto Life Science Laboratory
Tokyo
JAPAN

Vichai Tanphaichitr, MD, MSc (Med), PhD
Professor of Medicine and Chief, Division of Nutrition and Biochemical Medicine
Faculty of Medicine
Ramathibodi Hospital
Bangkok
THAILAND

Alice Thienprasert, MS
Graduate Student in Nutrition
Ramathibodi Hospital
Bangkok
THAILAND

M. Veyrac
Hopital Saint-Eloi
Montpellier
FRANCE

John Wahren, MD
Professor
Karolinska Institute
Department of Clinical Physiology
Huddinge University Hospital
Huddinge
SWEDEN

Mackenzie Walser, MD
Departments of Pharmacology and Medicine
School of Medicine
Johns Hopkins University
Baltimore, Maryland

Robert W. Wannemacher, Jr, PhD
United States Army Medical Research Institute of Infectious Diseases
Fort Detrick
Frederick, Maryland

Douglas W. Wilmore, MD
Associate Professor of Surgery
Harvard Medical School and
Associate Staff
Brigham and Women's Hospital
Boston, Massachusetts

Robert W. Winters, MD
Medical Director
Home Nutritional Support, Inc.
Verona, New Jersey

Marta H. Wolfe, MS, MPH
Massachusetts General Hospital
Shriners Burns Institute
Boston, Massachusetts

Richard J. Wurtman, MD
Professor of Neuroendocrine Regulation
Massachusetts Institute of Technology
Cambridge, Massachusetts

Vernon R. Young, PhD
Professor of Nutritional Biochemistry
Massachusetts Institute of Technology
Cambridge, Massachusetts

Yasumi Yugari, MD
Director
Ajinomoto Life Science Laboratory
Tokyo
JAPAN

Wilbur L. Zike, MD
Department of Surgery
College of Medicine
University of Iowa
Iowa City, Iowa

CONTENTS

Preface xix
George L. Blackburn

Acknowledgment xx

Introduction xxi
Mei Ohno

Section I **Physiology of Whole Body Amino Acid Metabolism**

1 **Metabolism and Functions of Amino Acids in Man—Overview and Synthesis** 1
Hamish N. Munro

2 **Modulation of Amino Acid Metabolism by Protein and Energy Intakes** 13
Vernon R. Young, Russell D. Yang, Carol Meredith, Dwight E. Matthews, Dennis M. Bier

3 **Developmental Aspects of Amino Acid Metabolism, with Reference to Sulfur Amino Acids** 29
John A. Sturman

4 **Aging: Amino Acid and Protein Metabolism** 37
Kent G. Lundholm

Communications

Whole Body Protein Turnover, Studied with ^{15}N-Glycine, During Weight Reduction by Moderate Energy Reduction 48
Leonard J. Hoffer, Bruce R. Bistrian, Stephen D. Phinney, George L. Blackburn, Vernon R. Young

Amino Acid Requirements of Japanese Young Men 55
Goro Inoue, Tatsushi Komatsu, Kyoichi Kishi, Yoshiaki Fujita

Section II **Metabolism of Amino Acids**

5 **Amino Acids and Gluconeogenesis 63**
Alan D. Cherrington, Kurt E. Steiner, William W. Lacy

6 **Urea Metabolism: Regulation and Sources of Nitrogen 77**
Mackenzie Walser

6A **Effects of Ketone Bodies on Leucine and Alanine Metabolism in Normal Man 89**
Morey W. Haymond, Steven L. Nissen, John M. Miles

Communications

Hormonal Regulation of Leucine Metabolism in the Conscious Dog 96
Naji N. Abumrad, Phillip E. Williams, William W. Lacy

Quantitation of Branched-Chain Amino and α-Ketoacids by HPLC 101
Steven L. Nissen, Carol Van Huysen, Morey W. Haymond

Section III **Amino Acid Interrelationships**

7 **Dispensable and Indispensable Amino Acid Interrelationships 105**
Alfred E. Harper

8 **Factors Influencing Utilization of Glycine, Glutamate and Aspartate in Clinical Products 123**
Lewis D. Stegink, Edward F. Bell, Tahia T. Daabees, Dean W. Andersen, Wilbur L. Zike, Lloyd J. Filer, Jr.

9 ***In Vivo* and *In Vitro* Branched-Chain Amino Acid Interactions 147**
Michael M. Meguid, Hanspeter Schwartz Dwight E. Matthews, Irene E. Karl, Vernon R. Young, Dennis M. Bier

Communications

Interrelationship Between Phenylalanine and Tyrosine Metabolism in the Postabsorptive Rat 155
Lyle L. Moldawer, Isao Kawamura,
Bruce R. Bistrian, George L. Blackburn

Relationship of Plasma Leucine and α-Ketoisocaproate ^{13}C Enrichment During a L-[1-^{13}C] Leucine Infusion in Man 159
Dwight E. Matthews, Hanspeter Schwartz
Russell D. Yang, Kathleen J. Motil,
Vernon R. Young, Dennis M. Bier

Section IV Amino Acid–Organ Interrelationships

LIVER

10 **Role of Amino Acid Availability in the Regulation of Liver Protein Synthesis 167**
Leonard S. Jefferson, Kathryn E. Flaim

11 **Amino Acid Metabolism as Studied in the Isolated Hepatocyte 183**
Khursheed N. Jeejeebhoy

Communications

The Effect of High Doses of Leucine on Protein Synthesis in Rat Tissues 188
Margaret A. McNurlan, Edward B. Fern,
Peter J. Garlick

A Possible Role for the Muscle in the Regulation and Oxidation of Branched-Chain Amino Acid in the Liver 191
Harbhajan S. Paul, Siamak A. Adibi

MUSCLE

12 **Factors Affecting Protein Balance in Skeletal Muscle in Normal and Pathological States 201**
Alfred L. Goldberg

Communication

Is the Liver or the Periphery Limiting for Hepatic Utilization of Amino Acids in Cancer-Induced Malnutrition? 212
Lars Ekman, Kent G. Lundholm

BRAIN

13 **Implications of Parenteral and Enteral Amino Acid Mixtures in Brain Function 219**
Richard J. Wurtman

14 **Amino Acids and the Regulation of Quantitative and Qualitative Aspects of Food Intake 225**
G. Harvey Anderson, N. Theresa Glanville, Edmund T.S. Li

Communication

Alterations in Amino Acid Transport Across Blood-Brain Barrier in Rats Following Portacaval Shunting 239
Richard A. Hawkins, Anke M. Mans, Julien F. Biebuyck

GASTROINTESTINAL

15 **Amino Acid and Peptide Absorption in Human Intestine: Implications for Enteral Nutrition 255**
Siamak A. Adibi

Section V Clinical Aspects of Amino Acid Metabolism

GENERAL CONSIDERATIONS

16 **An Evaluation of Techniques for Estimating Amino Acid Requirements in Hospitalized Patients 265**
George L. Blackburn, Lyle L. Moldawer

17 **Nutritional Consideration of Amino Acid Profiles in Clinical Therapy 291**
Calvin L. Long

18 **Enteral Administration of Amino Acids in Clinical Nutrition 309**
Yasumi Yugari, Ikuo Ohara, Hiroyuki Ohashi, Toru Takami

19 **Parenteral Amino Acid Nutrition in Infants 327**
Robert W. Winters, William C. Heird, Ralph B. Dell

20 **Nutritional Considerations and the Elderly Patient 333**
William P. Steffee

Communication

Urinary Excretion of Carnitine, A Lysine Catabolite, in Patients on Partial Parenteral Nutrition 342
Vichai Tanphaichitr, Alice Thienprasert, Siroj Kanjanapanjapol, Auchai Kanjanapitak

MALNUTRITION

21 **Clinical Impact of Protein Malnutrition on Organ Mass and Function 347**
John P. Grant

22 **Repletion of the Malnourished Patient 359**
David H. Elwyn

TRAUMA AND INFECTION

23 **Amino Acid Support in the Hypercatabolic Patient 377**
John M. Kinney

24 **Altered Amino Acid Concentrations and Flux Following Traumatic Injury 387**
Douglas W. Wilmore, David C. Brooks, Ferdinand Muhlbacher, C. Raja Kapadia, Thomas T. Aoki, Robert Smith

Communications

Protein Dynamics in Stress 396
Robert R. Wolfe, Richard D. Goodenough, John F. Burke, Marta H. Wolfe

Protein Turnover in Severely Ill Patients As Measured with ^{15}N-Glycine 401
Samuel D. Ang, T. Peter Stein

Nutritional and Metabolic Response to Intravenous Hyperalimentation in Severely Stressed Surgical Patients 406
Joel Faintuch, Jacob J. Faintuch, Marcel C.C. Machado, Arrigo A. Raia

Effect of Diet and Pneumococcal Infection on Protein Dynamics of Blood Lymphocytes in Cynomolgus Monkeys 414
Robert W. Wannemacher, Jr., George A. McNamee, Jr., Richard E. Dinterman, David L. Bunner

Intravenous Alanine Tolerance in Conscious Septic and Nonseptic Rats 417
John J. Spitzer, Gregory J. Bagby, Owen P. McGuinness, Charles H. Lang

Branched-Chain Amino Acid Solutions Enhance Nitrogen Accretion in Postoperative Cancer Patients 421
Michael M. Meguid, Aurora Landel, Chun-Chih Lo, Chun-Rong Chang, Daniel Debonis, L. Robert Hill

CANCER

25 **Protein and Amino Acid Metabolism in Cancer-Bearing Man: The Effects of Total Parenteral Nutrition on Alanine Kinetics 429**
Murray F. Brennan, Michael E. Burt

RENAL FAILURE

26 **Amino Acid Analogues: Metabolism and Use in Patients With Chronic Renal Failure 439**
William E. Mitch

27 **Amino Acid Metabolism in Chronic Renal Failure 451**
Joel D. Kopple

Communication

Purified Rat Kidney Branched-Chain Ketoacid Dehydrogenase Complex Contains Endogenous Kinase Activity 472
Richard Odessey

LIVER FAILURE

28 **Branched-Chain Amino Acids in Hepatic Encephalopathy 477**
H. Franklin Herlong, Anna Mae Diehl

Communications

Cystine and Tyrosine Requirements During the Nutritional Repletion of Cirrhotic Patients 484
Daniel Rudman, Rajender K. Chawla, Julie C. Bleier

Intravenous Administration of Branched-Chain Amino Acids in the Treatment of Hepatic Encephalopathy 497
John Wahren, Jaque Denis, Philippe Desurmont, Ljusk-Siw Eriksson, Jean-Marc Escoffier, A.P. Gauthier, Lars Hagenfeldt, Henri Michel, Pierre Opolon, J.C. Paris, M. Veyrac

Index 501

PREFACE

The proceedings of this conference report on newer aspects of research in the application of amino acid biochemistry to clinical medicine. This interaction between nutrition and medicine requires special definition. For example, we now realize that most amino acids, both dietary indispensable and dispensable, are required to meet the body's metabolic goals including the synthesis of body proteins important for host defense, wound healing, recovery from primary illness, and maintenance of individual tissue and organ function.

Advancement in the medical usage of amino acids depends, to a great extent, on a continuing effort to study several important clinical conditions such as trauma, sepsis, postsurgery, cancer, organ failure, and gastrointestinal dysfunction. Also important is the characterization of protein and amino acid requirements in neonates and in elderly patients. Special consideration must be given to the study of the metabolic changes that occur in disease, particularly the substrate–hormone interactions, the redistribution of body nutrients, and the physiology of malnutrition.

Studies in normal man and unstressed, uninjured animals are crucial to validate methodologies and to establish norms for healthy individuals. However, caution must be taken in extrapolating guidelines for the medical application of amino acids from such data. Clearly, there is the potential to exploit a variety of experimental approaches to elucidate total protein or individual amino acid requirements in diseased patients. Such approaches include investigation of cellular metabolism, nutrient balance studies, and cross-tissue studies such as measurement of arterial–venous concentrations and blood flow in the brain, splanchnic bed, and muscle tissue. These important experiments will form a basis for interpreting physiologic studies to test the use of amino acids in the integrated and functioning whole man.

The members of the organization committee deeply appreciate the efforts and promptness of the authors in submitting their manuscripts, thus allowing an early publication of these proceedings. A special note of thanks goes to the Ajinomoto Company for sponsoring this symposium in celebration of the opening of its first amino acid production plant in the United States.

We hope these proceedings will both facilitate the research efforts of investigators in the field and provide practitioners with an updated summary of progress in the medical applications of amino acids.

George L. Blackburn

ACKNOWLEDGMENT

The editors gratefully acknowledge Ajinomoto U.S.A., Inc. for sponsoring the international symposium:

"Amino Acids: Metabolism and Medical Applications,"
March 31–April 2, 1982, in Raleigh, North Carolina,

from which the contents of this book are drawn.

INTRODUCTION

It is with great pleasure that I have the opportunity to introduce this volume on amino acids metabolism and their medical applications. The articles that follow represent a culmination of many years of research by some of the world's foremost authorities on protein nutrition and amino acid metabolism.

Since the beginning of time, man has selected and refined useful materials for food. Although vast cultural differences remain throughout the world, mankind is unified in its pursuit of more efficient means to obtain the foodstuffs necessary for life. The studies on amino acid metabolism and their medical applications contained in this volume represent an extension of this endeavor.

In many ways, the history of amino acid production is a microcosm of the investigation into amino acid metabolism. The commercial production of amino acids has closely followed the increasing importance of individual amino acids as food supplements and, more recently, as medical products. It was 73 years ago that the Ajinomoto Company was founded to commercially isolate monosodium glutamate from the partial hydrolysis of wheat and soy protein to serve as a flavor enhancer. This represented the first case of industrial production of an amino acid in the world.

In the late 1920s, a joint venture in the United States with the Ajinomoto Company led to the first commercial production of an amino acid in this country. However, reliance on these "extraction" techniques was inadequate to isolate individual amino acids in quantities sufficient to meet the demands of a rapidly expanding field. It was only in the 1950s that fermentation research had progressed sufficiently to permit commercial production of amino acids. It was this single technological advance which was most important to the widespread availability of crystalline amino acids in quantities sufficient for agricultural feeds, for medical uses such as amino acid solutions, and for cosmetic and environmental applications. At the present time, for example, the worldwide production of glutamate exceeds 300,000 tons per year while for lysine the amount is 30,000 tons.

Amino acid synthesis by fermentation may take the form of direct fermentation by bacteria from a simple carbon source or the use of bacteria to enzymatically synthesize an amino acid from an intermediate. Although glutamate was and still continues to be fermented from a wild strain of bacteria, the more common practice today is to use either auxotrophic or regulatory mutants. By selecting a mutant that lacks a negative feedback mechanism, large quantities can be easily produced.

The next great frontier for commercial amino acid production is the application of recombinant DNA techniques. Production efficiency can be drastically increased by identification and isolation of the amino acid-producing enzymes using hybrid plasmid technology.

It is extremely satisfying to observe the profound advances that have been made in our understanding of amino acid metabolism and their medical applications. The editors of this symposium are to be congratulated for bringing together such an esteemed group of investigators to report on their current research achievements. Through increased availability of crystalline amino acids and further understanding of their metabolism and medical uses, progress will continue to be made for the treatment of hospitalized patients.

Mei Ohno, PhD
Ajinomoto Company, Inc.

SECTION I
Physiology of Whole Body Amino Acid Metabolism

1 Metabolism and Functions of Amino Acids in Man—Overview and Synthesis

Hamish N. Munro

This description of the metabolism and functions of amino acids in the body of man is intended to provide an overview of these processes in health and their distortion by some major diseases. The survey will first emphasize the integration of metabolic processes in various organs of the healthy person in order to show how these organs make special contributions to the overall picture of mammalian protein metabolism. This will be followed by an account of alterations in these metabolic processes caused by five diseases—diabetes, renal failure, hepatic cirrhosis, fever and sepsis, and cancer—which have an adverse effect on the integration of metabolism between organs. The integrated actions of organs are essential for the proper utilization of dietary nutrients. An understanding of these processes will surely lead to a rational approach to nutritional therapy of diseases involving specific organs.

AMINO ACID METABOLISM IN HEALTH

Dietary protein provides almost all the organic nitrogen available to the body from the environment. Consequently, it is not surprising that amino acids and their metabolites contribute to numerous pathways throughout the body. The metabolic fates of amino acids can nevertheless be conveniently grouped under three headings (Munro, 1964). *First,* they provide the basic materials for protein synthesis in all tissues. The amount of protein synthesized daily in the body of an adult man is about 300 g (Munro and Crim, 1980). Since this represents daily turnover of protein three times the intake of protein in the average diet, amino acids liberated as a result of breakdown of body protein must be extensively reutilized for synthesis of new tissue protein throughout the body. *Second,* amino acids provide precursors for the synthesis of numerous nitrogenous small molecules. Some of these pathways involve co-operation between tissues. For example, creatine synthesis begins with the formation in the kidney of guanidoacetic acid from arginine and glycine; the reaction product is then transferred to the liver where it is methylated to form creatine. The creatine so formed is next transported in the blood to muscle where it is concentrated. *Third,* amino acids in excess of requirements undergo degradation, the nitrogen moiety eventually forming urea by a reaction sequence located exclusively in the liver. In order to reach the liver, much of this nitrogen is transported from other tissues in the form of nonessential amino acids, notably alanine and glutamine.

These examples of interactions between organs involving amino acids and their metabolites alert us to the cooperative nature of amino acid metabolism. They emphasize that disease of a major organ must cause serious disruption of normal metabolism (Munro, 1982a). The importance of such interactions can be seen by tracing the changes that occur after the influx of amino acids following a meal of protein. Such a meal causes regulatory responses as illustrated in Figure 1-1. Following digestion of the protein in the meal, the resulting free amino acids and small peptides are absorbed into the mucosal cells where the peptides are resolved by peptidases into free amino acids (Kim and Freeman, 1977). In addition, certain amino acids also undergo metabolic changes within the mucosal cells. Thus, glutamic acid and glutamine are transaminated to form alanine, which is transferred via the portal

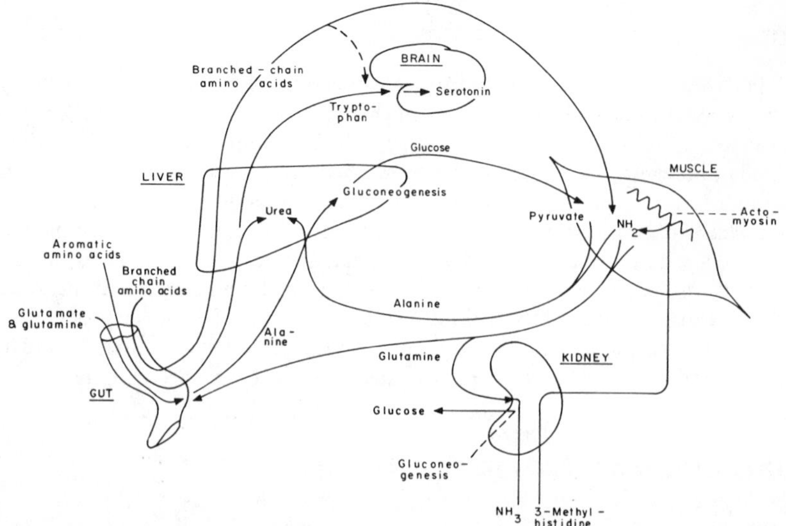

Figure 1-1 Interchanges of amino acids between organs (from Munro, 1982b with permission).

vein to the liver in order to provide carbon for gluconeogenesis while the nitrogen becomes urea. The same transamination reaction also utilizes glutamine coming from the peripheral tissues to form alanine (Windmueller and Spaeth, 1975).

On reaching the liver, the fate of incoming amino acids is determined by whether they are nutritionally essential or nonessential. If the essential amino acid is one of these (histidine, lysine, methionine, phenylalanine, threonine, tryptophan) for which the liver is the major site of catabolism (Miller, 1962), then the amount allowed to pass into the general circulation is regulated by the liver according to the needs of the body for that essential amino acid. Thus, intake of tryptophan beyond the amount needed by the tissues results in induction of the degradative liver enzyme tryptophan oxygenase (Young and Munro, 1973). On the other hand, branched-chain amino acids passing to the liver after a meal of protein are transferred intact to the systemic circulation and undergo transamination and degradation in the peripheral tissues such as muscle, kidney, adipose tissue, and brain. In consequence, the amino acid profile leaving the liver after consuming a large amount of protein is enriched in branched-chain amino acids because excess of the other essential amino acids and the nonessential amino acids have been selectively degraded by the liver. This has been confirmed quantitatively by comparing the flow of amino acids into and out of the liver of man during absorption of a meal (Wahren, Felig, and Hagenfeldt, 1976). This shows (Figure 1-2) that more than 70% of increase in free amino nitrogen leaving the liver after a large protein meal is accounted for by the branched-chain amino acids, compared with a concentration of 20% of these amino acids in the protein consumed in the meal.

This transfer of branched-chain enriched free amino acids to the peripheral tissues is accompanied by their uptake into the cells of muscle and adipose tissue. Arteriovenous catheterization of limb vessels (Wahren et al., 1976; Elia and Livesey, 1981) shows a selective uptake of these amino acids by the peripheral tissues of human subjects following a meal of protein. As Figure 1-2 illustrates, more than half the amino nitrogen removed from the circulation by leg tissues at 30 and 60 minutes after the protein meal were branched-chain amino acids, while at 90 through 180 minutes essentially all the amino acid nitrogen taken up could be accounted for by these amino acids. This entry into muscle and also adipose tissue is facilitated by insulin secreted in response to the carbohydrate and protein components of the meal (Munro, Black, and Thomson, 1959). This action of insulin was demonstrated by earlier experiments (Munro and Thomson, 1953) in which carbohydrate administration was shown to cause a reduction in plasma free amino acids that is least in the case of tryptophan and most extensive in the case of the branched-chain amino acids. These experiments thus indicate that branched-chain amino acids represent the major carriers of amino nitrogen from the viscera to the peripheral tissues. This raises an interesting question regarding the fate of this nitrogen. Branched-chain amino acids account for only 20% of the amino acids needed for muscle protein synthesis. Since the excess of branched-chain amino acids does not leave the muscle in the form of other nitrogenous compounds (Elia and Livesey, 1981), the excess amino nitrogen must be used to synthesize the nonessential amino acids needed for muscle protein synthesis during the absorptive period after the protein meal. The increased rate of catabolism of leucine following a large intake of protein is confirmed by the studies of Motil et al. (1981) on human subjects infused with 1-^{13}C-leucine.

Arteriovenous measurement across limbs and *in vitro* studies show that muscle releases large amounts of alanine and glutamine. Similar reactions occur in adipose

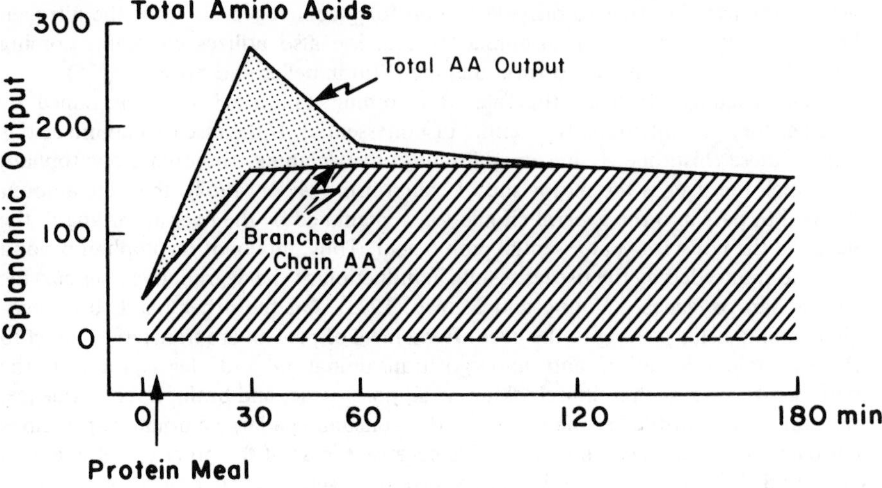

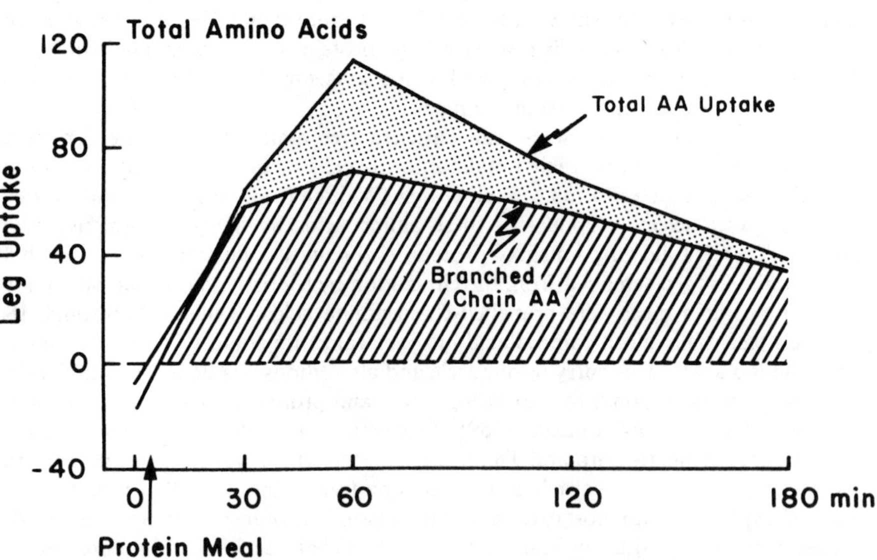

Figure 1-2 Effect of a meal of protein on splanchnic amino acid release (upper panel) and leg uptake of amino acids (lower panel). The exchanges are expressed in μmol/min. (adapted from DeFronzo and Felig, 1980).

tissue. Glutamine is a precursor of alanine in the mucosa of the small intestine and a source of ammonia for the kidney (Figure 1-1). The magnitude of alanine and glutamine release from muscle is considerable. Studies of arteriovenous differences across limbs (Felig, 1981) demonstrate that these two amino acids each account for about 30% to 40% of the total amino acid nitrogen released from the limbs of fasting subjects, thus greatly exceeding the proportions of these two amino acids in muscle protein and indicating their synthesis from precursors within muscle. About half the glutamine released from the peripheral tissues is transformed to alanine in the intestine and, along with alanine coming directly from the carcass, provides the substrate for gluconeogenesis by the liver. This glucose now becomes once more a carbon source available to muscle. This interchange of carbon between muscle and liver as alanine and between liver and muscle as glucose has been named the glucose–alanine cycle (Felig, 1973).

Several investigators have studied the relationship of branched-chain amino acid degradation by muscle and adipose tissue to release of alanine and glutamine by the peripheral tissues. By measuring arteriovenous differences across the arm, Elia and Livesey (1981) found that uptake of branched-chain amino acids following a large meal of meat does not affect glutamine output and actually reduces alanine output. On the other hand, infusion with only leucine resulted in increase output of glutamine from the tissues of the arm, while output of alanine remained unchanged. These studies are consistent with the conclusion of Felig (1981) that the carbon chain of alanine comes from glucose via pyruvate, the supply of which thus becomes rate-limiting for alanine synthesis by transamination, and emphasizes that release of alanine and of glutamine from muscle are independently regulated.

Under conditions of acidosis, the kidney is also a consumer of glutamine in order to provide ammonia for neutralization (Figure 1-1). The origin of this glutamine has been examined in rats made acidotic by a variety of procedures. By measuring amino acid exchange across the kidneys compared with exchange across muscle, liver and nonhepatic splanchnic organs (mainly gut), Schrock and Goldstein (1981) showed that, when acidosis was produced by administration of NH_4Cl or HCl, the increased uptake of glutamine by the acidotic kidney was balanced through increased release of this amino acid from muscle and liver, whereas uptake of glutamine by gut remained unaffected by acidosis. In these forms of acidosis, muscle contributed more total glutamine than did liver. When acidosis was caused experimentally by inducing diabetes in the rats, muscle was the only significant source of extra glutamine.

METABOLISM OF AMINO ACIDS AND ENERGY SUBSTRATES IN SELECTED DISEASES

The preceding section provides a profile of amino acid metabolism which focuses on the cooperative role of organs and tissues in its maintenance and regulation. This permits us in the present section to examine the consequences of malfunction of one or more of the participating organs. To make the picture complete, it is also necessary to recognize that energy metabolism also requires coordination of substrate flow between tissues, so that it is equally vulnerable to distortion by disease. A brief review of the role of different tissues and of hormones in the regulation of carbohydrate and fat metabolism is therefore appropriate before attempting an analysis of the metabolic consequences of disease. More detailed accounts of reactions involved in energy metabolism are provided by the reviews of Robinson and Williamson (1980) and of McGarry and Foster (1980).

Figure 1-3 summarizes the effects of feeding and fasting on metabolic interchanges between adipose tissue, liver and muscle. These are regulated by the plasma levels of insulin and glucagon. Following a meal, insulin level increases and causes

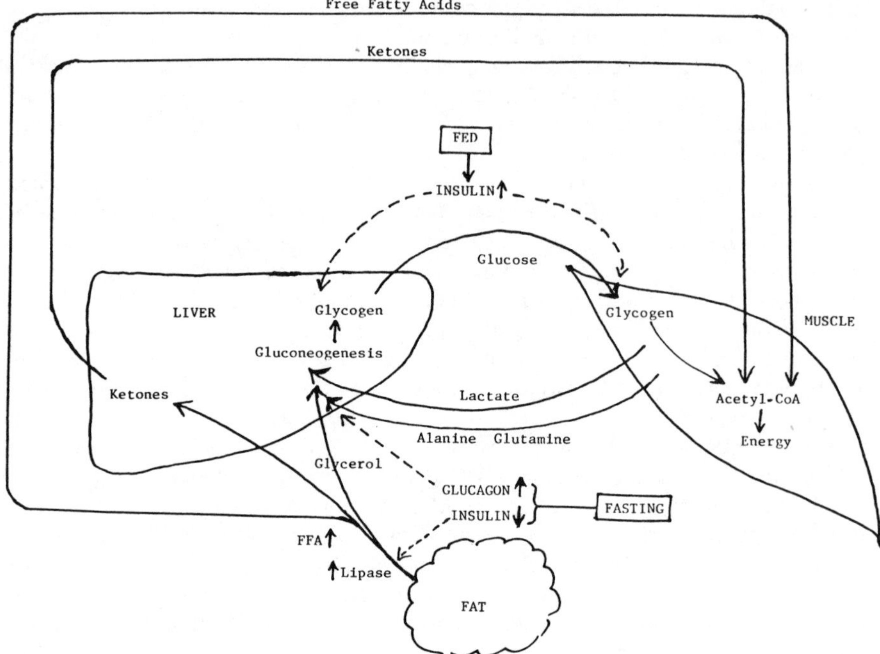

Figure 1-3 Role of liver and muscle in the metabolism of carbohydrate and fat in the fed and the fasted state.

deposition of glycogen in liver and muscle, carbohydrate thus becoming the dominant energy source in both tissues. In contrast, fasting not only lowers plasma insulin levels but increases the concentration of glucagon. The reduced insulin level results in less glycogen deposition, and in activation of adipose tissue lipase, causing release of free fatty acids and glycerol, while the increased level of glucagon promotes formation in the liver of ketone bodies from the incoming free fatty acids. In consequence, free fatty acids and ketone bodies replace glucose as the major fuel available to muscle during fasting.

One common factor in regulating the flow of metabolites of both energy and amino acids in response to fasting and feeding is insulin. In the case of energy metabolism, this hormone determines the type of energy metabolites (sugar versus fatty acids and ketones) available to the peripheral tissues, notably muscle (Figure 1-3). In the case of amino acid metabolism, insulin is also of particular significance, this time for the transfer of branched-chain amino acids into muscle cells and adipose tissue (Figure 1-1). It is therefore important to recognize that, in the five diseases to be discussed below, a recurring major factor is an aberration of function of insulin. This can take the form of insulin release in response to stimulation by a meal (diabetes) or excessive levels of insulin due to lack to regulation of plasma insulin as it passes through the liver (cirrhosis), or to insulin resistance of the tissues (renal failure, sepsis). These and other changes in the profiles of energy substrates and of amino acid utilization are summarized in Table 1-1 for five major diseases described in more detail below.

Table 1-1
Metabolic Profiles in Disease

Metabolite	Diabetes	Uremia	Cirrhosis	Sepsis	Cancer
Blood sugar	↑	↑		↑	↓
Insulin	↓	↑	↑	↑	
Glucagon				↑	
FFA				↓	
Ketones	↑			↓	
Plasma TG	↑	↑		↑	
VLDL	↑	↓			
Plasma BCAA	↑	↓	↓		
BCAA removal	↓	↑	↑	↑	↑
Glutamine release	↑			↑	±
Alanine release (muscle)	±	±		↑	↓
Alanine uptake (liver)	↑	±		↑	
Plasma alanine	↓	±			↓

Diabetes

Following administration of carbohydrate (Munro and Thomson, 1953), there is a rapid reduction in plasma free amino acids which is most marked for the branched-chain amino acids. This phenomenon is insulin-dependent and does not occur in diabetic rats. Measurements of amino acid exchange across the limbs of insulin-dependent diabetic humans also show that lack of insulin impairs uptake of branched-chain amino acids, which therefore increase in the plasma after a meal of protein (Wahren et al., 1976). Whereas alanine release from muscle is not affected by diabetes, extraction of this amino acid by the liver is increased (Wahren et al., 1976). Gluconeogenesis from lactate and pyruvate is also elevated in diabetics, thus contributing to a greater amount of glucose released from the liver when a meal of meat is fed to diabetics. Finally, lack of insulin secretion by the fed diabetic leads to higher levels of free fatty acids in the plasma as well as elevated levels of ketone bodies.

Renal Failure

Many of the metabolic changes occurring in uremia can be related to the intolerance for glucose in cases of chronic renal failure (DeFronzo et al., 1973). DeFronzo and Felig (1980) have shown, by studying uremic patients at a constant level of blood glucose, that such cases have higher insulin levels and lesser rates of removal of glucose from the blood than do nonuremic subjects, consistent with the insulin resistance of uremia. The elevation in insulin also appears to be responsible for the hypertriglyceridemia of uremics (Reaven et al., 1980). DeFronzo and Felig (1980) have explored the effect of the elevated plasma insulin levels in uremia on amino acid metabolism. When a comparison is made of amino acid metabolism in uremia and in insulin-dependent diabetes (Table 1-1), DeFronzo and Felig point out that both conditions exhibit hyperglycemia, although insulin levels are raised in uremia and depressed in diabetes. In diabetes, plasma levels of branched-chain amino acids are elevated due to reduced extraction by muscle and adipose tissue. In contrast, the levels of branched-chain amino acids in plasma are reduced in uremia and can be further depressed by infusion of insulin. Thus insulin resistance in uremic subjects applies only to glucose uptake by tissues which causes insulin secretion to increase. As a result of this persisting hyperinsulinemia in uremia, plasma concentrations of branched-chain amino acids are reduced from accelerated deposition in muscle. Unlike diabetes, there is no disturbance in alanine metabolism in the uremic patient (DeFronzo and Felig, 1980).

Liver Failure

Metabolic changes in cirrhosis of the liver are predictable on the basis of loss of metabolic control by the cirrhotic liver (Figure 1-4). Failure of the damaged liver to remove ammonia and amines formed by intestinal bacteria may contribute to hepatic coma. In addition, recent studies (e.g., Fernstrom et al., 1979) confirm the changed free amino acid patterns in the plasma of the cirrhotic subject, with elevation of the levels of aromatic amino acids (phenylalanine, tyrosine and tryptophan) contrasted with the depressed levels of the branched-chain amino acids. These changes can be explained as a result of loss of two regulatory functions peculiar to the liver. First, the normal liver regulates the passage of the aromatic amino acids into the general circulation. Second, half the insulin secreted by the pancreas is normally removed by the liver (Krass et al., 1974). In consequence, the peripheral plasma of cirrhotic subjects contains excessive levels of insulin, which thus causes increased uptake of branched-chain amino acids by muscle and consequent depression of their plasma levels. Because neutral amino acids compete for access to the brain, the reduction in branched-chain amino acid levels in the plasma of cirrhotic patients increases uptake of amino acid precursors of neurotransmitters such as tryptophan which is rate-limiting for serotonin biosynthesis. Thus, the occurence of elevated plasma levels of tryptophan and reduced levels of branched-chain amino acids in cirrhotics presumably causes overproduction of serotonin through increased uptake of its precursor tryptophan and may thus contribute to the drowsiness of hepatic coma (Munro et al., 1975).

Fever and Sepsis

Hormonal and metabolic changes related to the increased energy output of fever and sepsis are summarized by Beisel et al. (1980). These include elevation of plasma levels of glucocorticoids, glucagon, and especially insulin. The consequences can be interpreted in terms of changes in the metabolism of carbohydrate, fat and amino acids (Figure 1-5). Blood sugar and insulin levels are both elevated in fever and sepsis and the raised insulin level inhibits release of free fatty acids from adipose tissue and, in consequence, the substrate for ketone formation in the liver is reduced (Figure 1-5). For example, induction of sepsis in starving animals causes the ketosis of star-

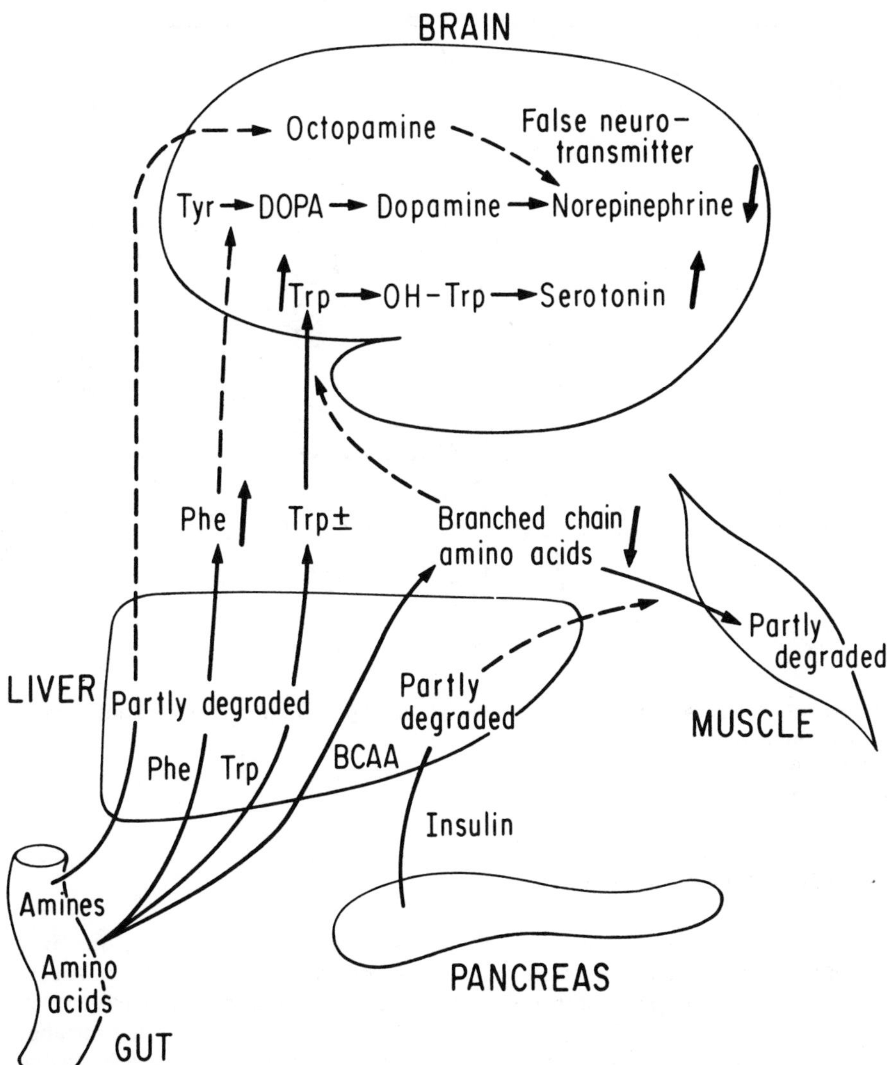

Figure 1-4 Relationship of changes in plasma amino acid imbalance in cirrhosis to brain neurotransmitter function (from Crim and Munro, 1977 with permission).

vation to disappear due to insulin secretion (Neufeld et al., 1976). Elevation of insulin also accelerates passage of branched-chain amino acids into muscle accompanied by an increased release of alanine and glutamine (Wannemacher, 1977). This permits accelerated gluconeogenesis for release of more glucose into the bloodstream (Figure 1-5).

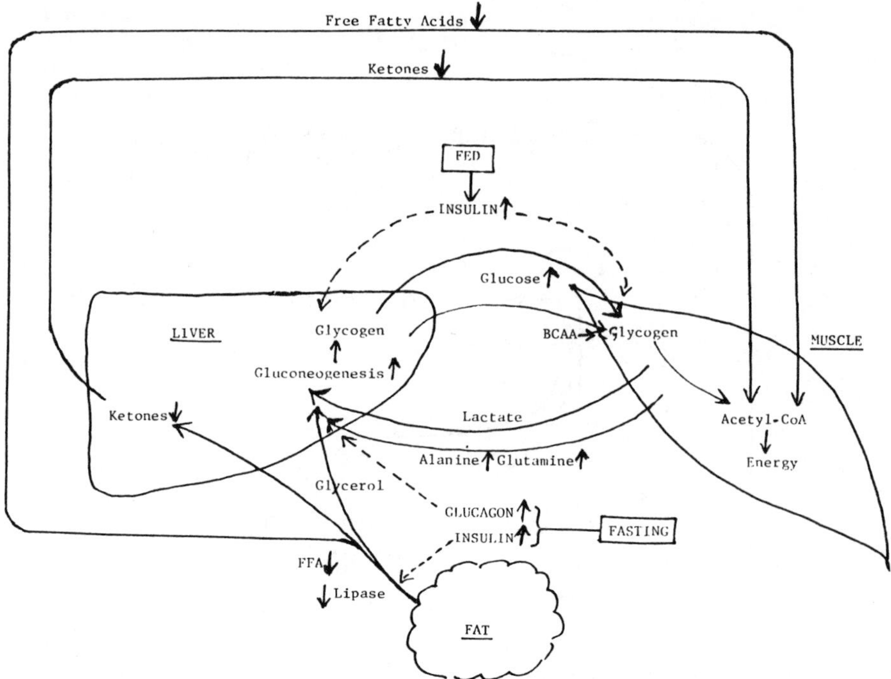

Figure 1-5 Changes in the interchange of energy-yielding substrates and amino acids between organs resulting from sepsis.

Host Metabolism in Cancer

Much of our evidence on the consequences of cancer on host metabolism comes from studies on animal models (see reviews by Goodlad, 1969; Munro, 1977). An experimental tumor takes up both amino acids and glucose and releases lactate, which can be reutilized by the liver for glucose through gluconeogenesis. Muscle metabolism is affected by the presence of the tumor. Both in man and animals, cachexia due to a tumor specifically causes loss of muscle (Munro, 1977). Goodlad and Clark (1980) used diaphragms excised from tumor-bearing rats to show that oxidation of leucine is increased whereas synthesis of muscle protein is diminished, while subsequent studies (Goodlad et al., 1981) showed that muscle protein breakdown is accelerated in the tumor-bearing animal. Although this increased breakdown of muscle protein results in increased release of essential amino acids under *in vitro* conditions, alanine release is depressed unless glucose is added to the medium (Goodlad and Clark, 1980), whereas glutamine output is not depressed and is not affected by addition of glucose to the medium. The reduced alanine release accounts for the low plasma alanine levels of patients with cancer (Clarke et al., 1972) and the low plasma glucose levels of tumor-bearing animals (Waterhouse et al., 1972), the latter indicative of depressed gluconeogenesis.

REFERENCES

Beisel, W.R., Wannemacher, R.W., Jr., and Neufeld, H.A. (1980): Relation of fever to energy expenditure. In: *Assessment of Energy Metabolism in Health and Disease* (ed: J.M. Kinney) pp. 144–150, Ross Laboratories, Columbus, Ohio.

Clarke, E.F., Lewis, A.M., and Waterhouse, C. (1980): Peripheral amino acid levels in patients with cancer. *Cancer* 42:2909–2913.

Crim, M.C., and Munro, H.N. (1977): Protein and amino acid requirements and metabolism in relation to defined formula diets. In: *Defined Formula Diets for Medical Purposes* (ed: M.E. Shils) pp. 5–15, American Medical Association, Chicago, IL.

DeFronzo, R.A., Andres, R., Edgar, P., and Walker, G.W. (1973): Carbohydrate metabolism in uremia: a review. *Medicine* 52:469.

DeFronzo, R.A., and Felig, P. (1980): Amino acid metabolism in uremia: insights gained from normal and diabetic man. In Symposium on Nutrition in Renal Disease, Proceedings of the Second International Congress on Nutrition in Renal Disease. *Am. J. Clin. Nutr.* 33:1378–1386.

Elia, M. and Livesey, G. (1981): Branched-chain amino acid and oxo acid metabolism in human and rat muscle. In: *Metabolism and Clinical Implications of Branched Chain Amino and Keto Acids* (eds. M. Walser and J.R. Williamson), pp. 257–262, Elsevier/North-Holland, New York.

Felig, P. (1973): The glucose-alanine cycle. *Metabolism* 22:179–207.

Felig, P. (1981): Inter-organ amino acid exchange, In: *Nitrogen Metabolism in Man,* (eds: J.C. Waterlow and J.M.L. Stephen), pp. 45–61, Appl. Sci. Publ., London.

Fernstrom, J.D., Wurtman, R.J., Hammarstrom-Wiklund, B., Rand, W.M., Munro, H.N., and Davidson, C.S. (1979): Diurnal variations in plasma neutral amino acid concentrations among patients with cirrhosis: effect of dietary protein. *Am. J. Clin. Nutr.* 32:1923–1933.

Goodlad, G.A.J. (1964): Protein metabolism and tumor growth. In: *Mammalian Protein Metabolism* (eds: H.N. Munro, and J.B. Allison), Vol.II., pp. 415–444, Academic Press, New York.

Goodlad, G.A.J., and Clark, C.M. (1980): Leucine metabolism in skeletal muscle of the tumor-bearing rat. *Europ. J. Cancer* 167:1153–1162.

Goodlad, G.A.J., Tee, M.K., and Clark, C.M. (1981): Leucine oxidation and protein degradation in the extensor digitorum longus and soleus of the tumour-bearing host. *Biochem. Med.* 26:143–147.

Kim, Y.S., and Freeman, H.J. (1977): The digestion and absorption of protein. In: *Clinical Nutrition Update: Amino Acids* (eds: H.L. Greene, M.A. Holliday, and H.N. Munro), pp. 135–141. American Medical Association, Chicago, IL.

Krass, E., Bittner, R., Meves, M., and Beger, H.G. (1974): Insulin-Konzentrationen im Pfortaderblut des Menschen nach Glucose-infusion. *Klin. Wschr.* 52:404–408.

McGarry, J.D., and Foster, D.W. (1980): Regulation of hepatic fatty acid oxidation and ketone body production. *Ann. Rev. Biochem.* 49:395–420.

Miller, L.L. (1962): The role of the liver and the non-hepatic tissues in the regulation of free amino acid levels in the blood. In: *Amino Acid Pools* (ed: J.T. Holden) pp. 708–721, Elsevier, Amsterdam.

Motil, K.J., Matthews, D.E., Bier, D.M., Burke, J.F., Munro, H.N., and Young, V.R. (1981): Whole body leucine and lysine metabolism studied simultaneously with [1-^{13}C]-leucine and [α-15N] lysine: response to altered dietary protein intake in young men. *Amer. J. Physiol.* 240, E712.

Munro, H.N. (1964): An introduction to biochemical aspects of protein metabolism In: *Mammalian Protein Metabolism,* (eds: H.N. Munro and J.B. Allison). Vol. I, pp. 31–34. Academic Press, New York.

Munro, H.N. (1977): Tumor-host competition for nutrients in the cancer patient. *J. Am. Dietetic Assoc.* 71:380–384.

Munro, H.N. (1982a): Metabolic integration of organs in health and disease, *J. PEN,* in press.

Munro, H.N. (1982b): Interaction of liver and muscle in the regulation of metabolism in response to nutritional and other factors. In: *The Liver: Biology and Pathobiology* (ed: I.M. Arias et al.). Raven Press, New York.

Munro, H.N. and Crim, M.C. (1980): The proteins and amino acids. In: *Modern Nutrition in Health and Disease* (eds: R.S. Goodhart and M.E. Shils). Sixth Ed., pp. 51–98. Lea and Febiger, Philadelphia.

Munro, H.N., and Thomson, W.S.T. (1953): Influence of glucose on amino acid metabolism. *Metabolism* 2:354–358.

Munro, H.N., Black, J.G., and Thomson, W.S.T. (1959): The mode of action of dietary carbohydrate on protein metabolism. *Brit. J. Nutr.* 13:475–485.

Munro, H.N., Fernstrom, J.D., and Wurtman, R.J. (1975): Insulin, plasma amino acid imbalance, and hepatic coma. *Lancet* 1:722–724.

Neufeld, H.A., Pace, J.A., and White, F.E. (1976): The effect of bacterial infections on ketone concentration in rat liver and blood and on free fatty acid concentrations in rat blood. *Metabolism* 25:877–884.

Reaven, G.M., Swenson, R.S., and Sanfelippo, M.L. (1980): An inquiry into the mechanism of hypertriglyceridemia in patients with chronic renal failure. In: Symposium on Nutrition in Renal Disease, Proceedings of the Second International Congress on Nutrition in Renal Disease. *Am. J. Clin. Nutr.* 33:1476–1484.

Robinson, A.M., and Williamson, D.H. (1980): Physiological roles of ketone bodies as substrates and signals in mammalian tissues. *Physiol. Rev.* 60:143–187.

Schröck, H., and Goldstein, L. (1981): Interorgan relationships for glutamine metabolism in normal and acidotic rats. *Amer. J. Physiol.* 240:E519–E525.

Wahren, J., Felig, P., and Hagenfeldt, J. (1976): Effect of protein ingestion on splanchnic and leg metabolism in normal man and diabetes mellitus. *J. Clin. Invest.* 57:978–999.

Wannemacher, R.W., Jr. (1977): Key role of various individual amino acids in host response to infection. *Am. J. Clin. Nutr.* 30:1269–1280.

Waterhouse, C., Jeanpetre, N., and Keilson, J. (1972): Gluconeogenesis from alanine in patients with progressive malignant disease. *Cancer Res.* 39:1968–1972.

Windmueller, H.G., and Spaeth, A.E. (1975): Intestinal metabolism of glutamine and glutamate from the lumen as compared to glutamine from blood. *Arch. Biochem. Biophys.* 171:662–672.

Young, V.R., and Munro, H.N. (1973): Plasma and tissue tryptophan levels in relation to tryptophan requirements of weanling and adult rats. *J. Nutr.* 103:1756–1763.

2 Modulation of Amino Acid Metabolism by Protein and Energy Intakes

Vernon R. Young
Russell D. Yang
Carol Meredith
Dwight E. Matthews
Dennis M. Bier

It is probably unnecessary here to emphasize that the status of organ and whole body amino acid metabolism are affected by many factors (Table 2-1); however, there are many influential diet and nutritional factors that require further attention. Critical assessment of the impact of disease and other pathological conditions on amino acid metabolism and the efficiency of body nitrogen utilization must be based on an understanding of how variations in protein, amino acid and energy intake confound interpretation of data from clinical studies.

Table 2-1
Some Factors Influencing Status of Whole Body Amino Acid Metabolism and Nutritional Requirement

Agent (Diet)	Host
N intake	Genetic
Amino acid intake	Physiological:
Energy supply	Metabolic state
and source	Age
Other nutrients	Hormonal condition
	Pathological:
	Organ, infection
	Trauma, cancer

As we begin to analyze how intake affects protein metabolism, we will explore briefly some aspects of the physiology of whole body amino acid and nitrogen metabolism, with particular reference to dietary nitrogen, amino acid and energy intakes. Because we have reviewed this topic on several recent occasions (Young, 1981; Young et al. 1981a,b; Young and Bier, 1981), here we focus on some new findings made in our laboratories in healthy adults. These may be of importance in the evaluation of the effects of pathological states on human nitrogen and amino acid metabolism and requirements. Our emphasis will be on the quantitative characteristics of whole body amino acid metabolism, a level of investigation of particular concern to the nutritionist. Elsewhere in this book, more specific considerations are given to the metabolism of amino acids in individual organs, to the interrelationships among organs in the maintenance of normal amino acid metabolism, and to the ways in which disease disturbs these features of amino acid metabolism. Finally, attention will be given to the metabolism of both indispensable and dispensable amino acids, since the nutritional requirement for protein consists of both indispensable (essential) amino acids and a utilizable source of nonspecific nitrogen, usually furnished as dispensable (nonessential) amino acids.

METABOLISM OF INDISPENSABLE AMINO ACIDS

Although the metabolic response of indispensable amino acids to dietary conditions may differ depending upon the amino acid in question, an index of change in metabolism for this class of amino acids can be obtained from the study of whole body leucine kinetics. Thus, it is worthwhile to examine how the whole body metabolism of leucine changes with alterations in the supply of dietary protein and energy.

Protein Intake

It is well known that the efficiency of retention of ingested protein (nitrogen) declines as the intake level approaches that required for maintenance of body N balance. Above this level, the fractional retention of nitrogen with further increments of intake is usually quite low (Young et al., 1973; Inoue et al., 1974; Hegsted, 1976) (Figure 2-1). To explore the metabolic alterations that account for these changes in the utilization of dietary nitrogen, we have used a continuous infusion, stable isotope model to quantify changes in whole body leucine kinetics when healthy young men were given diets varying in protein level within the submaintenance to supramaintenance range. Details of the model and its assumptions, have been discussed by Waterlow and colleagues (Golden and Waterlow, 1977; Waterlow et al., 1978) and by our group (Matthews et al., 1980).

In an earlier study (Motil et al., 1981a), we observed changes in the rate of leucine oxidation in the rate of disappearance of leucine from the plasma compartment into tissues (presumably due to protein synthesis) and in the entry of leucine into plasma (assumed to be a measure of body protein breakdown) when young men were given diets supplying protein intakes ranging between 0.1 and 1.5 g protein $kg^{-1}day^{-1}$. Furthermore, the magnitude of change in these components of whole body leucine metabolism depended upon whether protein intake levels were varied

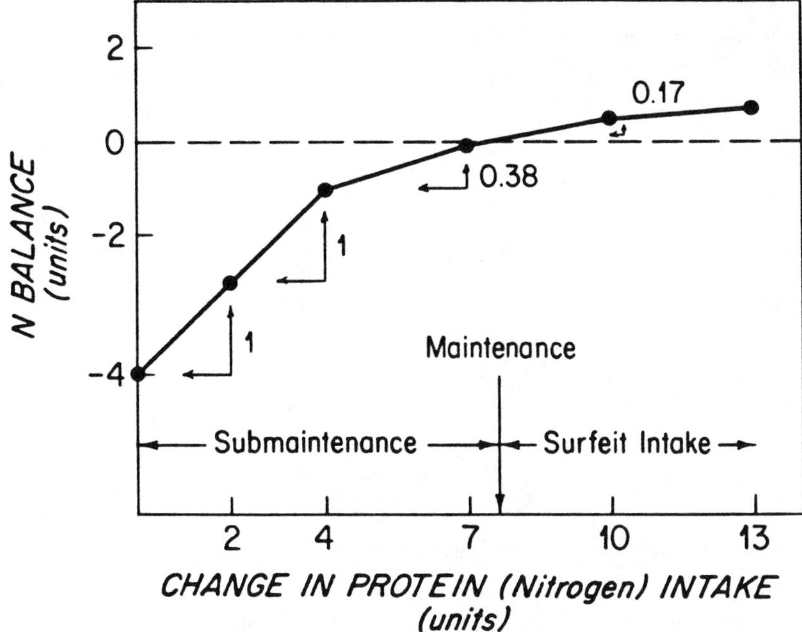

Figure 2-1 Schematic representation of the change in efficiency of dietary N retention with changes in the submaintenance and surfeit ranges of N (protein intake).

about the submaintenance or supramaintenance intake levels. To further examine responses of whole body leucine kinetics to changes in protein intake, we have carried out an additional study utilizing a design similar to that followed previously (Motil et al., 1981), but including a simultaneous investigation of the kinetics of alanine metabolism. These results are described below.

With respect to whole body leucine metabolism, Table 2-2 summarizes data for leucine oxidation, rate of incorporation into proteins (disappearance into tissues), and the balance between the rate of leucine incorporation into and release from whole body proteins. Four young men were studied after an overnight fast (postabsorption) or while consuming small isocaloric, isonitrogenous meals, following a seven-day period of adaptation to the experimental diets.

As shown in Table 2-2, leucine oxidation was relatively constant in the postabsorptive state irrespective of the prior protein intake, while in the fed state oxidation was significantly increased when meals supplying a generous protein intake (1.5 $g \cdot kg^{-1} \cdot day$) were consumed. Because 0.6 g protein/kg/day approximates the mean requirement for highly digested, good quality protein (Garza et al., 1976, 1977), this observation suggests that when the intake of protein, or leucine, exceeds the physiological requirement there is an enhanced rate of leucine oxidation during the period of amino acid absorption and distribution to tissues, which serves to maintain body leucine homeostasis. Reducing the intake of protein below that required does not cause further marked changes in leucine oxidation. However, rates of incorporation of leucine into and release from body proteins are significantly reduced with a decline in protein intake and there is, simultaneously, a less favorable balance between protein synthesis and breakdown.

Table 2-2
Mean Values for Parameters of Whole Body Leucine Metabolism at Various Protein Intakes*

Protein intake ($g \cdot kg^{-1} day^{-1}$)	Oxidation	Disappearance into tissues	Net retention or release
Post-Absorption		($\mu mol \cdot kg^{-1} h^{-1}$)	
1.5	10	88	−10
0.6	8.5	71	− 9
0.3	9.6	62*	− 9
0	8.2	66*	− 9
Fed			
1.5	22	107	+61
0.6	8†	85†	+25
0.3	7†	58†	+ 9
0	9†	57†	− 9

*Unpublished results of Yang et al., based on the use of 1-^{13}C-leucine (see Matthews et al., 1980).
†Significantly different from 1.5 g level ($p < 0.05$).

These observations confirm and extend those made earlier (Motil et al., 1981a) and suggest that there are a number of mechanisms responsible for the adaptive response of whole body leucine and protein metabolism to altered protein intake; at excess intakes of protein, or leucine, oxidative catabolism of leucine is significantly enhanced, whereas at low or inadequate intakes the intensity of body protein turnover (incorporation of leucine into and release from proteins) is diminished. Furthermore, these various mechanisms associated with maintenance of leucine homeostasis appear to operate in a way that might be linked to the total nitrogen and amino acid requirements of the host. Indeed, data obtained from studies in growing and adult rats (Brookes et al., 1972; Bergner et al., 1978; Simon et al., 1978; Kang-Lee and Harper, 1977, 1978) support this interpretation, which we will consider more extensively below.

RESPONSE TO MEALS

In addition to effects of past nutritional history on host whole body leucine kinetics, whole body leucine metabolism also responds to the immediate ingestion of food, as is indicated by the results shown in Table 2-2. Meal-dependent fluctuations in plasma amino acid concentrations have been described in humans (Hussein et al., 1971; Young et al., 1969; Fernstrom et al., 1979) and in liver and muscle protein turnover in experimental animals (Waterlow et al., 1978). Thus, it is worthwhile to review the available but limited data obtained in humans concerned with the dynamic status of whole body indispensable amino acid and protein metabolism in relation to the absorptive and postabsorptive phases of the daily feeding–fasting cycle.

From the data summarized earlier in Table 2-2, obtained using different groups of subjects for studies in the postabsorptive fed states, the rates of whole body protein were slightly, though not significantly, increased during ingestion of small meals supplying generous protein. However, we have observed that the rate of protein breakdown is significantly reduced when meals were consumed (e.g., Figure 2-2), suggesting that the economy of whole body nitrogen metabolism depends, at least in part, upon a modulation in the rate of whole body protein breakdown.

Using obese and lean subjects, Garlick and co-workers (Garlick et al., 1980; Clugston and Garlick, 1982) have observed that the rate of body protein synthesis is enhanced when subjects were given food following an overnight fast (Table 2-3). The possible reasons for the differences between our earlier observations and the more recent findings by Clugston and Garlick (1982) have been discussed by the latter investigators. Among the possible factors, is that in our studies separate subjects were

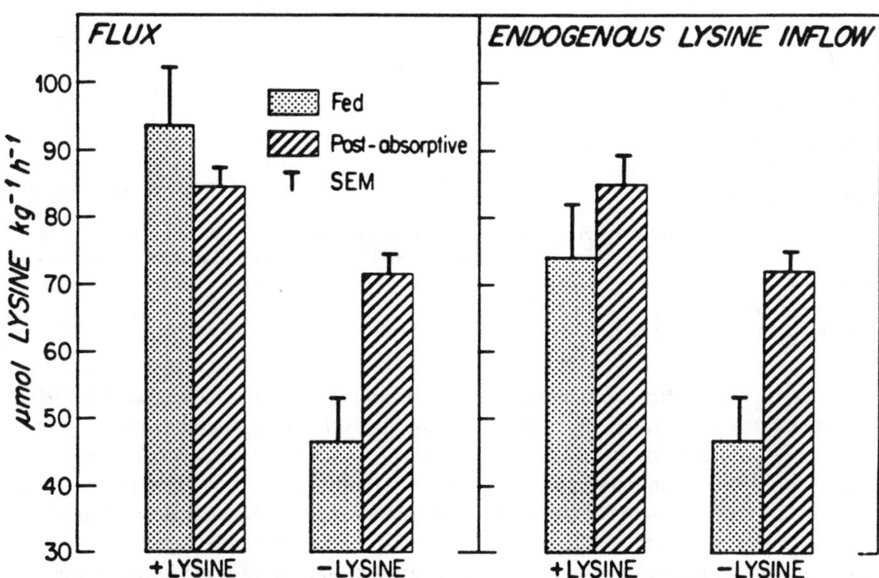

Figure 2-2 Comparison of rates of lysine release from body proteins during the fasted (postabsorptive) and fed states in young men adapted to a diet containing adequate lysine or one devoid in this amino acid. Drawn from Conway et al. (1980).

Table 2-3
Response of Leucine Metabolism to Food Intake, Studied with 24-Hour Infusion of 1-^{14}C-Leucine in Adult Men and Women*

Parameter	Fed	Fast	Fed/Fast†
		(mmol leucine•h^{-1})	(%)
Leucine:			
Intake	4.07	0	
Incorporation	5.70	4.15‡	140
Release from protein	3.82	5.11‡	75
Oxidation	2.19	0.96‡	228

*Summarized from Clugston and Garlick (1982).
†Subjects fed for first 12 hours and fasted remaining 12 hours.
‡Different from fed ($p < 0.01$).

used in the fed and postabsorptive states, whereas in the studies carried out by Garlick each subject was studied both in the fed and fasted states. A more recent experiment (R.D. Yang et al., unpublished) carried out in our laboratory suggests that this difference in experimental design might be important because, as summarized in Table 2-4, the rate of incorporation of leucine into whole body proteins was higher when studied in the same subjects, first after an overnight fast which was then followed by giving them meals.

Table 2-4
Whole Body Leucine Kinetics in Postabsorptive State Following an Overnight Fast and in Fed State (Hourly Meals)*

	Postabsorption	During Meals
Leucine intake	0	83.5
Leucine flux	86 ± 4†	117 ± 5‡
Incorporation	78 ± 3	95 ± 4‡
Release from breakdown	86 ± 4	34 ± 6‡
Oxidation	8 ± 1	22 ± 3‡

*Unpublished results of Yang et al., based on four young men studied during a continuous 10 hour infusion with 1-^{13}C-leucine. Meals given during final 6 hours, and results shown for last hour of each phase.
†Values are μmol kg^{-1}h^{-1}.
‡Differs significantly ($p < 0.01$) from postabsorption.

From these various observations, it is reasonable to conclude, therefore, that both the rate of leucine incorporation into and the release of leucine from body proteins are modulated by meal intake. The extent to which these two components of whole body leucine metabolism may be differentially affected by the size and composition of meals remains to be explored in further studies. Nevertheless, from these limited human studies it can be seen that the status of whole body amino acid metabolism, using ^{13}C-leucine as the index tracer, depends upon the prior dietary conditions of the host and the effects of meals. Furthermore, our findings indicate that the absorptive phase of amino acid metabolism reflects more dramatically the relationships between amino acid intake and changes in whole body amino acid kinetics. Together with the observations described above, suggesting that the maintenance of whole body leucine homeostasis is achieved by mechanisms that might be closely linked to nutritional requirements of the host, we have begun to assess whether use of stable isotope tracer techniques, to determine the kinetics of whole body amino acid metabolism, might offer an opportunity to determine the requirements for specific indispensable amino acids in human subjects. A summary of our studies, to date, is presented in the following section.

AMINO ACID METABOLISM IN RELATION TO AMINO ACID REQUIREMENTS

Studies in young rats have revealed, as mentioned above, that the rate of oxidation of a number of the indispensable amino acids remains low and relatively constant for intakes that are less than sufficient for supporting maximal rates of net body protein synthesis (or growth). This rate increases linearly when intakes are progressively raised above this requirement level (Figure 2-3). A similar response, although not as well defined, also occurs in adult rats (Figure 2-4). Adult human subjects may show similar patterns of change in the dynamics of whole body amino acid and N metabolism with graded intakes of speciic amino acids. Thus, distinct alterations in amino acid oxidation rates and/or in whole body protein turnover might occur when the dietary intake level of a given indispensable amino acid changes in the region approximating the minimal physiological need. If so, it should be possible to determine the requirement for the amino acid, using tracer techniques of the kind discussed above.

A series of experiments currently underway in our laboratories allow a partial evaluation of these possibilities. Our results for the rate of whole body lysine oxidation in young men receiving an amino acid diet supplying graded intakes of lysine are depicted in Figure 2-5, and the results for whole body leucine kinetics in young men receiving graded leucine intakes are shown in Figure 2-6. These data suggest that a marked change in the dynamics of whole body leucine metabolism, in this case shown for the rate of incorporation into body proteins, occurs at an intake of about 28 mg•kg^{-1}day^{-1} (Figure 2-6). For lysine, the changes in the oxidation response curve occur at about 35 mg•kg^{-1}day^{-1} (Figure 2-5). This "breakpoint"-type of response to

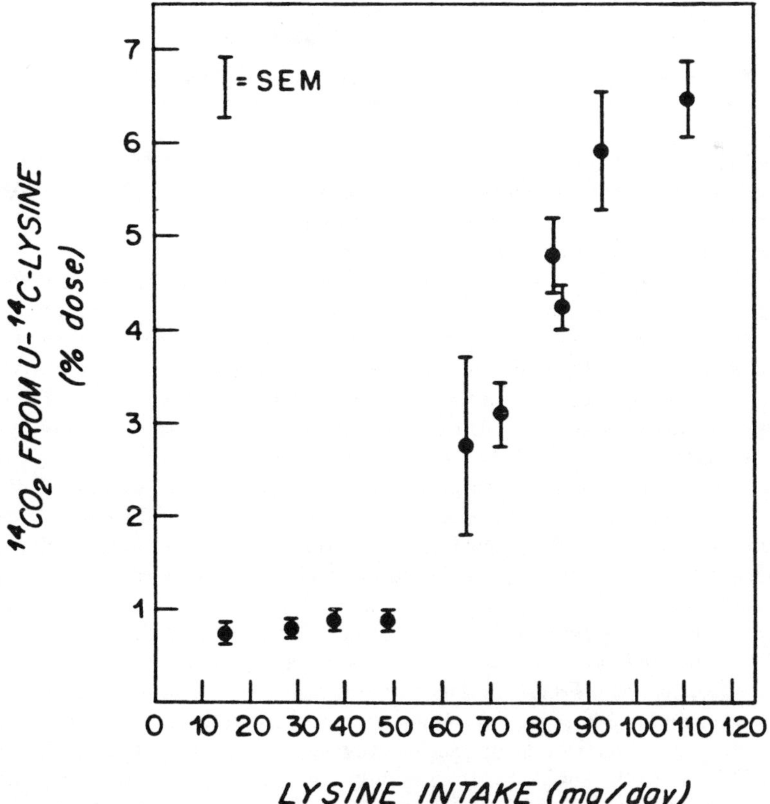

Figure 2-3 Relationship between lysine intake and oxidation in *growing* rats receiving varying intakes of dietary lysine. Drawn from Bergner et al. (1978).

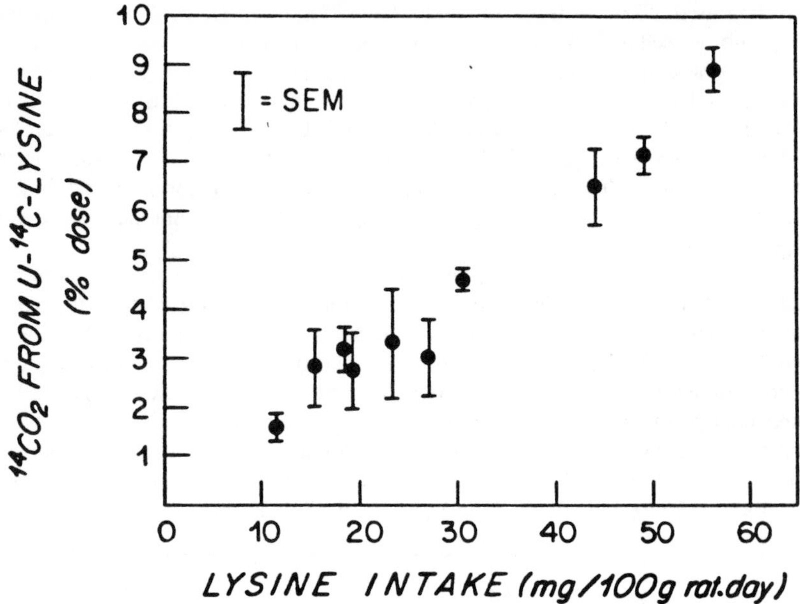

Figure 2-4 Relationship between lysine intake and oxidation in adult rats receiving various intakes of dietary lysine. Drawn from Simon et al. (1978).

graded intakes was unique to leucine and lysine. We did not find this same pattern of response in whole body valine kinetics to graded intakes of valine, as is shown in Figure 2-7 for the rate of valine incorporation into body proteins.

Plasma amino acid responses also were examined in our studies of whole body amino acid kinetics. By undertaking these various measurements it has been possible to evaluate further the results of the ^{13}C-tracer experiments. Our reason for measurement of plasma amino acid patterns is that they are known to be influenced by the level and adequacy of the amino acid intake (e.g., Young and Scrimshaw, 1978). Indeed, plasma amino acid responses have been used as a basis for identifying the limiting amino acids in food proteins and for quantifying dietary protein quality (Young and Scrimshaw, 1978). We found, in our studies, that amino acid-containing meals produce an increase in the plasma concentration of the nonlimiting dietary amino acids, as compared to the concentrations in plasma during the fasting state. In the case of the "limiting" amino acid, meal ingestion was associated with an increased concentration of the amino acid in plasma when meals contained an adequate supply of the amino acid. Below a specific dietary level, meal ingestion reduced the concentration of the limiting amino acid below fasting values. The intake level at which this altered plasma amino acid response occurs might be interpreted to reflect an inadequate intake. Based on these various considerations, results with lysine as the test amino acid (Figure 2-8) suggest that the amino acid requirement might approximate 35 $mg \cdot kg^{-1} day^{-1}$. This estimate is considerably higher than currently accepted values (FAO/WHO, 1973; NRC, 1974). Similarly, measurement of the responses of plasma-free leucine and valine levels to alterations in the dietary intake of these branched-chain amino acids revealed a marked increase in plasma valine when the leucine intake was reduced below about 30 $mg \cdot kg^{-1} day^{-1}$ (see Young et al., 1981).

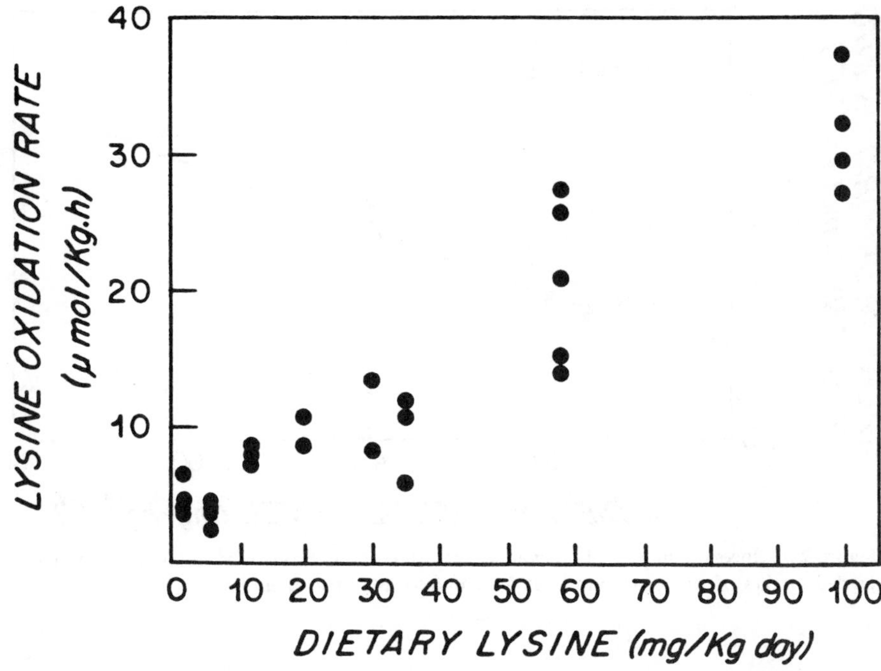

Figure 2-5 Lysine oxidation rate in healthy young men, receiving various intakes of dietary lysine, studied with the aid of 1-^{13}C-lysine during the fed state. Each point is a value for an individual subject. Unpublished MIT data of C. Meredith et al.

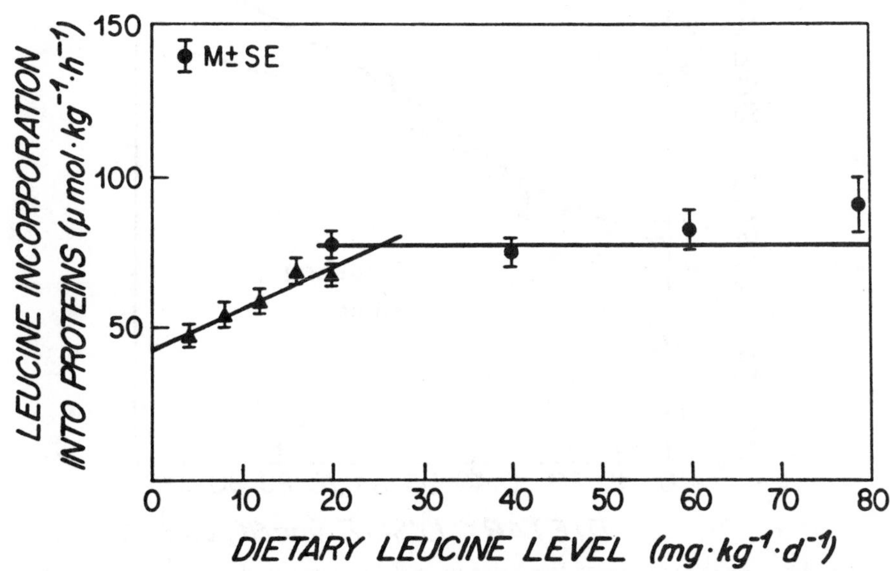

Figure 2-6 Rate of 1-^{13}C-leucine incorporation into whole body proteins in young men receiving various intakes of dietary leucine. Subjects were studied in the fed state. Unpublished MIT data of M. Meguid et al.

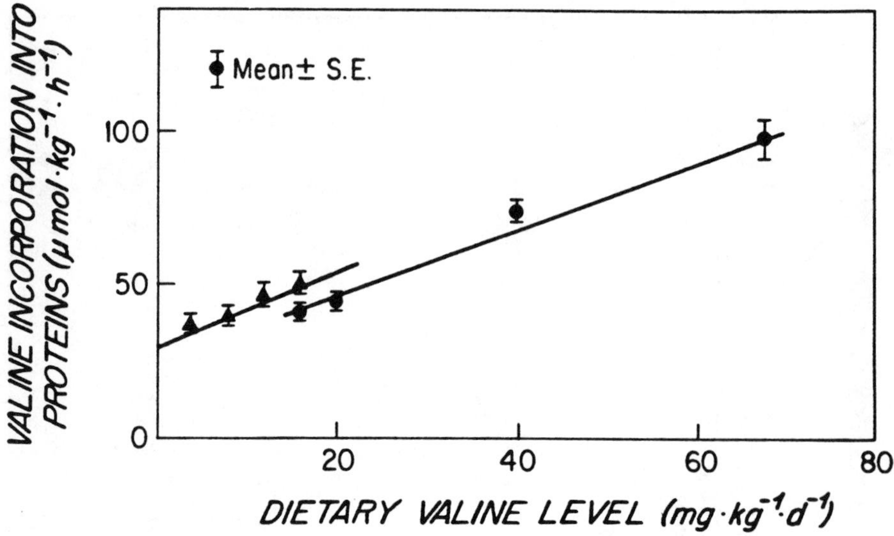

Figure 2-7 Incorporation of 1-^{13}C-valine into whole body proteins in young men receiving graded intakes of valine. Unpublished MIT data of M. Meguid et al.

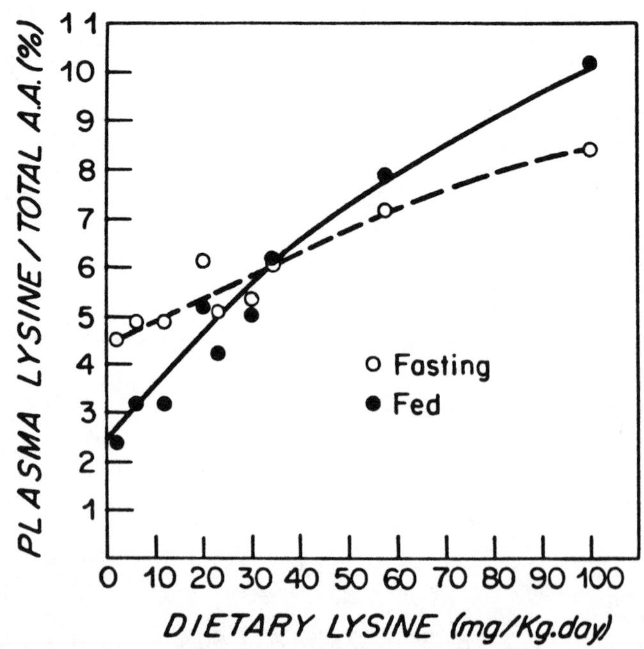

Figure 2-8 The ratio of plasma free lysine to total free amino acid concentration in young men receiving graded intakes of dietary lysine. Each value determined for a single subject and for plasma drawn after an overnight fast (fasting) or during consumption of small meals (fed). Unpublished MIT data of C. Meredith et al.

Also, a constant and low plasma valine concentration was achieved when the dietary supply of this amino acid was within the intake range of 0 to about 20 mg•kg^{-1}day.$^{-1}$ These intake levels of leucine and valine may reflect levels required for maintenance of a normal physiological state. Furthermore, these intakes approximate those estimates of required intakes based on interpretation of data for whole body amino acid kinetics.

Through these various studies involving the application of tracer methodology, in combination with measurements of plasma amino acid responses and body nitrogen balance over a wide range of intakes of test amino acids, we have arrived at a tentative and approximate estimate of the requirements for lysine (Table 2-5). Similarly derived estimates for leucine, valine and threonine are summarized in Table 2-6. It should be noted that interpretation of our results with respect to the requirements for these indispensable amino acids indicate considerably higher requirements than those established by Rose (1957) or those proposed by various expert groups (FAO/WHO, 1973; NRC, 1974). We have discussed previously the possible reasons for such marked differences in the estimated requirements for

Table 2-5
Lysine Requirements in Young Men Estimated by Different Metabolic Criteria*

Criterion	Estimated Lysine Requirement
	(mg•kg^{-1}•day^{-1})
N balance = 0†	17 ± 5
Plasma lysine concentration, Fed = Fasting	22 ± 8
Plasma lysine molar fraction, Fed = Fasting	33 ± 12
"Plasma amino acid score"‡ = 100	32 ± 10
Lysine oxidation breakpoint	~35
Plateau in rate of lysine disappearance into tissues (protein synthesis)	~35
Lysine flux, Fed = Fasting	~35

*Unpublished results of C. Meredith (MIT PhD Thesis, 1982).
†Nitrogen equilibrium defined at Ni = Nu + Nf + 5 mg N/kg•day.
‡Fed state plasma lysine concentration with experimental diet = Fasted state plasma lysine concentration with egg diet (McLaughlin and Illman, 1963).

Table 2-6
Comparison of Estimates of Requirements for Indispensable Amino Acids in Healthy Young Men

Requirement Based on	Amino Acid			
	Leu	*Val*	*Lys*	*Threo*
FAO/WHO 1973	14	10	12	7
MIT Studies				
N balance*	—	16	17	>20
Oxidation Rate	24	—	~35	>20
Plasma amino acids	~30	>20	~33	20–30
MIT/FAO-WHO	~2	2	2–3	2–3

*Assuming unmeasured losses of 5 mg N•kg^{-1}•day^{-1}.

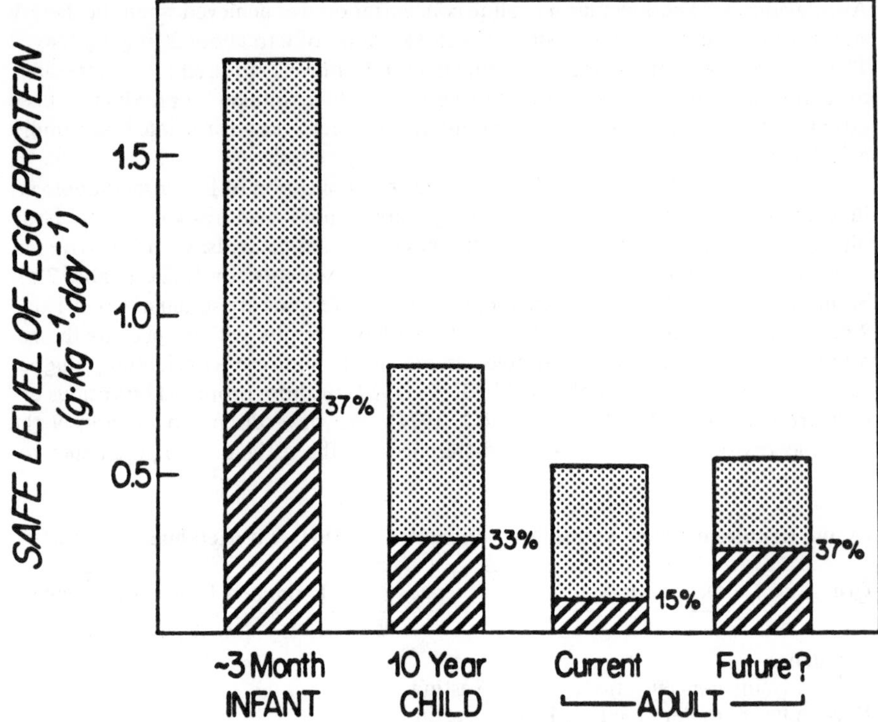

Figure 2-9 Schematic relationship between an adequate level of total protein intake and the requirement for total essential amino acids (cross-hatched portion of the total column, expressed also as a percent) for different age groups. Data for the adults show current relationship, as based on published data, and the possible relationship that might hold in the future with application of new methods, based upon use of stable isotope probes, as have been described in the text.

maintenance of protein nutritional status in healthy adults (Young et al., 1981; and Meredith et al., 1982). Thus, we are tempted to suggest that the current view about the relative rate of change in the amounts of total protein and indispensable amino acids required for the various age groups may not be correct (Figure 2-9). In the future, this picture may require modification.

METABOLISM OF DISPENSABLE AMINO ACIDS

The requirement for a source of nitrogen for the synthesis of dispensable amino acids represents a quantitatively important component of the total protein need. Furthermore, the nutritionally dispensable amino acids account for a significant proportion of the free amino-N pools in tissues. Also, they serve as precursors for the synthesis of numerous metabolically essential compounds, in addition to the role they play in protein synthesis. Thus, knowledge of the quantitative contribution of these amino acids to the economy of whole body nitrogen metabolism and the response of various dispensable amino acids to nutritional and hormonal factors is important to the understanding of human protein nutrition and metabolism.

Because alanine is a main nitrogen product of dietary glutamic acid, glutamine and aspartic acid and an important end product of nitrogen metabolism in heart and skeletal muscle (Lund, 1981), we have examined quantitative aspects of whole body alanine-nitrogen metabolism in healthy adults receiving various levels of protein and energy intake. By combining, in tracer infusion studies, use of an indispensable amino acid labeled with ^{13}C and ^{15}N-alanine, it has been possible to estimate rates of *de novo* alanine N formation (Robert et al., 1982). Results obtained in young adult men receiving varying intakes of protein for one week and studied after an overnight fast (postabsorption) or while consuming meals are summarized in Table 2-7.

In both metabolic states, alanine-N synthesis was enhanced when protein intakes were reduced below a requirement level of about 0.6 g protein $kg^{-1}day.^{-1}$ This observation contrasts with that obtained previously for glycine-N formation, which is reduced when protein intake is decreased (Gersovitz et al., 1980). Furthermore, energy intakes that are lower or higher than those required for body weight maintenance are associated with reduced and increased rates of alanine-N formation, respectively, as summarized in Table 2-8.

Finally, it is worth pointing out that urea formation, as reflected by changes in total urinary nitrogen output, did not parallel these changes in alanine-N formation. From these initial studies on whole body alanine kinetics, it is evident that the rate of endogenously formed alanine-N is not inevitably linked to the rate of urea-N formation. In view of the significance of alanine-N as a precursor of urea in man (Lund, 1981), it is clear that much further exploration of the role of alanine is warranted, as well as of other so-called dispensable amino acids, to determine their role in the regulation and maintenance of total body nitrogen economy. Furthermore, we (Young and Bier, 1981) have postulated previously that the increase in alanine turnover, as occurs in sepsis and trauma, might be responsible for a wasting of muscle and body nitrogen if the higher turnover of alanine promotes, under these

Table 2-7
Summary of Whole Body Alanine Kinetics at Different Protein Intakes in Young Men*

Protein ($g \cdot kg^{-1} \cdot day^{-1}$)	*De novo* Synthesis of alanine N	Reutilization† of alanine N
Postabsorption	($\mu mol \cdot kg^{-1} \cdot h^{-1}$)	
1.5	147	85 (34)‡
0.6	163	91 (31)
0.3	256§	205§ (61)
0.0	303§	236§ (59)
Fed		
1.5	346	216 (51)
0.6	379	303 (68)
0.3	458§	410§ (80)
0.0	439§	420§ (81)

*Unpublished results of Yang et al., based on use of ^{15}N-alanine model described by Robert et al. (1982).
†Reutilization of ala N = Qala-Ala for protein synthesis-Ala_N for urea.
‡Value in parenthesis is percent of flux of alanine N.
§Significantly different from 0.6 g level.

Table 2-8
Effect of Prior Energy Intake for 12 Days on Whole Body Alanine-^{15}N Kinetics During Postabsorptive State in Young Men*

	Energy Intake (% of maintenance)		
	75	*100*	*125*
Body wt change (kg)†	+0.9	+0.2	−1.1
Alanine N metabolism			
Flux	196§¶	283‡	369
From endogeneous protein	91	99	96
De novo synthesis	104‡§	185‡	273

*Unpublished data of Yang et al. Values are $\mu mol \cdot kg^{-1} \cdot h^{-1}$.
†Change during the diet period.
‡Significantly different ($p < 0.05$) from 125 % E.
§Significantly different ($p < 0.05$) from 100 % E.
¶Significantly different ($p < 0.005$) from 125 % E.

pathological conditions, an enhanced formation of urea. The interrelationships between nitrogen metabolism of the dispensable amino acids and ureagenesis deserve further examination.

SUMMATION AND CONCLUSION

In this chapter we have reviewed briefly some of our recent studies estimating whole body amino acid kinetics in healthy adult subjects. Particular attention has been given to the effects of protein, amino acid and energy intakes on the dynamics of whole body amino acid metabolism. Our work emphasizes not only the responsiveness of amino acid metabolism to acute and more chronic changes in diet, but also illustrates the need for standardization of nutritional factors when investigating the impact of disease on the metabolism of amino acids. An encouraging outgrowth of the experiments described here is that a more complete knowledge of the responses of whole body amino acid metabolism will lead to better estimates of nutritional requirements under various pathophysiological conditions. Finally, and although not discussed in detail in this short chapter, it must be pointed out that the stable isotope tracer models we have applied and which are now being used by an increasing number of investigators require further validation and improvement. This is particularly necessary if many aspects of whole body amino acid metabolism during acute and extensive changes in the internal and external environments are to be defined with confidence.

REFERENCES

Bergner, H., Simon, O., Adam, K. (1978): Lysinbedarsbestinning bei wachsenden Ratten anhand der Katabolisierungsrate von ^{14}C- and ^{15}n-Markiertem Lysin. *Arch. Tierernahrung* 28:21–29.

Brookes, I.M., Owens, F.N., Garrigus, U.S. (1972): Influence of amino acid level in the diet upon amino acid oxidation by the rat. *J. Nutr.* 102:27–36.

FAO/WHO (1973): Energy and protein requirements. WHO Technical Report Series No. 522. Geneva, World Health Organization.

Fernstrom, J.D., Wurtman, R.J., Hammerstraum-Wiklund, B., Rand, W.M., Munro, H.N., Davidson, C.S. (1979): Diurnal variations in plasma neural amino acid concentrations among patients with cirrhosis: effect of dietary protein. *Am. J. Clin. Nutr.* 32:1923–1933.

Garlick, P.J., Clugston, G.A., Swick, R.W., Waterlow, J.C. (1980): Diurnal pattern of protein and energy metabolism in man. *Am. J. Clin. Nutr.* 33:1983–1986.

Garza, C., Scrimshaw, N.S., Young, V.R. (1977): Human protein requirements: A long-term metabolic nitrogen balance study in young men to evaluate the 1973 FAO/WHO safe level of egg protein intake. *J. Nutr.* 107:335–352.

Garza, C., Scrimshaw, N.S., Young, V.R. (1976): Human protein requirements: The effect of variations in energy intake within the maintenance range. *Am. J. Clin. Nutr.* 29:280–287.

Gersovitz, M., Bier, D.M., Matthews, D.E., Udall, J., Munro, H.N., Young, V.R. (1980): Dynamic aspects of whole body glycine metabolism: Influence of protein intake in young adult and elderly males. *Metabolism* 29:1087–1094.

Glugston, G.A., Garlick, P.J. (1982): The response of protein and energy metabolism to food intake in lean and obese men. *Human Nutr. Clin. Nutr.* 36C:57–70.

Golden, M.H.N., Waterlow, J.C. (1977): Total protein synthesis in elderly people: A comparison of results with (^{15}N) glycine and (^{14}C) leucine. *Clin. Sci. Mol. Med.* 53:277–288.

Hegsted D.M. (1976): Balance Studies. *J. Nutr.* 106:307–311.

Hussein, M.A., Young, V.R., Murray, E., Scrimshaw, N.S. (1971): Daily fluctuation of plasma amino acid levels in adult men: Effect of dietary tryptophan intake and distribution of meals. *J. Nutr.* 101:61–70.

Inoue, G., Fujita, Y., Kishi, K., Yamomoto, S., Niiyama, Y. (1974): Nutritive values of egg protein and wheat gluten in young men. *Nutr. Rept. Intl.* 10:201–207.

Kang-Lee, T.A., Harper, A.E. (1977): Effect of histidine intake and hepatic histidase activity on the metabolism of histidine *in vivo. J. Nutr.* 107:1427–1443.

Kang-Lee, T.A., Harper, A.E. (1978): Threonine metabolism *in vivo:* effect of threonine intake and prior indication of threonine dehydratase in rats. *J. Nutr.* 108:163–175.

Lund P. (1981): Precursors of urea, in *Nitrogen Metabolism in Man,* (eds: Waterlow, J.C., and Stephen, J.M.L.) pp. 197–201. London, Applied Science Publishers.

Matthews, D.E., Motil, K.J., Rohrbaugh, D.K., Burke, J.F., Young, V.R., and Bier, D.M. (1980): Measurement of leucine metabolism in man from a primed continuous infusion of L-[1-^{13}C] leucine. *Am. J. Physiol.* 238:E473–E479.

Meredith, C., Bier, D.M., Meguid, M.M., Matthews, D.E., Wen, Z., Young, V.R. (1982): Whole body amino acid turnover with ^{13}C-tracers: A new approach for estimation of human amino acid requirements. *Proc. of the 3rd European Congress on Parenteral and Enteral Nutrition,* Maastricht, The Netherlands [In press].

Motil, K.J., Matthews, D.E., Bier, D.M., Burke, J.F., Munro, H.N., Young, V.R. (1981a): Whole body leucine and lysine metabolism: response to dietary protein intake in young men. *Am. J. Physiol.* 240:E712–E721.

NRC (1974): Improvement of protein nutriture. Washington, D.C. National Academy of Sciences.

Robert, J.J., Bier, D.M., Zhao, X.H., Matthews, D.E., Young, V.R. (1982): Glucose and insulin effects on *de novo* amino acid synthesis in young men: Studies with stable isotope labeled alanine, glycine, leucine and lysine. *Metabolism* [In press].

Rose, W.C. (1957): The amino acid requirements of adult man. *Nutr. Abstr. Rev.* 27:631–647.

Simon, O., Adam, K., Bergner, H. (1978): Stoffwechselorientierte Lysin-bedarfsbestimmung bei ausgewachsenden Ratten anhand der Katabolisierungsrate von ^{14}C- und ^{15}N-markiertem Lysin. *Arch. Tierernahrung* 28:609–617.

Waterlow, J.C., Garlick, P.J., Millward, D.J. (1977): *Protein Turnover in Mammalian Tissues and in the Whole Body,* p 804. Elsevier/North Holland Amsterdam and New York.

Young, V.R. (1981): Dynamics of human whole body amino acid metabolism: Use of stable isotope probes and relevance to nutritional requirements. *J. Nutr. Sci. Vitaminology* 27:395–413.

Young, V.R., Bier, D.M. (1981): Protein metabolism and nutritional state in man. *Proc. Nutr. Soc.* 40:343–359.

Young, V.R., Hussein, M.A., Murray, E., and Scrimshaw, N.S. (1969): Tryptophan intake, spacing of meals, and diurnal fluctuations of plasma tryptophan in men. *Am. J. Clin. Nutr.* 22:1563–1567.

Young, V.R., Meguid, M., Meredith. C., Matthews, D.E., Bier, D.M. (1981): Recent developments in knowledge of human amino acid requirements, in: *Nitrogen Metabolism in Man,* (eds: Waterlow, J.C., and Stephen, J.M.L.) pp. 133–153. London, Applied Science Publishers.

Young, V.R., Robert, J.J., Motil, K.J., Matthews, D.E., Bier, D.M.: Protein and energy intake in relation to protein turnover in man, in: *Nitrogen Metabolism in Man,* (eds: Waterlow, J.C., and Stephen, J.M.L.) pp. 419–447. London, Applied Science Publishers.

Young, V.R., Scrimshaw, N.S. (1978): Nutritional evaluation of proteins and protein requirements, in *Protein Resources and Technology* (eds: Milner, M., Scrimshaw, N.S., Wang, D.I.C.) pp. 136–173. Westport, Connecticut, AVI Publishing Co., Inc.

Young, V.R., Taylor, Y.S.M., Rand, W.M., Scrimshaw, N.S. (1973): Protein requirements of man: Efficiency of egg protein utilization at maintenance and submaintenance levels in young men. *J. Nutr.* 103:1164–1174.

3 Developmental Aspects of Amino Acid Metabolism, with Reference to Sulfur Amino Acids

John A. Sturman

Amino acids comprise an indispensable part of the nutrition requirements of the mature human. The detailed requirements of each of the amino acids has received much attention, including altered needs in a variety of clinical situations. The amino acid requirements are also altered in the developing human, both during gestation and after birth. In addition, failure of normal maturation of biochemical and physiological functions during fetal life caused by premature birth also imposes some extra demands. These changes are amply illustrated by the pathways of methionine metabolism (Figure 3-1) in which the activities of several key enzymes and the concentrations of many intermediates undergo considerable alterations during development.

METHIONINE-CYST(E)INE RELATIONSHIPS

Methionine has been demonstrated many times to be essential for growth in mammals, including man, whereas cyst(e)ine is nonessential, at least in mature mammals. The daily methionine requirement of young adult men was estimated to be 800 to 1100 mg in the absence of cystine (Rose et al., 1955). Of this, 80% to 89% could be replaced by cystine, suggesting that the transsulfuration pathway normally represents an important route for cyst(e)ine formation (Rose and Wixom, 1955). In 1970,

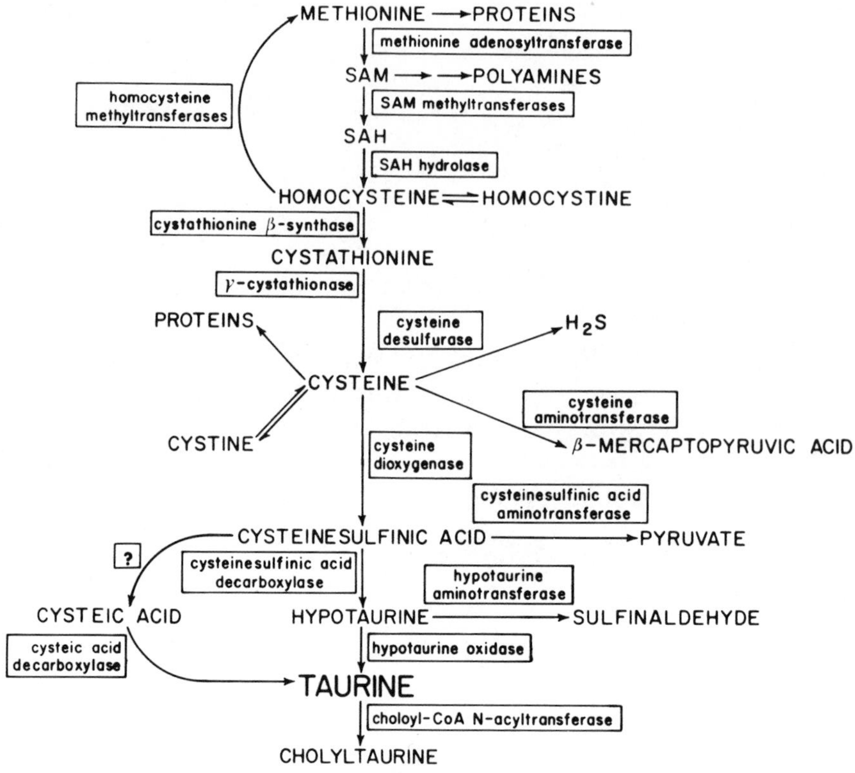

Figure 3-1 The transsulfuration pathway of methionine metabolism.

we reported that activity of cystathionase, the enzyme responsible for cleaving cystathionine to form cysteine, was not present in human fetal liver or brain (Sturman et al., 1970). Cystathionine synthase activity was present, although in smaller amounts than mature tissue, and cystathionine accumulated in fetal liver (Table 3-1). We also found that activity of cystathionase was absent from the liver of many preterm infants who died shortly after birth, and was low in normal term infants who died shortly after birth (Table 3-2). Our conclusion from these results was that development of human liver cystathionase activity was a postnatal phenomenon, and that cyst(e)ine was an essential amino acid for the human fetus, and possibly for prematurely born and even full-term infants for a short period after birth. A more recent study has confirmed that hepatic cystathionase activity in prematurely born infants is low, and that development of activity correlates significantly with postnatal age (Zlotkin and Anderson, 1982). In this study, development of hepatic cystathionase activity also correlated significantly with gestational age. They further reported that in full-term human infants, hepatic cystathionase activity increased rapidly after birth (Figure 3-2).

Table 3-1
Transsulfuration Enzymes and Cystathionine in Human Liver and Brain

	Cystathionine synthase	Cystathionine	Cystathionine
	(nmol/mg protein/h)		(μmol/100 g)
Liver			
Fetus (24)	21± 4	0	14 ± 2
Mature (9)	98 ± 12	126 ± 12	0
Brain			
Fetus (24)	12 ± 2	0	4.0 ± 0.6
Infant*	18	48	41

Data from Sturman et al., 1970.
*Occipital lobe from six-month-old infant.

Table 3-2
Cystathionase Activity in Human Liver[1]

Infant[2]		
680g;	24h	43
789g;	24h	0
830g;	11h	0
1000g;	8h	0
1060g;	14h	0
1260g;	3h	0
1500g;	96h	49
1650g;	216h	86
1780g;	72h	40
2250g;	24h	17
2600g;	144h	43
2730g;	96h	66
2950g;	24h	37
3450g;	7h	9
4000g;	96h	36
4250g;	72h	85
Adult		126 ± 12

Data from Gaull et al., 1972, 1973.
[1]Expressed as nmol cysteine/mg prot/h.
[2]Weight of infant at birth; time of death after birth.

Cystathionase activity correlates significantly with time of death after birth ($r = 0.776$), but not with weight at birth. Furthermore, correlation of cystathionase activity with time of death after birth and weight at birth as two independent variables does not add to the significance of the correlation with time of death after birth.

REQUIREMENT FOR CYST(E)INE

If cyst(e)ine is an essential amino acid for the human neonate, then it must be obtained from the mother's milk, or from a synthetic substitute. Human milk protein contains approximately 50% more cyst(e)ine than methionine, whereas cow's milk protein, from which most synthetic infants foods are prepared, contains more

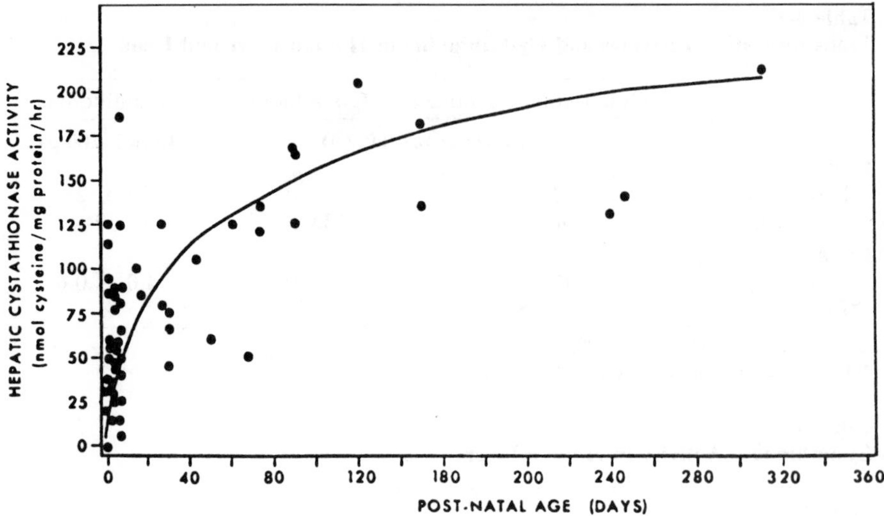

Figure 3-2 The effect of postnatal age on hepatic cystathionase activity in full-term infants. Data from Zlotkin and Anderson, 1982.

than twice as much methionine as cyst(e)ine (see Gaull et al., 1982, for review). Although cow's milk contains more protein than human milk on a volume basis, on a unit of protein basis it contains less than half the cyst(e)ine of human milk. Finally, newborn infants, both full-term and pre-term, that are unable to be fed by the oral route because of medical or surgical emergencies must be supplied with nutrition intravenously. Some studies have been performed on such infants, and the results provide some evidence that some cysteine should be provided during this form of nutrition (Pohlandt, 1974; Zlotkin et al., 1981; Zlotkin and Anderson, 1982).

The inability of the human fetus to biosynthesize cysteine means that it is dependent on the mother's circulation for this compound. Cyst(e)ine is unique among the free amino acids of plasma in that its concentration in maternal plasma is greater than or equal to that in fetal plasma. Most amino acids have a gradient of two- to threefold in favor of fetal plasma. Furthermore, increasing the concentration of cyst(e)ine in maternal plasma by infusion causes little increase in fetal plasma whereas for other amino acids the fetal–maternal gradient is maintained (Figure 3-3) (Gaull et al., 1973).

There are a number of possible reasons for this developmental change in the transsulfuration pathway. The human fetus conserves the carbon skeleton of methionine by remethylating homocysteine back to methionine, instead of losing it via the transsulfuration pathway. Methionine may be required to supply methyl groups for the increased methylation which occurs during development. In addition, greater decarboxylation of S-adenosylmethionine occurs in fetal liver than in mature liver, although the opposite change occurs in brain (Sturman and Gaull, 1974). The role of methionine metabolism in polyamine synthesis during development has been described elsewhere in greater detail (Sturman and Gaull, 1978). Cystathionine, a key intermediate in the transsulfuration pathway which is present in human brain in large concentrations, may not be needed until some time after birth. It should be noted here that although much information is available on this compound, its function is presently unknown (see Tallan et al., 1982, for review). Cysteine is a unique amino acid, largely by virtue of its sulfhydryl group. It is an important constituent of proteins in which it is largely responsible for their molecular configuration, either by forming disulfide bonds with other cysteine molecules incorporated into the same protein or by forming disulfide bonds with free cysteine. It can link together a number of separate proteins or polypeptides by forming disulfide bonds between cysteine residues in different molecules. Cyst(e)ine is an important precursor of the tripeptide, glutathione, and, theoretically, also of taurine, which may have an important role in development. This aspect has been discussed at length in recent reviews, and will not be considered further here (Sturman and Hayes, 1980; Hayes and Sturman, 1981). Finally, cysteine has been demonstrated to be toxic to developing brain (Olney and Ho, 1970; Olney et al., 1972). This latter observation may explain why the human fetus is protected from any excessive accumulation of cysteine, both by having a restricted synthesis and restricted placental transfer.

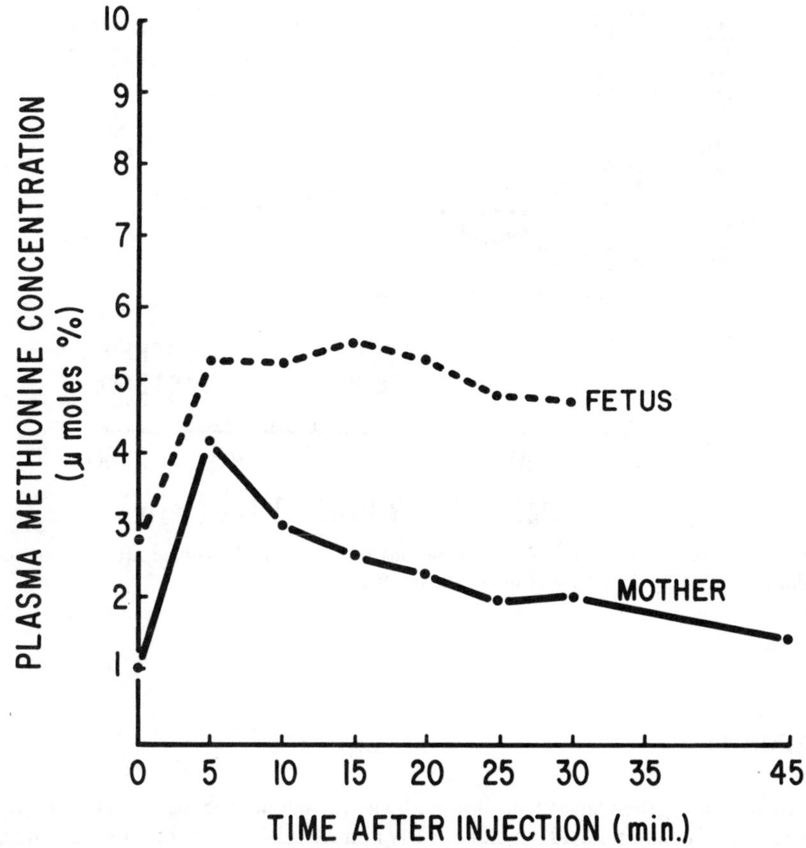

Figure 3-3A Fetal and maternal concentrations of methionine after intravenous administration of 0.5 mmol L-methionine to the mother.

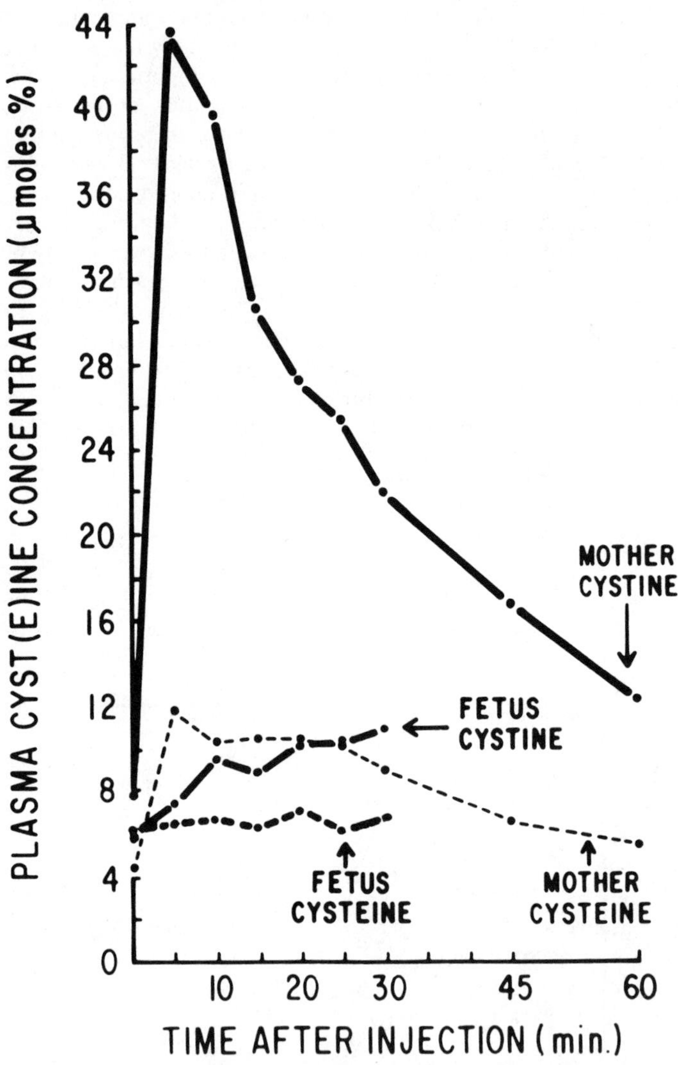

Figure 3-3B Fetal and maternal concentrations of cystine and cysteine after intravenous administration of 2.5 mmol L-cystine to the mother.

SUMMARY

In summary, the transsulfuration pathway of methionine metabolism provides an example of an amino acid which is clearly nonessential for the mature human and which is essential to the developing human fetus. In addition, it provides an example of a developmental metabolic change resulting in altered nutritional requirements.

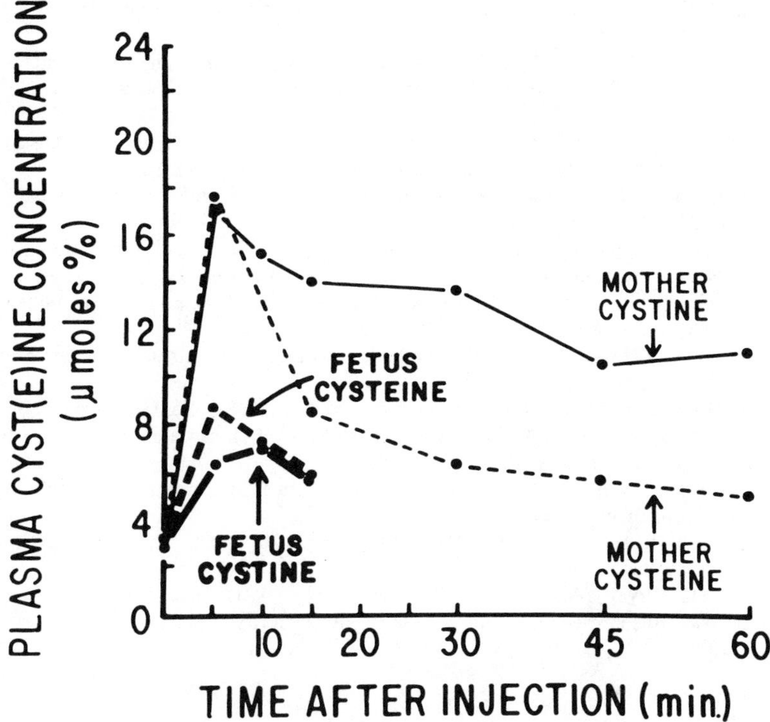

Figure 3-3C Fetal and maternal concentrations of cystine and cysteine after intravenous administration of 5.0 mmol L-cysteine to the mother. Data from Gaull et al., 1973.

ACKNOWLEDGMENT

The studies in the author's laboratory were supported by the New York State Office of Mental Retardation and Developmental Disabilities.

REFERENCES

Gaull, G.E., Jensen, R.G., Rassin, D.K. and Malloy, M.H. (1982): Human milk as food. In *Advances in Perinatal Medicine* (eds: A. Milunsky, E.A. Friedman, and L. Gluck) vol. 2, pp. 47–120, Plenum Publishing Corp., New York.

Gaull, G.E., Raiha, N.C.R., Saarikoski, S. and Sturman, J.A. (1973): Transfer of cyst(e)ine and methionine across the human placenta. *Pediat. Res.* 7:908–913.

Gaull, G., Sturman, J.A. and Raiha, N.C.R. (1972): Development of mammalian sulfur metabolism: Absence of cystathionase in human fetal tissues. *Pediat. Res.* 6:538–547.

Gaull, G.E., von Berg, W., Raiha, N.C.R. and Sturman, J.A. (1973): Development of methyltransferase activities of human fetal tissues. *Pediat. Res.* 7:527–533.

Hayes, K.C. and Sturman, J.A. (1981): Taurine in metabolism. *Ann. Rev. Nutr.* 1:401–425.

Olney, J.W. and Ho, O.L. (1970): Brain damage in infant mice following oral intake of glutamate, aspartate or cysteine. *Nature* 227:609–610.

Olney, J.W., Ho, O.L., Rhee, V. and Schainker, B. (1972): Cysteine-induced brain damage in infant and fetal rodents. *Brain Res.* 45:309–313.

Pohlandt, F. (1974): Cystine: A semi-essential amino acid in the newborn infant. *Acta. Paed. Scand.* 63:801–804.

Rose, W.C., Coon, M.J., Lockhart, H.B. and Lambert, G.F. (1955): The amino acid requirements of man. XI. The threonine and methionine requirements. *J. Biol. Chem.* 215:101–110.

Rose, W.C. and Wixom, R.L. (1955): The amino acid requirements of man. XIII. The sparing effect of cystine on the methionine requirement. *J. Biol. Chem.* 216:763–773.

Sturman, J.A. and Gaull, G.E. (1974): Polyamine biosynthesis in human fetal liver and brain. *Pediat. Res.* 8:231–237.

Sturman, J.A. and Gaull, G.E. (1978): Methionine and polyamine metabolism in the brain and liver of the developing human and rhesus monkey. *Adv. Polyamine Res.* 2:213–240.

Sturman, J.A., Gaull, G. and Raiha, N.C.R. (1970): Absence of cystathionase in human fetal liver: Is cystine essential? *Science* 169:74–76.

Sturman, J.A. and Hayes, K.C. (1980): The biology of taurine in nutrition and development. *Adv. Nutr. Res.* 3:231–299.

Tallan, H.H., Rassin, D.K., Sturman, J.A. and Gaull, G.E. (1982): Methionine metabolism in brain. In *Handbook of Neurochemistry* (ed: A. Lajtha) 2nd edition, vol. 2, Plenum Publishing Corp., New York, in press.

Zlotkin, H.S. and Anderson, G.H. (1982): The development of cystathionase activity during the first year of life. *Pediat. Res.* 16:65–68.

Zlotkin, S.H. and Anderson, G.H. (1982): Sulphur balances in intravenously fed infants: Effects of cysteine supplementation. *Am. J. Clin. Nutr.* in press.

Zlotkin, S.H., Bryan, M.H. and Anderson, G.H. (1981): Cysteine supplementation to cysteine-free intravenous feeding regimens in newborn infants. *Am. J. Clin. Nutr.* 34: 914–923.

4 Aging: Amino Acid and Protein Metabolism

Kent G. Lundholm

The process of aging is associated with structural and functional impairments, which occur in the living organism and are expressed in gradual deterioration and decline in performance (Shock, 1972). The manifestation of aging is multiple, probably occurring at several levels of structure and function with different rates in species of various life spans, but not markedly different when maximum life span is normalized (Sacher, 1980). Several studies have explored the maintenance of the accuracy of protein synthesis and its relevance to aging (Ogrodnik et al., 1975; Rubinson et al., 1976). Such studies have been based on theories and results emphasizing modifications of gene structure and gene expression, essentially based on animal models and cell cultures. Human studies have shown qualitative and quantitative changes in body and tissue composition with age (Munro and Young, 1978), but it has been difficult to correlate such changes directly to impaired organ function.

Dynamic studies of whole body protein metabolism in man have suggested reduced rate of protein turnover in relation to body weight, associated with an internal redistribution of protein synthesis as adult life progresses (Uauy et al., 1978a). Whole body protein kinetics in human studies have not been aimed at distinguishing among changes of protein metabolism in different tissues and organs. Therefore, this presentation emphasizes protein synthesis in human liver and skeletal muscles and evaluates specifically the liver and muscle tissue capacity of protein synthesis in relationship to age. The stimulatory effect of endogenous and exogenous insulin and amino acids on protein synthesis *in vitro* has been measured, as well as liver and muscle tissue content of lysosomal, glycolytic and oxidative enzyme activities (V_{max}) among middle-aged and elderly hospitalized patients.

MATERIAL AND METHODS

Patients

Males and females of different ages (range 17 to 86 years), have been selected on clinical grounds. The patients were hospitalized for operation of uncomplicated gallstone disease. Informed consent was obtained from all patients and the protocols were approved by the Ethical Committee of the University of Gothenburg. All metabolic measurements were performed after a 12-hour fast. All patients ate a free-choice, balanced hospital diet but of similar overall fat, protein and carbohydrate composition for a minimum of two days before the studies were performed. No complications arose due to the biopsy procedures.

Tissue Experiments

The procedures for taking biopsies, the handling of the tissues and the incubation procedures of liver and muscle tissue have been published elsewhere (Lundholm et al., 1975, 1977, 1981; Lundholm and Scherstén, 1975, 1977, 1979). The limitations of the *in vitro* systems have been discussed (Lundholm and Scherstén, 1979; Lundholm et al., 1981). Measurements of enzyme activities (V_{max}) were as described elsewhere (Scherstén and Lundholm, 1972; Bjorkerud et al., 1967; Bylund et al., 1976).

RESULTS

The mean age in all patient groups was about 45 years with the S.E. varying from four to eight years among the different groups for whom are given in Tables 4-1 through 4-7. Hepatic lysosomal enzyme activities, evaluated as acid phosphotase, aryl sulphatase, B-glucuronidase and Cathepsin D showed a positive correlation with age ($r = 0.49$, $p < 0.05$; $r = 0.45$, $p < 0.025$; $r = 0.38$, $p < 0.05$; $r = 0.35$; $p < 0.025$), as calculated from measurements on 80 patients with the age range 17 to 86 years. Table 4-1 summarizes the activities of different lysosomal enzymes measured on fresh liver biopsy specimens taken at operation. Patients older than 60 years had significantly higher enzyme activities compared with younger patients. Cathepsin D activity was also significantly increased in skeletal muscle tissue from elderly patients, while acid phosphatase and B-glucuronidase did not change with age (Table 4-2).

Patients older than 60 years had elevated hepatic protein synthesis *in vitro,* measured as leucine incorporation into acid precipitable proteins. The incorporation rate into hepatic immunoreactive albumin was unchanged at advanced age, and the hepatic content of RNA was similar in individuals younger and older than 60 years (Table 4-3).

Leucine incorporation into skeletal muscle proteins, in relationship to RNA, is shown in Table 4-4. Isolated muscle fibers from elderly patients had a higher incorporation rate of leucine, in spite of an RNA similar to that for tissue from younger patients. The results shown in Table 4-4 were obtained with isolated muscle fibers that were incubated in buffer solution supplemented with high concentrations of amino acids. Table 4-5 shows the influence of insulin and amino acids in excess on protein synthesis as compared with that of muscle fibers incubated in buffer with amino acids at normal plasma concentration only. Addition of insulin and of high concentrations of amino acids stimulated significantly muscle protein synthesis *in vitro* equally in muscle fibers from elderly and younger patients. The stimulation by insulin given *in vivo* on protein synthesis measured *in vitro* is shown in Table 4-6. Patients received 0.9% saline or 10% D-glucose with an intravenous infusion rate of about 2 mg glucose/min $\times$ kg body weight for at least two hours before the biopsies were taken. This procedure raised plasma insulin from fasting levels (7 $\pm$ 1 μU/ml) to a level of 14 $\pm$ 2 μU/ml. This procedure stimulated *in vitro* protein synthesis by 38 $\pm$ 7% in middle-aged patients and 52 $\pm$ 6% ($p < 0.10$) in elderly patients.

Table 4-7 shows the results from measurements of key enzymes that are important for the transfer of energy in skeletal muscle tissue from middle-aged (45 $\pm$ 12, mean $\pm$ S.D.) and elderly patients 69 $\pm$ 8 years.

DISCUSSION

The intensity of body and tissue protein metabolism declines with increased adult body size in mammals. The declining protein turnover parallels a similar decline in the intensity of energy metabolism. These changes are accompanied by a continuous loss of lean body mass, leading to an altered body composition in the senescence (Munro, 1981).

In aging organisms several examples are available of continuously changing organ function and alterations in tissue composition associated with structural and functional impairments. Such examples are: loss of muscle mass (Bruce et al., 1980),

Table 4-1
Hepatic Lysosomal Enzyme Activities (V_{max})
Measured on Fresh Liver Biopsies from Healthy Individuals
Operated on for Uncomplicated Gallstone Disease

Age	Cathepsin D	Acid phosphatase	B-glucuronidase
		nmol/min/mg protein	
< 60 years	17.1 $\pm$ 1.8(7)	11.5 $\pm$ 0.6(7)	16.9 $\pm$ 1.6(7)
> 60 years	22.5 $\pm$ 1.7(9)	11.7 $\pm$ 1.1(9)	23.4 $\pm$ 2.3(9)
	$p < 0.025$		$p < 0.025$

The enzymes were measured in the postmitochondrial supernatant after solubilization with Triton X-100. All enzymes were measured in aliquots from each supernatant. Mean $\pm$ S.E. Number of patients within parenthesis.

Table 4-2
Lysosomal Enzyme Activities (V_{max}) Measured on Fresh Skeletal Muscle Biopsies (Rectus Abdominis Muscle) from Healthy Individuals Operated on for Uncomplicated Gallstone Disease

	Cathepsin D	Acid phosphatase	B-glucuronidase	Protein
Age		*nmol/min/mg protein*		*mg/ml*
< 60 years	2.13 ± 0.22(22)	0.52 ± 0.05(14)	0.12 ± 0.003(13)	3.9 ± 0.1(22)
> 60 years	2.95 ± 0.31(19)	0.52 ± 0.02(11)	0.13 ± 0.010(8)	3.8 ± 0.1(19)
	$p < 0.025$			

The enzymes were measured on the post-mitochondrial supernatant after solubilization by Triton X-100. "Protein" is protein content in the enzyme fraction. Mean ± S.E. Number of patients within parenthesis.

Table 4-3
Protein Synthesis Measured as Incorporation Rate of Leucine into Acid Precipitable Proteins and into Immunoreactive Albumin in Relationship to Hepatic Content of RNA

	Leucine incorporation into protein (nmol/h/mg protein)			
			Albumin	
Age	*Hepatic acid precipitable proteins*	*Immunoreactive albumin*	*Hepatic protein*	Hepatic RNA content mg/g
< 60 years	0.390 ± 0.04(20)	5.83 ± 0.99(11)	19.7 ± 2.9	5.1 ± 0.2(14)
> 60 years	0.550 ± 0.06(11)	6.31 ± 1.19(9)	17.8 ± 1.7	5.3 ± 0.2(13)
	$p < 0.025$			

The experiments were performed on incubated liver slices from patients operated on for uncomplicated gallstone disease. Immunoreactive albumin was isolated from the liver cells at the end of the incubation. Therefore, it includes proalbumin. Mean ± S.E. Number of patients within parenthesis.

accumulation of trace elements in aging cells (Sugarman et al., 1980; Sugarman and Munro, 1980a,b), altered levels of cerebral neurotransmitters (Samorajski, 1977), decreased hormonal-receptor sensitivity and responsiveness (Roth, 1979; Parchman et al., 1978; Bolla, 1980), impaired hormonal regulation of enzyme activities during aging, (Adelman, 1975; Miller and Bolla, 1981), inactive enzyme molecules in aging

Table 4-4
Protein Synthesis in Relationship to RNA Content in Skeletal Muscle Tissue (Rectus Abdominis Muscle)

Age	Leucine incorporation into muscle proteins (nmol/h/mg protein)	RNA content mg/g
< 60 years	0.180 ± 0.01(27)	0.67 ± 0.03(13)
> 60 years	0.244 ± 0.02(24)	0.68 ± 0.03(10)
	p< 0.01	

Isolated muscle fibers were incubated as described in the text. RNA was measured on fresh muscle biopsies. Mean ± S.E. Number of patients within parenthesis.

Table 4-5
The Stimulatory Effect on Protein Synthesis *In Vitro* by Insulin and by High Concentrations of Amino Acids

	Leucine incorporation into muscle proteins nmol/h/mg protein		
Age	*Basal rate*	†*Insulin in vitro (25 U/l)*	†*Amino acids in vitro 10 times normal plasma conc.*
< 60 years	0.123 ± 0.015(7)	0.137 ± 0.020(7)*	0.220 ± 0.025(7)†
> 60 years	0.120 ± 0.015(8)	0.152 ± 0.025(8)*	0.232 ± 0.026(8)†

*p < 0.05 versus basal rate
†p < 0.01 versus basal rate

Table 4-6
Protein Synthesis *In Vitro* after Stimulating by Endogenous Insulin

	Leucine incorporation into muscle proteins nmol/h/mg protein		
Age	*0.9% Sodium chloride*	*10% D-Glucose*	*Stimulatory effect %*
< 60 years	0.117 ± 0.018(0)	0.161 ± 0.009(24)	38 ± 7
> 60 years	0.131 ± 0.019(9)	0.199 ± 0.012(25)	52 ± 6
		p < 0.01	

Patients received intravenous infusion of 0.9% saline or 10% D-glucose (2 mg glucose/min /kg bwt) for at least 2 h prior to when the biopsies were taken (rectus abdominis muscle). The experiments were performed as described in the text. Isolated muscle fibers were incubated in buffer supplemented with amino acids at human plasma concentration. Mean ± S.E. Number of patients within parenthesis.

Table 4-7
Activities of Key Enzymes (V_{max}) Involved in Glycogen Metabolism, Glycolysis and Oxidative Metabolism of Skeletal Muscles (Rectus Abdominis Muscle)

Age	GLS		GP	HK	PFK	LDH	GPDH	ACDH	CS	Cytox	Prot.
	I	II									
< 60 years	2.8±	16.2±	81±	41.6±	804±	3144±	1.4±	59.6±	21.6±	10.1±	191±
	0.6	5.7	8	2.2	54	319	0.2	9.9	2.7	1.1	5
	(5)	(5)	(11)	(11)	(11)	(11)	(8)	(6)	(6)	(11)	(11)
> 60 years	2.9±	12.6±	73±	37.2±	758±	2443±	2.2±	62.0±	23.3±	10.1±	196±
	0.7	1.9	9	3.1	69	231	0.3	8.0	2.3	0.9	4
	(6)	(5)	(8)	(9)	(9)	(9)	(4)	(7)	(7)	(9)	(9)
						$p < 0.025$					

GLS I, II: glycogen synthase active form (I) and total form (II); GP: glycogen phosphorylase, HK: hexokinase, PFK: phosphofructokinase, LDH: lactate dehydrogenase, GPDH: glucose-6-phosphate dehydrogenase, ACDH: 3-OH-acyl-CoAdehydrogenase, CS: citrate synthase, Cytox: cytochrome C oxidase, Prot: protein content in muscle tissue. The enzyme activities have been related to the protein content of the tissue specimens. Number of patients within parenthesis.

organisms (Zeelon et al., 1973; Gershon and Gershon, 1970), and altered composition of collagen (Miyahara et al., 1978; Eyre and Muir, 1977), and eye lens proteins (Bando et al., 1976), as well as qualitative changes with age of proteoglycans of human lumbar discs (Adams and Muir, 1976). All of these changes could, theoretically, be due to an increase in the inaccuracy of protein synthesis with aging. Therefore, it is an attractive hypothesis that aging is intimately related to disturbances of the protein synthesis machinery both at translational and transcriptional level (Martin, 1980). In support of this theory is evidence of loss of genes coding for ribosomal RNA in aging brain cells from animals (Johnson and Strehler, 1972) and of age-dependent structural changes in human neuronal chromatin (Ermini et al., 1978). The hypothesis of "the error catastrophy" of protein synthesis in aging has been suggested based on such discoveries. However, few data are available that correlate decreased accuracy of protein synthesis to functional disturbances as the cause of aging and death. In contrast, it has been emphasized that enzyme abnormalities in old animals and in cultured old cells closely resemble those demonstrated to be post-translational modifications, as in the case of human glucose-6-phosphate dehydrogenase (Kahn et al., 1974).

At a clinical level it is, at present, more reasonable to explore the effects of aging and altered protein metabolism at a more unsophisticated level of investigation. That is, to consider the role in protein metabolism played by physiological and other factors such as declining food intake, perhaps secondary to altered food regulation associated with changed metabolism of central neurotransmitters; alterred availability, requirements and efficiency of utilization of dietary proteins and calories.

It is well known that food intake declines continuously with increasing age (Munro, 1981). However, it is difficult to assess whether or not this phenomenon is the cause of a fall in body cell mass or rather a consequence of the altered body composition *per se.* Studies of energy intake among adult young and old subjects in Sweden have shown that food composition and the relative distribution of fat, carbohydrates, protein and trace elements, etc. were the same in young and old people (Steen and Svanborg, 1975). Elderly subjects seemed to have a lower absolute intake of proteins per body weight (0.69 g/kg bwt/day) compared with young people (0.91 g/kg bwt/day). However, these results may not be really different considering the expected depressed lean body mass in the elderly subjects. Interestingly, several Scandinavian studies have shown that elderly men and woman habitually consumed 0.65–0.70 g protein/kg bwt/day, corresponding to 13% to 14% of their dietary caloric intake. These figures agree with reported and calculated needs of protein requirements for elderly women (0.83 g/kg bwt/day) in other studies providing about 12% to 14% protein calories (Uauy et al., 1978b). Therefore, it seems that old subjects who had free access to a well-balanced diet consumed the amount that is predicted to be sufficient to maintain nitrogen balance. Young people with larger lean body mass had slightly higher spontaneous intake of proteins and seemed to have a correspondingly higher requirement of daily protein intake for their nitrogen balance (Cheng et al., 1978). These results may suggest that regulation of food intake is adequately maintained in senescense. However, in this respect it is apparent that we are dealing with quite subtle or almost immeasurable differences. This is obvious when it is realized that the loss of 12 to 13 kg of muscles from between 25 and 70 years of age can be calculated to correspond to a daily negative nitrogen balance in between 20 to 30 μmol of nitrogen. This difference is technically impossible to measure over short time periods not realistic to assess by studies of nitrogen balance in man. Therefore, in our future efforts to identify the changes and mechanisms related to the effects of the aging process on protein metabolism and in measurements of differences among young and old subjects, we will need to use methods that offer high precision of assessment at the nanomolar level.

Previous studies have shown an age-related decline of whole body protein turnover in elderly subjects, even when related to body weight (g protein/kg bwt/day) (Uauy et al., 1978a; Young et al., 1975). However, a careful analysis of these results have shown that whole body protein turnover in elderly males and females was rather increased than decreased when related to the estimates of the whole body protein mass ($p < 0.10$) (Uauy et al, 1978a). Studies of whole body protein turnover in elderly have suggested reduced rates of whole body protein turnover coupled with an internal redistribution of whole body protein synthesis; the contribution of skeletal muscles to whole body protein turnover was reduced. More recent studies of albumin turnover in old patients have suggested that albumin synthesis in young people, but not in the elderly, was sensitive to changes in protein intake (Gersovitz et al., 1980).

The investigators concluded that albumin synthesis in the elderly is controlled at a lower set point, which prevented the response of albumin synthesis to high protein intakes. The results in that study were obtained from comparatively complicated *in vivo* kinetics based on use of stable isotopes. Our direct measurements of albumin and total hepatic protein synthesis in an unselected group of hospitalized patients are in support of the reported *in vivo* studies (Table 4-3). The significantly elevated hepatic protein synthesis *in vitro* suggests that the internal redistribution of protein synthesis in old subjects is associated with elevated synthesis of hepatic-derived proteins other than albumin. Such proteins may have some connection with the lysosomal system in the liver, since several lysosomal enzymes had increased maximum activities, as discussed above.

In man, age-dependent changes in the rate of myofibrillar protein degradation, assessed by 3-methylhistidine and creatinine excretion, have suggested that little, if any, alteration in myofibrillar protein degradation occurs after 20 to 30 years of age (Tomas et al., 1979). This suggests that whole muscle protein turnover is essentially unchanged under the progress of adult life. However, it seemed likely that muscles account for a lower proportion of whole body turnover in old people, and that a lower proportion of obligatory N-losses originates from the muscles (Uauy et al., 1978a). This probably means that a higher proportion of obligatory nitrogen losses arise from nitrogen turnover in visceral organs. This led Uauy and coworkers to conclude that protein metabolism in skeletal muscles might be especially vulnerable to the aging processes in man. However, our direct measurements of protein synthesis in isolated human muscle fibers from the rectus abdominus muscle argue against this conclusion. Muscle fibers of this comparatively white muscle obtained from unselected elderly subjects showed a higher rate of protein synthesis per unit of RNA, compared with that of middle-aged subjects (Table 4-4). The stimulatory effect of insulin on protein synthesis was also maintained in elderly subjects when the muscle tissue was subjected to insulin stimulation *in vivo* as well as *in vitro* (Tables 4-5, 4-6). Therefore, it is unlikely that minor nutritional changes among aging subjects could lead to significant impairments in the protein synthesis machinery in skeletal muscles. However, the decreasing muscle mass, must by definition be explained by a net negative nitrogen balance in skeletal muscles as the process of aging continues. It is clear that the mechanism remains to be determined.

In conclusion, the adaptation of protein metabolism in aging subjects is obvious in terms of altered body composition and loss of muscle mass. The mechanism(s) for these changes remain unclear and are probably multifactorial. Major factors may be of neuroendocrine origin. It can be anticipated that such factors will be extremely difficult to identify due to the fact that age-dependent changes in protein metabolism proceed continuously over several decades.

REFERENCES

Adams, P. and Muir, H. (1976). Qualitative changes with age of proteoglycans of human lumbar discs. *Ann. Rheum. Dis.* 35:289–296.

Adelman, R.C. (1975): Impaired hormonal regulation of enzyme activity during aging. *Fed. Proc.* 34:179–182.

Bando, M., Ishii, Y. and Nakajima, A. (1976): Changes in blue fluorescence intensity and coloration of human lens protein with normal lens aging and nuclear cataract. *Ophthalmic Res.* 8:456–463.

Björkerud, S., Björntorp, P. and Scherstén, T. (1967): Lysosomal enzyme activity in human liver in relation to the age of the patient and in cases with obstructive jaundice. *Scand. J. Clin. Lab. Invest.* 20:224–230.

Bolla, R. (1980): Age-dependent changes in rat liver steroid hormone receptor proteins. *Mechanisms of Aging and Development* 12:249–259.

Bruce, A., Andersson, M., Arvidsson, B. and Isaksson, B. (1980): Body composition. Prediction of normal body potassium, body water and body fat in adults on the basis of body height, body weight and age. *Scand. J. Clin. Lab. Invest.* 40:461–473.

Bylund, A-C., Holm, J., Lundholm, K. and Scherstén, T. (1976): Incorporation rate of glucose carbon, palmitate carbon and leucine carbon into metabolites in relation to enzyme activities and RNA levels in human skeletal muscles. *Enzyme* 21:39–52.

Cheng, A.H.R., Gomez, A., Bergan, J.G., Lee, T-C., Monckeberg, F. and Chichester, C.O. (1978): Comparative nitrogen balance study between young and aged adults using three levels of protein intake from a combination wheat-soy-milk mixture. *Am. J. Clin. Nutr.* 31:12–22.

Ermini, M., Moret, M-L., Reichmeier, K. and Dunne, T. (1978): Age-dependent structural changes in human neuronal chromatin. *Akt. Gerontol.* 8:675–680.

Eyre, D.R. and Muir, H. (1977): Quantitative analysis of types I and II collagens in human intervertebral discs at various ages. *Biochimica. et Biophysica Acta* 492:29–42.

Gershon, H. and Gershon, D. (1970): Detection of inactive enzyme molecules in aging organisms. *Nature* 227:1214–1217.

Gershon, H. and Gershon, D. (1973): Inactive enzyme molecules in aging mice: Liver aldolase. *Proc. Nat. Acad. Sci.* 70:909–913.

Gersovitz, M., Munro, H.N., Udall, J. and Young, V.R. (1980): Albumin synthesis in young and elderly subjects using a new stable isotope methodology: Response to level of protein intake. *Metabolism* 29:1075–1086.

Johnson, R. and Strehler, B.L. (1972): Loss of genes coding for ribosomal RNA in aging brain cells. *Nature* 240:412–414.

Kahn, A., Boivin, P., Vibert, M., Cottheau, D. and Dreyfus, J.C. (1974): Post-translational modifications of human glucose-6-phosphate dehydrogenase. *Biochimie.* 56:1395–1407.

Lundholm, K., Bylund, A-C., Holm, J., Smeds, S. and Scherstén, T. (1975): Metabolic studies in human skeletal muscle tissue. *Europ. Surg. Res.* 7:65–82.

Lundholm, K., Edström, S., Ekman, L., Karlberg, I., Walker, P. and Scherstén, T. (1981): Protein degradation in human skeletal muscle tissue: the effect of insulin, leucine, amino acids and ions. *Clin. Science* 60:319–326.

Lundholm, K. and Scherstén, T. (1975): Determination in vitro of the rate of protein synthesis and degradation in human-skeletal-muscle tissue. *Europ. J. Biochem.* 60:181–186.

Lundholm, K. and Schersten, T. (1977): Protein synthesis in human skeletal muscle tissue: influence of insulin and amino acids. *Europ. J. Clin. Invest.* 7:531–536.

Lundholm, K. and Scherstén, T. (1979): Protein synthesis in isolated human skeletal muscle tissue: evaluation of an experimental model. *Clin. Science* 57:221–223.

Lundholm, K., Scherstén, T., Lindstedt, G. and Lundberg, P-A. (1977): Studies on the biosynthesis of albumin and proteins in human liver tissue. *Europ. J. Clin. Invest.* 7:275–282.

Martin, G.M. (1980): Genotropic theories of aging. An overview. In: *Advances in Pathobiology, 7: Aging, Cancer and Cell Membranes* (Eds: C. Borek, C.M. Fenoglio and D.W. King) pp. 5–20, Georg Thieme Verlag, Stuttgart.

Miller, J.K. and Bolla, R. (1981): Influence of steroid-hormone-receptor-protein complexes on initiation of ribonucleic acid synthesis in liver nuclei isolated from rats of various ages. *Biochem. J.* 196:373–375.

Miyahara, T., Shiozawa, S. and Murai, A. (1978): The effect of age on amino acid composition of human skin collagen. *J. Geront.* 33:498–503.

Munro, H.N. and Young, V.R. (1973): Protein metabolism in the elderly. *Postgrad. Med.* 63: 143–152.

Munro, H.N. (1981): Nutrition and ageing. *Brit. Med. Bull.* 37:83–88.

Ogrodnik, J.P., Wulf, J.H. and Cutler, R.G. (1975): Altered protein hypothesis of mammalian ageing processes. II. Discrimination ratio of methionine vs. ethionine in the synthesis of ribosomal protein and RNA of C57BL/6J mouse liver. *Exp. Geront.* 10:119–136.

Parchman, L.G., Cake, M.H. and Litwack, G. (1978): Functionality of the liver glucocorticoid receptor during the life cycle and development of a low-affinity membrane binding site. *Mechanisms of Aging and Development* 7:227–240.

Roth, G.S. (1979): Hormone receptor changes during adulthood and senescence: Significance for aging research. *Fed. Proc.* 38:1910–1914.

Rubinson, H., Kahn, A., Boivin, P., Schapira, F., Gregori, C. and Dreyfus, J-C. (1976): Aging and accuracy of protein synthesis in man: Search for inactive enzymatic cross-reacting material in granulocytes of aged people. *Gerontology* 22:438–448.

Sacher, G.A. (1980): Mammalian life histories: Their evolution and molecular-genetic mechanisms. In: *Advances in Pathobiology, 7: Aging, Cancer and Cell Membranes* (Eds: C. Borek, C.M. Fenoglio and D.W. King), pp. 21–42, George Thieme Verlag.

Samorajski, T. (1977): Central neurotransmitter substances and aging: A review. *J. Am. Ger. Soc.* 25:337–348.

Scherstén, T. and Lundholm, K. (1972): Lysosomal enzyme activity in muscle tissue from patients with malignant tumor. *Cancer* 30:1246–1251.

Shock, N.W. (1972): Energy metabolism, caloric intake and physical activity of the aging. Symposia of the Swedish Nutrition Foundation, X, Nutrition in old age (Ed: Lars A. Carlsson), pp. 12–22, Almqvist and Wiksell, Uppsala, Sweden.

Steen, B., and Svanborg, A., (1975): *Nordisk Gerontologi, Andra Nordiska Kongressen i Gerontologi, Göteborg,* pp. 233–263. Astra Läkemedel AB, Södertälje, Sweden.

Sugarman, B. and Munro, H.N. (1980a): Altered [^{65}Zn] chloride accumulation by aged rats' adipocytes in vitro. *J. Nutr.* 110:2317–2320.

Sugarman, B. and Munro, H.N. (1980b): [^{14}C]-pantothenate accumulation by isolated adipocytes from adult rats of different ages. *J. Nutr.* 110:2297–2301.

Sugarman, B. and Munro, H.N. (1980c): Altered accumulation of zinc by aging human fibroblasts in culture. *Life Sciences* 26:915–920.

Tomas, F.M., Ballard, F.J. and Pope, L.M. (1979): Age-dependent changes in the rate of myofibrillar protein degradation in human as assessed by 3-methylhistidine and creatinine excretion. *Clin. Science* 56:341–346.

Uauy, R., Scrimshaw, N.S. and Young, V.R. (1978b): Human protein requirements: nitrogen balance response to graded levels of egg protein in elderly men and women. *Am. J. Clin. Nutr.* 31:779–785.

Uauy, R., Winterer, J.C., Bilmazes, C., Haverberg, L.N., Scrimshaw, N.S., Munro, H.N. and Young, V.R. (1978a): The changing pattern of whole body protein metabolism in aging humans. *J. Geront.* 33:663–671.

Young, V.R., Steffee, W.P., Pencharz, P.B., Winterer, J.C. and Scrimshaw, N.S. (1975): Total human body protein synthesis in relation to protein requirements at various ages. *Nature* 253:192–193.

Zeelon, P., Gershon, H. and Gershon, D. (1973): Inactive enzyme molecules in aging organisms. Nematode fructose-1,6-diphosphate aldolase. *Biochem. J.* 12:1743–1750.

Whole Body Protein Turnover, Studied With ^{15}N-Glycine, During Weight Reduction by Moderate Energy Restriction

Leonard J. Hoffer, Bruce R. Bistrian, Stephen D. Phinney, George L. Blackburn, Vernon R. Young

Obesity is not new, nor are weight reduction diets. Attempts to define effective, nutritionally sound weight loss diets go back to the turn of the century (Dapper, 1898). From the beginning, a major interest has been the effect of dietary energy restriction on protein metabolism: a controversial area then (Keeton et al., 1931) and now (DeHaven et al., 1980; Bistrian, 1980; Blackburn, 1980).

Out of a large body of research in many species has come clear evidence that protein and energy independently influence the efficiency of body protein retention (Munro, 1951; Committee on Dietary Allowances, 1980). When calories are restricted, nitrogen balance worsens; increasing the protein intake under these conditions improves the nitrogen balance (Calloway, 1975). A detailed picture of this phenomenon has been made possible by the administration of tracer amino acids, allowing an estimate of the rates of body protein turnover. Using ^{15}N-glycine and the Picou Taylor-Roberts model for whole body protein kinetics (Picou and Taylor-Roberts, 1969), protein turnover rate and inferred protein synthesis and breakdown were maintained at normal rates in healthy, moderately obese women after three weeks on a diet consisting only of high quality animal protein, 1.5 g/kg of ideal body weight (Winterer et al., 1980) providing only 440 kcal/day. A similar diet with protein in United States recommended dietary allowance (RDA) levels (0.8 g/kg ideal body weight) and made isocaloric by adding glucose, led to important declines in turnover, synthesis, and breakdown compared to baseline rates (Bistrian et al., 1981). It would appear, if normal rates of protein synthesis and breakdown are desirable, that protein intake at RDA levels was inadequate for these subjects on very low calorie diets, a finding which might have been predicted from the earlier evidence mentioned. In fact, nitrogen equilibrium was attained after three weeks on the protein-only diet but remained approximately − 2 g/day on the RDA-level protein diet, a mild but significant rate of protein loss.

In order to explore this relationship further, we have tested a diet still providing approximately RDA levels of protein and clearly in the hypocaloric range but with 400 calories more than the semistarvation diets studied before. It was wondered if protein synthesis and breakdown would be well maintained on a diet now approaching conventional balanced diets in energy and calories, and how this would relate to the nitrogen balance.

MATERIALS AND METHODS

The study diet was a dried product which supplied protein from calcium caseinate, dry milk powder, yeast extract and soy, giving 49 g protein, 138 g carbohydrate, 8 g fat, 2.2 g potassium, 2.3 g sodium and 820 kcal/day. RDA of vitamins and essential minerals were also supplied (Demical, Richardson-Vicks). This diet was preceded by four days on a baseline meat-free commercial liquid formula diet calculated to provide energy at 130% the basal expenditure (kcal 1959 ± 211, sd) and 1.5 g/kg IBW protein (Ensure, Ross Laboratories, supplemented as necessary with egg white protein).

Table 1
Patient Characteristics

Patient	Age	Height (cm)	Weight on Baseline Diet (kg)	Percent Ideal Body Weight	Weight loss After 14 days (kg)
MB	23	168	103.1	177	4.6
LF	37	166	88.8	156	4.4
SF	21	173	73.8	119	1.8
GH	23	160	92.2	175	2.9
RM	28	168	94.0	162	4.6

The subjects were five moderately obese healthy women admitted to the General Clinical Research Center of the Massachusetts Institute of Technology (Table 1). Candidate subjects underwent a medical evaluation which included history, physical examination, blood chemistry, urinalysis, chest x-ray and electrocardiogram. Informed consent was obtained under a protocol approved by the M.I.T. Committee on the Use of Humans as Experimental Subjects. Subjects were allowed to continue their normal daily activity, but received their diet under supervision and lived in the C.R.C. Dietary compliance was monitored by daily interview, qualitative urine ketones using the nitroprusside reaction, venous whole-blood beta-hydroxybutyrate (Bergmeyer, 1971) and by urinary potassium and urea nitrogen excretion. The completeness of urine collections was verified by urinary creatinine and potassium excretion. All urine and stool was collected throughout the study. Fecal collections were pooled weekly using stool markers, and stool and urine nitrogen determined spectrophotometrically after Kjeldahl digestion (Munro and Fleck, 1969). Daily nitrogen balance was calculated including estimated integumental losses of 5 mg N/kg (Joint FAO/WHO Committee, 1973). During the second to fourth days of the baseline diet, whole body protein turnover was estimated by the continuous oral administration of ^{15}N-glycine with simultaneous timed urine collections for determination of the enrichment in urinary urea. The study diet was then given for 14 days; during the last three days the ^{15}N-glycine study was repeated.

The tracer studies were conducted according to the Picou Taylor-Roberts model for whole body protein turnover (Q), synthesis (S), breakdown to amino acids (B), urinary excretion as byproducts of amino acid catabolism (E) and dietary intake (I) (Picou and Taylor-Roberts, 1969). The model assumes a single homogenous metabolic pool into which amino acids enter from the diet and from the breakdown of body proteins (I) + (B); and from which they leave, either by incorporation into body proteins or by oxidation, with resultant excretion as nitrogenous products in the urine (S) + (E). Under steady state conditions, the rates of entry and exit from the pool are equal, and are termed the flux, (Q). Thus, (Q) = (I) + (B) = (E) + (S).

Previous studies (Steffee et al., 1976; Matthews et al., 1981) have shown that when ^{15}N-glycine is given continuously or at three-hour intervals, by 60 hours the isotope has equilibrated in the metabolic nitrogen pool, so that the fraction of the administered isotope excreted as ^{15}N in urea may be taken to equal the fraction of all amino acid nitrogen entering the pool and excreted as urea. Knowing the rate of isotope administration, its rate of excretion in urea, and the rate of total urea excretion, the rate of entry of amino acid nitrogen into the pool, (Q), may immediately be calculated by the principle of isotope dilution.

^{15}N-glycine (99% enriched) provided in an amount sufficient to provide approximately 0.5 mg ^{15}N/kg body weight, was given as 20 equal oral doses at precise three-hour intervals for 60 hours. The urine was collected at three-hour intervals for analysis of ^{15}N-enrichment of urinary urea nitrogen by isotope ratio mass spectrometry. The achievement of isotopic plateau was confirmed and the plateau value for enrichment determined by inspection, permitting a calculation of (Q). (I) being known and (E) being the total urinary nitrogen, (S) and (B) were calculated from the Picou Taylor-Roberts equation.

RESULTS

The diet was tolerated well by the subjects whose average weight loss during the test diet period was kg 3.7 ± 1.3 SD (Table 1). Ketonuria developed in the first few days and was persistent throughout the study; venous whole-blood beta-hydroxybutyrate was 0.71 ± 0.50 mM. During the baseline diet, the average daily nitrogen balance was − 0.8 ± 0.4g, not significantly different from zero. During the first week on the study diet, nitrogen balance was − 3.6 ± 1.0 g/day but improved to − 2.2 ± 0.5 during the second week. Four subjects continued on the same diet for a further two weeks; for these subjects, the average daily nitrogen balance during the fourth week of the diet was − 1.5 ± 0.2 g/day. All values are significantly less than the baseline ($p < 0.05$).

The results obtained from the ^{15}N-glycine studies are shown in Table 2, which also shows (I) and (E) for each subject. The dietary manipulation decreased the protein intake by 38 g/day. In response, (Q) decreased by 49 g, a change of 16% ($p < 0.02$). (S) and (B) decreased by 7% and 5%, but these small changes are not statistically significant, and neither, therefore, is the difference between the fall in (I) and (Q). It thus appears that there was a decrease in protein flux corresponding to the decrease in the protein intake, with a parallel decrease in the rate of amino acid catabolism (E). Considering fecal and integumental losses, the nitrogen balance was significantly negative on the study diet, but whole body protein synthesis and catabolism were maintained.

DISCUSSION

The results are clear-cut. In a previous study by Bistrian et al. (1981) a diet providing approximately 44 g protein and 440 kcal was insufficient to support normal rates of (Q), (S), and (B), which all fell by roughly 30%. The present diet, providing almost the same protein intake (49 g) and only 400 kcal more, maintained these parameters. It is noteworthy that nitrogen balance was not improved, being − 2.1 ± 0.9 g/day the week of the turnover study on the 400 kcal diet and − 2.2 ± 0.5 in the present one.

Table 2
Protein Turnover (g/protein/day)

Subject	Diet	(I)	(E)	(Q)	(S)	(B)
MB	baseline diet	87	81	309	228	222
	study diet	49	55	274	218	224
LF	baseline diet	90	86	334	248	244
	study diet	49	54	265	211	216
SF	baseline diet	93	77	334	257	241
	study diet	49	46	250	204	201
RM	baseline diet	86	102	280	179	195
	study diet	49	54	265	211	216
BH	baseline diet	79	75	322	247	243
	study diet	49	46	280	234	231
Average	(mean ± sd)	87 ± 5	84 ± 11	316 ± 22	232 ± 31	229 ± 21
		49 ± 0	51 ± 5	267 ± 11	216 ± 11	218 ± 11
Significant change		–	$p < 0.001$	$p < 0.02$	ns	ns

It cannot be determined from these studies if it is physiologically desirable to maintain normal rates of (Q) and (S). However, protein recycling at the observed rates—about four times the dietary intake rate—is energetically expensive (Flatt, 1978), and this suggests that it may be regulated. Using the Picou Taylor-Roberts model, Steffee et al. (1976) found in normal volunteers that (Q) fell only 8% in response to a 75% decrease in protein intake when an ample energy intake was maintained; the flux was maintained by increases in (B) and (S). It could be argued that the increased energy expenditure entailed in maintaining (Q) under these conditions was supportable because exogenous energy was amply present. Similarly, (Q), (S), and (B) were maintained in a study of obese women on a diet in which the energy intake was dropped to about 25% of maintenance but the protein intake kept high. In contrast, (Q), (S), and (B) were markedly lowered with hypocaloric, protein-free diets (Garlick et al., 1980) and in manifest protein-calorie malnutrition (Waterlow, 1977). In total fasting, (Q), and (S), were observed to decline but (B) did not (Winterer et al., 1980). Within the context of this particular model, a situation reminiscent of the effect of energy and protein on nitrogen balance may be formulated. Some protein intake is essential, but when the protein intake is low (Q) and (S) are maintained provided there is ample dietary energy. When the energy intake is limited, a higher protein intake then becomes necessary, such that below critical combinations of protein and energy intake, (Q), (S), and (B) are not maintained. The decrease in (Q), (S), and (B) observed with a RDA-protein level, 440 kcal diet (Bistrian et al., 1981) would then represent either a failure of regulation or a down-regulation of whole body protein kinetics. Either might be undesirable and could be prevented either by giving more calories, as was done in the present study, or—more desirable in a weight reduction regimen—simply more protein (Winterer et al., 1980).

Garlick et al. (1980) have drawn different conclusions from these in their study of protein kinetics in obese subjects on a diet providing 50 g protein and 500 kcal. In three subjects studied using the Picou Taylor-Roberts model, (Q), (S), and (B) remained at baseline values after three weeks on this diet; it was therefore concluded that, provided some protein is included in the diet, changes in energy over a wide range do not influence (S) and (B). There is no ready explanation for the difference in these results and those of Bistrian et al. (1981) except to note that in all these studies the number of subjects studied has been small and biological variability is great (Williams, 1956). It is possible that the protein and energy intakes in the study by Garlick et al. (1980), falling slightly above those used by Bistrian et al. (1981) were still in a range acceptable for the maintenance of (Q). Altogether, the results of recent studies (Winterer et al., 1980; Bistrian et al., 1981) would not be incompatible with the conclusion of Garlick et al. (1980), but would place a "safe" protein intake rather higher than theirs, approximately 75 g/day for women on highly energy-restricted diets (Winterer et al., 1980).

The differences among nitrogen balance, (S) and (B) deserve comment. In our calculations, as in those of others (Garlick et al., 1980), fecal and estimated integumental losses are ignored in the Picou Taylor-Roberts model. This may be defended on the grounds that these products of protein breakdown are not participants in the homogenous metabolic nitrogen pool assumed by the model. Yet, these losses are not negligible, amounting in combination to some 1 g N/day. It should also be recognized that there is not a necessary fixed relationship between turnover on the one hand, and nitrogen balance on the other, although from the Picou

Taylor-Roberts equation, (I) - (E), which is nitrogen balance, equals (S) - (B). For example, in the study by Garlick et al. (1980) the three subjects studied maintained (Q), (S), and (B) at baseline rates, yet analysis of their data (assuming fecal nitrogen losses of 0.5 g/day) gives an average nitrogen balance of approximately −3 g/day during the turnover study. Also, as mentioned above, (Q), (S), and (B) were maintained in the present study and decreased in the study of Bistrian et al. (1981), while nitrogen balance was the same, mildly negative, in both. The maintenance of normal (S) and (B) does not necessarily imply that the body protein mass is being maintained, because fecal and miscellaneous losses must be considered and perhaps because at high cycling rates small, methodologically indiscernible differences between (S) and (B) may become important when the protein intake is low or moderate. It may be that high rates of (S) and (B) are incompatible with maximal efficiency in protein sparing when energy is simultaneously restricted.

It is instructive to compare the kinetic parameters of various studies carried out during a baseline maintenance diet. While absolute values for (Q), (S), and (B) are quite variable from one study to another, the mean values are in close agreement when normalized by the creatinine excretion (Table 3). Since publication of two of the studies (Winterer et al., 1980; Bistrian et al., 1981), it has been determined that the enrichment of the glycine used was some 12% to 14% higher than initially determined. Therefore, values for these studies more correctly are some 10% to 15% higher than shown in the table. Despite this, excellent agreement across these several studies is maintained. Forbes et al. (1976) have shown that urinary creatinine excretion correlates well with the lean body mass as determined by total body potassium, so it would be anticipated that protein turnover rates would be related to the creatinine excretion. Nevertheless, normalizing in this way does not invariably decrease the considerable intersubject variability. Other factors, as yet undetermined, play an important role in determining absolute whole body protein kinetic parameters.

Table 3
Whole Body Protein Turnover Parameters in Obese Subjects on Baseline Diets in Four Studies

	Present Study	Winterer et al. (1980)	Bistrian et al. (1981)	Garlick et al. (1980)
(Q) g protein/g creatinine•day	182 ± 42	188 ± 29	187 ± 24	193 ± 19
(S) g protein/g creatinine•day	134 ± 38	128 ± 26	129 ± 19	134 ± 34
(B) g protein/g creatinine•day	132 ± 33	125 ± 22	131 ± 21	146 ± 29

ACKNOWLEDGMENT

The authors thank Marta Wolfe, Shriners Burns Institute, Boston, for performing the mass spectrometric analyses.

Supported in part by a grant from Richardson-Vicks Inc., and NIH grants

AM-26349, awarded by the National Institute of Arthritis, Metabolism, and Digestive Diseases and RR-88, awarded by the Research Resources Division, National Institutes of Health. Dr. Hoffer is a Fellow of the Medical Research Council of Canada.

REFERENCES

Bergmeyer, H.V. (1971): *Methods of Enzymatic Analysis*. Academic Press, New York.

Bistrian, B.R. (1980): Low-calorie versus mixed diet. *N. Engl. J. Med.* 303:157–158.

Bistrian, B.R., Sherman, M., and Young, V. (1981): The mechanisms of nitrogen sparing to fasting supplemented by protein and carbohydrate. *J. Clin. Endocrinol. Metab.* 53:874–878.

Blackburn, G.L. (1980): Low-calorie versus mixed diet. *N. Engl. J. Med.* 303:158.

Calloway, D.H. (1975): Nitrogen balance of men with marginal intakes of protein and energy. *J. Nutr.* 105:914–923.

Committee on Dietary Allowances, Food and Nutrition Board (1980): *Recommended Dietary Allowances*. National Academy of Science, Washington, D.C.

Dapper, C. (1898): Ueber Entfettungskuren. *Arch. F. Verdauungskrankheiten* 3:1–18.

DeHaven, J., Sherwin, R., Hendler, R., and Felig, P. (1980): Nitrogen and sodium balance and sympathetic-nervous system activity in obese subjects treated with a low-calorie protein or mixed diet. *N. Engl. J. Med.* 302:477–482.

Forbes, G.B., and Bruining, G.J. (1976): Urinary creatinine excretion and lean body mass. *Am. J. Clin. Nutr.* 29:1359–1366.

Flatt, J.P. (1978): The biochemistry of energy expenditure. In: *Recent Advances in Obesity Research: II* (ed: G.A. Bray), pp. 379–384, Newman Publishing, London.

Garlick, P.J., Clugston, G.A., and Waterlow, J.C. (1980): Influence of low-energy diets on whole-body protein turnover in obese subjects. *Am. J. Physiol.* 238:E235–E244.

Joint FAO/WHO Expert Committee (1973): *Energy and Protein Requirements*. World Health Organization, Geneva (WHO Technical Report Series No. 522).

Keeton, R.W., MacKenzie, H., Olson, S., and Pickens, L. (1931): The influence of varying amounts of carbohydrate, fat, protein, and water on the weight loss of hogs in undernutrition. *Am. J. Physiol.* 97:473–490.

Matthews, D.E., Conway, J.M., Young, V.R., and Bier, D.M. (1981): Glycine nitrogen metabolism in man. *Metabolism* 30:886–893.

Munro, H.N. (1951): Carbohydrate and fat as factors in protein utilization and metabolism. *Physiol. Rev.* 31:449–488.

Munro, H.N., and Fleck, A. (1969): Analysis of tissues and body fluids for nitrogenous constituents. In: *Mammalian Protein Metabolism* (ed: H.N. Munro), Vol. 3, pp. 423–525, Academic Press, New York.

Picou, D., and Taylor-Roberts, T. (1969): The measurement of total protein synthesis and catabolism and nitrogen turnover in infants in different nutritional states and receiving different amounts of dietary protein. *Clin. Sci.* 36:283–296.

Steffee, W.P., Goldsmith, R.S., Pencharz, P.B., Scrimshaw, N.W., and Young, V.R. (1976): Dietary protein intake and dynamic aspects of whole body nitrogen metabolism in adult humans. *Metabolism* 25:281–297.

Waterlow, J.C., Golden, M., and Picou, D. (1977): The measurement of rates of protein turnover, synthesis, and breakdown in man and the effects of nutritional status and surgical injury. *Am. J. Clin. Nutr.* 30:1333–1339.

Williams, R.J. (1956): *Biochemical Individuality*. John Wiley and Sons, New York.

Winterer, J., Bistrian, B.R., Bilmazes, C., Blackburn, G.L., and Young, V.R. (1980): Whole body protein turnover studied with ^{15}N-glycine and muscle protein breakdown in mildly obese subjects during a protein-sparing diet and a brief total fast. *Metabolism* 29:575–581.

Amino Acid Requirements of Japanese Young Men

Goro Inoue, Tatsushi Komatsu, Kyoichi Kishi, and Yoshiaki Fujita

The amino acid requirements of Japanese young men have been studied using a synthetic diet containing *L*-amino acid mixture. The general procedures were the modifications of Rose's short-term nitrogen balance technique. Throughout the experimental periods, energy intake was kept on approximately maintenance level of 44 ± 2 kcal/kg body weight.

Exp. 1: *Essential amino acid (EAA) requirements for the prevention of single amino acid deficiency.*

Throughout the experimental periods, total N intake for 26 subjects was constant at a level of 0.16 g/kg with 35% EAA-N of Rose's pattern (Table 1A). Figure 1 shows one example of leucine experiment. When high urinary nitrogen excretion was observed in pre-experimental free-feeding period, an excess energy of 50 kcal/kg B. W. was given for the first few days and then energy intake of 44 kcal/kg was allowed to attain zero balance in basal diet period. In the experimental period, the intake of one of eight EAAs changed in three deficient levels with each five to seven days period by ascending design. The nitrogen balance was calculated using urinary nitrogen excretions of the last two to three days of each amino acid-deficient diet period. The results of eight EAAs are given in Figure 2A and Figure 2B showing the relation between intake of each EAA and nitrogen balance. The maintenance requirement of each EAA can be estimated from the respective regression line. Table 2 shows the regression equations and the maintenance requirements of eight EAAs. In expressing the mean requirement of an EAA as E/A ratio, no great differences were observed between our results and those of Rose, although the ratios of methionine and tryptophan tended to be lower and those of valine and threonine to be higher than Rose's figures. Furthermore, total EAA requirement of 105 mg/kg/day as mean + 1 SD is comparable with 91 mg/kg/day (recalculated as 70 kg of body weight) obtained by Rose under excess energy supply. This agreement in EAA requirement indicates that excess energy has no beneficial effect on nitrogen losses caused by single amino acid deficiency. This finding is in striking contrast to the protein-sparing effect of excess energy observed in protein deficiency.

Exp. 2: *Total N requirement of amino acid mixture simulating egg protein.*

After one week of standard habitual diet with N intake of 200 mgN/kg/day and about 45 kcal/kg/day of energy, a synthetic diet with amino acid mixture simulating egg protein (Table 1B) was given for two weeks. N intakes were 60 mgN/kg/day for five subjects, 75 mgN/kg/day for ten subjects and 100 mgN/kg/day for three subjects. Figure 3 shows the results of N intake of 75 mgN/kg/day. In order to examine the effect of nitrogen sources, egg protein was given isonitrogenously in place of

Table 1
Composition of Amino Acid Mixture

A Experiment 1
(in case of subj. MK weighed 62.5 kg)

	As used	*N content*
	g/day	mg/day
EAA		
L-ILE	3.356	358
L-LEU	5.274	563
L-LYS.HCl	4.791	735
L-MET	5.274	495
L-PHE	5.274	447
L-THR	2.397	281
L-TRP	1.198	164
L-VAL	3.836	459
Total	31.400	3,503
NEAA		
L-ARG.HCl	2.000	532
L-HIS	1.000	200
L-GLU	25.000	2,393
L-GLU.Na	27.000	2,235
GLY	4.000	746
Total	59.000	6,106
Unknown N		400
Grand total	90.400	10,009

Total N intake: 0.16 gN/kg
Content of EAA-N with Rose's pattern was 35% of total N.

B Experiment 2
(AA mix. with egg pattern*)

	As AA	*As N*
	g/100g	mg/100g
EAA		
ILE	6.08	649
LEU	8.53	911
LYS	6.75	1,293
MET	6.18	580
PHE	9.21	781
THR	4.95	582
TRP	1.44	198
VAL	6.63	793
Total	49.77	5,787
ARG	5.90	1,898
HIS	2.35	636
ALA	5.73	901
ASP	9.30	979
GLU	12.32	1,173
GLY	3.20	597
PRO	4.02	489
SER	7.40	986
Total	50.22	7,659
Grand total	99.99	13,446

Content of EAA-N with egg pattern was 43% of total N.
*Referred to "Amino-acid content of foods", FAO, 1970.

Table 2
Maintenance Requirements of Eight EEAs Estimated from Pooled and Individual Data

		Pooled Data[1]					Individual Data[2]			
		Regression Equation[3]			*Maintenance intake*					
	Subj. No.	*Slope*	*Y-intercept*	*r*	*Mean*	*SD*	*Maintenance intake*			
			(mgN/kg)		(mg/kg)				(mg/kg)	
ILE	3	4.55	−47.61	0.95	10.5	1.61		9.9	10.6	10.9
LEU	3	2.77	−35.53	0.70	12.8	4.69		10.2	13.5	13.5
LYS	3	2.64	−30.85	0.78	11.7	2.95		8.8	12.1	13.1
MET	3	1.62	−17.28	0.90	10.7	1.82		10.2	11.0	11.1
PHE	3	2.05	−29.09	0.80	14.2	3.85		11.3	13.4	17.2
THR	3	4.11	−33.66	0.80	8.2	2.05		7.0	7.9	9.3
TRP	4	5.75	−14.50	0.80	2.5	1.34	1.9	2.1	2.3	3.2
VAL	4	1.71	−23.27	0.90	13.6	2.23	12.3	13.2	14.0	15.9
				(Total)	84.2	20.54				94.2

[1]In pooled data, regression equation was calculated using 9 and 12 data obtained in 3 and 4 subjects.
[2]In individual data, the equation was calculated using 3 and 4 data obtained each subject.
[3]Regression equation was calculated between essential amino acid intake (X: mg/kg) and N balance (Y: mgN/kg).

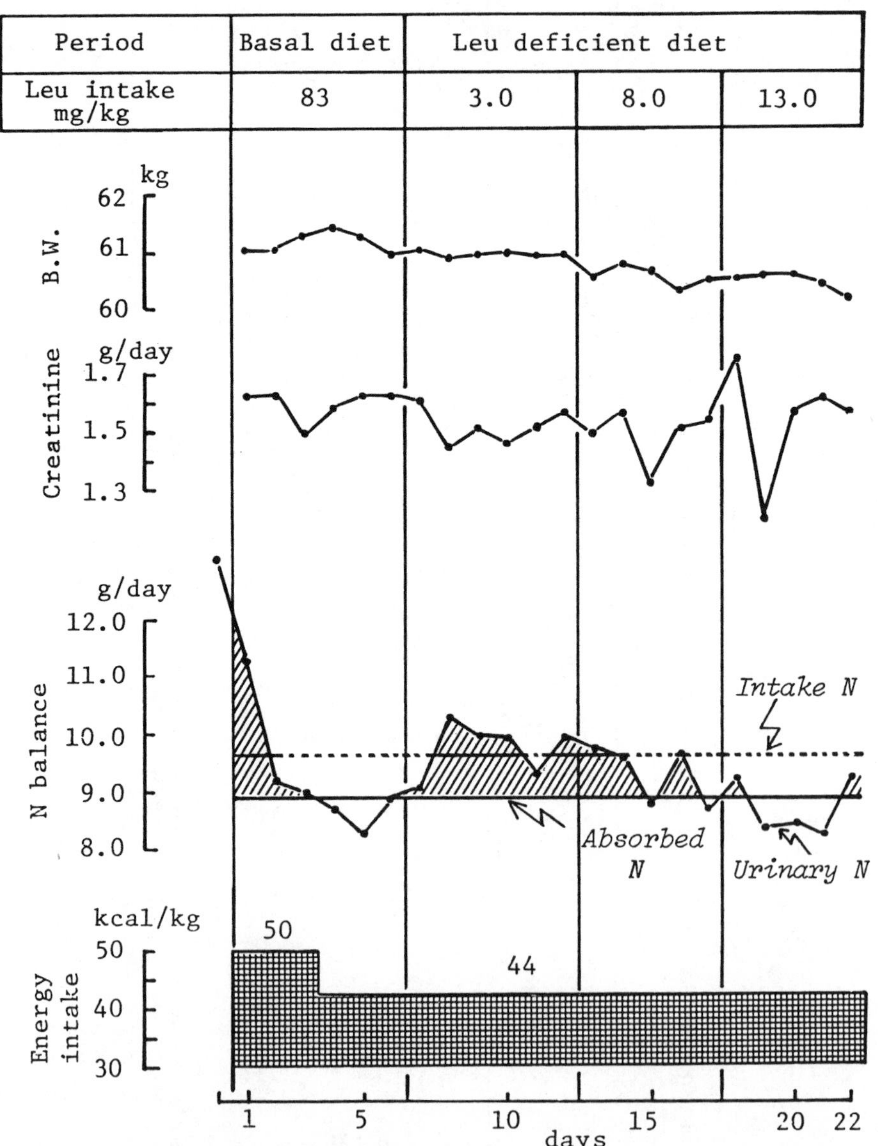

Figure 1 N balance with low leucine intake.

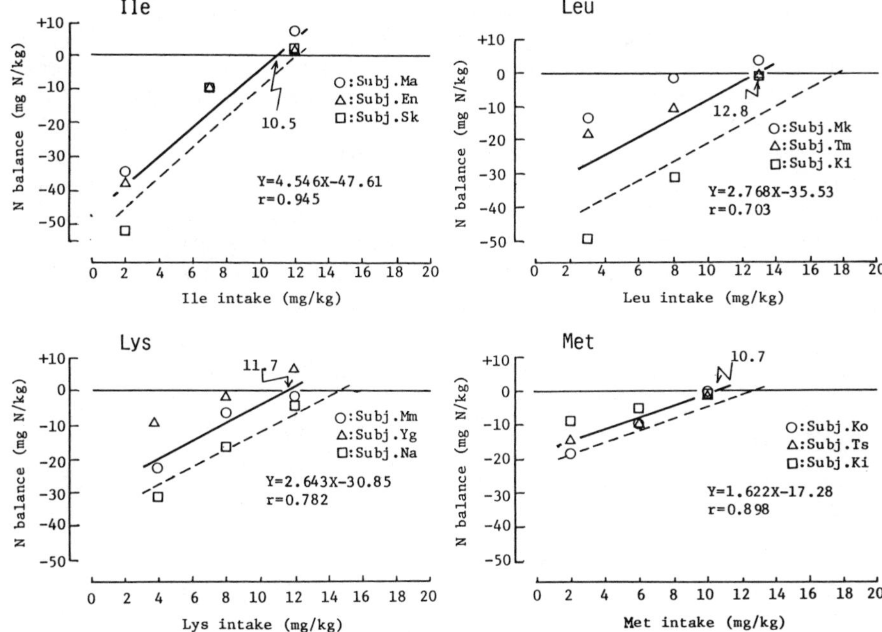

Figure 2A Regression lines obtained with each EAA (Ile, Leu, Lys, Met).

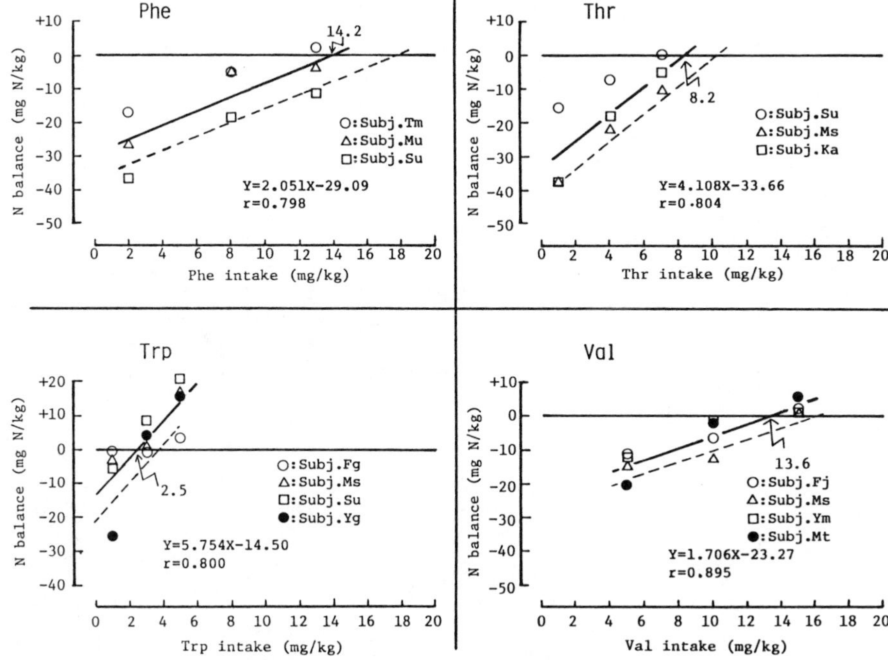

Figure 2B Regression lines obtained with each EAA (Phe, Thr, Trp, Val).

amino acid mixture for one week after the amino acid diet period. The results are shown in Table 3. Linear regression equation obtained between total amino acid N intake (X: mgN/kg/day) and nitrogen balance (Y: mgN/kg/day) was as follows; $Y = 0.276X - 25.11$ (Figure 4). No significant difference was observed between this equation and that obtained previously with whole egg protein, that is, $Y = 0.411X - 37.03$. Mean maintenance requirement of total amino acid N was 91.0 mgN/kg/day which was equivalent to egg protein requirement. The same conclusion can be made from the observations as shown in Table 3 that urinary nitrogen excretion and nitrogen balance showed no significant difference in changing amino acid diet to egg protein diet. It can be said that the amino acid mixture had similar nutritive value to intact egg protein under the present experimental conditions. Further studies are

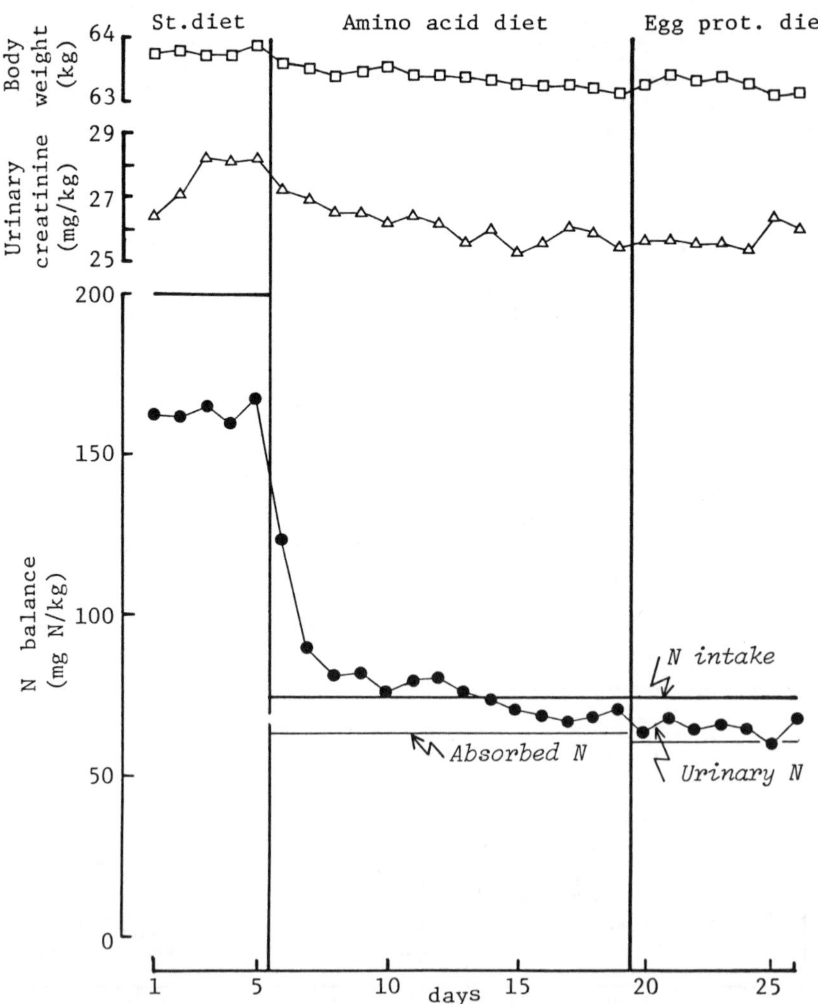

Figure 3 Daily changes in mean urinary N excretion and body weight of 10 subjects fed a diet of 75 mgN/kg of amino acid mixture.

Table 3
Nitrogen Balance Data at Three Levels of N Intake from Amino Acid Diet and Egg Protein Diet

	N level	60	75	100
	Subject No.	*5*	*10*	*3*
			(mg/kg)	
Amino acid mix[1]	N intake	59.4 ± 0.43	74.8 ± 0.67	99.9 ± 0.84
	Urinary N	57.7 ± 5.61[2]	69.2 ± 7.87[2]	84.8 ± 2.12[2]
	Fecal N	10.2 ± 1.08	10.4 ± 1.09*	12.1 ± 2.93
	N balance	− 8.5 ± 6.00	− 4.8 ± 7.60	+ 3.0 ± 2.64
Egg protein	N intake		74.8 ± 0.67	99.9 ± 0.84
	Urinary N		64.9 ± 11.37[3]	86.0 ± 2.01[3]
	Fecal N		12.2 ± 1.28*	15.7 ± 3.93*
	N balance		− 2.3 ± 10.84	− 1.8 ± 3.73

*Significantly different between amino acid and protein diets.
[1]Amino acid mixture was simulated egg protein pattern.
[2]Average of last 5 days of each experimental period of 2 weeks.
[3]Average of last 3 days of each experimental period of a week.

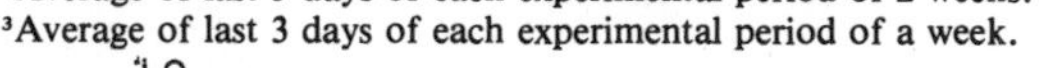

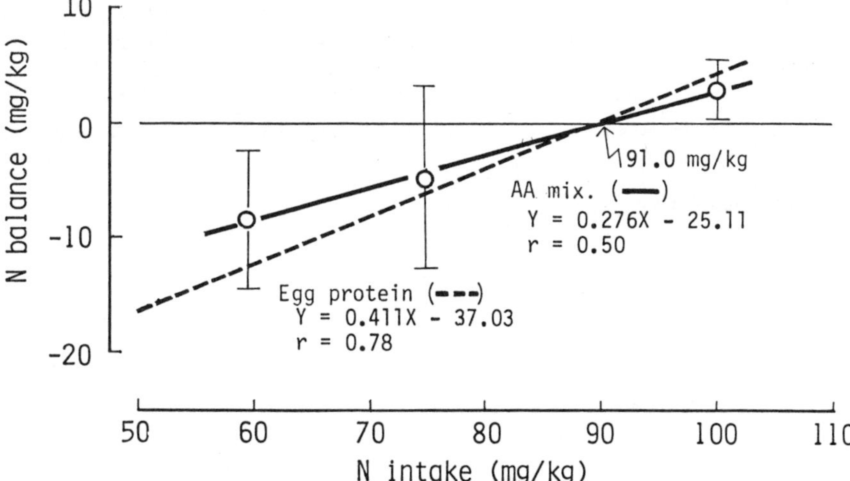

Figure 4 Comparison of the regression lines obtained with amino acid mixture diet and egg protein diet. Note: 1) There is no significant difference between the two regression lines. 2) Energy intake in both experiments was nearly equal at approximate maintenance intake. 3) Result of egg protein was reported in *J. Nutr.* 103:1673, 1973.

needed to clarify the nutritive efficiencies of intact protein, peptides and amino acid mixture.

In a pilot study (Table 4) we reinvestigated the amino acid requirement of 3.50 gN/day with 1.46 gN of EAA reported by Rose et al. Nitrogen balance observed in that study was almost zero with excess energy intake of 44 kcal/kg/day, while it remained strongly negative with 45 kcal/kg/day. This result suggests that we should not supply excess energy in the experiment on amino acid requirements as well as protein requirements.

In summary: 1) Total amino acid N requirement was similar to egg protein N being about 90 mgN/kg/day (Exp. 2) and therefore the N requirement of 3.5 gN/day (that is, 50 mgN/kg/day as 70 kg of body weight) reported by Rose et al. might be too low. 2) EAA-N requirement obtained in Exp. 1 was 14.7 mgN/kg/day being 16% of total amino acid N requirement of 90 mgN/kg/day (that is, E/T ratio of 1.37) and the Rose's figure of 10.4 mgN/kg/day corresponds to 12% of total N (that is, E/T ratio of 1.00). On the other hand, the EAA-N content of egg protein is 43% and E/T ratio is 3.70. However, Drs. Scrimshaw and Young showed that EAA content of egg protein could be diluted by nonspecific nitrogen sources to 25—21% of total N (E/T ratio of 2.16–1.85) without affecting their nutritive value. The problem of E/T ratio should be examined further with amino acid mixture diet.

Table 4
Effect of Excess Energy on Utilization of Amino Acid Nitrogen in Pilot Study[1]

Energy level (kcal/kg)		45	55
Number of subj.		3	4
Mean body weight (kg)		61.3 ± 9.2	63.7 ± 8.9
N intake[2]	(g/day)	3.50	3.50
	(mg/kg)	58.0 ± 9.0	55.8 ± 8.5
Fecal N	(mg/kg)	12.3 ± 0.4	12.8 ± 1.1
Urinary N[3]	(mg/kg)	68.3 ± 9.1	49.8 ± 13.6
N balance	(mg/kg)	– 22.6 ± 10.6	– 6.8 ± 8.2

[1]Experimental period was 10 days in each diet. Free feeding of 3 days between two energy intake periods was inserted.
[2]Containing 1.46 gN of EAA with egg pattern.
[3]Average of last 4 days.

SECTION II
Metabolism of Amino Acids

5 Amino Acids and Gluconeogenesis

Alan D. Cherrington
Kurt E. Steiner
William W. Lacy

Gluconeogenesis is the process by which lactate, pyruvate, glycerol and certain amino acids are converted to glucose. Two organs of the body, the liver and kidney, possess the full enzymic machinery necessary to accomplish this. Under most circumstances, however, it is only the liver that plays a significant role in the synthesis of glucose and so the present discussion will focus on that organ.

Figure 5-1 depicts the various components of the gluconeogenic process and serves to illustrate the main ways in which it can be regulated. Control can be exerted at three points: the supply of gluconeogenic precursors coming from peripheral tissues, their uptake by the liver, and their subsequent conversion to glucose within the liver. The purpose of this paper is to review our understanding of the way in which physiologic increments in insulin, glucagon and catecholamines regulate these processes *in vivo*, giving particular emphasis to recent studies carried out in our laboratories.

Before attempting to define the role of hormones in the regulation of gluconeogenesis *in vivo,* it is important to review the biochemical steps involved in the conversion of gluconeogenic substrates to glucose within the liver. Figure 5-2 outlines the gluconeogenic pathway and illustrates the three sites at which the process can be regulated. These regulatory loci were first determined by Exton and his coworkers

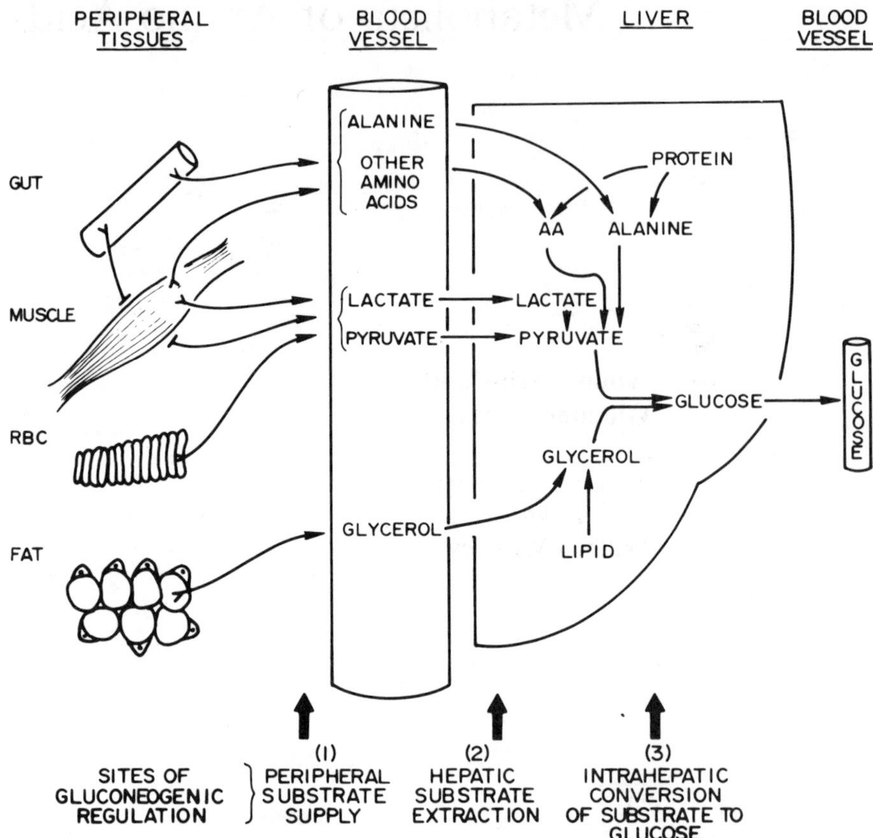

Figure 5-1 Schematic representation of the sites of gluconeogenic regulation within a whole animal. (Reproduced with permission; Cherrington, 1981).

(1972) from measurements of the intracellular levels of various metabolites in the liver before and after hormone treatment. Subsequent work has firmly established the location of regulatory sites between pyruvate and phosphoenol pyruvate, between fructose 1-6 diphosphate and fructose-6-phosphate, and between glucose-6-phosphate and glucose. Details of the enzymic regulation involved at these sites are beyond the scope of this paper and readers are directed to the reviews of Cherrington, 1981, and Claus and Pilkis, 1981, for a summary of the latest work in this area.

MEASUREMENT OF GLUCONEOGENESIS *IN VIVO*

Both tracer and arteriovenous (AV) difference techniques have been used to assess gluconeogenesis in man and whole animals. The AV difference technique involves the measurement of the concentration of a given gluconeogenic precursor in the blood entering and leaving the liver, and multiplication of this difference by the hepatic blood flow. It should be noted that in man, because of the difficulty in obtaining portal blood, it is splanchnic rather than hepatic uptake which is calculated.

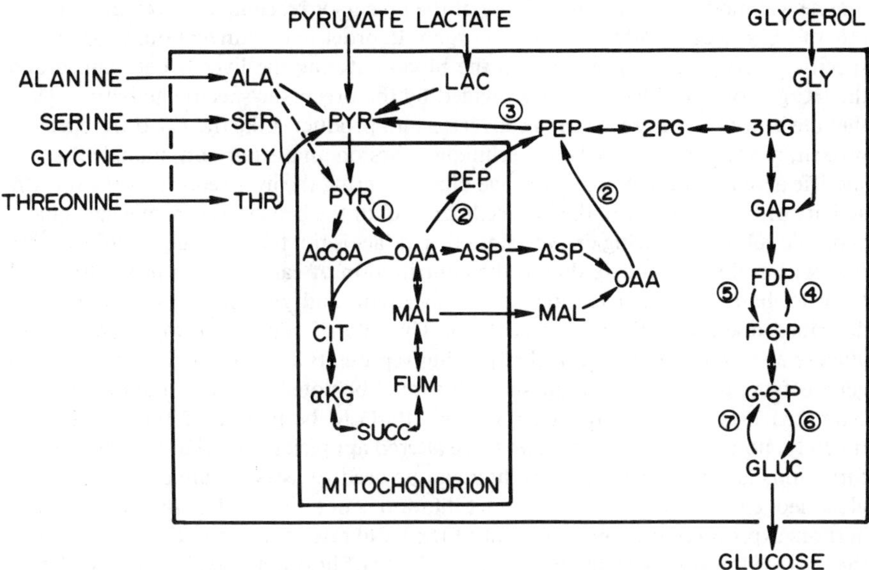

Figure 5-2 Schematic representation of the gluconeogenic process within the hepatocyte, ALA (alanine), SER (serine), GLY (glycine), THR (threonine), PYR (pyruvate), LAC (lactate), AcCoA (acetyl CoA), CIT (citrate), αKG (α-ketoglutarate), SUCC (succinate), FUM (fumarate), MAL (malate), OAA (oxaloacetate), PEP (phosphoeneolpyruvate), ASP (aspartate), 2PG (2-phosphoglycerate), 3PG (3-phosphoglycerate), GLY (glycerol), GAP (glyceraldehyde phosphate), FDP (fructose diphosphate), F-6-P (fructose-6-phosphate), G-6-P (glucose-6-phosphate), GLUC (glucose). The numbers refer to rate-limiting enzymes in the gluconeogenic and glycolytic sequence: (1) pyruvate carboxylase, (2) phosphoenolpyruvate carboxykinase (this enzyme can be mitochondrial or cytosolic), (3) pyruvate kinase, (4) phosphofructokinase, (5) fructose diphosphatase, (6) glucose-6-phosphatase, and (7) glucokinase. The dotted line taking alanine into the mitochondrion reflects the potential conversion of alanine to pyruvate within the subcellular organelle. (Reproduced with permission; Cherrington, 1981).

Implicit in the use of this approach to quantitate gluconeogenesis is the assumption that all of the precursor being taken up is converted to glucose. In fact, this is not the case, and thus one cannot use the AV difference approach to accurately quantitate gluconeogenesis *in vivo*. One can, however, use this method to calculate the maximal contribution that a given precursor can make to glucose production. The AV difference technique also can be used to calculate the hepatic fractional extraction of a given precursor by dividing the amount of precursor extracted by the amount delivered to the liver. Such a calculation allows determination of whether changes in hepatic uptake are due to a change in the load of the precursor reaching the liver or to a change in the ability of the liver to extract the precursor.

The tracer technique involves the infusion of a ^{14}C-labeled gluconeogenic precursor and measurement of the rate of ^{14}C-labeled glucose production by the liver. The latter can itself be determined using a tracer technique (^{3}H-glucose infusion) or an AV difference method. Obviously the rate of ^{14}C glucose production by the liver will be controlled not only by hepatic events but also by peripheral events, since a change in the rate of release of the particular substrate in question from fat or muscle will modify the specific activity of the precursor reaching the liver and thus the rate of ^{14}C glucose production by that organ. In order to circumvent this problem the specific activity of the precursor in the blood entering the liver is determined and the ^{14}C glucose production rate is divided by the precursor-specific activity to yield the rate at which the precursor is converted into product. Like the AV difference approach, the validity of the tracer technique relies on an assumption, namely that the specific activity of the precursor in the blood entering the liver represents the specific activity of the precursor in the intracellular pool of the hepatocyte from which gluconeogenic substrate is being drawn. Since this in fact is not the case, the specific activity falls within the hepatocyte due to the contribution of carbon from proteolysis and from exchange between carbon in the glycolytic and gluconeogenic pathways as described elsewhere (Krebs et al., 1966). The rate of conversion of a substrate to glucose as determined by this technique thus represents a minimum rate of gluconeogenesis from the substrate in question. It should be noted that this dilution has been estimated using ^{14}C-bicarbonate (Hetenyi, 1981) to be between 2.0 and 2.8. Fortunately, however, it does not seem to be altered appreciably by acute hormonal perturbations and thus the tracer method can be used to assess relative changes in the gluconeogenic process even if the exact dilution is not known. For this reason, most authors express conversion as percent of the basal rate, not attempting to quantitate the process but simply trying to assess the ability of hormones to change it. It should be noted that under conditions in which glycogen deposition might occur it is necessary to biopsy the liver at the end of the study (or to flush out the glycogen using glucagon) in order to determine how much of the gluconeogenically derived carbon was stored as glycogen rather than released by the liver. In this way the ^{14}C glucose stored as glycogen can be assessed and added to the ^{14}C glucose released by the liver to yield the true hepatic ^{14}C glucose formation rate.

A change in conversion will occur whether a particular hormone has its effect on peripheral tissues, intrahepatic enzymes or transport at the hepatocyte plasma membrane. This is particularly important to remember when amino acids are used as gluconeogenic precursors since their hepatic uptake can be regulated at the transport level (Donner et al., 1978). It is possible, using the tracer technique, to separate the intrahepatic effects from the others by calculating the fraction of the extracted ^{14}C precursor which is converted to glucose. A change in this fraction should denote an intrahepatic event. Obviously, no method used to assess gluconeogenesis *in vivo* is perfect; however, when the various methods are combined they can give a useful assessment of the hormonal control of the process. Accurate quantitation awaits definitive determination of the magnitude and stability of the dilution of the precursor-specific activity within the liver.

In our studies we used ^{14}C alanine as the gluconeogenic precursor and measured the following: 1) net hepatic alanine uptake; 2) the fractional extraction of alanine by the liver; 3) the rate of conversion of alanine to glucose by the liver; and 4) the fraction of the extracted ^{14}C alanine which was converted to ^{14}C glucose. It should be noted that alanine, like the other gluconeogenic amino acids (serine, glycine, and threonine), enters the gluconeogenic pathway as pyruvate (Exton et al., 1972) after entering the hepatocytes via a specific transport system (Donner et al., 1978). Thus, unlike lactate which also enters the gluconeogenic pathway as pyruvate but without the involvement of a carrier, amino acid gluconeogenesis can be hormonally regulated by control of its transport rate across the plasma membrane.

Assessment of the regulation of any process *in vivo* requires careful control of the factors modulating the process so that in any particular experiment only one variable is altered. A valuable tool in this regard has been somatostatin. This peptide is a potent inhibitor of both insulin and glucagon secretion (Cherrington et al., 1976) and by its infusion through a peripheral vein one can rapidly turn off the endocrine pancreas. If at the same time one quantitatively compensates for the deficiency of endogenous insulin and glucagon by infusing the two hormones through a previously inserted portal catheter one ends up with an animal which is metabolically normal, which has normal insulin and glucagon levels in the peripheral and portal circulations, but which has no feedback control over its rate of insulin and glucagon release. An isolated change can thus be brought about in the level of either pancreatic hormone or a catecholamine and its "pure" metabolic effect can be discerned.

HORMONAL ACTIONS ON GLUCONEOGENESIS

Control Studies

Figure 5-3 indicates that the model we used to assess gluconeogenesis *in vivo* is valid. Overnight fasted conscious dogs were infused with somatostatin and basal replacement amounts of insulin and glucagon through a previously inserted portal catheter. After a 90-minute titration period during which the infusion rate of insulin was adjusted to maintain euglycemia, there was a 40-minute control period followed by a 3-hour test period. The infusion rates of insulin and glucagon remained basal and unaltered throughout the course of the experiment and, as a result, the plasma levels of the two hormones remained fixed at 5 μU/ml and 63 pg/ml respectively. Under this circumstance, the uptake and fractional extraction of alanine by the liver were approximately 4 μmol/kg-min and 0.35 respectively during the study. The rate at which alanine was converted to glucose (0.9 μmol/kg-min) rose by 65% over the course of the study. This change can be viewed as a consequence of the slow progression of the dog into the fasted state. It should be noted that according to the tracer method only 22% of the extracted alanine was converted to glucose during the control period. Neither the plasma alanine level nor the rate of appearance of alanine in the circulation (data not shown) changed over the course of the experiment, indicating that the supply of the amino acid from muscle was constant, as was its rate of uptake by the liver, but that the enzymic machinery within the hepatocyte slowly adapted to the ensuing fast.

Since the above findings were identical to those obtained in saline-infused dogs it can be concluded that when effects of somatostatin on insulin and glucagon secretion are offset the peptide has no effects on alanine metabolism or on the gluconeogenic process *per se,* and thus it can validly be used as a tool to study gluconeogenesis *in vivo.*

Effects of Glucagon

Figure 5-4 shows data from a representative experiment in which the effects of selective hyperglucagonemia were assessed. Somatostatin was used to control the

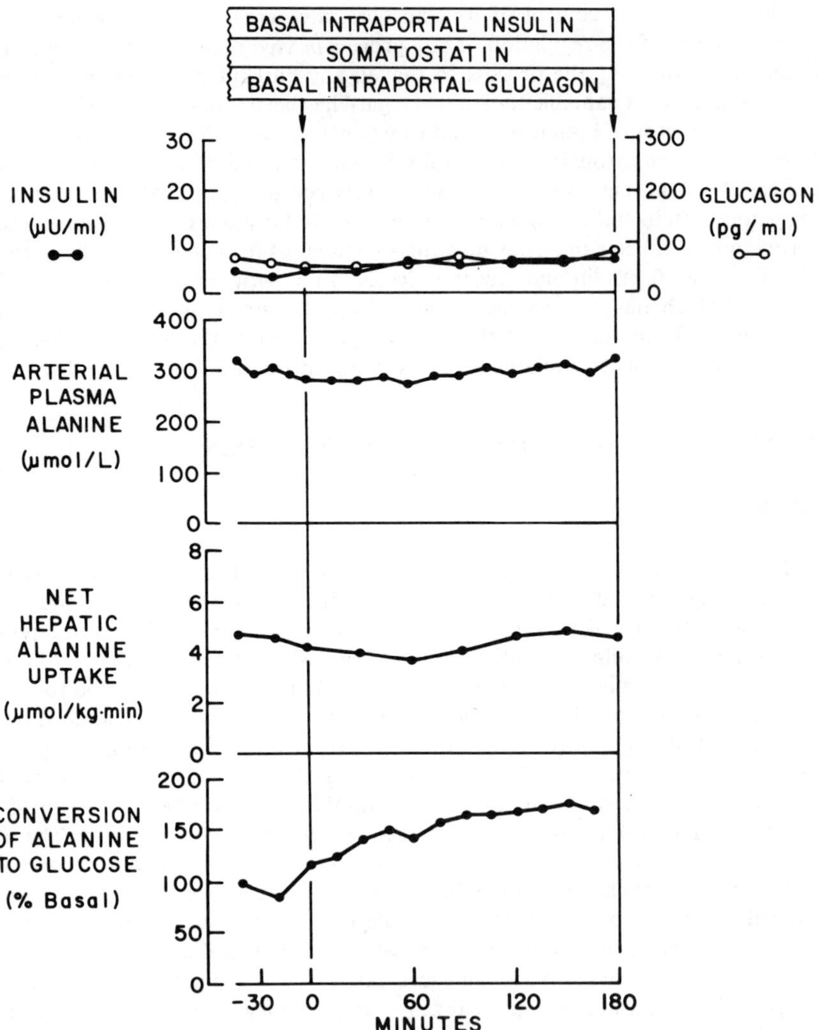

Figure 5-3 The effects of infusion of somatostatin (0.08 μg/kg-min) and basal amounts of glucagon (0.65 ng/kg-min) and insulin (125 μU/kg-min) on insulin, glucagon and arterial plasma alanine levels, net hepatic alanine uptake and conversion of alanine to glucose in an overnight fasted conscious dog. These data are taken from a representative experiment of a group of five dogs. (Manuscript in preparation, Steiner et al.)

endocrine pancreas as described earlier. After a control period in which the insulin (8 μU/ml) and glucagon (92 pg/ml) levels were basal, the infusion rate of glucagon was increased fourfold and its level rose to an average of 362 pg/mg. In response to this selective rise in glucagon the plasma alanine level fell markedly as a result of the increase in net hepatic alanine uptake. The fall in the plasma alanine concentration eventually limited the increase in uptake such that a new steady state was reached in which the net uptake of alanine by the liver was increased by 100%. The full effect of glucagon on hepatic alanine uptake can best be appreciated by examining the frac-

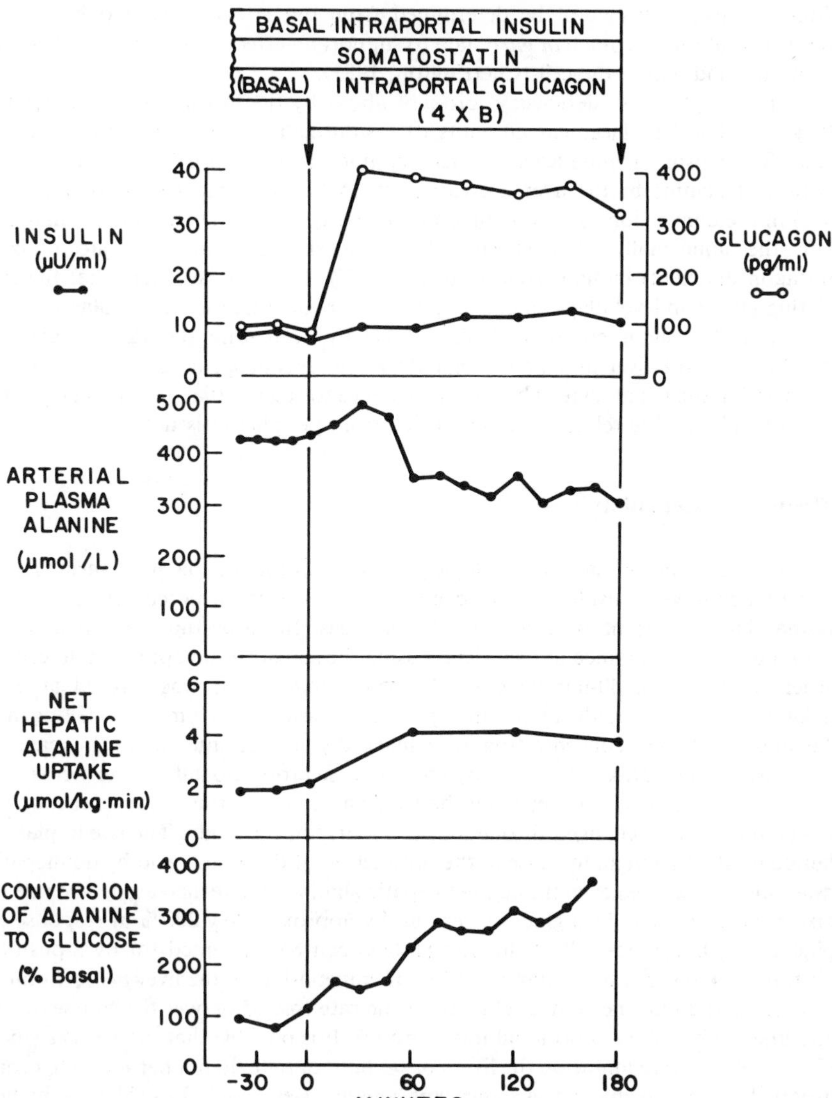

Figure 5-4 The effects of infusion of somatostatin (0.08 μg/kg-min), basal amounts of insulin (200 μU/kg-min) and four times basal amounts of glucagon (2.6 ng/kg-min) on insulin, glucagon and arterial plasma alanine levels, net hepatic alanine uptake and conversion of alanine to glucose in an overnight fasted conscious dog. These data are taken from a representative experiment of a group of four dogs. (Manuscript in preparation, Steiner et al.)

tional extraction of the amino acid by the liver which increased from 0.26 to 0.79 over the course of the study. The effect of glucagon on the conversion of alanine into glucose increased progressively with time such that after three hours it was elevated by more than threefold. Whether the increase in gluconeogenesis was primarily attributable to the increase in alanine uptake or to an effect of glucagon on enzymes within the liver cell cannot be determined from our study. It should be noted, however, that there is much *in vitro* data to support an effect of glucagon both at the membrane and within the cell (Cherrington, 1981).

Selective glucagon deficiency, brought about by the infusion of somatostatin along with basal replacement amounts of insulin caused the opposite changes to occur. The plasma alanine level rose (Δ 230 μmol/L over 4.5 h), the fractional extraction of alanine by the liver decreased (by 35%) and a slight decrease (10% to 20%) in the conversion rate of alanine to glucose occurred. These findings may explain the abnormally high plasma alanine level found in pancreatectomized (glucagon deficient) humans (Barnes et al., 1977). It is thus apparent that the circulating glucagon level plays an important role in regulating the plasma alanine concentration. Glucagon controls alanine levels by regulating the rate of alanine transport into the liver and/or by regulating the gluconeogenic and glycolytic enzymes within the hepatocyte. There is no evidence to suggest that glucagon plays any role in regulating the release of amino acids from peripheral tissues.

Effects of Catecholamines

Figure 5-5 shows that a physiologic increment in the plasma epinephrine level, brought about with insulin and glucagon fixed, also has a potent effect on the plasma alanine concentration and gluconeogenesis. In these studies the pancreatic hormones were maintained at basal levels using the somatostatin approach described earlier. Following a 40-minute control period, epinephrine was infused at 0.04 μg/kg/min and as a result the plasma epinephrine level rose from 73 to 433 pg/ml. The plasma alanine concentration rose markedly in response to the increase in epinephrine. The uptake of alanine by the liver rose proportionally to the increase in the load of the amino acid reaching the liver and thus the fractional extraction of alanine remained unchanged throughout the course of the study. The rise in plasma alanine resulted from an increase in the production of the amino acid by nonhepatic tissue since it occurred even though net hepatic alanine uptake increased. The rate of conversion of alanine into glucose went up by approximately 200% in response to epinephrine, but almost all of this rise (150%) can be accounted for by a push of substrate to the liver rather than an effect of epinephrine on the liver *per se* (it must be remembered that the control gluconeogenic rate rose 65% over the course of the experiment without any hormonal intervention). It is possible that there was a small effect of the catecholamine on the liver *per se,* but our data do not permit such a conclusion. It is conceivable that a significant hepatic effect would be evident at higher epinephrine concentrations.

It thus appears that four- to sixfold increments in the plasma level of glucagon or epinephrine significantly increase the uptake of alanine by the liver. Glucagon brings about its effect in the presence of hypoalaninemia by regulating the gluconeogenic process and/or the amino acid transport system in the liver. Epinephrine, on the other hand, brings about its effect in the presence of hyperalaninemia primarily by regulating the production of alanine by nonhepatic tissue and consequently the supply of substrate to the liver.

When the norepinephrine level (data not shown) was increased in a manner similar to epinephrine, again with insulin and glucagon fixed, there was a small drift down in the plasma alanine level (79 μmol/L over 3 h), a small increase (5%) in

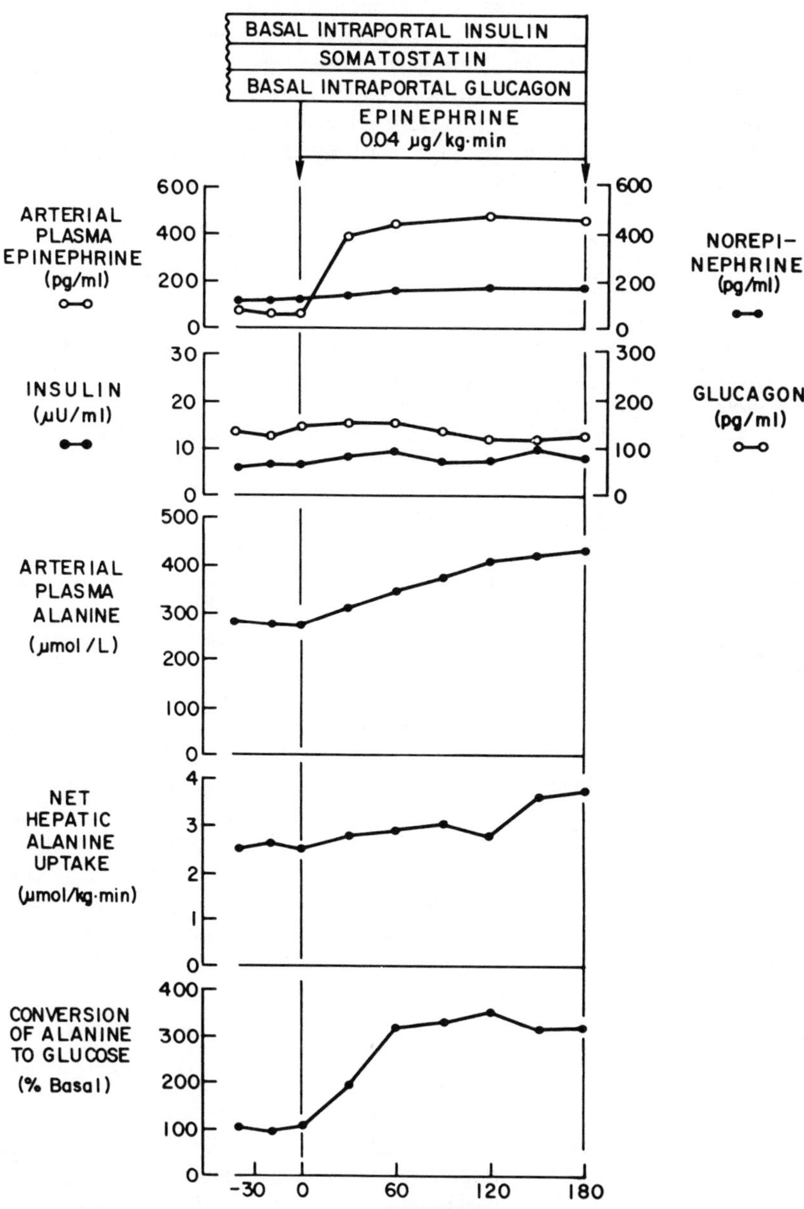

Figure 5-5 The effects of infusion of somatostatin (0.08 μg/kg-min), basal amounts of insulin (150 μU/kg-min), glucagon (0.65 ng/kg-min) and epinephrine (0.04 μg/kg-min) on insulin, glucagon, epinephrine, norepinephrine and arterial plasma alanine levels, net hepatic alanine uptake and conversion of alanine to glucose in an overnight fasted conscious dog. These data are taken from a representative experiment of a group of six dogs. (Manuscript in preparation, Cherrington et al.)

hepatic alanine uptake, a small increase (0.06) in the fractional extraction of the amino acid by the liver and a small increase in the conversion of alanine into glucose (a 120% increase as opposed to a 65% increase in the control experiments). It would thus appear that norepinephrine has a slight stimulatory effect on gluconeogenesis directly at the liver presumably mediated in a similar manner as any that might be caused by epinephrine. It occurs, however, in the absence of any peripheral effects on alanine metabolism and thus the plasma alanine level tends to decline in parallel with the small increase in hepatic alanine uptake.

Effects of Insulin

Figure 5-6 shows data from an experiment in which a selective rise in plasma insulin was brought about. Following a control period in which plasma insulin and glucagon were kept at basal levels using the "pancreatic clamp" technique the insulin infusion rate was increased fourfold. Consequently, the plasma insulin level rose from 10 to 38 μU/ml. Glucose was infused in order to keep the plasma glucose level from changing. In response to this selective hyperinsulinemia there was a substantial fall in the plasma alanine level (304 to 196 μmol/L after 3 h) which was presumably associated with a decrease in the release of the amino acid from peripheral tissues. This finding is supported by the fact that net hepatic alanine uptake failed to change significantly, thus preventing it from offering an explanation for the change in the alanine level. In addition the tracer-determined appearance rate of alanine in the circulation increased. There was a small increase in the fractional extraction of alanine by the liver and a slight decrease in the apparent conversion rate of alanine to glucose. The latter decrease did not represent a true intrahepatic inhibition of gluconeogenesis, however, since the deficit in ^{14}C glucose produced could be accounted for by an increase in the amount of ^{14}C glucose deposited in liver glycogen. It would thus appear that in overnight fasted dogs small selective changes in plasma insulin 1) do not affect hepatic gluconeogenesis, 2) slightly increase the fractional extraction of alanine by the liver, and 3) slow the release of alanine from the periphery. Work in man (Chiasson et al., 1981) and dogs (Chiasson et al., 1976) have shown, however, that large increases in insulin (Δ 220 μU/ml) can suppress intrahepatic gluconeogenesis. Such insulin levels, however, are at the extreme limits of the physiologic range.

Interaction of Insulin and Glucagon

Interestingly, the effects of concurrent increases in insulin and glucagon on the plasma alanine level are additive (Figure 5-7). The plasma alanine level drops further in three hours when both hormones increase (338 to 110 μmol/L) than with an increase in either hormone alone. This large drop can be explained by the addition of the inhibition of alanine release from peripheral tissues attributable to insulin to the augmentation of alanine extraction by the liver attributable to glucagon. With regard to the effects of glucagon, it is evident that the fractional extraction of alanine by the liver went up normally in response to glucagon and thus, despite the reduced load of the amino acid reaching the liver, the amount which was extracted remained

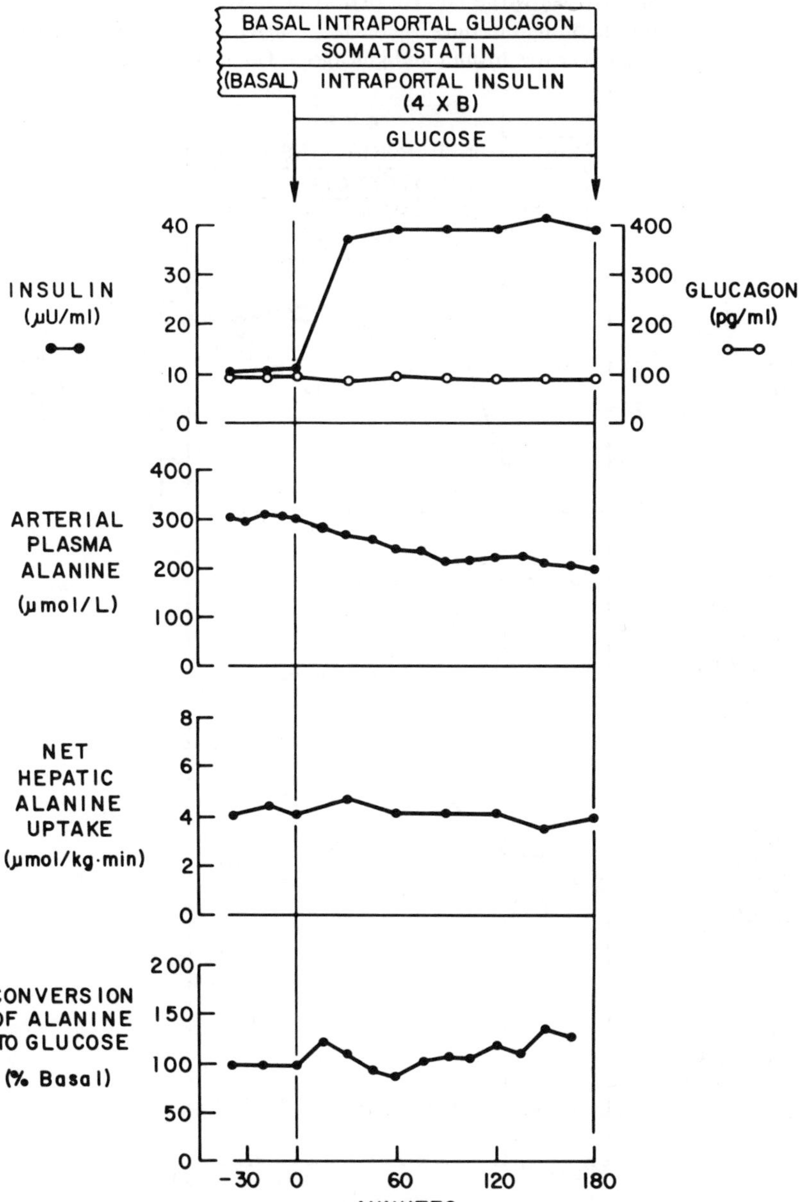

Figure 5-6 The effects of infusion of somatostatin (0.08 μg/kg-min), basal amounts of glucagon (0.65 ng/kg-min) and four times basal amounts of insulin (1170 μU/kg-min) on glucagon, insulin, and arterial plasma alanine levels, net hepatic alanine uptake and conversion of alanine to glucose in an overnight fasted conscious dog. These data are taken from a representative experiment of a group of six dogs. (Manuscript in preparation, Steiner et al.)

unaltered. The ability of the increase in glucagon to stimulate gluconeogenesis within the hepatocyte was completely blocked by the rise in insulin but the gluconeogenic rate was not depressed below the control period rate. This combination of events probably occurs during protein feeding when a large surfeit of amino acids reaches the liver at the same time as extra insulin and glucagon. The increase in the level of the

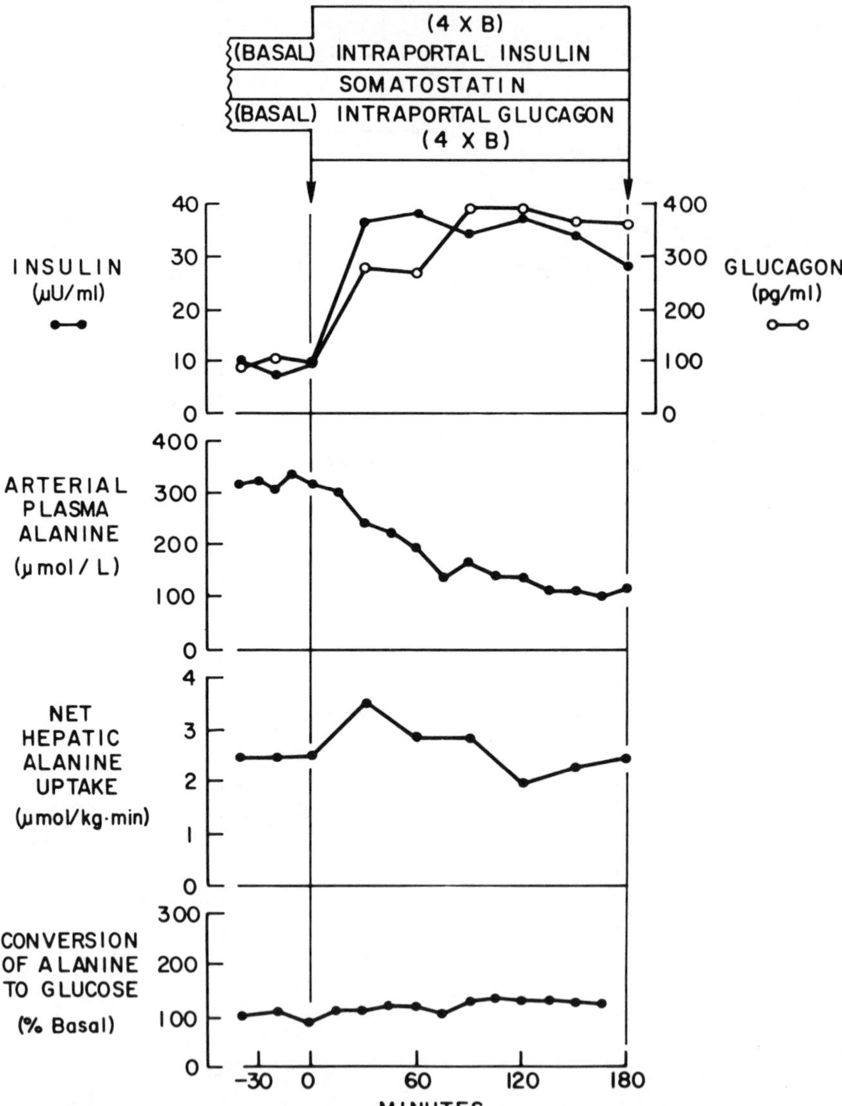

Figure 5-7 The effects of infusion of somatostatin (0.08 µg/kg-min), and four times basal amounts of both insulin (1100 µU/kg-min) and glucagon (2.6 ng/kg-min) on insulin, glucagon and arterial plasma alanine levels, net hepatic alanine uptake and conversion of alanine to glucose in an overnight fasted conscious dog. These data are taken from a representative experiment of a group of five dogs. (Manuscript in preparation, Steiner et al.)

amino acids and an augmentation of transport due to glucagon results in a marked increase in hepatic amino acid uptake. There is no inhibition of the gluconeogenic pathway within the liver so the increase in hepatic uptake of amino acids produces an almost proportional rise in their overall gluconeogenic conversion to glucose. Some of this glucose is released into the circulation while some is stored as glycogen within the liver. Thus, as a result of the coordinate regulation of insulin and glucagon, a carnivore can consume a diet very low in carbohydrate and yet can still store glycogen both in muscle and liver.

REFERENCES

Barnes, A.J., Bloom, S. R., and Mashiter, K. (1977): Persistent metabolic abnormalities in diabetes in the absence of glucagon. *Diabetologia* 13:71–75.

Cherrington, A.D., Chiasson, J.L., Liljenquist, J.E., Jennings, A.S., Keller, U., and Lacy, W.W. (1976): The role of insulin and glucagon in the regulation of basal glucose production in the postabsorptive dog. *J. Clin. Invest.* 58:1407–1418.

Cherrington, A.D. (1981): Gluconeogenesis: its regulation by insulin and glucagon. In: *Diabetes Mellitus* (ed: M. Brownless), pp. 49–117. Garland Press, New York.

Claus, T., and Pilkis, S.J. (1981): Hormonal control of hepatic gluconeogenesis. In: *Biochemical Actions of Hormones* (ed: J. Litwack), Vol. 8, pp. 209–271. Academic Press, New York.

Chiasson, J.L., Liljenquist, J.E., Finger, F.E., and Lacy, W.W. (1976): Differential sensitivity of glycogenolysis and gluconeogenesis to insulin infusion in dogs. *Diabetes* 25:283–291.

Chiasson, J.L., Atkinson, R.L., and Cherrington, A.D. (1980): Insulin regulation of gluconeogenesis from alanine in man. *Metabolism* 20:810–818.

Donner, D.B., Nakayama, K., and Lutz, U. (1978): The effects of bioregulators upon amino acid transport and protein synthesis in isolated rat hepatocytes. *Biochim. Biophys. Acta* 507:322–336.

Hetenyi, G., Jr. (1981): Calculation of the rate of gluconeogenesis *in vivo.* In: *Carbohydrate Metabolism* (ed: C. Cobelli and R.N. Bergman), pp. 201–219. J. Wiley and Sons Ltd., London.

Krebs, H.A., Hems, R., Weidemann, J., and Speake, R.N. (1966): The fate of isotopic carbon in the kidney cortex synthesizing glucose from lactate. *Biochem. J.* 101:242–249.

6 Urea Metabolism: Regulation and Sources of Nitrogen

Mackenzie Walser

The biosynthesis of urea involves a series of enzymatic reactions of high capacity that plays a central role in the N economy of ureotelic organisms. Its purpose has often been defined as ridding the organism of ammonia, owing to the fact that impairment of ureagenesis is characterized by hyperammonemic symptoms. However, a better definition of its purpose might be the removal of N in excess of the organism's needs. Thus, for example, patients with hyperornithinemia secondary to hereditary deficiency of ornithine aminotransferase exhibit continuous *hypo*ammonemia (Valle et al., 1980) but are nevertheless able to grow and maintain N balance normally; functions that require appropriate regulation of ureagenesis. In such patients, regulation of blood ammonia by the urea cycle is defective owing to hyperornithinemia, but regulation of the circulating level of free amino acids is evidently not significantly impaired.

Ureagenesis has traditionally been viewed as having no effect on acid-base balance. However, Bean and Atkinson (1981) have recently questioned this view and have ascribed to the urea cycle the function of removing excess bicarbonate ions derived from oxidative metabolism. While it is true that the biosynthesis of urea consumes bicarbonate ions, it also consumes ammonium ions. The loss of a bicarbonate ion from the body is equivalent in its effect on acid-base balance to the gain of a proton, while the loss of an ammonium ion is equivalent in its effect on acid-base balance to the loss of a proton. Ureagenesis can be viewed as consuming two ammonium ions for each bicarbonate ion, but also yields a proton, as can be seen by writing the overall stoichiometry as follows:

$$2NH_4^+ + HCO_3^- \rightleftharpoons H_2NCONH_2 + 2H_2O + H^+$$

This simplified equation for the overall reaction omits ATP, ADP, AMP, and P_i, and also substitutes one NH_4^+ for the difference between one aspartate, which is consumed, and one fumarate, which is produced. The difference between the empiric formula for the aspartate ion, $H_6C_4O_4N^-$, and the empiric formula for the fumarate ion, $H_2C_4O_4^=$, is equal to NH_4^+ and therefore can be equated with a second ammonium ion. Hence, the net effect of ureagenesis on acid-base balance should be nil.

This conclusion is further borne out by observation of infants lacking a complete urea cycle, in whom no urea is synthesized except that produced from arginine by the action of arginase. No disturbance in acid-base balance in these patients has been identified (Walser, 1982a).

Study of these infants has also made clear that the urea cycle is not essential to the survival of ureotelic organisms. When maintained on a low protein diet supplemented by N-free analogues of essential amino acids, ten patients with complete enzyme defects have grown normally for months or years (Walser, 1982a). One boy with complete ornithine carbamoyltransferase deficiency is now almost five years old and growing normally on this regimen, plus sodium benzoate, though severely retarded as a result of earlier episodes of hyperammonemia (Michels et al., 1978). These observations support the view that the principal role of the urea cycle is the removal of N taken in beyond the requirements of the organism.

UREAGENESIS IN RELATION TO N ECONOMY

Since ureagenesis, in subjects with an intact urea cycle, is the largest component of total N excretion, it is obvious that the rate of ureagenesis is a major determinant of N balance. However, it is not the total rate of urea N generation that affects N balance but rather the difference between urea production and urea hydrolysis by gut bacteria. In normal subjects, about 20% of the produced urea is destroyed by intestinal urease (Table 6-1). The difference between urea production and urea metabolism has been termed urea appearance (Walser et al., 1973). It can be measured as the sum of urinary urea excretion and the rate of change of the body urea pool. The body urea pool can be estimated as the product of blood urea concentration and total body water, since urea is almost uniformly distributed throughout total body water.

Urea N appearance, calculated in this manner, is closely correlated with total N excretion (Grodstein et al., 1980). Indeed, the difference between these quantities, which is equal to the rate of excretion of N in all forms other than urea, shows only a weak dependence on the rate of total N excretion. The average value for the difference between these two quantities is about 2 g per day. It follows that total N excretion can be roughly estimated as urea N appearance plus 2 g per day. This is far simpler than measuring total N in urine and stool.

Urea degradation was at first thought to be of major nutritional importance as a source of N for protein synthesis. The concept of urea N reutilization arose from

Table 6-1
Urea Metabolism in Normal Human Subjects

Reference	No. of subjects	Degradation gN/day	Extrarenal clearance liters/day
Walser and Bodenlos, 1959	3	3.5	14
Jones et al., 1969	2	3.4	19
Murdaugh, 1970	2	2.6	36
Walser and Dlabl, 1974	6	4.9	27
Varcoe et al., 1975	6	1.5	18
Gibson et al., 1976			
40 g protein	6	2.9	31
100 g protein	6	5.1	31
Long et al., 1978	3	3.2	22
Vilstrup, 1980	6	2.4	9
Mean		3.3	23

studies of urea utilization by ruminants. In these animals, urea is highly effective as a source of dietary N for protein synthesis (Briggs, 1967). Bacteria in the rumen hydrolyze the ingested urea and then incorporate the ammonia via microbial action, into amino acids. When it was found that urea is also degraded in the human gut (Walser and Bodenlos, 1959), it was not far-fetched to suggest that the ammonia so formed could become a source of N for synthesis of nonessential amino acids, or for the conversion of ingested keto-analogues to the corresponding essential amino acids (Richards et al., 1967).

REUTILIZATION OF UREA N

The evidence that was first adduced to support this concept was based on a misconception. Labeled ammonia (or labeled urea N) was shown to become incorporated into proteins in patients (Richards et al., 1967). This does not prove urea N reutilization but is in fact an inevitable consequence of the biochemical reactions in which ammonia is known to participate. The most important of these is the reaction catalyzed by glutamate dehydrogenase:

$$\text{glutamate} \rightleftharpoons \text{ammonium} + \alpha\text{-ketoglutarate}$$

It was not appreciated that even when this reaction is at equilibrium, addition of labeled ammonia will lead to the appearance of labeled glutamate, and then by transamination reactions to the appearance of labeled N in all of the amino acids except lysine and threonine.

How then, can urea N reutilization be detected? One way is to study the effect of suppressing urea degradation. If this is done under conditions such that N intake is limiting for N balance, then suppressing urea breakdown in the gut by antibiotics should lead to a deterioration of N balance, manifested as an increase in urea N appearance.

In chronic uremic patients given oral neomycin or kanamycin at a time when total N intake was near the lower limit for N balance, urea N appearance did not increase and N balance improved rather than deteriorated (Mitch et al., 1977; Mitch and Walser, 1977). This is strong evidence against the idea of urea N reutilization.

We have also examined this question in rats by placing them on a nutritional formula containing little N but ample calories and keto-analogues of essential amino acids (Abras and Walser, 1982a). This mixture was administered into the stomach via an implanted catheter for 25 days. The fraction of dietary N utilized for growth in these rats was substantially higher than has been previously reported, 67%. We then reinfused 90% of each day's urine into the stomach, thus causing a progressive accumulation of urea N (Abras and Walser, 1982b). The fraction of exogenous N utilized for growth (excluding the reinfused urea N) remained the same, 67%. Again this suggests that urea N is not utilized synthetically even under these conditions of limited N intake.

Despite this evidence, the concept of urea N reutilization is still prevalent. This may be because there is some evidence for urea N *utilization* in man, even though there is no evidence for urea N *reutilization*. Evidence for urea N utilization comes from studies of normal subjects fed urea. Under some conditions improved N balance results (Tripathy et al., 1970; Snyderman et al., 1962). It remains a mystery why reutilization does not occur, if in fact utilization can occur.

The main significance of urea degradation may lie in its role in urea toxicity. As Johnson and associates (1972) have shown, by adding urea to the dialysis bath in patients on regular hemodialysis, symptoms such as tremor, nausea, vomiting, headache and lethargy are induced as blood urea N rises above 150 mg per dl. They did not measure blood ammonia nor did they determine whether these symptoms could be suppressed by oral antibiotics. Nevertheless, it is possible that these were in fact symptoms of hyperammonemia, caused by an increased rate of urea hydrolysis in the gut.

PRECURSORS OF UREA N

The two N atoms used in urea biosynthesis come directly from ammonium and from aspartate. However, both of these precursors derive their N from glutamate. Mitochondrial glutamate dehydrogenase is responsible for the conversion of glutamate to ammonium, while aspartate-oxaloacetate aminotransferase is responsible for the transfer of glutamate N to aspartate (Meijer et al., 1975). Thus, glutamate is indirectly the source of both N atoms in urea.

The principal extrahepatic sources of N for urea biosynthesis are portal ammonia, which can be estimated to comprise about 25% in normal man (Walser, 1980), glutamine, and alanine. Glutamine N is taken up by the gut and released into the portal vein as ammonia, citrulline, alanine, and proline (Weber et al., 1977), all of which are precursors of urea. Other amino acids are also metabolized in the liver, yielding ammonia that becomes channeled into urea biosynthesis (Krebs et al., 1978). Branched-chain amino acids are also metabolized by the liver to some extent (Felig, 1982), contrary to earlier views that no hepatic uptake of these compounds occurs. All of these amino acids presumably transfer their N to glutamate and thence to ammonium and aspartate.

REGULATION OF UREA PRODUCTION

The most important factor determining the rate of urea synthesis is the circulating concentrations of substrates, i.e., amino acids and ammonium. When a protein load is ingested concentrations of all amino acids in the arterial blood rise, as does portal ammonia concentration, and urea production promptly increases. Several groups of workers have examined the rate of urea synthesis following protein loads in normal subjects. In the first study of this type, Rudman and associates (1973a) reported that a maximal rate of urea synthesis was reached in normal subjects given large nitrogen loads. However, a later report (Rypins et al., 1979) from the same laboratory in which an improved technique for measuring urea production was used led to the conclusion that no maximal rate of urea synthesis is demonstrable in normal subjects. Rafoth and Onstad (1975) reached the same conclusion. These workers measured total plasma α-amino N during protein loading and observed a linear relationship between urea production and this quantity. There was no tendency for urea production to reach a plateau, and the approximately linear relationship had a significant extrapolated intercept on the horizontal axis. This means that increments in total amino acid concentration produce proportionately greater increments in the rate of urea synthesis. Furthermore, the relationship suggests that urea synthesis might cease at a low level of circulating amino acids. This might be a useful property of this regulatory system. If urea production were proportional to amino acid concentration, i.e., if there were no intercept on this graph, N excretion as urea would continue even during periods of protein deprivation, and the circulating levels of amino acids would fall so far that protein synthesis would become impaired. A relationship with this shape serves to protect the free amino acid pool from depletion. It also serves to rid the body of excess N rapidly. Thus, this might be termed an autoregulatory mechanism. Vilstrup (1980) has performed similar experiments in normal subjects infused with a complete amino acid solution, and has induced even higher rates of urea production in this way without reaching a maximal rate. Again, there was a statistically significant extrapolated intercept on the horizontal axis in these data at a total amino acid concentration of about 2 mmol/L. From the slope of this approximately linear relationship one can calculate a hepatic urea N "clearance." This turns out to be about 400 ml per minute—approaching hepatic blood flow via hepatic artery plus portal vein. In cirrhotics as well as in normal subjects, Vilstrup (1980) found that hepatic urea N "clearance" is correlated with other quantitative measures of hepatic function such as antipyrine clearance or galactose elimination capacity.

We have explored the biochemical basis for this short-term autoregulation of urea biosynthesis. Clearly it cannot be enzyme adaptation, because the turnover times of the urea cycle enzymes are too slow (Das and Waterlow, 1974; Nicoletti et al., 1977). The possibility that mitochondrial carbamoyl phosphate synthetase (CPS) might play a role in regulating the rate of ureagenesis was first suggested when it was found (Marshall et al., 1961); Shigesada and Tatibana, 1971a) that N-acetylglutamate (AGA) was required for the activation of this enzyme. Thus, rapid changes in AGA concentration would bring about rapid changes in the activity of CPS and hence in the rate of ureagenesis (Shigesada et al., 1978). Studies by others had also suggested that this might be the case (Meijer and Van Woerkom, 1978; Saheki et al., 1977).

In order to explore this possible mechanism, we administered a complete mixture of amino acids intraperitoneally in rats (Stewart and Walser, 1980). The concentration of all amino acids in plasma rose rapidly, as did plasma ammonia, especially at higher doses of the amino acid mixture. CPS activity, assayed in intact mitochondria with their endogenous AGA content, increased rapidly in a dose-dependent manner, finally reaching the maximal activity as measured in disrupted mitochondria exposed to saturating concentrations of AGA. Mitochondrial AGA content also increased rapidly in a dose-dependent manner, thereby causing CPS activation.

The rapid response of mitochondrial AGA content to amino acid loading was apparently a substrate effect on AGA synthetase caused by an increase in mitochondrial glutamate. Thus, glutamate serves not only as the indirect precursor of both N atoms that become incorporated into urea, but also brings about an activation of the urea cycle, thus facilitating its own disposal.

Although the rate of ureagenesis was not measured in these experiments, it is probable that it changed in parallel to the measured changes in CPS activity of intact mitochondria. When this activity is plotted as a function of the plasma amino acid concentration of the animals just before sacrifice (Figure 6-1), a curve is seen that is similar in shape to the curves described by Rafoth and Onstad (1975) and Vilstrup (1980). Again, an increment in amino acid concentration brings about a proportionately greater increment in the activity of CPS and therefore presumably in the rate of ureagenesis. At high doses of the amino acid mixture, CPS activity becomes maximal and hyperammonemia then supervenes.

The role of enzyme adaptation (Schimke, 1962) in the regulation of ureagenesis

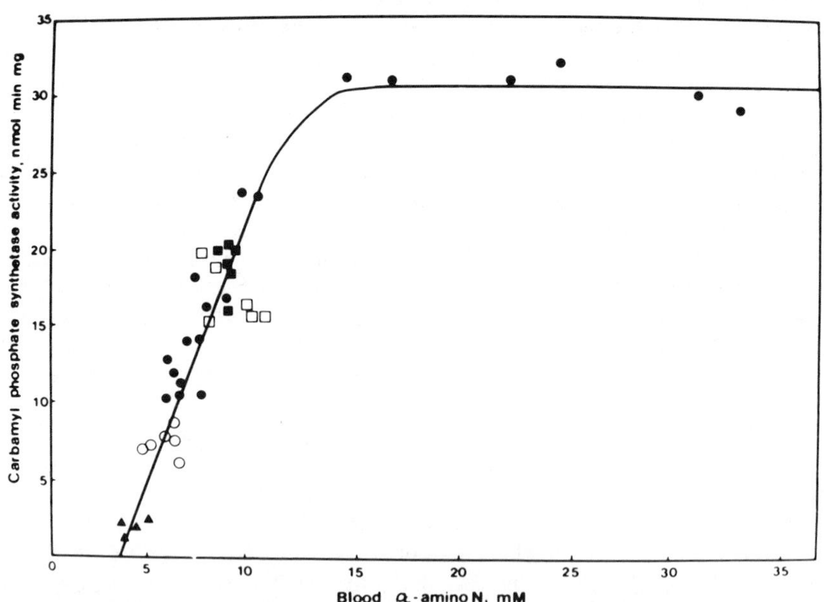

Figure 6-1 The relationship of carbamoyl phosphate synthetase activity in intact mitochondria to blood alpha-amino nitrogen in amino acid-loaded rats. Values obtained with various doses of amino acids injected intraperitoneally with or without arginine at 15 min (●); values in control rats (○); values at t = 5 min with and without arginine (□); values at t = 30 min with and without arginine (■). (Plotted from data of Stewart and Walser, 1980). Rats fed ad libitum on 20% dextrose for a day (▲). Reprinted by permission from Walser, 1981.

also may be to stabilize the concentration of circulating amino acids. A high protein diet will tend to steepen the linear portion of this relationship and to raise the plateau, thereby hastening the return of amino acid concentration to the usual level. A low protein diet will lower the slope, making ureagenesis even lower and helping to preserve the amino acid pool from depletion.

In all of these experiments, the total concentration of amino acids has been taken into consideration. This is not unreasonable, because the concentrations of all the amino acids in plasma rise following a protein meal (Palmer et al., 1973). However, the rate of ureagenesis is clearly influenced more by certain amino acids than by others. Branched-chain amino acids are probably the least effective in this regard, and leucine inhibits urea production in isolated liver (Buttery and Boorman, 1971; Mendes-Mourao et al., 1975). Arginine, ornithine, glutamate, and aspartate have all been viewed as particularly effective in stimulating ureagenesis, but definitive comparisons have rarely been made. In the studies cited above (Stewart and Walser, 1980) of CPS activity in intact hepatic mitochondria of rats injected with amino acid mixtures, no difference in the response of this enzyme system could be detected when arginine was omitted from the mixture (even though plasma ammonia was appreciably higher in these animals). However, arginine does stimulate acetylglutamate synthetase (Shigesada and Tatibana, 1971b), and could in theory augment ureagenesis by this mechanism. There is no doubt that arginine is particularly effective in combating hyperammonemia in a variety of clinical situations (Fahey et al., 1957; Dudrick et al., 1972), but again comparisons of arginine versus ornithine have rarely been reported. This effect of arginine may simply reflect correction of arginine deficiency, which is known to be associated with hyperammonemia, for reasons that are still obscure (Walser, 1982b).

Some animal species are especially susceptible to the hyperammonemia of arginine deficiency. The domestic cat, for example, may develop fatal hyperammonemic coma following a single arginine-free meal (Morris and Rogers, 1978). No satisfactory explanation for this phenomenon has been found, other than the fact that affected cats exhibit extremely low hepatic ornithine levels, which could impair ureagenesis (Stewart et al., 1981).

The stimulatory effect of ornithine on ureagenesis is also poorly understood. It is readily observed *in vitro,* particularly when ornithine levels in the liver are depleted before it is added (Krebs et al., 1973; Saheki and Katunuma, 1975; Krebs and Henseleit, 1932; Hems et al., 1966; Meijer et al., 1975; Briggs and Freedland, 1976). It was previously believed that ornithine had little direct effect on the CPS I reaction, and that this reaction was effectively irreversible because of the high K_i for product inhibition by carbamoyl phosphate (10–19 mM, Elliott, 1976). Thus, if the CPS reaction determines the rate of ureagenesis, it would be difficult to explain how ornithine could stimulate urea production. However, recent evidence shows that the carbamoyl phosphate concentration in the liver during ornithine deficiency may easily become high enough to cause product inhibition of the reaction (Cohen et al., 1980). Furthermore, Powers (1981) has recently found that ornithine at 5 mM does stimulate the CPS reaction when traces of heavy metals are present in the assay system. She attributes this effect to removal by ornithine of the inhibitory effect of these heavy metals on the reaction, secondary to their association with ornithine.

Other amino acids were even more effective than ornithine in this system (Powers, 1981), perhaps owing to their greater affinity for zinc, copper, and cadmium. The degree of activation of CPS caused by 1 mM of individual amino acids was in the following sequence: cysteine > histidine > asparagine > aspartate > threonine = valine > lysine > glutamate > methionine > tryptophan = tyrosine > leucine > isoleucine > serine > proline. At this concentration (1 mM) arginine, ornithine, glutamine, phenylalanine, alanine, and cystine caused no activation.

An entirely different sequence is seen when individual amino acids are compared with respect to their tendency to induce hyperammonemia in patients with hepatic encephalopathy (Rudman et al., 1973b): a group comprising arginine, aspartate, glutamate and tryptophan had the least effect to raise blood ammonia; a group comprising the branched-chain amino acids, aromatic amino acids, alanine and proline was intermediate in causing this effect; and glycine, serine, threonine, glutamine, histidine, lysine and asparagine were the most effective. The authors suggested that the "ammonigenic" property of these last-named amino acids was explained by the production of ammonia rather than aspartate during their metabolism.

Impairment of ureagenesis is most commonly manifested as hyperammonemia and hyperaminoacidemia. Indeed, it seems reasonable to infer that ureagenesis is defective in every case of hyperammonemia, since an increased rate of urea production would certainly relieve the problem. In portal-systemic shunting, hyperammonemia is seen without generalized hyperaminoacidemia, and could be relieved by increased ureagenesis only at the expense of some degree of hypoaminoacidemia. Whether this would be deleterious is uncertain. The converse situation, hypoammonemia without hypoaminoacidemia, is seen in ornithine aminotransferase deficiency, as noted in the introductory paragraph. Excessive ureagenesis, manifested as hypoaminoacidemia, is apparently seen in only one clinical situation, *viz.*, glucagonomas. Here the stimulatory effect of glucagon on ureagenesis (Yamazaki and Graetz, 1977) is probably responsible. Glucagon administration reduces the concentration of all of the circulating amino acids except the branched-chain amino acids, as shown by administering it to diabetic subjects (Liljenquist et al., 1981). In nondiabetics a secondary increase in insulin levels brings about a fall in the concentrations of these amino acids as well.

SUMMARY AND CONCLUSIONS

In summary, ureagenesis serves to rid the body of N ingested in excess of needs. Urea N recycling appears to be of little nutritional importance. Regulation of ureagenesis is mediated chiefly by variations in substrate concentrations and exhibits an autoregulatory character. This is apparently achieved by glutamate-induced modulation of mitochondrial acetylglutamate levels in the liver. The different effects of individual amino acids on ureagenesis and hyperammonemia remain largely unexplained.

ACKNOWLEDGMENT

Supported by a U.S. Public Health Service Grant (AM 28527).

REFERENCES

Abras, E., and Walser, M. (1982a): Growth of rats fed by a continuous intragastric infusion containing amino acids and ketoacids. *Am. J. Clin. Nutr.* in press.

Abras, E., and Walser, M. (1982b): Growth of rats with severe renal insufficiency fed a formula designed to minimize urinary solutes. *Am. J. Clin. Nutr.* in press.

Bean, E.S., and Atkinson, D.E. (1981): Urea synthesis and pH regulation. *Fed. Proc.* 40:1619.

Briggs, M.H. (1967): *Urea as a Protein Supplement.* Pergamon Press, Oxford.

Briggs, S., and Freedland, R.A. (1976): Effect of ornithine and lactate on urea synthesis in isolated hepatocytes. *Biochem. J.* 160:205–209.

Buttery, P.J., and Boorman, K.N. (1971): The inhibition of urea synthesis by leucine in the perfused rat liver. *Biochem. J.* 122:55P–56P.

Cohen, N.S., Cheung, C.W., and Raijman, L. (1980): The effects of ornithine on mitochondrial carbamyl phosphate synthesis. *J. Biol. Chem.* 255:10248–10255.

Das, T.K., and Waterlow, J.C. (1974): The rate of adaptation of urea cycle enzymes, aminotransferases and glutamic dehydrogenase to changes in dietary protein intake. *Br. J. Nutr.* 32:353–373.

Dudrick, S.J., Macfayden, B.V., Jr., Van Buren, C.Y., Ruberg, R.L., and Maynard, A.T. (1972): Parenteral hyperalimentation: metabolic problems and solutions. *Ann. Surg.* 176: 259–264.

Elliott, K.R.F. (1976): Kinetic studies on mammalian liver carbamyl phosphate synthetase. In: *The Urea Cycle* (eds: S. Grisolia, R. Baguena, F. Mayor), pp. 123–131. John Wiley and Sons, New York.

Fahey, J.L., Nathans, D., and Rairigh, D. (1957): Effect of L-arginine on elevated blood ammonia levels in man. *Am. J. Med.* 22:860–869.

Gibson, J.A., Sladen, G.E., and Dawson, A.M. (1976): Protein absorption and ammonia production: the effects of dietary protein and removal of the colon. *Br. J. Nutr.* 35:61–65.

Grodstein, G.P., Blumenkrantz, M.J., and Kopple, J.D. (1980): Nutritional and metabolic response to catabolic stress in uremia. *Am. J. Clin. Nutr.* 3:1411–1416.

Hems, R., Ross, B.D., Berry, M.N., and Krebs, H.A. (1966): Gluconeogenesis in the perfused rat liver. *Biochem. J.* 101:284–292.

Johnson, W.J., Hagge, W.W., Wagoner, R.D., Dinapoli, R.P., and Rosevear, J.W. (1972): Effects of urea loading in patients with far-advanced renal failure. *Mayo Clin. Proc.* 47: 21–29.

Jones, E.A., Smallwood, R.A., Craigie, A., and Rosenoer, V.M. (1969): The enterohepatic circulation of urea nitrogen. *Clin. Sci.* 37:825–836.

Krebs, H.A., and Henseleit, K. (1932): Untersuchungen über die Harnstoff-bildung im Tierkörper. *Hoppe-Seyler's Z. Physiol. Chem.* 210:33–66.

Krebs, H.A., Hems, R., and Lund, P. (1973): Some regulatory mechanisms in the synthesis of urea in the mammalian liver. *Adv. Enzyme Reg.* 11:361–377.

Krebs, H.A., Hems, R., Lund, P., Halliday, D., and Read, W.W.C. (1978): Sources of ammonia for mammalian urea synthesis. *Biochem. J.* 176:733–737.

Liljenquist, J.E., Lewis, S.B., Cherrington, A.D., Sinclair-Smith, B.C., and Lacy, W.W. (1981): Effects of pharmacologic hyperglucagonemia on plasma amino acid concentrations in normal and diabetic man. *Metabolism* 30:1195–1199.

Long, C.L., Jeevanandam, M., and Kinney, J.M. (1978): Metabolism and the recycling of urea in man. *Am. J. Clin. Nutr.* 31:1367–1382.

Marshall, M., Metzenberg, R.L., and Cohen, P.P. (1961): Physical and kinetic properties of carbamyl phosphate synthetase from frog liver. *J. Biol. Chem.* 236:2229–2237.

Meijer, A.J., Gimpel, J.A., Deleeuw, G.A., Tager, J.M., and Williamson, J.R. (1975): Role of anion translocation across the mitochondrial membrane in the regulation of urea synthesis from ammonia by isolated rat hepatocytes. *J. Biol. Chem.* 250:7728–7738.

Meijer, A.J., and Van Woerkom, G.M. (1978): Control of the rate of citrulline synthesis by short-term changes in N-acetylglutamate levels in isolated rat-liver mitochondria. *FEBS Lett.* 86:117–121.

Mendes-Mourao, J., McGivan, J.D., and Chappell, J.B. (1975): The effect of L-leucine on the synthesis of urea, glutamate and glutamine by isolated rat liver cells. *Biochem. J.* 146: 457–464.

Michels, V.V., Beaudet, A., Batshaw, M., and Walser, M. (1978): Dietary therapy of ornithine transcarbamylase (OTC) deficiency. *Pediat. Res.* 12:454.

Mitch, W.E., Lietman, P.S., and Walser, M. (1977): Effects of oral neomycin and kanamycin in chronic uremic patients. I. Urea metabolism. *Kid. Internat.* 11:116–122.

Mitch, W.E., and Walser, M. (1977): Effects of oral neomycin and kanamycin in chronic uremic patients. II. Nitrogen balance. *Kid. Internat.* 11:123–127.

Morris, J.G., and Rogers, Q.R. (1978): Ammonia intoxication in the near-adult cat as a result of dietary deficiency of arginine. *Science* 199:431–432.

Murdaugh, H.V., Jr. (1970): Urea metabolism during low protein intake: studies in man and dog. In: *Urea and the Kidney* (eds: B. Schmidt-Nielsen and D.W.S. Kerr), pp. 471–477. Excerpta Medica Foundation, Amsterdam.

Nicoletti, M., Guerri, C., and Grisolia, S. (1977): Turnover of carbamyl-phosphate synthetase, of other mitochondrial enzymes and of rat tissues: effect of diet and of thyroidectomy. *Eur. J. Biochem.* 75:583–592.

Palmer, T., Rossiter, M.A., Levin, B., and Oberholzer, V.G. (1973): The effect of protein loads on plasma amino acid levels. *Clin. Sci. Mol. Med.* 45:827–832.

Powers, S.G. (1981): Regulation of rat liver carbamyl phosphate synthetase I. Inhibition by metal ions and activation by amino acids and other chelating agents. *J Biol. Chem.* 256: 11160–11165.

Rafoth, R.J., and Onstad, G.R. (1975): Urea synthesis after oral protein ingestion in man. *J. Clin. Invest.* 56:1170:1174.

Richards, P., Metcalfe-Gibson, A., Ward, E.E., Wrong, O., and Houghton, B.J. (1967): Utilisation of ammonia nitrogen for protein synthesis in man, and the effect of protein restriction and uraemia. *Lancet* 2:845–849.

Rudman, D., DiFulco, T.J., Galambos, J.T., Smith, R.B., III, Salam, A.A., and Warren, W.D. (1973a): Maximal rates of excretion and synthesis of urea in normal and cirrhotic subjects. *J. Clin. Invest.* 52:2241–2249.

Rudman, D., Galambos, J.T., Smith, R.B., III, Salam, A.A., and Warren, W.D. (1973b): Comparison of the effect of various amino acids upon the blood ammonia concentration of patients with liver disease. *Am. J. Clin. Nutr.* 26:916–925.

Rypins, E.B., Henderson, J.M., Fulenwider, J.T., Warren, W.D., and Rudman, D. (1979): Pharmacokinetic method for measuring urea synthesis rates. *Surg. Forum* 30:390–393.

Saheki, T., and Katunuma, N. (1975): Analysis of regulatory factors for urea synthesis by isolated perfused rat liver. I. Urea synthesis with ammonia and glutamine as nitrogen sources. *J. Biochem.* 77:659–669.

Saheki, T., Katsunuma, T., and Sase, M. (1977): Regulation of urea synthesis in rat liver. Changes of ornithine and acetylglutamate concentrations in the livers of rats subjected to dietary transitions. *J. Biochem.* 82:551–558.

Schimke, R.T. (1962): Adaptive characteristics of urea cycle enzymes in the rat. *J. Biol. Chem.* 237:459–468.

Shigesada, K., and Tatibana, M. (1971a): Role of acetylglutamate in ureotelism. *J. Biol. Chem.* 246:5588–5595.

Shigesada, K., and Tatibana, M. (1971b): Enzymatic synthesis of acetylglutamate by mammalian liver preparations and its stimulation by arginine. *Biochem. Biophys. Res. Comm.* 44:1117–1124.

Shigesada, K., Aoyagi, K., and Tatibana, M. (1978): Role of acetylglutamate in ureotelism. Variations in acetylglutamate level and its possible significance in control of urea synthesis in mammalian liver. *Eur. J. Biochem.* 85:385–391.

Snyderman, S.E., Holt, L.E., Jr., Dancis, J., Roitman, E., Boyer, A., and Balis, M.E. (1962): "Unessential" nitrogen: a limiting factor for human growth. *J. Nutr.* 78:57–72.

Stewart, P.M., and Walser, M. (1980): Short term regulation of ureagenesis. *J. Biol. Chem.* 255:5270–5280.

Stewart, P.M., Batshaw, M., Valle, D., and Walser, M. (1981): Effects of arginine-free meals on ureagenesis in cats. *Am. J. Physiol.* 241:E310–E315.

Tripathy, K., Klahr, S., and Lotero, H. (1970): Utilization of exogenous urea nitrogen in malnourished adults. *Metabolism* 19:253–262.

Valle, D., Walser, M., Brusilow, S.W., and Kaiser-Kupfer, M. (1980): Gyrate atrophy of the choroid and retina: amino acid metabolism and correction of hyperornithinemia with an arginine-deficient diet. *J. Clin. Invest.* 65:371–378.

Varcoe, R., Halliday, D., Carson, E.R., Richards, P., and Tavill, A.S. (1975): Efficiency of utilization of urea nitrogen for albumin synthesis by chronically uraemic and normal man. *Clin. Sci. Mol. Med.* 48:379–390.

Vilstrup, H. (1980): Synthesis of urea after stimulation with amino acids: relation to liver function. *Gut* 21:990–995.

Walser, M., and Bodenlos, L.J. (1959): Urea metabolism in man. *J. Clin. Invest.* 38:1617–1626.

Walser, M., Coulter, A.W., Dighe, S., and Crantz, F.R. (1973): The effect of keto-analogues of essential amino acids in severe chronic uremia. *J. Clin. Invest.* 52:678–690.

Walser, M. (1980): Determinants of ureagenesis, with particular reference to renal failure. *Kid. Internat.* 17:709–721.

Walser, M. (1981): Regulation of nitrogen catabolism. In: *Nutritional Factors: Modulating Effects on Metabolic Processes* (eds: R.F. Beers, Jr., and E.G. Bassett), pp. 355–370. Raven Press, New York.

Walser, M. (1982a): Urea cycle disorders and other hereditary hyperammonemic syndromes. In: *Metabolic Basis of Inherited Disease* (eds: J.B. Stanbury, J.B. Wyngaarden, D.S. Fredrickson, J.L. Goldstein, and M.S. Brown) 5th edition. McGraw Hill Book Company, New York, in press.

Walser, M. (1982b): Urea cycle enzymopathies. *Sem. Liver Dis.* in press.

Walser, M., and Dlabl, P. (1974): Urea metabolism. In: *Proceedings of a Conference on the Adequacy of Dialysis,* sponsored by the Artificial Kidney-Chronic Uremia Program, National Institute of Arthritis, Metabolism and Digestive Diseases, Monterey, California, March 20–22.

Weber, F.L., Jr., Maddrey, W.C., and Walser, M. (1977): Amino acid metabolism of dog jejunum before and during absorption of keto-analogues. *Am. J. Physiol.* 232:F210–F214.

Yamazaki, R.K., and G.S. Graetz (1977): Glucagon stimulation of citrulline formation in isolated hepatic mitochondria. *Arch. Biochem. Biophys.* 178:19–25.

6A Effects of Ketone Bodies on Leucine and Alanine Metabolism in Normal Man

Morey W. Haymond
Steven L. Nissen
John M. Miles

The branched-chain amino acids, leucine, isoleucine and valine, are essential amino acids because their carbon skeletons cannot be synthesized in mammalian tissues. Therefore, diet and endogenous proteolysis are the only sources of these amino acids for ongoing protein synthesis. During periods of limited or no dietary protein intake, precise regulation of the catabolism of individual essential amino acids, such as the branched-chain amino acids (BCAA), derived from endogenous protein must occur to prevent depletion of amino acids required for ongoing synthesis of body proteins. The initial step in BCAA metabolism is a reversible transamination with α-ketoglutarate, forming glutamate and the respective branched-chain α-ketocids (Odessey et al., 1979). Subsequently, the branched-chain α-ketoacids may undergo irreversible decarboxylation by branched-chain α-ketoacid dehydrogenase, resulting in loss of these essential amino acids (Manchester et al., 1965). Thus, BCAA carbon could be conserved by decreasing proteolysis [protein breakdown (Waterlow et al., 1977)], by decreasing their rate of transamination (a prerequisite to oxidation), or by decreasing the activity of the branched-chain α-ketoacid dehydrogenase.

The substrate and hormonal factors responsible for the complex metabolic changes associated with fasting are not completely understood. During caloric deprivation in man, rates of nitrogen loss decrease, indicating decreased amino acid catabolism and evidence of a protein-sparing adaptation to fasting (Cahill et al., 1966). During fasting, fatty acid oxidation becomes the primary source of cellular energy. Thus, fatty acid and/or products of their oxidation (i.e., ketone bodies) may decrease the oxidation (and thus irreversible loss) of essential amino acids resulting in relative protein sparing.

Utilizing leucine as a paradigm of an essential amino acid, the effect of fatty acids on amino acid oxidation has been examined in rat muscle. Octanoate, which is freely oxidized by mitochondria and is not subject to transport regulation as are long chain fatty acids (McGarry et al., 1977), does not have a consistent effect on leucine oxidation in rat muscle. Waymach et al. (1980) observed an octanoate-dependent decrease in leucine oxidation in perfused rat heart, while this fatty acid stimulated leucine oxidation in rat heart (Buse et al., 1972), and in perfused rat hindquarters (Spydevold and Hokland, 1982). Addition of carnityl fatty acid esters (C_6 to C_{16}) decreases leucine oxidation in mitochondria derived from heart and skeletal muscle (Bremer and Davis, 1978). In contrast, palmitate had no effect on leucine oxidation in rat diaphragm (Odessey and Goldberg, 1972) or rat heart (Buse et al., 1972). These studies suggest that in rat muscle, fatty acids have no consistent effect on the oxidation of the BCAA.

In addition to fatty acids, ketone bodies have been implicated in the protein sparing observed with fasting (Sherwin et al., 1975). As was observed with fatty acids, no uniform response to ketone bodies has been reported in rat skeletal muscle. A decrease in leucine oxidation was observed with a β-hydroxybutyrate alone (Buse et al., 1972) or in combination with acetoacetate (Zapalowski et al., 1981). In contrast, Paul and Adibi (1978) observed a stimulation of leucine oxidation with acetoacetate but not β-hydroxybutyrate, while others observed no effect of β-hydroxybutyrate on leucine oxidation (Odessey and Goldberg, 1972), proteolysis (Fulks et al., 1975; Tischler et al., 1982) or protein synthesis (Tischler et al., 1982).

Leucine carbon oxidation has been measured *in vivo* in 14- and 96-hour fasted dogs, utilizing a combined infusion of tritiated leucine and ^{14}C-α-ketoisocaproate, the α-ketoacid of leucine (Nissen and Haymond, 1981). Fasting resulted in a decrease in total leucine carbon entry, reflecting a decrease in proteolysis. In addition, a parallel decrease in the conversion of leucine to α-ketoisocaproate (KIC) was observed, suggesting a decreased rate of leucine transamination with fasting. This apparent decrease in the rate of leucine transamination provides a mechanism which may, in part, account for the decreased urinary nitrogen losses observed with caloric restriction. The irreversible loss of KIC, which is assumed to reflect the rate of leucine carbon oxidation, decreased in the 96-hour fasting dog. The decrease in conversion of leucine to KIC and in leucine carbon oxidation is evidence for conservation of the essential carbon structure of leucine. These data are in agreement with the observed decrease in leucine oxidation in muscle of short-term fasted rabbit (Ryan et al., 1974), but stand in contrast to *in vivo* (Meikle and Klair, 1972) and *in vitro* (Hutson et al., 1978; Goldberg and Odessey, 1972; Tischler and Goldberg, 1980: Paul and Adibi, 1978; Buse et al., 1973) oxidation studies in rats which suggest increased catabolism of BCAA with starvation. Whether species, tissue studied, or relative state of protein and/or caloric restriction contribute to these differences remains to be determined.

In man, during short-term fasting, plasma concentrations of glucose and alanine (a potential gluconeogenic substrate) and urinary nitrogen excretion decrease, while plasma BCAA, FFA, and ketone body concentrations increase

(Cahill et al., 1966). Assessment of the effects of FFA on BCAA metabolism have not been carried out in man; however, ingestion of a diet high in fat content results in increased plasma concentrations of the BCAA (Adibi et al., 1970). Whether this increase in plasma BCAA concentration is the result of decreased utilization or increased production has yet to be determined.

It has been proposed that utilization of ketone bodies by brain (Owen et al., 1967) may have an indirect protein-sparing effect by decreasing the need for glucose, which during fasting is derived in large part from amino acids via gluconeogenesis (Cahill et al., 1966). In addition, it has been suggested that ketone bodies may have a direct protein sparing effect on muscle in man (Sherwin et al., 1975). The available data relating to this hypothesis, however, are contradictory. Infusion of sodium D,L-β-hydroxybutyrate (Sherwin et al., 1975) or sodium acetoacetate (Fery and Balasse, 1980) in overnight fasted subjects decreases plasma glucose and alanine concentrations in the absence of any change in plasma insulin concentrations; prolonged infusion of sodium β-hydroxybutyrate in fasting obese adults decreases urinary nitrogen excretion (Sherwin et al., 1975). These data suggest that hyperketonemia *per se* might be protein sparing. Other studies suggest that the decrease in plasma alanine concentrations during ketone body infusion is due to a change in acid-base balance rather than a direct effect of ketone bodies *per se,* since an equimolar infusion of sodium bicarbonate decreases plasma alanine concentrations (Fery and Balasse, 1980). In the same studies, infusion of acetoacetic acid increased plasma alanine, lactate and glutamate concentrations in the absence of any change in blood pH, suggesting that hyperketonemia directly stimulates alanine release or alters its utilization.

A close relationship between the metabolism of the BCAA and alanine has been suspected since alanine release from rat muscle increases in response to added BCAA (Odessey et al., 1974; Garber et al., 1976; Goldberg and Chang, 1978), suggesting a role of BCAA as nitrogen donors for alanine synthesis. Recent studies have confirmed the role of BCAA as nitrogen donors for alanine synthesis in postabsorptive dogs (Ben Galim et al., 1980) and man (Haymond and Miles, 1982), using ^{15}N to trace the incorporation of leucine nitrogen into alanine. In these studies, under steady state conditions, only 40% of alanine flux was derived from proteolysis. Therefore, changes in the plasma concentration and/or flux of alanine may not be good predictors of alterations in protein metabolism.

In the studies of Fery and Balasse (1980) and Sherwin et al. (1975), only plasma concentrations of alanine were measured. Therefore, it is not known whether the changes in plasma alanine concentrations observed during the infusion of sodium β-hydroxybutyrate or sodium bicarbonate were the result of an alteration in the rate of alanine production or utilization. We undertook studies to determine whether infusion of sodium D,L-β-hydroxybutyrate or of sodium bicarbonate altered the rates of production and utilization of leucine and alanine. Since leucine is an essential amino acid, a decrease in the rate of appearance of leucine would be consistent with decreased proteolysis, whereas an increase in leucine utilization would be compatible with an increase in protein synthesis and/or leucine oxidation. In addition, rates of leucine nitrogen transfer to alanine were estimated to determine the effects of ketosis and alkalosis on the rate of alanine synthesis and release from muscle.

Normal volunteers were infused with L-[^{15}N] leucine, L-[6,6,6-$^{2}H_3$] leucine and L-[2,3,3,3-$^{2}H_4$] alanine, as previously described (Haymond and Miles, 1982). Following baseline determinations, subjects were infused for three hours with sodium-D, β-hydroxybutyrate or sodium bicarbonate at 15 μmol/kg•min and plasma obtained at frequent intervals for the determination of plasma amino acids, ketone body and hormone concentrations. Isotopic enrichment in leucine and alanine were determined as previously described (Haymond and Miles, 1982). Near steady state conditions were achieved during the baseline period and during the last 60 minutes of the three-hour ketone body infusion. Rates of amino acid flux and interconversion were calculated using steady state assumptions.

During the infusion of sodium β-hydroxybutyrate, plasma ketone body concentrations increased from 0.2 to 2.3 mM. Plasma leucine concentrations increased by 15 μM, whereas plasma alanine concentrations decreased by 40 μM, changes similar to those reported by Sherwin et al. (1975). Rather than observing a decrease in alanine flux as speculated by Sherwin et al. (1975), alanine flux increased by 50%, from 5.5 to 7.7 μmol/kg•min, comparing the basal period to the final 60 minutes of ketone body infusion. The metabolic clearance of alanine increased from approximately 20 to 35 ml/kg•min over the course of study. Infusion of β-hydroxybutyrate increased leucine nitrogen flux from 2.6 to 3.1 μmol/kg•min, whereas the flux of leucine carbon (1.7 to 1.8 μmol/kg•min) was not significantly increased. During the 180 minutes of infusion, the rate of transfer of leucine nitrogen to alanine nearly doubled from 0.7 to 1.3 μmol/kg•min.

Infusion of $NaHCO_3$ resulted in a similar degree of alkalemia as observed following infusion of Na-β-hydroxybutyrate (pH = 7.52). Alkalosis decreased plasma alanine concentration by increasing its metabolic clearance rate since alanine flux did not change. Neither the flux of leucine carbon (Table 6A-1) nor the transfer of leucine nitrogen to alanine was affected by infusion of $NaHCO_3$ (data not shown).

Table 6A-1
Mean Flux Rates (μmol/kg•min) of Alanine and Leucine Before and After Infusion of β-hydroxybutyrate or Sodium Bicarbonate in Man

	β-hydroxybutyrate		Bicarbonate	
	Before	After	Before	After
Alanine flux	5.5	7.7	5.1	4.9
Leucine carbon	1.7	1.8	1.5	1.5
Leucine nitrogen	2.6	3.1	2.6	2.9

Under these experimental conditions, several factors relating to the isotopes employed must be considered. Recycling of the [^{15}N] leucine, [$^{2}H_3$] leucine or [$^{2}H_4$] alanine labels out of protein over the course of study could lead to an underestimation of the alanine and leucine carbon or leucine nitrogen fluxes. The absence of change in the alanine and leucine carbon flux during sodium bicarbonate infusion would suggest that this is not a significant problem over the five to six hours of isotope infusion. However, recycling of the ^{15}N label back into the leucine pool may have resulted in a significant underestimation of the leucine N flux and thus the rate of transfer of leucine N to alanine. The [$^{2}H_4$] alanine, on the other hand, should provide a reasonable estimate of the rate of transamination of alanine (since transamination of this label will result in the loss of the C-2 deuterium), but may overestimate the true rate of alanine carbon flux. In contrast, use of a carbon label of alanine would most likely underestimate the rate of alanine transamination (and thus, *de novo* synthesis of alanine), but could also underestimate alanine carbon flux because of recycling of the label back from both the glucose and protein pools.

From the data presented above, the infusion of ketone bodies in man results in an increase in the flux of alanine (both rate of appearance and disappearance); however, since the plasma concentration decreased, the rate of utilization must have exceeded the rate of appearance of alanine during the ketone body infusion. In the absence of an increase in the rate of appearance of leucine carbon, i.e., increased proteolysis, and in view of the increased rate of leucine nitrogen incorporation into alanine, the increase in alanine flux must be primarily the result of increased *de novo* synthesis. The increase in alanine utilization is at least in part due to the alkalosis induced by ketone body infusion, and most likely contributed to the decrease in the plasma concentrations of alanine. This hypothesis is in keeping with the dramatic increase in plasma alanine concentrations observed during the infusion of acetoacetic acid in humans which did not alter the plasma pH, and the decrease in plasma alanine during the infusion of sodium acetoacetate which did cause alkalemia (Fery and Balasse, 1980). As a result, it may be concluded that alkalosis *per se* alters the relative efficiency of removal of alanine, independent of its rate of appearance; therefore, a change in plasma alanine concentration is a poor indicator of alterations in its rate of appearance or disappearance, let alone extrapolation to the regulation of protein metabolism.

These studies demonstrate that ketone bodies *per se* have little effect on the rate of proteolysis or leucine utilization in man since the rate of leucine carbon flux was not altered by ketone body infusion. Whether the hyperketonemia *per se* altered in a reciprocal fashion the rates of leucine oxidation and protein synthesis cannot be determined. Nevertheless, these results are consistent with rat muscle studies demonstrating no effect of β-hydroxybutyrate on leucine oxidation (Odessey and Goldberg, 1972), proteolysis (Fulks et al., 1975), or protein synthesis (Tischler et al., 1982). The dissociation between the rates of leucine nitrogen and carbon flux during ketone body infusion is compatible with augmented recycling of the leucine carbon skeleton through α-ketoisocaproate. Whether this mechanism provides a subtle means for nitrogen sparing, facilitating the redistribution of amino acid nitrogen during fasting, cannot be determined by the present studies. However, the augmented transfer of leucine nitrogen to alanine in response to hyperketonemia is consistent with such a hypothesis.

ACKNOWLEDGMENTS

These studies were supported by the Juvenile Diabetes Foundation, Wasie Foundation, Mayo Foundation, and National Institutes of Health, AM-26989. We would like to thank Mr. Pete Berg, Ms. Collette Schmidt, Mrs. Joan Aikens and Mrs. Carol Van Huysen for their technical assistance, and Mrs. Marylee Campion for her secretarial help.

REFERENCES

Adibi, S.A., Drash, A.L., Livi, E.D. (1970): Hormone and amino acid levels in altered nutritional states. *J. Lab. Clin. Med.* 76:722–732.

Ben Galim, E., Hruska, K., Bier, D.M., Matthews, D.E., Haymond, M.W. (1980): Branched chain amino acid nitrogen transfer to alanine in vivo in dogs: Direct isotopic determination with [^{15}N] leucine. *J. Clin. Invest.* 66:1295–1304.

Brewer, J., Davis, E.J. (1978): The effect of acylcarnitines on the oxidation of branched chain α-ketoacids in mitochondria. *Biochim. Biophys. Acta* 528:269–275.

Buse, M.G., Biggers, J.F., Drier, C., Buse, J.F. (1973): The effect of epinephrine, glucagon, and the nutritional state on the oxidation of branched chain amino acids and pyruvate by isolated hearts and diaphragms in the rat. *J. Biol. Chem.* 248:697–706.

Buse, M.G., Biggers, J.F., Friderici, K.H., Buse, J.F. (1972): Oxidation of branched chain amino acids by isolated hearts and diaphragms of the rat: The effects of fatty acids, glucose and pyruvate respiration. *J. Biol. Chem.* 247:8085–8096.

Cahill, G.F., Herrera, M.G., Morgan, A.P., Soeldner, J., Steinke, J., Levy, P.L., Richards, G.A., Kipnis, D.M. (1966): Hormone fuel interrelationship during fasting. *J. Clin. Invest.* 45:1751–1759.

Fery, F., Balasse, E.O. (1980): Differential effects of sodium acetoacetate and acetoacetic acid infusions on alanine and glutamine metabolism in man. *J. Clin. Invest.* 66:323–331.

Fulks, R.M., Li, J.B., and Goldberg, A.L. (1975): Effects of insulin, glucose, and amino acids on protein turnover in rat diaphragm. *J. Biol. Chem.* 250:290–298.

Garber, A.J., Karl, I.E., Kipnis, D.M. (1976): Alanine and glutamine synthesis and release from skeletal muscle. I. Glycolysis and amino acid release. *J. Biol. Chem.* 251:826–835, 1976.

Goldberg, A.L., Chang, T.W. (1978): Regulation and significance of amino acid metabolism in skeletal muscle. *Fed. Proc.* 37:2301–2307.

Goldberg, A.L., Odessey R. (1972): Oxidation of amino acids by diaphragms from fed and fasted rats. *Am. J. Physiol.* 223:1384–1391.

Golden, M.H.N., Waterlow, J.C. (1977): Total protein synthesis in elderly people: a comparison of results with [^{15}N] glycine and [^{14}C] leucine. *Clin. Sci. Mol. Med.* 53:277–288.

Haymond, M.W., Miles, J.M. (1982): Branched chain amino acids as a major source of alanine nitrogen in man. *Diabetes* 31:186–189.

Hutson, S.M., Cree, T.C., Harper, A.E. (1978): Regulation of leucine and α-ketoisocaproate metabolism in skeletal muscle. *J. Biol. Chem.* 253:8126–8133.

Manchester, K.L. (1965): Oxidation of amino acids by isolated rat diaphragm and the influence of insulin. *Biochim. Biophys. Acta* 100:295–298.

Matthews, D.E., Motil, K.J., Rohrbaugh, D.K., Burke, J.E., Young, V.R., Bier, D.M. (1980): Measurement of leucine metabolism in man from a primed continuous infusion of L-[1-^{13}C] leucine. *Am. J. Physiol.* 238:E473–E479.

McGarry, J.D., Manaerts, G.P., Foster, D.W. (1977): A possible role for malonyl-CoA in the regulation of hepatic fatty oxidation and ketogenesis. *J. Clin. Invest.* 60:265–270.

Meikle, A.W., Klain, G.J. (1972): Effect of fasting and fasting-refeeding on conversion of leucine into CO_2 and lipids in rats. *Am. J. Physiol.* 222:1246–1250.

Nissen, S. and Haymond, M.W. (1981): Effects of fasting on flux and interconversion of leucine and α-ketoisocaproate in vivo. *Am. J. Physiol.* 241:E72–E75.

Odessey, R., Goldberg, A.L. (1972): Oxidation of leucine by rat skeletal muscle. *Am. J. Physiol.* 223:1376–1383.

Odessey, R., Goldberg, A.L. (1979): Leucine degradation in cell-free extracts of skeletal muscle. *Biochem. J.* 178:475–489.

Odessey, R., Khairallah, E.A., Goldberg, A.L. (1974): Origin and possible significance of alanine production by skeletal muscle. *J. Biol. Chem.* 249:7623–7629.

Owen, O.E., Morgan, A.P., Kemp, H.G., Sullivan, J.M., Herrera, M.G., Cahill, G.F., Jr. (1967): Brain metabolism during fasting. *J. Clin. Invest.* 46:1589–1595.

Paul, H.S., Adibi, S.A. (1978): Leucine oxidation in diabetes and starvation: effects of ketone bodies on branched chain amino acid oxidation in vitro. *Metabolism* 27:185–200.

Ryan, N.T., George, B.C., Odessey, R., Egdahl, R.H. (1974): Effect of hemorrhagic shock, fasting, and corticosterone administration on leucine oxidation and incorporation into protein by skeletal muscle. *Metabolism* 23:901–904.

Sherwin, R.S., Hendler, R.G., Felip, P. (1975): Effect of ketone infusion on amino acid and nitrogen metabolism in man. *J. Clin. Invest.* 55:1382–1390.

Spydevold, O., Hokland, B. (1981): Oxidation of branched-chain amino acids in skeletal muscle and liver of rat, effects of octanoate and energy state. *Biochem. Biophys. Acta* 679:279–288.

Tischler, M.E., DeSautels, M., Goldberg, A.L. (1982): Does leucine Leucyl-tRNA, or some metabolite of leucine regulate protein synthesis and degradation in skeletal and cardiac muscle. *J. Biol. Chem.* 257:1613–1621.

Tischler, M.E., Goldberg, A.L. (1980): Amino acid degradation and effect of leucine on pyruvate oxidation in rat atrial muscle. *Am. J. Physiol.* 238:E480–E486.

Waterlow, J.C., Golden, M., Picou, D. (1977): The measurement of rates of protein turnover: the effects of nutritional status and surgical injury. *Am. J. Clin. Nutr.* 30:1333–1339.

Waymach, P.P., Buysere, M.S., Olson, M.S. (1980): Studies on the activation and inactivation of branched chain α-veto dehydrogenase in the perfused rat heart. *J. Biol. Chem.* 255:9773–9781.

Zapalowski, C., Hutson, S.M., Harper, A.E. (1981): Effects of starvation and diabetes on leucine and valine metabolism in the perfused rat hindquarter. In: *Metabolism and Clinical Implications of Branched Chain and Amino and Ketoacids* (eds: M. Walser and J. Williamson), pp. 239–244, Elsevier/North Holland, The Netherlands.

Hormonal Regulation of Leucine Metabolism in the Conscious Dog

Naji N. Abumrad, Phillip E. Williams, and William W. Lacy

The purpose of this report is to summarize some aspects of the metabolism of the branched-chain amino acids and their control by the endocrine system. We have previously observed a differential effect of basal insulin on the rates of entry and exit of leucine through the plasma compartment of the conscious animal (Abumrad et al., 1982). In the present study we will explore the effects of selective changes in glucagon and glucocorticoids on the flux of the essential amino acid, leucine, in conscious overnight-fasted dogs. This amino acid was used as a prototype because of its unique ability to stimulate protein synthesis, inhibit protein breakdown, and spare glucose utilization in muscle preparations, and to inhibit urea production *in vivo* and in rat liver perfusion studies (Goldberg and Tischler, 1981).

Experiments were carried out on 21 conscious dogs (21 to 26 kg) with silastic catheters placed in the femoral artery as previously described (Abumrad et al., 1981). On the day of the study, and after an 18-hour fast, all animals received an infusion of 4,5-[^{3}H]-leucine for 7.5 hours for the measurement of leucine kinetics. After three hours of isotopic equilibration, blood samples were obtained during a half-hour basal period and a four-hour experimental period during which hormonal perturbations were induced as follows: Group 1 (control) received saline. Group 2 (4 $\times$ basal glucagon-IRG) received a peripheral infusion of somatostatin (SRIF) plus intraportal replacement of basal INS (300 μU/kg/min) and IRG at 3 ng/kg/min to produce selective fourfold increase in peripheral IRG levels. The last two groups (3 and 4) received an infusion of ACTH (1 μU/min) throughout the experimental period; Group 4 received additional pretreatment with ACTH (500 μU/d for four days) given intramuscularly.

The effect of hormonal perturbations on plasma leucine, its rate of appearance and clearance during both the basal period and the last hour of the experimental period are shown in Figures 1–3. Physiologic elevations of glucagon, to fourfold levels, had no effect on either plasma leucine concentration or flux. Glucocorticoid excess caused significant changes in leucine depending on the duration of the ACTH treatment. After four hours of hypercortisolemia, there was a 17% rise in plasma leucine (from 117 $\pm$ 4 μM to 137 $\pm$ 8, $p < 0.01$), a 31% decline in its clearance from plasma (from 26 $\pm$ 2 to 18 $\pm$ 3 ml/kg/min, $p < 0.001$) without a change in its rate of appearance. Prolonged, but comparable, levels of hypercortisolemia resulted in a more sustained elevation in plasma leucine during both basal and experimental periods; Ra was 47% higher (3.0 $\pm$ 0.1 to 4.4 $\pm$ 0.2 μmol/kg/min, $p < 0.001$) and Cl was 42% lower (15 $\pm$ 2 ml/kg/min, $p < 0.001$) than control levels.

In the present study we measured the effect of different hormonal changes on the flux of unlabeled leucine through the plasma compartment from all sources. It is assumed that during the 7.5-hour period of leucine infusion, the amount of labeled leucine recycled into and out of protein is quite minimal (Garlick, 1978). Thus, the method used allows a qualitative estimate of the rates of protein turnover *in vivo*

(Abumrad, 1982). In the absence of exogenous intake, Ra reflects changes in whole body protein breakdown, while Rd (the rate of utilization) reflects changes in whole body protein synthesis and/or oxidation (James et al., 1976).

The effect of hyperglucagonemia, to levels comparable to those seen after the ingestion (Aoki et al., 1976) of a protein meal or an infusion (Abumrad et al., 1982) of an amino acid load, on leucine kinetics is quite negligible. Yet blood alanine levels fell by 25% and its uptake across the hepatic bed increased by 85% (data not shown) suggesting increased gluconeogenesis *in vivo* (Cherrington et al., 1982). Glucagon has been shown to have no demonstrable effect on forearm metabolism of 12-hour or 60-hour fasted man (Pozefsky et al., 1976) or on isolated rat skeletal muscle preparations (Ruderman, 1975). However, it has been shown to increase the percentage of protein degradation in hepatocytes (Ballard, 1980) and in perfused rat livers (Woodside et al., 1974), via a cAMP-dependent mechanism (Ballard, 1980). Yet, this effect of glucagon on protein breakdown is inhibited in the presence of physiologic levels of insulin, despite the observed elevation of cAMP (Ballard, 1980). Thus, it is possible to speculate that the prevailing basal insulin protected the animals against the catabolic effects of glucagon.

The effect of glucocorticoid excess on total body leucine kinetics is that of net catabolism. The elevated plasma leucine observed with acute hypercortisolemia was primarily due to a decrease in the efflux of leucine out of the plasma compartment, while with more prolonged glucocorticoid excess, it was due to a combination of increased influx and a further decrease in efflux of leucine through the plasma compartment. With comparable levels of hypercortisolemia to those seen in the present study, we recently observed increased rates of leucine oxidation in both man and the

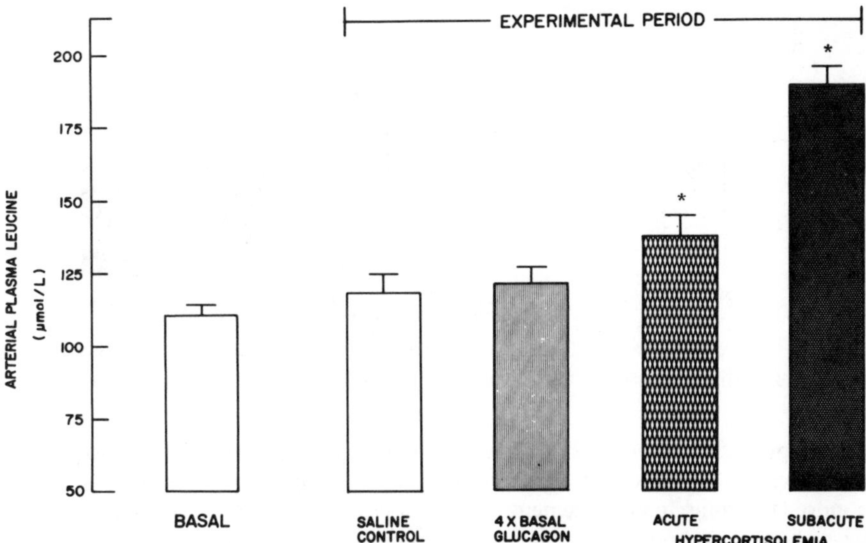

Figure 1 The effect of excess glucagon and cortisol on arterial plasma leucine concentration in overnight (18-hour) fasted dogs. The values in the basal period, represent an average of four samples per dog for 16 dogs. The values in the experimental period represent an average of two samples per dog for each of the group. Refer to the text for the hormonal perturbations during the experimental period. * Represents significance from basal with $p < 0.05$.

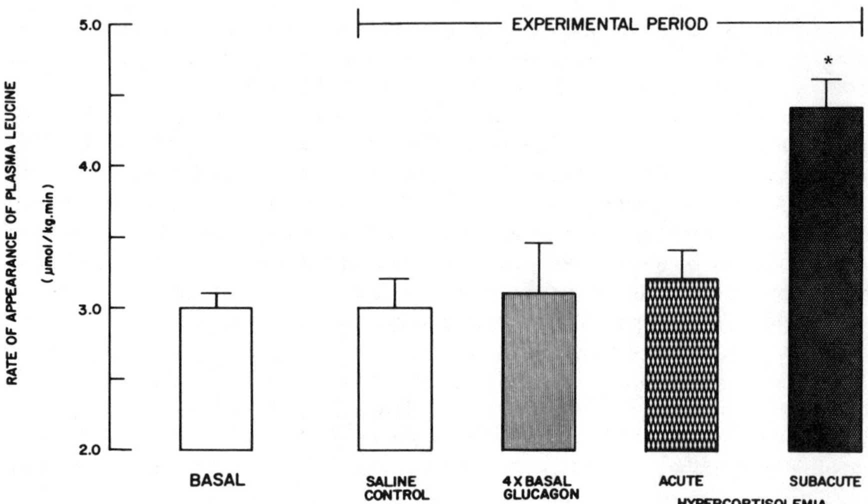

Figure 2 The effect of excess glucagon and cortisol on the rate of appearance of leucine into the plasma compartment in overnight (18-hour) fasted dogs. *Represents significance from basal with $p < 0.05$.

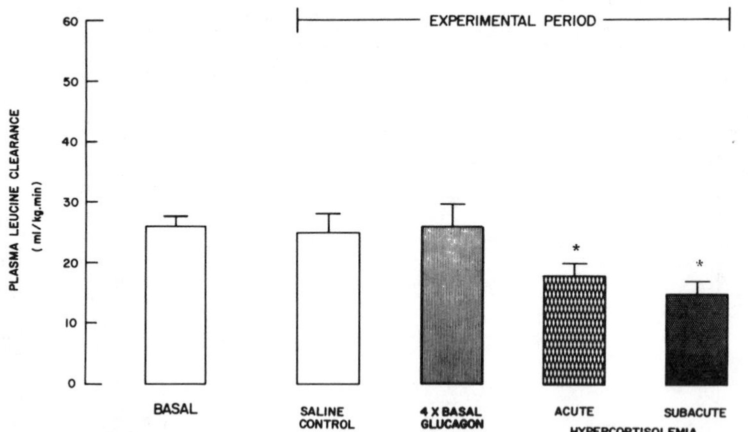

Figure 3 The effect of excess glucagon and cortisol on the rate of clearance of plasma leucine in overnight (18-hour) fasted dogs. *Represents significance from basal with $p < 0.05$.

dog (unpublished observations). Based on these data, it is then reasonable to assume that excess glucocorticoid results, early on, in a reduction of protein synthesis, and at a more later time, in enhancement of protein degradation. Previous *in vivo* studies have shown an increase in urinary excretion of 3-methylhistidine in glucocorticoid-treated rats (Tomas et al., 1979) suggestive of increased protein degradation. On the other hand, studies done on skeletal muscle preparations obtained from glucocorticoid-treated rats, showed either a decrease in protein synthesis alone (Rannels et al., 1978) or a combined decrease in protein synthesis and an increase in protein degradation (Goldberg et al., 1980).

The mechanism by which glucocorticoids exert their effects on protein turnover cannot be identified from the present study. Because the effects of a nonpeptide hormone are generally related to the number of receptors present (Butler and O'Malley, 1976), it is then reasonable to suggest that the effects of glucocorticoids on protein turnover *in vivo* are dependent on the number and activation of available receptors. Recent observations indicate that receptors proliferate during hormone administration in a dose- and a time-dependent fashion (Max, 1980). Thus, it is possible to speculate that a more prolonged exposure and a higher number of glucocorticoid receptors, are required for the activation of protein breakdown than those required for the inhibition of protein synthesis. It is also possible that the receptor density and affinity are dependent on the presence of other hormones, most notably insulin.

The level of insulin is probably the most important factor in regulating total body protein turnover. We have previously shown that in the basal postabsorptive state, selective, acute insulin withdrawal, brought about by the concurrent infusion of somatostatin and intraportal replacement of basal glucagon for four hours, resulted in a significant elevation of plasma leucine which was not attributed to a change in its rate of appearance into the plasma compartment, suggesting a preferential effect of basal insulin on the routes of disposal of leucine, namely protein synthesis. On the other hand, physiologic elevations of plasma insulin to twice basal levels, brought about with concurrent infusion of SRIF and intraportal replacement of twice basal insulin, resulted in a significant reduction in plasma leucine which was secondary to a stimulation of protein synthesis and inhibition of protein breakdown (Abumrad et al., 1982). These findings in the intact animal agree with the *in vitro* data showing that the inhibitory effects of insulin on protein breakdown were only observed at concentrations three to ten orders of magnitude higher than physiologic levels (Jefferson et al., 1977).

In summary, acute elevations of glucagon to four times basal levels had no effect on either leucine entry or exit through the plasma compartment. However, glucocorticoid excess resulted initially in a reduction of leucine exit from the plasma compartment and later on a stimulation of its entry into plasma, suggesting an early inhibition of protein synthesis and a later stimulation of protein breakdown.

ACKNOWLEDGMENTS

The authors would like to acknowledge the excellent technical assistance of S.L. Rannels, C.L. McKinley, L.L. Brown and D.B. Lacy, and are most grateful for the excellent secretarial skills of Rose A. Hornsby.

This investigation was supported by Juvenile Diabetes Foundation Grant #80R010 and NIH Grant #AM30515 and Diabetes Research and Training Center Grant #AM20593.

REFERENCES

Abumrad, N., et al. (1981): The effect of starvation on leucine kinetics in the conscious dog. In: *Metabolism and Clinical Implications of Branched Chain Amino Acids and Ketoacids* (eds: M. Walser and J.R. Williamson) p. 335–360, Elsevier/North-Holland, New York.

Abumrad, N., et al. (1982): The role of insulin in the regulation of leucine kinetics in the conscious dog. *J. Clin. Invest.* (In Press).

Abumrad, N., et al. (1982): The disposal of an intravenously administered amino acid load across the human forearm. *Metabolism* (In Press).

Aoki, T., et al. (1976): Amino acid levels across the normal forearm muscle and splanchnic bed after a protein meal. *Am. J. Clin. Nutr.* 29:340–350.

Ballard, J.F. (1980): Hormonal control of protein degradation in liver and isolated cells. In: *Biochemical Actions of Hormones* (eds: Litwack and Gerald) vol. VII, p. 91–117, Academic Press, New York.

Butler, R.E. and O'Malley, B.W. (1976): The biology and mechanism of steriod hormone receptor interaction with the eukaryote nucleus. *Biochem. Pharmacol.* 25:1–12.

Cherrington, A.D., et al., (1983): Amino acid and gluconeogenesis. In *Amino Acids* (eds: G.L. Blackburn, J.P. Grant, V.R. Young), John Wright • PSG Inc., Boston.

Garlick, P.J. (1978): An analysis of errors in estimation of the rate of protein synthesis by constant infusion of labeled amino acid. *Biochem. J.* 176:402–405.

Goldberg, A.L., et al. (1980): Hormonal regulation of protein degradation and synthesis in skeletal muscle. *Fed. Proc.* 39:31–36.

Goldberg, A.L. and Tischler, M.E. (1981): Regulatory effects of leucine on carbohydrate and protein metabolism. In: *Metabolism and Clinical Implications of Branched Chain Amino and Ketoacids* (eds: M. Walser and J.R. Williamson) pp. 205–216. Elsevier/North-Holland, New York.

James, W.P.T., et al. (1976): Studies of amino acid and protein metabolism in normal man with L-[$U^{14}C$]-tyrosine. *Clin. Sci. Mol. Med.* 50:525–532.

Jefferson, L.S., et al. (1977): Regulation by insulin of amino acid release and protein turnover in the perfused rat hemicorpus. *J. Biol. Chem.* 252:1476–1483.

Max, S.R. (1980): Effect of estrogen on denervated muscle. *Society for Neuroscience* Abstracts 6:90.

McNamara, D.J. and Webb, T.E. (1974): Glucagon-mediated changes in the concentration of rat hepatic tyrosine transaminase: An immunochemical analysis. *Arch. Biochem. Biophys.* 163:777–783.

Pozefsky, G., et al. (1976): Metabolism of forearm tissues in man. Studies with glucagon. *Diabetes* 25:128–135.

Rannels, S.R., et al. (1978): Glucocorticoid effects on peptide-chain initiation in skeletal muscle and heart. *Am. J. Physiol.* 4:E134–E139.

Ruderman, N.B. (1975): Muscle amino acid metabolism and gluconeogenesis. *Ann. Rev. Med.* 26:245–258.

Tomas, F.M., et al. (1979): Effect of glucocorticoid administration on the rate of muscle protein breakdown in vivo in rats, as measured by urinary excretion of N^{+}-methylhistidine. *Biochem. J.* 178:139–146.

Woodside, K.H., et al. (1974): Effects of glucagon on general protein degradation and synthesis in perfused rat liver. *J. Biol. Chem.* 249:5458–5463.

Quantitation of Branched-Chain Amino and α-Ketoacids by HPLC

Steven L. Nissen, Carol Van Huysen, and Morey W. Haymond

Branched-chain amino acid metabolism is closely linked to the metabolism of their respective branched-chain α-ketoacids, often requiring quantitation of both the amino and α-ketoacids. Gas liquid chromatography was the first practical method for the measurement of plasma branched-chain α-ketoacids (Cree et al., 1979) which was laborious and time consuming. High performance liquid chromatographic (HPLC) methods for the quantitation of BCKA (Nissen et al., 1981; Hayashi et al., 1981) were subsequently published, but none were able to quantitate all three BCKA in physiological fluids.

Quantitation of the branched-chain amino acids (BCAA) in plasma has usually required ion exchange chromatographic methods. HPLC methods have the potential for decreasing the time and expense involved in amino acid analysis, but most are not suitable for routine quantitation of plasma BCAA due to poor peak resolution and instability (Shuster, 1980; Hill et al., 1979). The present manuscript describes a HPLC method for the quantitation of all three BCKA and BCAA in small plasma samples (Nissen et al., 1982). In addition, this method is adaptable to automated HPLC analysis and can be used to isolate compounds of interest.

MATERIALS

Solvents (HPLC grade) were obtained from Fisher Chemical. Norleucine (Pierce Chemical) and calibrated amino acid standards (Hamilton) were obtained from commercial sources. Alpha-ketoisocaproate, α-ketomethylvalerate, α-ketoisovalerate, α-ketocaproate, amino acid oxidase, catalase and all other chemicals were obtained from Sigma Chemical Company.

HPLC was accomplished using a 5 μ, C-18 silica column (Altex) and a Varian Liquid Chromatograph (Model 5060) interfaced with an integrator (Varian 401) and a UV detection (Model 441, Waters) at 214 nm. The HPLC running buffer (1.4 ml/min) consisted of 0.05 M sodium phosphate, pH 7.0, and aceteonitrile (90:10). Between each sample the column was flushed for one minute with methanol and re-equilibrated with running buffer. All injections were made with an automatic sample injector (WISP, Waters). Plasma BCAA concentrations were independently determined using a Beckman 119 CL Amino Acid Analyzer (Schmidt et al., 1982).

METHODS

Plasma samples (1 ml) are adjusted to pH ~1 with 1 N HC1 (~200 μl) and the internal standards, α-ketocaproate (20 nmol for ketoacid analysis) and norleucine (50 nmol for amino acid analysis) are added to each tube. Standard solutions of the BCAA (50 to 500 μM) and BCKA (5 to 50 μM) are processed along with each set of plasma samples. Plasma is then transferred to a 1 × 5 cm column (Isolab) containing 2 ml of a 50% aqueous solution of cation exchange resin, H+ form (BioRad). The column is washed with aliquots of 0.01 N HCL, and the effluent plus washings collected in 25 mm × 150 mm glass screw-capped tubes for BCKA analysis. The amino acids are eluted from the washed column with 4 ml of 4 M ammonium hydroxide into 17 × 60 mm screw-cap vials (Kimble) and frozen for subsequent analysis (see below).

The effluent from the columns containing the BCKA is extracted once with 35 ml of methylene chloride, centrifuged, and the supernate (aqueous layer) discarded. The methylene chloride layer (infranate) is transferred to a clean 25 mm × 150 mm tube and back-extracted with 350 μl of 0.1 M sodium phosphate buffer (pH 7.0). After centrifugation, the aqueous layer is transferred to 250 μl centrifuge tubes, briefly centrifuged (Beckman Microfuge) and 200 μl of the aqueous solution injected into the HPLC system. Plasma BCKA concentrations are calculated from a standard curve of the peak height ratios of the standard solutions of BCKA and the internal standard, α-ketocaproate.

The ammonia effluent is lyophilized and 1 ml of a solution containing amino acid oxidase and catalase (0.1 mg amino acid oxidase and .05 mg catalase in 1 ml of 0.5 M tris buffer, pH 7.6) is added. The sample is flushed with oxygen, capped, and placed in a shaking water bath at 37° for 1.5 hours. 1 N HCl (~150 μl) is then added to lower the pH to < 1.0, and subsequently processed as described above for the BCKA. Plasma BCAA concentrations are calculated from the peak height ratios of the BCAA standards and the internal standard, norleucine.

RESULTS AND DISCUSSION

BCKA Analysis

Figure 1 presents the chromatograms derived from standard BCKA solutions (dotted line) and human plasma (solid line). Using this method, a sample can be analyzed every ten minutes from as little as 50 μl of plasma.

The standard curves of α-ketoisocaproate, α-ketomethylvalerate and α-ketoisovalerate are linear over a range of 5 to 30 μM and the recovery of α-ketoisocaproate, α-ketomethylvalerate, and α-ketoisovalerate added to plasma was linear and parallel to the standard curves. The coefficient of variation for replicate analyses was 3% for each of the α-ketoacids.

BCAA Analysis

Figure 2 illustrates the HPLC chromatograms derived from a standard solution of BCAA (dotted line) and plasma after treatment with amino acid oxidase and analysis as α-ketoacids. In addition to quantitation of the BCAA, it appears methionine can also be analyzed as its α-ketoacid (α-ketomethiolbutyrate). The standard curve of all amino acids were linear and were parallel when added to plasma curves, indicating quantitative recovery of leucine from plasma.

The correlation between leucine concentration measured by the amino acid analyzer and the HPLC procedure described here, indicated close agreement (r = .986). Isoleucine and valine have similar correlations (r = .92, r = .85, respectively).

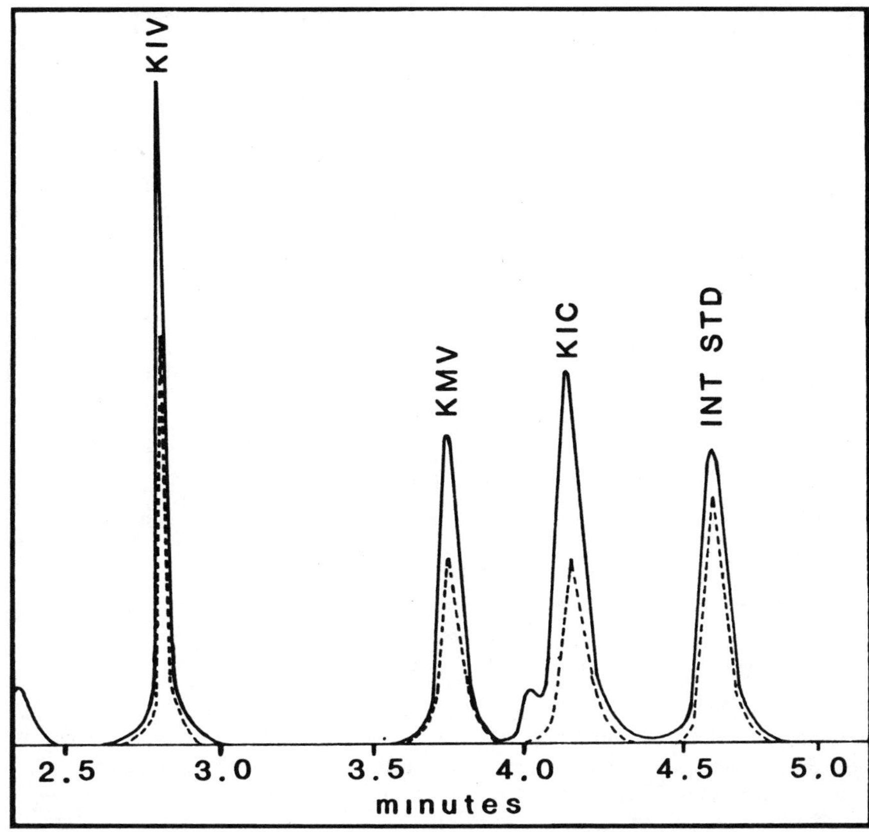

Figure 1 Chromatogram of α-ketoacid standards (broken line) and a plasma extract (solid line); KIV, α-ketoisovalerate; KMV, α-ketomethylvalerate; KIC, α-ketoisocaproate; and Int Std, α-ketocaproate. Reproduced with permission of the *J Chromatography* (in press).

Analysis of the BCAA by HPLC requires approximately ten minutes per sample compared to a minimum of two hours by conventional amino acid analyzer techniques. In addition to being as accurate as the amino acid analyzer, this HPLC technique can also be automated. The α-ketoacids derived directly from plasma or from the BCAA were stable for at least eight hours at room temperature in the automatic injector sample deck.

ACKNOWLEDGMENTS

The authors are indebted to Collette Schmidt for technical assistance and to Marylee Campion for her secretarial help. This investigation was supported by the Wassie and Mayo Foundations and U.S. Public Health Service Grant AM-26989. Dr. Nissen is supported by Diabetes Training Grant AM-7352C.

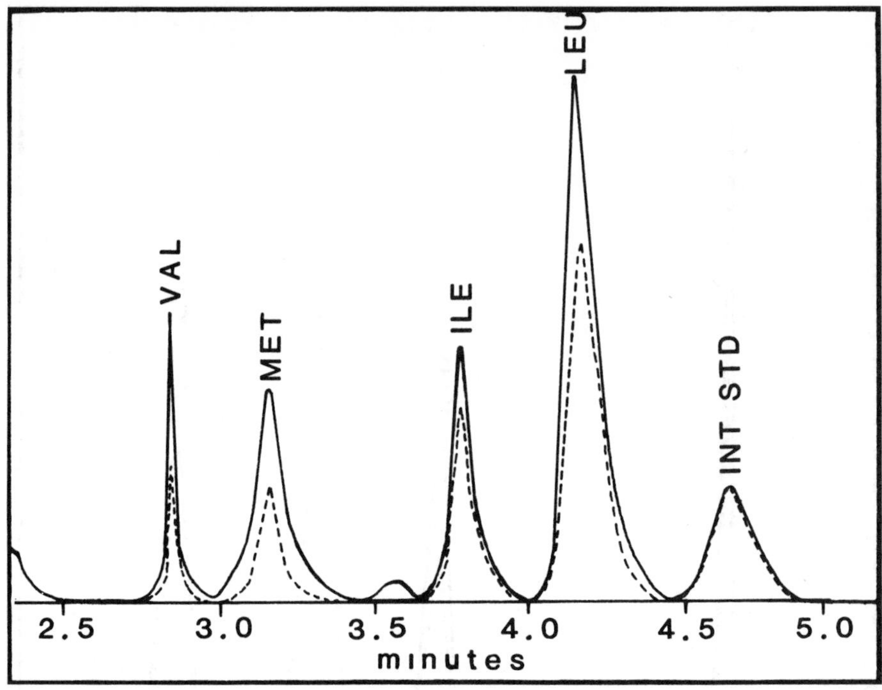

Figure 2 Chromatograms of the branched-chain amino acids standards (broken line) and a plasma extract (solid line); Val, valine; Met, methionine; Ile, isoleucine; Leu, leucine; Int Std, norleucine. Samples are deaminated with amino acid oxidase and subsequently chromatographed as their respective α-ketoacids. Reproduced with permission from the *J Chromatography* (in press).

REFERENCES

Cree, T.C., Hutson, S.M., Harper, A.E. (1979): Gas-liquid chromatography of α-ketoacids: Quantification of the branched chain α-ketoacids from physiological sources. *Anal. Biochem.* 92:156–163.

Hayashi, T., Todoriki, H., Narusa, H. (1981): High performance liquid chromatographic determinations of α-ketoacids. *J. Chrom.* 224:197–204.

Hill, D.W., Walters, F.G., Wilson, T.D., Stuart, D. (1979): High performance liquid chromatographic determinations of amino acids in the picomole range. *Anal. Chem.* 51:1339–1341.

Nissen, S., Van Huysen, C., Haymond, M.W. (1981): Measurement of plasma α-ketoisocaproate and specific radioactivity by high-performance liquid chromatography. *Anal. Biochem.* 110:389–392.

Nissen, S., Van Huysen, C., Haymond, M.W. (1982): Measurement of branched chain amino acids and branched chain α-ketoacids in plasma by HPLC. *J. Chrom.* In press.

Schmidt, C., Berg, P., and Haymond, M. (1982): Use of α-glucosaminic acid as an internal standard in single column accelerated amino acid analysis of physiological fluids. *Anal. Biochem.* 123:74–77.

Shuster, R. (1980): Determination of the amino acids by high performance liquid chromatography. *Anal. Chem.* 52:617–620.

SECTION III
Amino Acid Interrelationships

7 Dispensable and Indispensable Amino Acid Interrelationships

Alfred E. Harper

For the most part, interrelationships between the dispensable and indispensable amino acids are taken for granted. They are rarely discussed in a general way. Once amino acids have been consumed in adequate amounts in the diet, interrelationships are not between the dispensable and indispensable amino acids but occur between pairs and among groups of amino acids, independently of their nutritional essentiality. This, I think, emphasizes that the distinction between dispensable and indispensable amino acids is strictly nutritional. It has little significance or meaning metabolically, except that one group can be synthesized by mammals and the other cannot.

Nutritional classification of the amino acids of proteins as dispensable (nonessential) or indispensable (essential) could not be completed until after the discovery of threonine by McCoy et al. (1935). This discovery enabled preparation of diets, in which the protein was replaced by a mixture of amino acids, that would support growth of rats and maintenance of human subjects (Rose, 1938, 1957). Then by deleting one amino acid after another from these diets and feeding the diets devoid of one amino acid to rats and to human volunteers, Rose and his associates were able to distinguish between amino acids that could and those that could not be synthesized by mammals. In the late 1930s, they were able to complete the list of amino acids that were essential nutrients—a list that was begun in 1906 when Willcock and Hopkins (1906) discovered that tryptophan was required preformed in the diet by rodents, a finding that was subsequently confirmed by Osborne and Mendel (1914) who also demonstrated the nutritional essentiality of lysine and sulfur-containing amino acids.

NUTRITIONAL CLASSIFICATION OF AMINO ACIDS

The studies of Rose and his associates (Rose 1938) led to the nutritional classification of amino acids shown in Table 7-1. A few amino acids did not fit either the dispensable or indispensable category satisfactorily. These were amino acids such as arginine which, although they could be synthesized in the body, were not synthesized by the young of most species in amounts sufficient to meet physiological needs. Cystine and tyrosine, which are synthesized only from methionine and phenylalanine, respectively, have the characteristics of indispensable amino acids if their precursors are not present in a diet in adequate amounts or if there is a defect in the pathway by which they are synthesized. Such amino acids have been classified as "semi-essential" or "semi-indispensable" (Block and Bolling, 1944), terms that are self-contradictory and, therefore, unsatisfactory. Rudman (1982) proposed recently that an amino acid which is ordinarily nutritionally dispensable be classified as "conditionally" indispensable (or essential) when, owing to either metabolic impairment or the physiological state of the organism, the need for the amino acid exceeds the synthetic capacity of the body.

When young rats are fed a diet that contains a high proportion of indispensable amino acids, as is shown in Table 7-2, the so-called "nonessential" amino acids are synthesized from the essentials at too slow a rate to support maximum growth (Rose et al., 1949; Lardy and Feldott, 1950; Stucki and Harper, 1962; Rogers et al., 1970). Snyderman et al. (1962) have reported that "unessential" nitrogen can become limiting for the growth of human infants with a low intake of high quality protein. Under these conditions, the so-called "nonessential" amino acids become conditionally indispensable or essential. It, therefore, seems more appropriate to call them "dispensable" rather than nonessential, as this term does not carry the implication

Table 7-1
Nutritional Classification of Amino Acids

Dispensable	Conditionally Indispensable		Indispensable
Arg (human)	Arg (most mammals)		Arg (birds)
Gly	Gly (birds)		Trp
Ala			Thr
Ser			His
Asp	Cys	Tau	Met
Glu			Val
Pro			Ile
Asn			Leu
Gln	Tyr		Phe
			Lys

Table 7-2
Weight Gain of Weanling Rats Fed Different Proportions of Indispensable and Dispensable Amino Acids for 17 Days

Diet (2.4% N)		
Indispensable	*Dispensable*	Weight Gain (17 Days)
%	%	gm
100	—	21
75	25	57
50	50	68

After Stucki and Harper, 1962.

that such amino acids are literally "nonessential" (Harper, 1974). The nutritional classification of amino acids (Table 7-1) takes these observations and commentaries into account.

Many amino acids that are present in foods, such as hydroxyproline, trimethyllysine, carboxyglutamate and 3-methylhistidine can be used by mammals, if they are used at all, only as sources of energy. These and the many nonprotein amino acids found in plants might truly be called nutritionally "nonessential". It might also be noted that indispensable amino acids other than lysine or threonine can be replaced in diets by their α-ketoacid analogues (Berg, 1959). Thus, lysine and threonine are the only amino acids that are truly nutritionally essential.

OVERVIEW OF INTERRELATIONSHIPS BETWEEN DISPENSABLE AND INDISPENSABLE AMINO ACIDS

Sites where interrelationships may occur between the dispensable and indispensable amino acids during the course of their metabolism are indicated schematically in Figure 7-1. First, during absorption from the intestine or during transport into cells of organs and tissues anywhere in the body, interactions between some members of these two groups of amino acids can occur through competition for a component of a common carrier system.

Second, interrelationships between these two groups of amino acids occur during the synthesis of proteins. The primary need for amino acids is for synthesis of proteins and for synthesis of small nitrogen-containing molecules. As all amino acids are required together at the same time for protein synthesis, a shortage of an amino acid from either group will result in reduced efficiency of utilization of all of the others.

Third, probably the main interrelationships in the synthesis of small molecules occur in the use of nitrogen from the indispensable amino acids for synthesis of dispensable amino acids. Also, nitrogen from the dispensable amino acids may be used for resynthesis of indispensable amino acids from their α-ketoacid precursors.

Fourth, the most complex and highly integrated series of interactions between these two groups of amino acids undoubtedly occurs during the course of degradation of surpluses of amino acids that are not used for protein synthesis or are released as the result of protein degradation. Interactions during degradation become

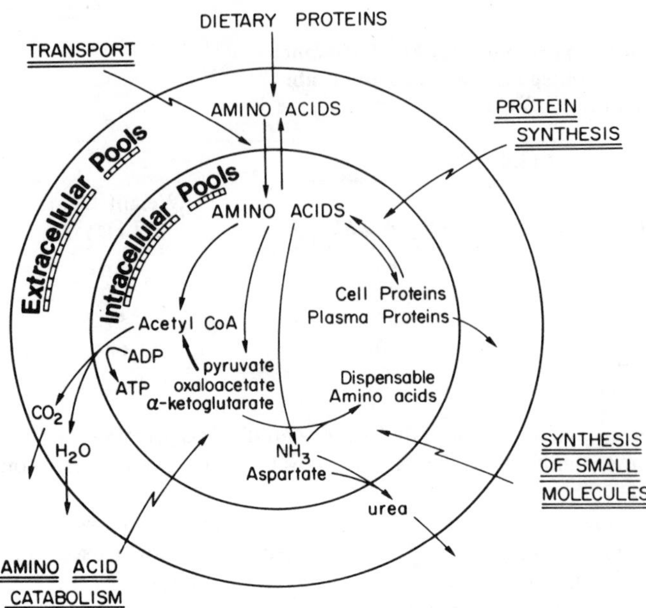

Figure 7-1 Schematic representation of sites of interrelationships in the metabolism of the dispensable and indispensable amino acids.

quantitatively of increasing importance the greater the amounts of amino acids in the diet are above the amounts required for protein synthesis and the greater the proportion of total energy they provide.

During the degradation of excesses of amino acids, interrelationships between the dispensable and indispensable amino acids occur in connection with: 1) removal of the nitrogen from the indispensable amino acids as the initial step in making the carbon skeletons available for gluconeogenesis, lipogenesis, ketogenesis or direct oxidation; 2) transfer of the nitrogen from one amino acid to another in cells to form compounds that traverse membranes readily and function in the interorgan transport of nitrogen between organs and, ultimately, to the liver; 3) incorporation of nitrogen from amino acids into urea, a nontoxic compound, that can be transported from the liver to the kidney for disposal by excretion in urine.

AMINO ACID POOLS

Values for postprandial concentrations of total dispensable and total indispensable amino acids in plasma, liver, muscle and brain of young rats fed ad libitum for 10 days purified diets differing in protein content are shown in Table 7-3 (Tews and Harper, 1982). In blood plasma, the total concentrations of these two groups of amino acids are fairly similar; in tissues, the concentrations of the dispensable amino acids are much higher than those of the indispensables. In muscle the difference in concentration between the two groups of amino acids is less than in other tissues but, as lysine and threonine together make up from 80% to 90% of the total indispensable concentration, if these two amino acids were excluded from the comparison, the

Table 7-3
Postprandial Plasma and Tissue Concentrations of Total Dispensable and Total Indispensable Amino Acids in Young Rats Fed for 10 Days *ad Libitum*

	Plasma	Liver	Muscle	Brain
	μmol/ml		μmol/g	
Dispensable (minus glutamine)				
6% lactalbumin	2.2	12.6	13.3	21.2*
15% lactalbumin	1.7	15.7	10.7	20.5*
50% lactalbumin	1.7	11.7	9.5	20.4*
Indispensable				
6% lactalbumin	1.6	1.8	4.5†	1.5
15% lactalbumin	3.1	2.9	8.0†	2.2
50% lactalbumin	4.0	3.0	6.3†	1.4

*about 60% glutamate.
†60% to 70% lysine; 20% to 30% threonine.

From Tews and Harper, unpublished. Glutamine was not measured in this experiment. Glutamine concentration in plasma is about 0.5 mM; in liver, 3 mM; in muscle, 2 to 4 mM; in brain, 4 mM.

ratio of dispensable to the remaining indispensable amino acids would resemble that for the brain.

The concentration of total dispensable amino acids (DAA) in plasma and tissues is influenced very little by differences in protein intake, whereas the concentration of total indispensable amino acids (IAA) rises sharply when the lactalbumin content of the diet ingested is increased from 6% to 15%. Increasing the lactalbumin content of the diet further, from 15% to 50%, results in some additional rise in plasma total IAA concentration, but no change in liver, and decreases in muscle and brain concentrations.

The changes in the concentration of IAA when the dietary protein content was increased from 6% to 15% were the result of increases generally in the concentrations of amino acids in this group. The greatest part of the change, nevertheless, could be accounted for by increases in the concentrations of lysine and threonine and the branched-chain amino acids (BCAA), as shown in Table 7-4. When the dietary lactalbumin content was increased further, from 15% to 50%, the IAA concentration changes observed—an increase in plasma, no change in liver, and decreases in muscle and brain were striking. These are accounted for mainly by reciprocal changes in the concentrations of lysine and threonine and the BCAA—decreases in the former and increases in the latter. The decreases in the concentrations of most IAA, especially lysine and threonine when rats are fed a high protein diet, occur in association with increases observed within a few days in the enzymes for IAA degradation in liver (Kang-Lee and Harper, 1978; Soliman and Harper, 1971). The opposite trend is observed only for the BCAA (Table 7-4); the activities of enzymes for degradation of this group of amino acids do not increase significantly in animals fed high protein diets (Harper and Zapalowski, 1981).

The concentrations of dispensable amino acids respond much less to changes in protein intake. The most striking changes, which account for most of the declines observed in the concentrations of the DAA (Table 7-3), were in glycine and serine (Table 7-4), the concentrations of which fell in plasma and tissues with increasing protein intake.

The total free pools of most of the indispensable amino acids are small (30 to 200 μM). Also, it is evident that these pools do not increase as protein intake increases from adequate to excessive, but may actually fall. The free pools of dispensable amino acids are much larger than those of the indispensables (often greater than 1 mM). These, too, do not increase in response to increases in protein intake above the adequate level. As tissue protein does not accumulate in response to increasing protein intake, surpluses of both groups of amino acids are evidently oxidized rapidly. There is thus no reserve of free amino acids. A question that may be raised from examination of the large quantities of alanine, glumate, aspartate and glutamine in tissue pools is: Do the high concentrations of these amino acids contribute to conservation of the indispensable amino acids by shifting the steady-state of transamination reactions in the direction that favors amination of the α-keto acids of the IAA?

Table 7-4
Postprandial Plasma and Tissue Concentrations of Selected Groups of Amino Acids in Young Rats Fed *ad Libitum* for 10 Days

	Plasma	Liver	Muscle	Brain
	μmol/ml		μmol/g	
Lys + Thr				
6% albumin	1.1	1.0	4.2	1.1
15% albumin	2.1	1.7	7.1	1.7
50% albumin	1.9	0.9	4.8	1.1
BCAA				
6% albumin	0.23	0.38	0.16	0.12
15% albumin	0.52	0.54	0.29	0.15
50% albumin	1.5	1.3	0.73	0.21
Gly + Ser				
6% albumin	1.0	3.8	6.9	2.4
15% albumin	0.6	2.5	4.1	1.9
50% albumin	0.5	1.1	2.1	1.8

From Tews and Harper, unpublished.

PROTEIN SYNTHESIS

The primary need for amino acids is for synthesis of tissue proteins. Dispensable and indispensable amino acids are required in close to equal amounts during periods of rapid growth. In the young rat and in the chick it has been shown that a satisfactory rate of growth cannot be maintained with diets containing only the IAA, even at double the required levels (Table 7-2). Under these conditions the dispensable amino acids become conditionally indispensable. Evidently they cannot be synthesized from the indispensable amino acids rapidly enough to supply the needs for tissue formation when growth is rapid. There is no evidence of a unique need for any one of them; each can be omitted in turn from a complete diet without growth being impaired. On the other hand, they do differ in effectiveness as supplements to a diet containing only indispensable amino acids (Rogers et al., 1970). Glutamate is nearly, but not quite, as effective as the entire mixture of dispensables, with glycine and serine being least effective.

It is scarely necessary to mention that even if the dispensable amino acids are either provided or synthesized in excess of the amounts required, net protein synthesis will be limited if any one of the indispensable amino acids is not provided in an adequate amount. Unlike the dispensable amino acids which, as was shown before, are maintained at nearly constant concentrations in plasma and tissues whether the protein content of the diet is low or high, the pools of the indispensables are depleted when protein intake or the intake of a specific amino acid is low (Kang-Lee and Harper, 1977). Under such conditions, the efficiency of utilization and retention of the limiting indispensable amino acid is high. This can be seen from Figure 7-2, which shows the rate of oxidation of histidine in relation to intake. Only after the needs for protein synthesis have been met does an appreciable proportion of dietary histidine become available for the synthesis of the dispensable amino acids. From measurements of oxidation of histidine and other amino acids (Kang-Lee and Harper, 1977, 1978), it would appear that the young growing animal can retain close to 90% of the dietary IAA supply when the amount provided is inadequate.

A question arises as to whether the high tissue concentrations of the dispensable amino acids contribute to this conservation. Swendseid et al. (1960) have been able to maintain some adult human subjects in nitrogen equilibrium with amounts of egg protein that provided barely the minimum requirements of indispensable amino acids if the dispensable amino acids were added to provide 6.5 or 10.0 g of nitrogen. Similar observations have been made by Clark et al. (1963) and Kies et al. (1965). Scrimshaw and associates (1969) have observed that substitution of nonspecific

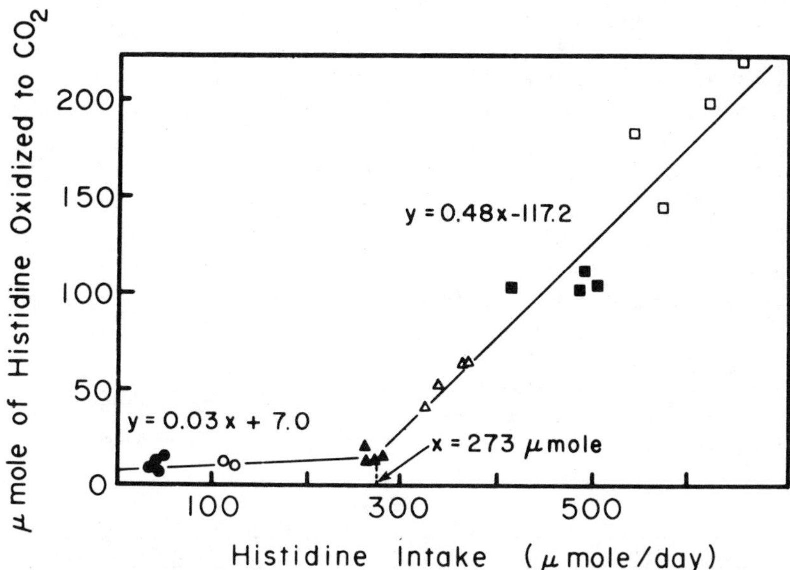

Figure 7-2 Oxidation of histidine to carbon dioxide by the rat: effect of histidine intake. (Reproduced from Kang-Lee and Harper, 1977, with permission.)

nitrogen sources for part of the dietary protein improved nitrogen balance of young men receiving diets containing somewhat subadequate amounts of milk, meat or egg proteins. Snyderman et al. (1962) have reported that as protein content was reduced in formulas fed to infants, a growth response to addition of nonspecific sources of nitrogen occurred. The basis for these effects remains to be established, but the possibility that the DAA contribute to conservation of IAA through reamination of the α-ketoacids of IAA is a possibility that deserves consideration.

SYNTHESIS OF SMALL MOLECULES

The possibility that the dispensable amino acids contribute to high efficiency of re-utilization of the carbon skeletons of the indispensables when intake of protein is low, leads logically to consideration of the dispensable amino acids as amino donors and the ready reversibility of transamination reactions. Transamination, as illustrated for the branched-chain amino (BCAA) and ketoacids (BCKA) in Figure 7-3, provides a mechanism whereby carbon skeletons of several of the indispensable amino acids can be conserved. Glutamate is the major participant among the dispensable amino acids in transamination reactions. It is present in cells in concentrations many fold higher than the indispensable amino acids that participate in transamination reactions. Besides being in high concentration in cells, glutamate can be generated from α-ketoglutarate through transamination with either alanine or aspartate, both of which are also in high concentration in most cells.

It is striking that the two indispensable amino acids in highest concentration in the free tissue pools (Table 7-4), lysine and threonine, are the two that do not participate in transamination reactions. They are also the two that rise most in concentration when protein intake is increased. They are also the two that cannot be conserved by reamination reactions.

Krebs and Lund (1977) predicted from kinetic and thermodynamic considerations that, with the high intracellular glutamate concentration in muscle 1 to 2 mM (lower than in liver, 4 mM; or brain, 12 mM), the concentrations of the α-ketoacids

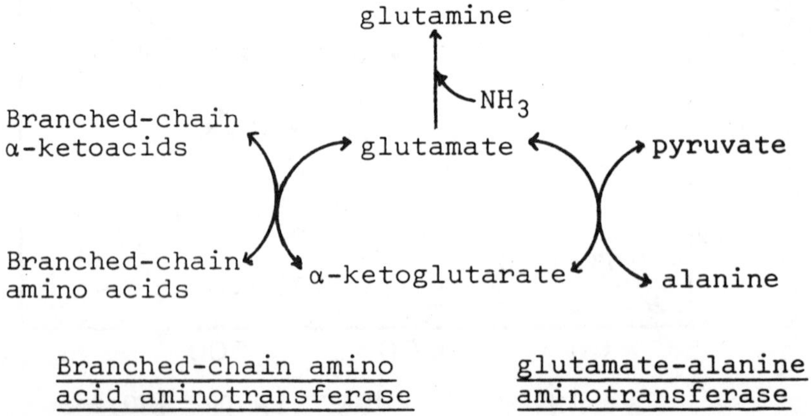

glutamine

NH_3

Branched-chain α-ketoacids ↔ glutamate ↔ pyruvate

Branched-chain amino acids ↔ α-ketoglutarate ↔ alanine

Branched-chain amino acid aminotransferase

glutamate-alanine aminotransferase

Figure 7-3 Relationships among branched-chain α-amino and α-ketoacids, glutamate, glutamine and alanine.

of the BCAA that undergo transamination with α-ketoglutarate would be one-fifteenth to one-twentieth those of the BCAA. This proved to be the case with BCAA concentrations in muscle being about 0.1 mM and BCKA concentrations being about 5 to 8 μM (Hutson and Harper, 1981). Nissen and Haymond (1981) and Matthews et al. (1981), using amino acids doubly labeled with heavy isotopes of hydrogen, nitrogen or carbon have obtained evidence for reamination of the carbon skeletons of the BCAA (Figure 7-3).

Amination of the BCKA is readily demonstrated by the use of α-keto analogues of several amino acids in the diets of animals (Chawla et al., 1975) and as traps for amino nitrogen in the treatment of renal patients and patients with metabolic defects of urea synthesis (Close, 1974). The formation of leucine from α-ketoisocaproate (α-KIC) has been shown to occur readily in the perfused hindquarter (Hutson et al., 1978). Cooper and Meister (1974) have suggested that glutamine aminotransferase, which will use many α-ketoacids as substrates, may function in the salvage of the α-ketoacids of tyrosine, phenylalanine and methionine.

AMINO ACID DEGRADATION

The most complex and integrated series of interactions and interrelationships between the dispensable and indispensable amino acids occurs during the course of degradation of surpluses of amino acids that are not used for protein synthesis or that have been released through tissue protein degradation. Degradation of amino acids involves removal of the nitrogen for eventual conversion to urea and then the carbon skeleton can be either oxidized directly to carbon dioxide with the release of energy or be converted to glucose or fatty acids and ketone bodies.

The indispensable amino acids undergo either transamination, as shown in Figure 7-3 for the reaction of the branched-chain amino acid aminotransferase, with the transfer of the amino group to α-ketoglutarate to form glutamate; or, as for example threonine, deamination with the release of ammonia. The ammonia can be used directly in urea synthesis or can be used directly in the glutamate dehydrogenase reaction, to form glutamic acid. Both of these pathways can, thus, give rise to glutamate which can then undergo further transamination with oxaloacetate or pyruvate, thereby, giving rise to aspartate and alanine.

During the course of degradation, certain of the indispensable amino acids serve directly as precursors of specific dispensable amino acids. Methionine, for example, is a precursor of homocysteine, homoserine, cysteine and taurine. In the series of reactions involved in generation of homoserine and cysteine, serine a dispensable amino acid, undergoes transulfuration with homocysteine. Phenylalanine is a precursor of tyrosine; lysine, of carnitine; and threonine of glycine (White et al. 1978).

Enzymes for the degradation of indispensable amino acids are not uniformly distributed in organs and tissues. Miller (1962) demonstrated in studies in which he used the isolated perfused liver and the isolated perfused eviscerated rat carcass, that most of the indispensable amino acids were degraded almost exclusively in the liver. The branched-chain amino acids were exceptions. They and the dispensable amino acids are degraded in most tissues and organs including liver. For amino acids that are degraded in nonhepatic sites, the nitrogen must still be transported to the liver for conversion to urea. Glutamate, the initial acceptor of the amino group from BCAA, is not readily transported across cell membranes so there must, therefore, be a system for transfer of the nitrogen to a readily transportable form. Extensive studies of the metabolism of the branched-chain amino acids in muscle have revealed that the nitrogen from them leaves the cell in the form of either alanine or glutamine. The amino group of glutamate can be transferred to pyruvate to form alanine or be released from glutamate as ammonia which, in turn, can combine with glutamate to form glutamine. These nitrogen-containing products, alanine and glutamine, can then be readily transported from the cell to the blood stream and, thence, to the liver.

There is thus extensive interorgan transport of the nitrogen from the branched-chain amino acids which depends upon a series of interrelationships between the dispensable and indispensable amino acids, as illustrated in Figure 7-4 (Harper and Zapalowski, 1981). Amino acids absorbed from the intestine pass initially to the liver. Most of the indispensable amino acids are metabolized by that organ. The branched-chain amino acids are exceptions. They are removed less by the liver than are most of the IAA and are distributed to other organs. Muscle is a major site for metabolism of this group of amino acids but they can also be metabolized in most, if not all, organs. The interactions shown in Figure 7-2 occur in muscle, giving rise to alanine. A part of the alanine may be transported to the liver and some may be distributed to other organs. Glutamine is also released from muscle. It may be transported to kidney which utilizes it readily or to the small intestine which can use

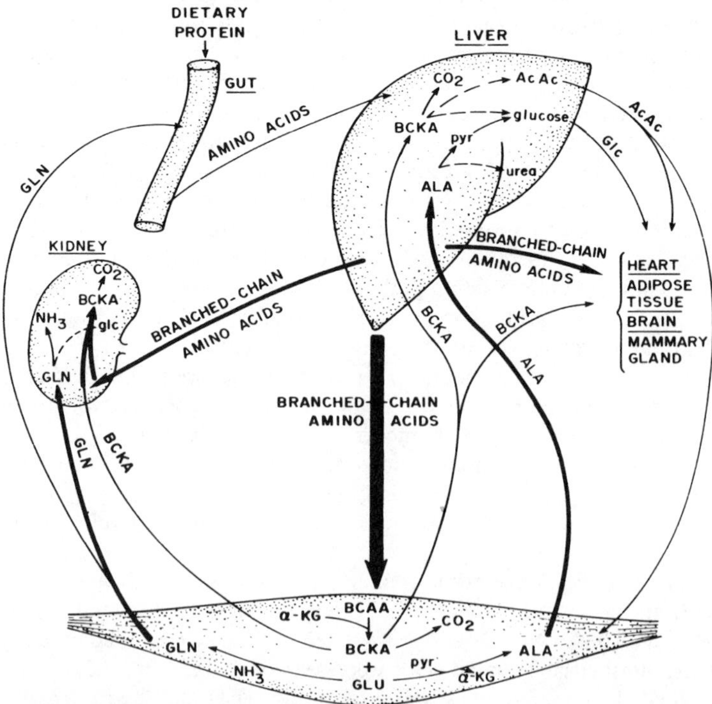

Figure 7-4 Interorgan relationships in the metabolism of branched-chain amino and α-ketoacids. (Reproduced from Harper and Zapalowski, 1981, with permission.)

it as a source of energy. Both of these organs may release alanine, which again serves as a vehicle for the transport of nitrogen to the liver (Felig, 1982). Thus, synthesis of dispensable amino acids, from the nitrogen of the branched-chain amino acids and carbon skeletons from carbohydrate, provides nontoxic, readily transportable nitrogen-containing compounds.

The final disposal of surplus nitrogen also involves a series of interrelationships between the dispensable and indispensable amino acids as shown in Figure 7-5. Ammonia is released directly from the indispensable amino acids threonine and histidine and from methionine via homoserine. It is also released from the dispensable amino acids glycine and serine, which were not included in the diagram. Methionine and tryptophan can undergo transamination with pyruvate to give rise to alanine. The nitrogen from the branched-chain amino acids, as has already been discussed, is used in peripheral tissues to form alanine, which serves as the vehicle for transporting nitrogen from the BCAA, leucine, isoleucine and valine, to the liver. In the liver, alanine can undergo transamination with α-ketoglutarate to give rise to glutamate. Methionine, tyrosine, lysine and the branched-chain amino acids also give rise directly to glutamate in the liver. Thus, the nitrogen from both of these groups of amino acids is used for synthesis of glutamate, which undergoes further transamination to yield aspartate.

Ammonia and aspartate provide nitrogen for synthesis of urea through the series of reactions shown in Figure 7-5, representing the urea cycle. In this, the nitrogen from the various indispensable amino acids is used for the synthesis of two other dispensable amino acids, citrulline and arginine. Arginine is then degraded to ornithine and urea. This extensive series of interactions between the dispensable and indispensable amino acids serves to convert the highly toxic compound, ammonia, into the relatively nontoxic compound, urea. The latter can then be transported readily to the kidneys for excretion in the urine.

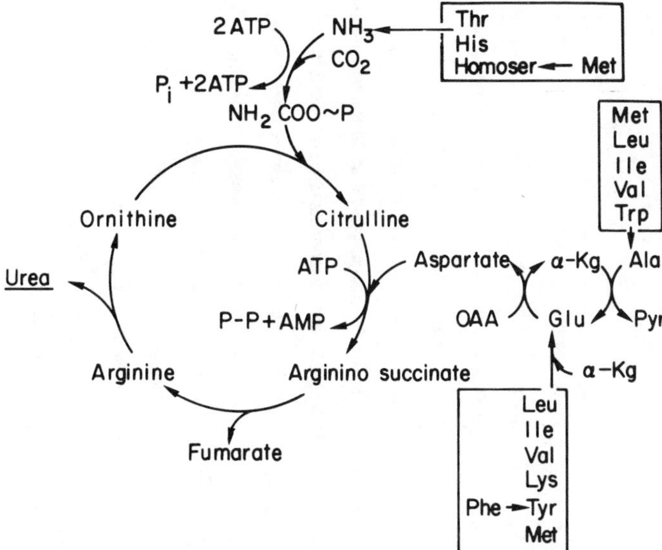

Figure 7-5 Relationships between dispensable and indispensable amino acids in the synthesis of arginine and incorporation of α-amino nitrogen into urea.

INTERACTIONS IN TRANSPORT

There is also the potential for interactions between the dispensable and indispensable amino acids in membrane transport. This has been an interest of ours, arising from studies of relationships among diet, blood and brain amino acids and feeding behavior (Peng et al., 1972; Peters and Harper, 1981). We have observed a close association between depletion of the brain pool of a single indispensable amino acid and depression of food intake. This type of alteration in the brain amino acid pool is also associated with a preference of the young rat for a diet with a balanced amino acid pattern or one containing no protein over a diet with an imbalance of amino acids that leads to depletion of the brain amino acid pool. In earlier studies of our own (Peng et al., 1972; Lutz et al., 1975) and in studies by Fernstrom and Wurtman (1972) depletion of the brain pool was shown to be the result of the competition among amino acids in a particular transport system for uptake into brain.

One of the techniques we have used as a guide in formulating diets that will result in depletion of an indispensable amino acid from brain is by assessing competition among amino acids for uptake into brain slices (Lutz et al., 1975). Threonine uptake into brain slices, for example, is inhibited by several amino acids (Figure 7-6) but most effectively by the small neutral amino acids alanine and serine (Tews et al.,

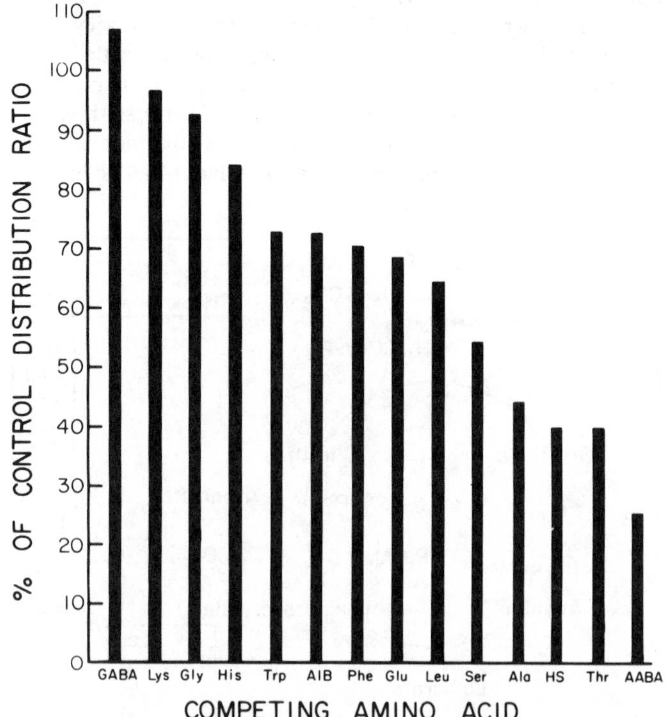

Figure 7-6 Effects of various amino acids on uptake of threonine by brain slices.

$$\text{Distribution ratio} = \frac{\text{intracellular } ^{14}\text{C threonine}}{\text{extracellular } ^{14}\text{C threonine}}$$

after incubation of slices for 60 minutes (Reproduced from Tews et al., 1978, with permission.)

1978, 1980). Glycine does not inhibit uptake of threonine into brain slices but, as it is readily converted to serine in the body, it can contribute indirectly to such competition. The branched-chain amino acids will also inhibit threonine uptake into brain slices but the inhibition is less than that observed with the small neutral, dispensable amino acids. All of these amino acids apparently share some common transport systems.

As shown in Table 7-5, addition of a mixture of the small neutral amino acids will depress the food intake of the young rat. This depression of food intake is associated with depletion of the brain pool of threonine (Table 7-6). The branched-chain amino acids are as effective as the small neutral amino acids, alanine and serine, in producing this effect. All of the effects are prevented if additional threonine is provided (Tews et al., 1979).

Table 7-5
Effects of Dietary Additions of Small Neutral (SN) and Large Neutral (LN) Amino Acids on Growth and Food Intake of Rats Fed a Low Protein (6% casein + L-met), Threonine-limiting Diet

Diet	Wt. Gain (5 days)	Food Intake (5 days)
Basal (B)	14	56
B + 4.5% SN	3	40
B + 4.5% LN	−1	40
B + SN + LN	−5	29
B + SN + LN + Thr	19	53

From Tews, Kim and Harper, 1979, with permission.

Table 7-6
Effects of Dietary Additions of Small Neutral (SN) and Large Neutral (LN) Amino Acids on Plasma and Brain Threonine Content of Rats Fed Low Protein (6% casein + L-met), Threonine-limiting Diet for One Day

Diet	Threonine Plasma	Concentration Brain
	μmol/ml	μmol/g
Basal (B)*	0.10	0.15
B + 4.5% SN	0.05	0.07
B + 4.5% LN	0.07	0.09
B + SN + LN	0.05	0.07
B + SN + LN + Thr	0.11	0.20

*6% casein + 0.2% L-met. Threonine is limiting for the growth of rats fed this diet. From Tews, Kim and Harper, 1980, with permission.

When threonine uptake is plotted against the plasma threonine to small neutral amino acid concentration ratio, what might be called a competition ratio or an inhibition ratio, there is a direct relationship between threonine uptake into brain and the ratio of threonine to small neutral amino acids in the blood that is highly significant (Figure 7-7).

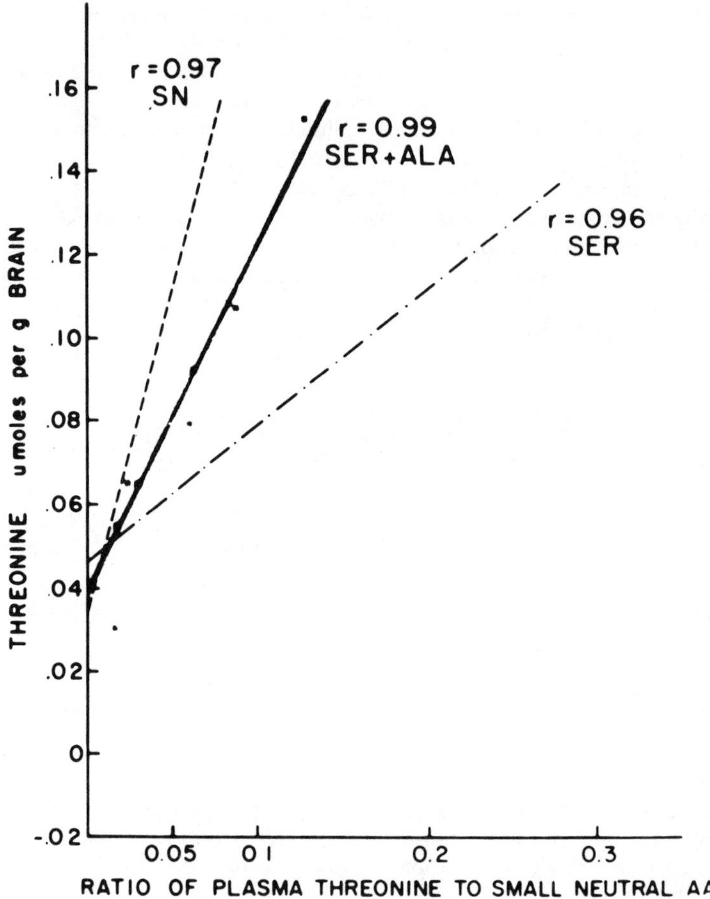

Figure 7-7 Relationship between brain concentration of threonine and ratio of threonine to small neutral (SN) amino acids in plasma (After Tews et al., 1978.)

Similar observations have been made with the indispensable amino acid lysine and the dispensable amino acids arginine and ornithine. The effect is smaller in this case, as lysine is taken up more slowly than threonine by brain. Also, arginine is metabolized rapidly in the body so that concentration tends to rise less than that of many other amino acids. Nevertheless, it is possible to demonstrate that excess arginine and ornithine in the diet will lead to depletion of the brain lysine pool which is associated with reduced food intake (Tews et al., 1981) Thus, there is potential for interactions between the dispensable amino acids and the indispensable amino acids at sites of transport into brain and for effects of this type of interaction on behavior (Wurtman, 1982; Anderson, 1982). This type of inhibition of transport can be demonstrated in other tissues *in vitro,* but the physiological significance of such effects *in vivo* has not been established.

CONCLUSIONS

In conclusion then, the dispensable amino acids are not nonessential. Their conditional indispensability can be readily demonstrated as is indicated in Table 7-2. Their metabolic essentiality, as I hope I have illustrated, is great. If, then, we return to Figure 7-1, it is evident that interrelationships between the dispensable and indispensable amino acids occur during the synthesis of proteins, during the synthesis of many smalll nitrogen-containing molecules, during the course of degradation of surpluses of the indispensable amino acids and during absorption and transport.

REFERENCES

Anderson, G.H. (1982): Amino acids and the regulation of food intake. In press.

Berg, C.P. (1959): Utilization of D-amino acids. In: *Protein and Amino Acid Nutrition* (ed: A.A. Albanese), pp. 57–96, Academic Press, New York.

Block, R.J., and Bolling, D. (1944): Nutritional opportunities with amino acids. *J. Am. Diet. Assoc.* 20:69–76.

Chawla, R.K., Stackhouse, W.J., and Wadsworth, A.E. (1975): Efficiency of α-ketoisocaproic acid as a substitute for leucine in the diet of the growing rat. *J. Nutr.* 105:798.

Clark, H.E., Kenney, M.A., Goodwin, A.F., Goyal, K., and Mertz, E.T. (1963): Effect of certain factors on nitrogen retention and lysine requirements of adult human subjects. IV. Total nitrogen intake. *J. Nutr.* 81:223–229.

Close, J.H. (1974): The use of amino acid precursors in nitrogen-accumulation diseases. *New Engl. J. Med.* 290:663.

Cooper, A.J.L., and Meister, A. (1974): Isolation and properties of a new glutamine transaminase from rat kidney. *J. Biol. Chem.* 249:2554–2561.

Felig, P. (1982): Impact of hormones on amino acid metabolism in various tissues. In press.

Fernstrom, J.D., and Wurtman, R.J. (1972): Brain serotonin content: physiological regulation by plasma neutral amino acids. *Science* 178:414–416.

Harper, A.E. (1974): "Nonessential" amino acids. *J. Nutr.* 104:965–967.

Harper, A.E., and Zapalowski, C. (1981): Interorgan relationships in the metabolism of the branched-chain amino and α-ketoacids. In: *Metabolism and Clinical Implications of Branched Chain Amino and Ketoacids* (eds: M. Walser and J.R. Williamson), pp. 195–203, Elsevier/North Holland, Inc., New York.

Hutson, S.M., Cree, T.C., and Harper, A.E. (1978): Regulation of leucine and α-ketoisocaproate metabolism in skeletal muscle. *J. Biol. Chem.* 253:8126–8133.

Hutson, S.M., and Harper, A.E. (1981): Blood and tissue branched-chain amino and α-keto acid concentrations: Effect of diet, starvation and disease. *Am. J. Clin. Nutr.* 34:173–183.

Kang-Lee, Y.A., and Harper, A.E. (1977): Effect of histidine intake and hepatic histidase activity on the metabolism of histidine *in vivo*. *J. Nutr.* 107:1427–1443.

Kang-Lee, Y.A., and Harper, A.E. (1978): Threonine metabolism *in vivo:* Effect of threonine intake and prior induction of threonine dehydratase in rats. *J. Nutr.* 108:163–175.

Kies, C., Williams, E., and Fox, H.M. (1965): Effect of "non-specific" nitrogen intake on adequacy of cereal proteins for nitrogen retention in human adults. *J. Nutr.* 86:357–361.

Krebs, H.A., and Lund, P. (1977): Aspects of the regulation of the branched-chain amino acids. *Adv. Enz. Regul.* 15:375–394.

Lardy, H.A., and Feldott, G. (1950): The net utilization of ammonium nitrogen by the growing rat. *J. Biol. Chem.* 186:85–91.

Lutz, J., Tews, J.K., and Harper, A.E. (1975): Simulated amino acid imbalance and histidine transport in rat brain slices. *Am. J. Physiol.* 229:229–234.

Matthews, et al (1981): Modeling leucine metabolism in man. In: *Metabolism and Clinical Implications of Branched Chain Amino and Ketoacids* (eds: M. Walser and J.R. Williamson), pp. 313–316, Elsevier/North Holland, New York.

McCoy, R.H., Meyer, C.E., and Rose, W.C. (1935): Feeding experiments with mixtures of highly purified amino acids. VIII. isolation and identification of a new amino acid. *J. Biol. Chem.* 112:283–302.

Miller, L.L. (1962): The role of the liver and the non-hepatic tissues in the regulation of free amino acid levels in the blood. In: *Amino Acid Pools* (ed: J.T. Holden), pp. 708–721, Elsevier/North Holland, New York.

Nissen, S., and Haymond, M.W. (1981): Use of dual isotope techniques in determining the flux and interconversion of leucine and α-ketoisocaproate in vivo. In: *Metabolism and Clinical Implications of Branched Chain Amino and Ketoacids* (eds: M. Walser and J.R. Williamson), pp. 301–306, Elsevier/North Holland, New York.

Osborne, T.B., and Mendel, L.B. (1914): Amino acids in nutrition and growth. *J. Biol. Chem.* 17:325–349.

Peng, Y., Tews, J.K., and Harper, A.E. (1972): Amino acid imbalance, protein intake, and changes in rat brain and plasma amino acids. *Am. J. Physiol.* 222:314–321.

Peters, J.C., and Harper, A.E. (1981): Protein and energy consumption, plasma amino acid ratios, and brain neurotransmitter concentrations. *Physiol. and Behavior* 27:287–298.

Rogers, Q.R., Chen, D. M-Y., and Harper, A.E. (1970): The importance of dispensable amino acids for maximal growth in the rat. *Proc. Soc. Exp. Biol. Med.* 134:517–522.

Rose, W.C. (1938): The nutritive significance of the amino acids. *Physiol. Rev.* 18:109–136.

Rose, W.C. (1957): The amino acid requirements of adult man. *Nutr. Abstr. Rev.* 27:631–647.

Rose, W.C., Smith, L.C., Womack, M., and Shane, M. (1949): The utilization of the nitrogen of ammonium salts, urea and certain other compounds in the synthesis of non-essential amino acids *in vivo*. *J. Biol. Chem.* 181:307–316.

Rudman, D. (1982): Overview: Deficiencies of essential nutrients, clinical and biochemical manifestations. *Am. J. Clin. Nutr.* In press.

Scrimshaw, N.S., Young, V.R., Huang, P.C., Thanangkul, O., and Cholakos, B.V. (1969): Partial dietary replacement of milk protein by nonspecific nitrogen in young men. *J. Nutr.* 98:9–17.

Snyderman, S.E., Holt, L.E., Jr., Dancis, J., Roitman, E., Boyer, A., and Balis, M.E. (1962): "Unessential" nitrogen: a limiting factor for human growth. *J. Nutr.* 78:57–72.

Soliman, A-G, and Harper, A.E. (1971): Effect of protein content of diet on lysine oxidation by the rat. *Biochem. Biophys. Acta* 244:146–154.

Stucki, W.P., and Harper, A.E. (1962): Effects of altering the ratio of indispensable to dispensable amino acids in diets for rats. *J. Nutr.* 78:278–286.

Swendseid, M.E., Harris, C.L., and Tuttle, S.G. (1960): The effect of sources of non-essential nitrogen on nitrogen balance in young adults. *J. Nutr.* 71:105–108.

Tews, J.K., Bradford, A.M., and Harper, A.E. (1981): Induction of lysine imbalance in rats: Relationships between tissue amino acids and diet. *J. Nutr.* 111:968–978.

Tews, J.K., Good, S.S., and Harper, A.E. (1978): Transport of threonine and tryptophan by rat brain slices: Relation to other amino acids and concentrations found in plasma. *J. Neurochem.* 31:581–589.

Tews, J.K., and Harper, A.E. (1982): Effects of protein intake on plasma and tissue amino acid pools. Unpublished data.

Tews, J.K., Kim, Y-W.L., and Harper, A.E. (1979): Induction of threonine imbalance by dispensable amino acids: Relation to competition for amino acid transport into brain. *J. Nutr.* 109:304–315.

Tews, J.K., Kim, Y-W.L., and Harper, A.E. (1980): Induction of threonine imbalance by dispensable amino acids: Relationships between tissue amino acids and diet in rats. *J. Nutr.* 110:394–408.

White, A., Handler, P., Smith, E.L., Hill, R.L., Lehman, I.R. (1978): *Principles of Biochemistry.* (6th Edition), pp. 677–755, McGraw-Hill, New York.

Willcock, E.G., and Hopkins, F.G. (1906): The importance of individual amino acids in metabolism; observations on the effect of adding tryptophan to a dietary in which zein is the sole nitrogenous constituent. *J. Physiol. (London)* 35:88–102.

Wurtman, R.J. (1982): Amino acids as neurotransmitter precursors. This volume, in press.

8 Factors Influencing Utilization of Glycine, Glutamate and Aspartate in Clinical Products

Lewis D. Stegink
Edward F. Bell
Tahia T. Daabees
Dean W. Andersen
Wilbur L. Zike
Lloyd J. Filer, Jr.

Man usually ingests amino acids required for normal function as dietary protein. Such proteins provide both indispensable amino acids and dispensable amino acids. It is important to remember that the latter, although listed as dispensable, are important sources of nitrogen for many synthetic processes occurring in the body.

We have been asked to discuss the use of glycine, glutamate and aspartate as sources of dispensable amino acid nitrogen in clinical products. As shown in Table 8-1, these amino acids are major sources of dispensable amino acid nitrogen in the "typical protein" man ingests for food. The data shown in Table 8-1 are amino acid composition values for "typical proteins" recalculated from data presented by Jukes et al. (1975) and by Doolittle (1981). The information used for these calculations was obtained from completely sequenced proteins. Thus, the distribution of total glutamate between glutamine and glutamate, and total aspartate between asparagine and aspartate is known. This contrasts with earlier reports of amino acid composition, such as those compiled by Orr and Watt (1957), where values for total glutamate and aspartate include glutamine and asparagine respectively. The compilation of Jukes et al. (1975) included 47 eukaryotic, 17 prokaryotic and four virus proteins. Only one representative of each "family" of proteins, such as the globins, was included. Doolittle (1981) carried out similar calculations using the Atlas of Protein Sequence and Structure (Dayhoff, 1978) and an accumulation of published sequences assembled by Doolittle called Newat.

Table 8-1
Amino Acid Composition of a Typical Protein (Mole Percent)

Amino Acid	Jukes et al. (1975)	Doolittle (1981) *Atlas*	Doolittle (1981) *Newat*	Average
Dispensable	%	%	%	
Alanine	8.69	8.4	7.8	8.3
Arginine	4.26	4.4	5.2	4.6
Asparagine	4.92	3.9	4.1	4.3
Aspartate	5.90	5.1	5.6	5.5
Cysteine	2.13	3.3	2.0	2.5
Glutamine	3.93	3.6	3.7	3.7
Glutamate	5.40	5.4	6.8	5.9
Glycine	7.85	9.0	8.1	8.3
Proline	4.10	5.4	5.0	4.8
Serine	7.38	7.4	6.2	7.0
Tyrosine	3.77	3.4	3.4	3.5
Indispensable				
Histidine	2.30	2.4	2.3	2.3
Isoleucine	5.08	4.0	5.1	4.7
Leucine	7.70	7.5	8.6	7.9
Lysine	6.72	7.0	6.3	6.70
Methionine	1.80	1.6	2.1	1.8
Phenylalanine	3.77	4.0	4.0	3.9
Threonine	6.07	6.1	5.5	5.9
Tryptophan	1.31	1.2	1.5	1.3
Valine	6.89	6.4	6.1	6.5
Total	99.97	99.5	99.4	99.4

In the "average protein" described in Table 8-1, 58.4% of the total amino acids is present as dispensable amino acids. Glutamate, aspartate, and glycine comprise about 34% of this dispensable nitrogen. However, dietary protein-bound glutamine and asparagine may undergo deamination during processing and cooking, forming glutamate and aspartate in the process. Further, glutamine and asparagine are metabolized by conversion to glutamate and aspartate in mucosal cells (Windmueller and Spaeth, 1975, 1976, 1980). If glutamine and asparagine are considered sources of dietary glutamate and aspartate, these five amino acids provide approximately 47% of the dispensable amino acid nitrogen in a typical protein. Thus, it is logical to consider these amino acids as major sources of dispensable amino acids when formulating amino acid preparations for enteral and parenteral use.

In practice, however, most amino acid formulations intended for clinical use avoid glutamate and aspartate because of fear of potential neurotoxicity (Olney et al., 1973a). Instead, most preparations use glycine as a major source of dispensable amino acid nitrogen in quantities much larger than the amount provided by a typical dietary protein (Table 8-2). The three most widely used solutions of amino acids in the United States (Aminosyn, Abbott Laboratories; Travasol, Baxter-Travenol; FreAmine II or III, McGaw Laboratories) do not contain glutamate and aspartate. Glycine provides 21 to 33 mole percent of the total amino acid mixture in these proteins. In contrast, Neopham, recently introduced by Cutter Laboratories, contains relatively large amounts of glutamate and aspartate, and much less glycine than the

Table 8-2
Amino Acid Composition of Parenteral Solutions in use in the United States (Mole Percent)

Amino Acid	Aminosyn	Travasol	Freamine		Neopham	Average Protein
			II	*III*		
Dispensable						
Alanine	12.0	18.7	6.3	9.6	13.7	8.3
Arginine	7.0	7.1	2.5	6.7	4.3	4.6
Asparagine	0	0	0	0	0	4.3
Aspartate	0	0	0	0	6.0	5.5
Cysteine	0	0	0	0	1.6	2.5
Glutamine	0	0	0	0	0	3.7
Glutamate	0	0	0	0	10.4	5.9
Glycine	21.2	33.1	31.7	22.7	5.5	8.3
Proline	9.4	4.3	11.6	11.8	9.4	4.8
Serine	5.1	0	6.7	6.8	7.0	7.0
Tyrosine	0.4	0.3	0.0	0.0	0.5	3.5
Indispensable						
Histidine	2.4	3.4	2.2	2.2	2.6	2.3
Isoleucine	6.9	4.4	6.3	6.5	4.6	4.7
Leucine	8.9	5.7	8.2	8.4	10.4	7.9
Lysine	5.0	3.8	4.8	4.9	6.0	6.7
Methionine	3.3	4.6	4.2	4.3	1.7	1.8
Phenylalanine	3.3	4.5	4.1	4.2	3.2	3.9
Threonine	5.5	4.2	4.0	4.1	5.9	5.9
Tryptophan	1.1	1.1	0.9	0.9	1.3	1.3
Valine	8.5	4.7	6.7	6.8	6.0	6.5
Total	100.0	99.9	100.2	100.1	100.1	99.4

other solutions. Its mole percent composition is similar to that calculated for the "average protein" described in Table 8-1.

In an attempt to demonstrate that glutamate and aspartate should be considered as appropriate sources of dispensable amino acid nitrogen for clinical products, the effects of dietary loads of glutamate, aspartate and glycine upon plasma concentrations will be discussed.

ENTERAL NUTRITION

Since glycine, glutamate, and aspartate account for a significant percentage of the total amino acids present in dietary protein, it is important to consider how oral ingestion of these amino acids in protein-bound form affects plasma concentrations. This is particularly important for the dicarboxylic amino acids, glutamate and aspartate, since neurotoxicity is only noted when plasma levels of these amino acids are grossly elevated (Stegink, et al., 1974; O'hara and Takasaki, 1979; Okaniwa et al., 1979; Daabees et al., 1982). Neurotoxicity is not reported from ingestion of the protein-bound glutamate and aspartate present in meals. Thus, background data obtained from meal studies will be essential whenever we consider how infusion of parenteral solutions containing amino acids in free form affects plasma concentrations.

The absorption of glycine, glutamate and aspartate in the intestinal lumen differs, depending on whether these amino acids are ingested in free or peptide-bound form. When ingested as free amino acids, they are absorbed from the intestinal lumen by active transport processes. When ingested in protein-bound form, the glycine-, aspartate- and glutamate-containing peptides produced by proteolysis enter mucosal cells directly, where they are hydrolyzed to their constituent amino acids by specific intracellular peptidases (Matthews, 1975). Thus, the effect of dietary ingestion of these amino acids on plasma concentrations may differ depending upon the form in which the amino acid is ingested.

Protein meal studies in man (Nixon and Mawer, 1970a, 1970b) strongly suggest that only protein-bound neutral and dibasic amino acids are quantitatively absorbed as free amino acids. The amino acids (proline and hydroxyproline), glycine, glutamate and aspartate all appear to enter mucosal cells as constituents of small peptides. These small peptides apparently are hydrolyzed within the mucosal cells to release their constituent free amino acids. Although large amounts of protein-bound glycine, glutamate, and aspartate are absorbed in peptide-bound form, the gut also has specific transport sites for the free forms of these amino acids. Thus, these amino acids are readily absorbed whether presented in free or peptide-bound form.

We have been interested in the role of the gastrointestinal tract in amino acid metabolism for some time. First, we wished to know how alterations in the route of alimentation, such as parenteral nutrition, affect amino acid metabolism. Second, we wished to know why the ingestion of large amounts of dicarboxylic amino acids with food prevents neurotoxicity. Although large doses of glutamate and aspartate given to infant mice without food produce hypothalamic neuronal necrosis (Olney, 1969; Olney and Ho, 1970; Lemkey-Johnston and Reynolds, 1974; Takasaki, 1978a; Okaniwa et al., 1979; Daabees et al., 1982), administration of large amounts of glutamate in the diet does not produce neuronal necrosis (Takasaki, 1978b; Anantharaman, 1979).

When amino acids are ingested in protein-bound form, proteolysis produces a relatively slow release of constituent amino acids and peptides to the absorptive process. Maximal plasma levels of most amino acids in peripheral blood are not reached until two to six hours after meal ingestion. In contrast, ingestion of an equivalent quantity of free amino acid produces a more rapid increase in plasma concentration. Thus, the form in which amino acids are ingested may affect plasma concentrations.

Over the past several years, we have administered a variety of meals to normal volunteers, measuring the effect of protein ingestion upon plasma amino acid levels. The meals studied include a beverage meal providing no nutrients, Sustagen, a formula meal providing 0.4 g protein/kg body weight (Stegink et al., 1982a), an egg-milk custard meal providing 1 g protein/kg body weight (Filer et al., 1979), and a hamburger–milk shake meal that also provided protein at 1 g/kg body weight (Stegink et al., 1982b). Table 8-3 lists the protein content of these meals as well as the estimated quantity of glycine, glutamate, aspartate and valine provided.

Before considering how the oral intake of glycine, glutamate and aspartate affects plasma concentrations, let us consider how variations in the intake of a typical essential amino acid, such as valine, affect plasma concentrations. When normal subjects ingest a beverage providing no protein, plasma valine levels remain unchanged or decrease slightly (Figure 8-1). When these subjects ingest a Sustagen meal providing 0.4 g protein and 28 mg valine/kg body weight, plasma valine concentrations increase 30 minutes after meal ingestion, and remain at an increased level over six hours (Stegink et al., 1982a). When subjects ingest larger quantities of protein (1 g protein/kg body weight providing 56 or 71 mg valine/kg body weight), changes in plasma valine concentration are greater (Filer et al., 1979; Stegink et al., 1982b). Plasma valine concentration increases slowly with time, reaching maximal values three to six hours after ingestion of the hamburger–milk shake meal. In general, the peak plasma concentrations and the areas under the plasma concentration-time-curve increase in proportion to the quantity of valine ingested.

Figure 8-2 shows plasma glycine concentrations in these same subjects. Plasma glycine levels remained constant or decreased slightly after meals providing glycine at 0 (not shown), 8, or 24 mg/kg body weight. A significant increase in peak plasma glycine concentration and the area under the plasma concentration-time-curve was only noted when glycine intake increased to 57 mg/kg body weight.

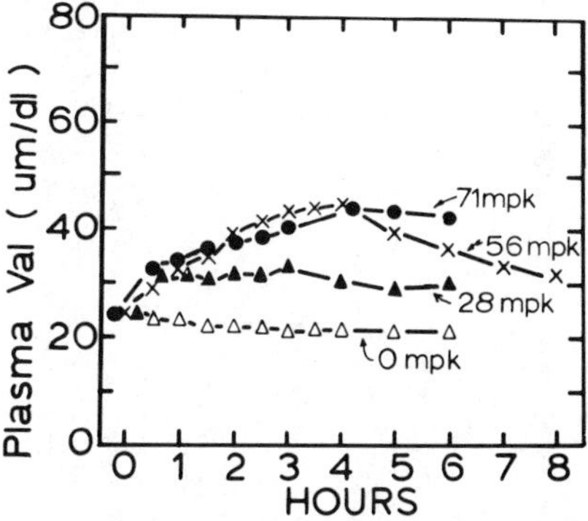

Figure 8-1 Mean plasma valine (val) concentrations in normal adults (n = 6/group) fed either a beverage meal providing no protein (△), a Sustagen meal providing 0.4 g protein and 28 mg valine/kg body weight (▲), a hamburger meal providing 1 g protein and 56 mg valine/kg body weight (X), or a custard meal providing 1 g protein and 71 mg valine per kg body weight (●). The valine content of the meals was calculated from the data of Orr and Watt (1957).

Table 8-3
Protein, Glycine, Glutamate and Aspartate Content of the Meals Studied

Meal	Protein g/kg	Glycine mg/kg	Total Glutamate mg/kg	Total Aspartate mg/kg	Estimated* Glutamate mg/kg	Estimated Aspartate mg/kg	Valine mg/kg
Beverage	0	0	0	0	0	0	0
Sustagen	0.4	8	95	29	55	16	28
Custard	1.0	24	207	73	120	40	71
Hamburger–Milk Shake	1.0	57	162	82	94	46	56

*The total glutamate and aspartate values reported by Orr and Watt (1957) were obtained after acid hydrolysis, and thus include glutamine and asparagine. The approximate quantities of glutamate and aspartate present were calculated using the estimate of Jukes et al. (1975) that 58% of the total glutamate and 55% of the total aspartate are actually present as those amino acids.

Plasma concentrations of glutamate and aspartate (Figures 8-3 and 8-4) respond only slightly to the ingestion of large amounts of protein-bound glutamate and aspartate. Glutamate loads of 55 to 120 mg/kg body weight produced only a small increase (3 to 6 μmol/dl) in mean peak plasma glutamate levels above baseline values (Figure 8-3), and had only a minimal effect on the area under the plasma glutamate concentration-time-curve. Similarly, aspartate loads of 40 to 46 mg/kg body weight increased the mean peak plasma aspartate concentration by only 0.53 to 0.81 μmol/dl over baseline values (Figure 8-4). These data indicate that orally administered, protein-bound glutamate and aspartate are metabolized more rapidly than valine, and that ingestion of large amounts of these amino acids as part of a meal produces only a small elevation in the peripheral plasma concentration.

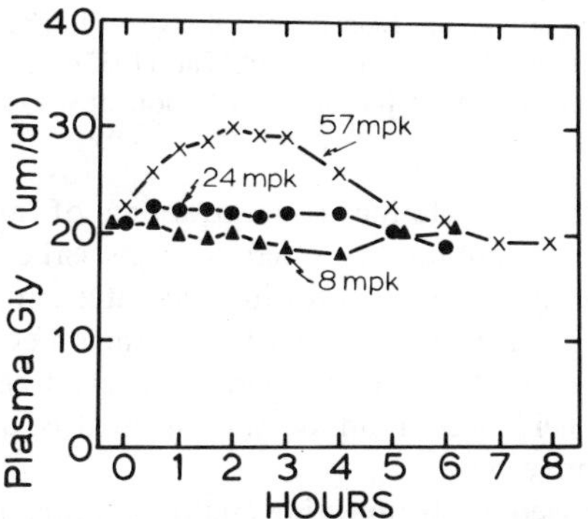

Figure 8-2 Mean plasma glycine (gly) concentrations in normal adults (n = 6/group) fed either a Sustagen meal providing 0.4 g protein and 8 mg glycine/kg body weight (▲), a custard meal providing 1 g protein and 24 mg glycine/kg body weight (●), or a hamburger meal providing 1 g protein and 57 mg glycine/kg body weight (X). The glycine content of the meals was calculated from the data of Orr and Watt (1957).

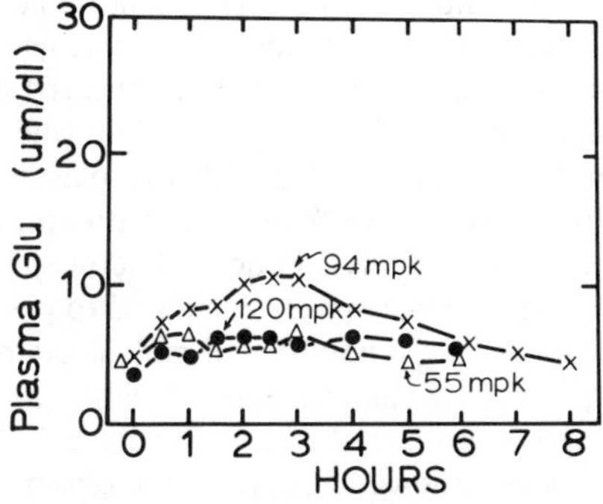

Figure 8-3 Mean plasma glutamate (glu) concentrations in normal adults (n = 6/group) fed either a Sustagen meal providing 0.4 g protein and 55 mg glutamate/kg body weight (△), a hamburger meal providing 1 g protein and 94 mg glutamate/kg body weight (X), or a custard meal providing 1 g protein and 120 mg glutamate/kg body weight. (●). The glutamate content of the meals was calculated from the data of Orr and Watt (1957) and corrected for glutamine using the values published by Jukes et al. (1975) for the glutamate to glutamine distribution of a typical protein.

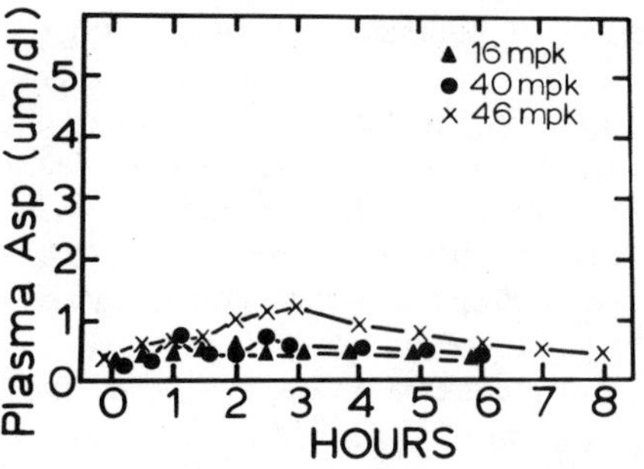

Figure 8-4 Mean plasma aspartate (asp) concentrations in normal adults (n = 6/group) fed either a Sustagen meal providing 0.4 g protein and 16 mg aspartate/kg body weight (▲), a custard meal providing 1 g protein and 40 mg aspartate/kg body weight (●), or a hamburger meal providing 1 g protein and 46 mg aspartate/kg body weight (X). The aspartate content of the meals was calculated from the data of Orr and Watt (1957). The values were corrected for asparagine using the asparagine to aspartate distribution of a typical protein published by Jukes et al., (1975).

The small increase in plasma concentrations of glycine, aspartate, and glutamate relative to the amount ingested suggests either: (a) a higher rate of catabolism for those amino acids than for indispensable amino acids like valine; (b) that some component of the meal may be affecting their metabolism and/or absorption; (c) that ingestion of these amino acids in protein-bound form produces a smaller plasma amino acid effect than ingestion as the free amino acid; or (d) some combination of the above.

Studies in rats, carried out by injecting mixtures of amino acids into loops of intestine, suggest that the absorption of free aspartate and glutamate is much slower than that of other amino acids (Gitler, 1964). Similar findings in humans were reported by Adibi et al. (1967) using an intubation technique to perfuse the jejunum with equimolar amounts of free amino acids. Again, glutamate and aspartate were the slowest to be absorbed. Silk et al. (1973) extended this work to the absorption of peptides containing aspartate and glutamate. They reported that free glutamate, and especially free aspartate were only slowly absorbed, whereas the same amino acids from peptides present in a tryptic digest of casein appeared better absorbed.

However, these data may be somewhat misleading when extrapolated to meal feeding. Thus, we decided to evaluate factors affecting plasma amino acid levels during meal ingestion. In these studies we focused our attention on glutamate. In the first experiment, plasma glutamate levels in normal adult subjects administered 100 mg glutamate/kg body weight in water were compared to plasma amino acid values noted in normal subjects ingesting a hamburger–milk shake meal that provided approximately the same quantity of glutamate in protein-bound form (Stegink et al., 1979a). The results of this study are shown in Figure 8-5. Subjects ingesting 100 mg/kg free glutamate in water showed a rapid rise in plasma glutamate levels, with values reaching a mean peak concentration of 50 μmol/dl. The mean area under the plasma glutamate concentration-time-curve was 2220 units over the eight-hour time period. This contrasts with the mean peak plasma glutamate level of only 10.8 μmol/dl and an eight-hour area under the curve of 1152 units when the equivalent quantity of protein-bound glutamate was ingested with a meal.

These data suggest that some meal component affected plasma glutamate concentrations. To test this, we selected a low protein diet (0.4 g/kg body weight) that

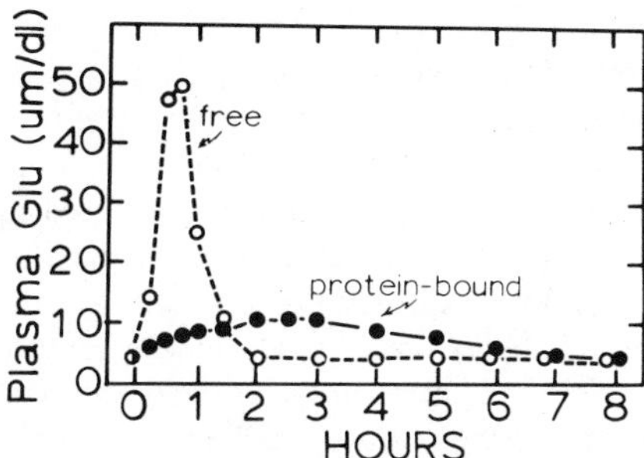

Figure 8-5 Mean plasma glutamate (glu) concentrations in normal adults (n = 6/group) ingesting either 100 mg glutamate/kg body weight dissolved in 4.2 ml/kg water (○), or a hamburger meal providing 1 g protein, 94 mg protein-bound glutamate, and 68 mg of protein-bound glutamine/kg body weight (●).

provided only minimal quantities of protein-bound glutamate (55 mg/kg body weight). Normal subjects were given Sustagen, a formula meal, with and without added free glutamate (100 mg/kg) to see whether meal ingestion affected free glutamate as well as protein-bound glutamate. Sustagen alone provided 0.4 g protein, 1.12 g carbohydrate, 0.06 g fat and 55 mg protein-bound glutamate/kg body weight. Sustagen with added glutamate provided 55 mg protein-bound glutamate and 100 mg free glutamate/kg body weight. The effect of these two feedings on plasma glutamate concentration is shown in Figure 8-6. For comparative purposes the response to 100 mg glutamate/kg body weight administered in water is also shown. Ingestion of glutamate in water increased plasma glutamate levels to a mean peak value of 50 μmol/dl. When Sustagen was ingested the mean peak plasma glutamate concentration was 6.7 μmol/dl. The addition of free glutamate (100 mg/kg body weight) to Sustagen had only a small effect on plasma glutamate concentration beyond that produced by the meal alone. The mean peak plasma glutamate concentration was 11.2 μmol/dl, significantly less ($p < 0.05$) than values noted when glutamate was ingested with water. The area under the plasma glutamate concentration-time-curve values showed similar results. The mean six-hour area under the curve value when 100 mg/kg body weight glutamate was ingested in water was significantly larger than the value noted after ingestion of the meal alone or the meal with added glutamate.

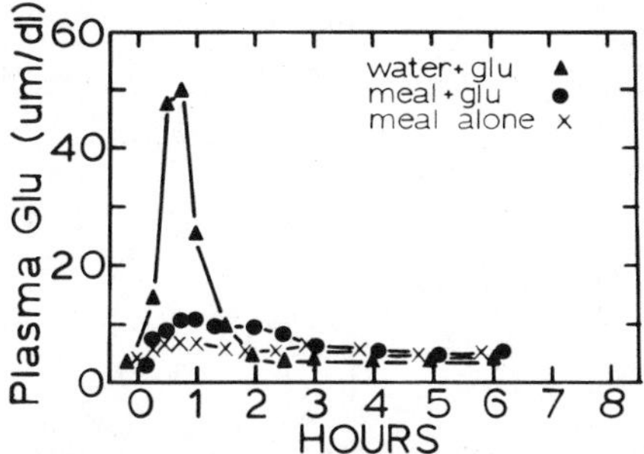

Figure 8-6 Mean plasma glutamate (glu) concentrations in normal adults ingesting either a Sustagen meal providing 0.4 g protein and 55 mg protein-bound glutamate (X), a Sustagen meal with added free glutamate (100 mg/kg body weight) (●), or water providing 100 mg glutamate/kg body weight (▲).

These data suggest that glutamate is metabolized more rapidly when ingested with meals than with water. However, it was not clear from these studies whether the meal or one of its components modulated the absorption and/or metabolism of glutamate. A slower rate of absorption would permit greater catabolism of glutamate by the intestinal mucosa, resulting in a decreased release of glutamate to the portal blood. Alternatively, carbohydrate present in Sustagen could serve as a source of pyruvate, thereby facilitating the transamination of glutamate to α-ketoglutarate and increasing the rate of glutamate catabolism in the intestinal mucosa (Figure 8-7). We have previously pointed out on theoretical grounds (Stegink, 1976), that dietary carbohydrate was likely to affect the rate of glutamate transamination in mucosal cells, since the quantity of administered glutamate appearing in portal blood as alanine or glutamate depends both upon the glutamate load administered and the availability of glucose. Neame and Wiseman (1957, 1958) showed that the quantity of glutamate appearing in the portal blood as glutamate or alanine varied with the glutamate load. A comparison of Parsons and Volman-Mitchell's data (1974) with data from Ramaswamy and Radhakrishnan (1970) suggests the importance of carbohydrate. Both research groups used similar methods; glutamate was circulated in a Krebs-Ringer solution through the lumen of rat intestinal segments *in vitro*. The "sweat" secreted at the serosal side of the segment was collected at regular time intervals, and the glutamate, α-ketoglutarate and alanine content determined. Parsons and Volman-Mitchell (1974) added 28 mM glucose to the perfusion solution and noted the presence of a large amounts of alanine in serosal "sweat." Ramaswamy and Radhakrishnan (1970) did not add glucose, and found glutamate as the major amino acid in serosal "sweat," with little alanine. These data suggest that the percentage of alanine appearing at the serosal surface of the intestinal segment after glutamate administration increases greatly when glucose is present in the lumen.

To test this hypothesis, normal adult subjects were given 100 mg/kg body weight glutamate dissolved either in water, or in water containing sufficient carbohydrate to provide a 1.12 g/kg body weight carbohydrate dose (Stegink et al., 1979a). The carbohydrate was administered as Polycose (Ross Laboratories, Columbus, Ohio), a partially hydrolyzed corn starch preparation. The response of a normal adult subject to ingestion of 100 mg glutamate/kg body weight in either water or Polycose is illustrated in Figure 8-8. It is clear that the addition of car-

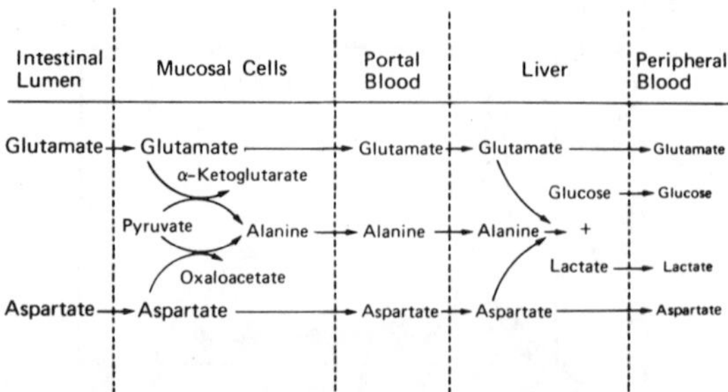

Figure 8-7 Dicarboxylic amino acid absorption from the intestinal lumen, showing mucosal cell transamination to yield alanine and hepatic conversion of those amino acids to glucose and lactate as factors modulating peripheral plasma levels. (Reprinted with permission from Stegink, 1976.)

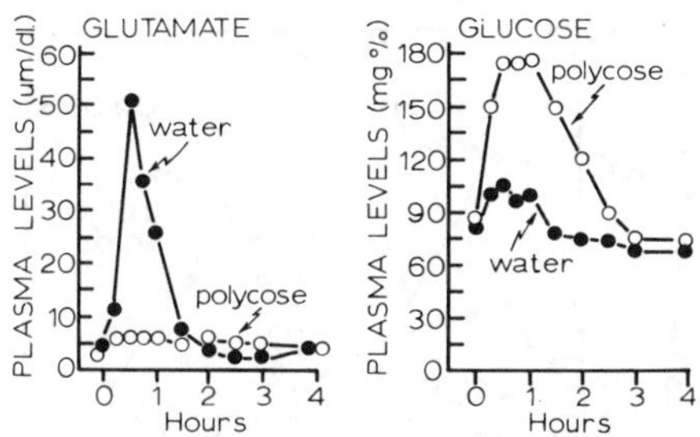

Figure 8-8 Plasma glutamate and glucose levels in a single normal male subject administered glutamate at 100 mg/kg body weight dissolved either in water or in a water solution providing 1.12 g Polycose/kg body weight. (Reprinted with permission from Stegink et al., 1979a.)

bohydrate had a striking effect on plasma glutamate concentration. Changes in blood glucose and glutamate levels indicate that gastric emptying has occurred. It seems likely that the rapid metabolism of glutamate after ingestion with meals reflects in part the carbohydrate content of the meal. Presumably carbohydrate is absorbed into the intestinal mucosa and converted to glucose and pyruvate, ultimately facilitating the transamination and metabolism of glutamate by mucosal cells.

However, it was possible that other meal components (protein?) affected mucosal cell metabolism, or that Polycose affected glutamate metabolism in other ways, such as by blocking glutamate uptake. For example, Polycose addition would increase the viscosity of the solution and might alter the rate of glutamate absorption. To test this hypothesis, feeding tubes were placed in the jejunum of young pigs through gastrostomy openings. Portal vein catheters were chronically implanted through abdominal incisions. Following recovery from surgery, the animals were administered 500 mg of glutamate/kg body weight dissolved in four different solutions. Glutamate was administered in: (a) water (4.2 ml/kg); (b) a water solution providing 1.12 g Polycose/kg body weight; (c) a water solution providing an amino acid mixture (0.4 g/kg; Aminosyn, Abbott Laboratories) not containing glutamate or aspartate; and (d) a water solution providing 1.12 g of a nonmetabolizable carbohydrate per kg body weight (β-cellobiose, Abbott Laboratories). The β-cellobiose was added to test whether increased viscosity resulting from Polycose addition affected the rate of glutamate absorption rather than facilitating its metabolism. Plasma glutamate concentrations in portal blood of these animals are shown in Figure 8-9. Mean plasma glutamate concentration in portal blood peaked at: 120 μmol/dl when glutamate was administered in water, 115 μmol/dl when glutamate was administered with cellobiose, and 52 μmol/dl when glutamate was administered with Polycose. The addition of amino acids (0.4 g/kg) slightly decreased the mean peak plasma glutamate concentration of portal blood (95 μmol/dl). When amino acids were present, there was greater animal-to-animal variability in time at which peak plasma glutamate concentration was attained. Each animal developed a peak plasma glutamate concentration in portal blood approximating 100 to 115 μmol/dl, but the time at which peak values were observed varied from 30 to 90 minutes. This resulted in a lower overall mean peak value.

These data support the conclusion that carbohydrate exerts a metabolic effect on glutamate metabolism in the intestinal mucosa. Other data demonstrate that carbohydrate ingestion with glutamate not only affects portal plasma glutamate concentrations in the pig, but also increases hepatic glutamate metabolism.

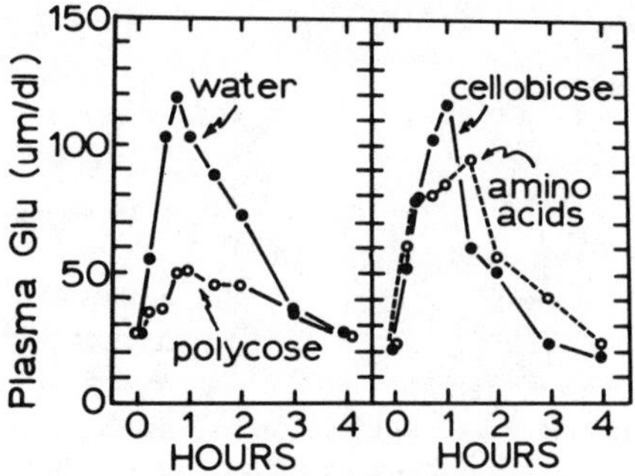

Figure 8-9 Mean portal plasma glutamate (glu) concentrations in young pigs administered 500 mg glutamate/kg body weight either in water (●, left panel), in a water solution also providing 1.12 g Polycose/kg body weight (○, left panel), in a water solution also providing 1.12 g cellobiose/kg body weight (●, right panel), or in a water solution also providing 0.4 g of an amino acid mixture (○, right panel).

In considering these data, it is important to realize that the effect of metabolizable carbohydrate on glutamate metabolism may be greater in man than other species. We have compared the ability of Polycose to alter the peak plasma glutamate concentration resulting from a glutamate load in man, mice and pigs. To carry out this study it is necessary to use a glutamate dose that would produce a similar mean peak plasma glutamate response in all three groups when administered in water. A glutamate load was selected for each species that would produce a mean peak plasma glutamate response of 50 to 70 μmol/dl. Since humans metabolize glutamate less rapidly than mice or monkeys (Stegink et al., 1979b), a 100 mg/kg body weight dose was used in man, and a 300 mg/kg body weight dose was used in mice and pigs. Although simultaneous administration of carbohydrate with glutamate had a dramatic effect on plasma glutamate concentrations in man, a much smaller effect was noted in mice and pigs (Figure 8-10).

These data demonstrate that while glutamate ingested in water produces a rapid, large increase in plasma glutamate concentration, ingestion with a meal or with carbohydrate produces a lower plasma response in men, mice and pigs.

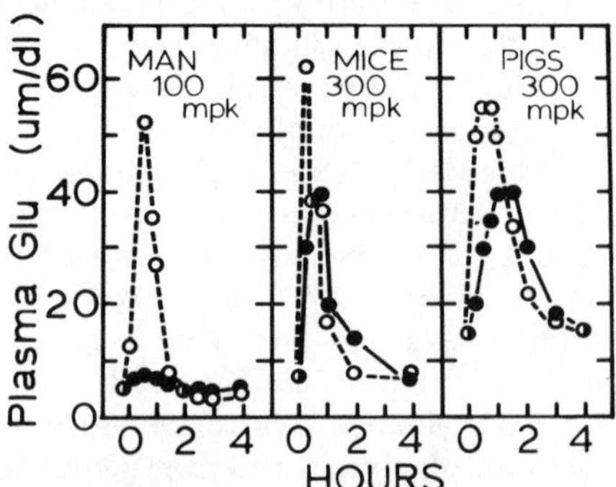

Figure 8-10 Mean plasma glutamate (glu) concentrations in adult humans, infant mice, and young pigs administered glutamate dissolved in water (○), or in a water solution also providing 1.12 g Polycose/kg body weight (●). Humans were administered glutamate at 100 mg/kg body weight, while mice and pigs were administered glutamate at 300 mg/kg body weight.

USE OF GLYCINE, GLUTAMATE AND ASPARTATE IN PARENTERAL AMINO ACID SOLUTIONS

In designing amino acid solutions for use in parenteral nutrition, it would seem appropriate to balance the quantities of amino acids present in such a way as to allow man to maintain plasma amino acid concentrations approximating normal postprandial values. It would also seem logical to consider glutamate and aspartate as potential sources of dispensable amino acid nitrogen, since these amino acids are present in considerable amounts in dietary protein. Eliminating these amino acids from amino acid mixtures requires the addition of disproportionate amounts of other dispensable amino acids to appropriately balance the mixture.

Although protein hydrolysates containing glutamate and aspartate were used during the development of parenteral nutrition for infants (Shohl et al., 1939; Cox et al., 1947; Wilmore and Dudrick, 1968; Wilmore et al., 1969; Filler et al., 1969), most solutions of crystalline amino acids currently used in the United States do not contain these amino acids. As a result, many solutions contain much larger quantities of glycine than would be found in a dietary protein (see Table 8-2).

The large quantities of glycine present in some parenteral solutions may result in gross elevation of plasma glycine concentrations when these solutions are infused in infants. This is illustrated by Figure 8-11 redrawn from the data of Winters et al. (1977). Winters correlated plasma glycine values with glycine intake in young infants infused with different parenteral solutions of amino acids. These preparations contained widely varying quantities of glycine. They noted a direct relationship between the amount of glycine infused and the plasma glycine concentration. Gross elevations of plasma glycine concentration occurred when large quantities of glycine present in some parenteral solutions were infused. It is not known whether sustained gross elevation of plasma glycine concentration has a deleterious effect in human infants. However, animals fed disproportionate amounts of glycine develop adverse effects (Harper et al., 1970). Children born with defects in their ability to metabolize glycine have elevated plasma glycine concentrations, may have hyperammonemia, and are often mentally retarded (Nyhan, 1978; Wada et al., 1972). Thus, it seems appropriate to limit the glycine content of parenteral amino acid formulations.

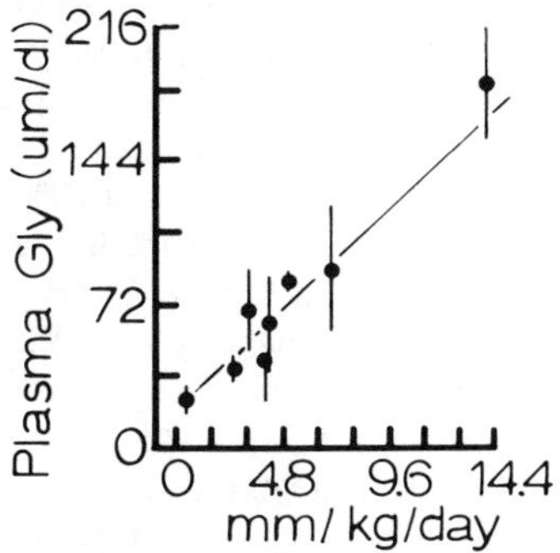

Figure 8-11 Plasma glycine (gly) concentrations in young infants fed parenterally with different amino acid solutions plotted against glycine intake (mmol/kg body weight/day). (Data redrawn from the data of Winters et al., 1977). The mean (± SD) normal postprandial glycine concentration is 33.7 ± 8.2 μmol/dl. (From Filer et al., 1977b).

The reasons for omitting glutamate and aspartate from parenteral solutions concern the potential neurotoxicity of these amino acids in some infant animals. When administered at high levels, glutamate and aspartate are neurotoxic to neonatal animals of susceptible species. Oral ingestion, as well as intraperitoneal or subcutaneous injections of glutamate- and/or aspartate-containing solutions produce hypothalamic neuronal necrosis in neonatal rodents (Olney, 1969; Olney and Ho, 1970; Lemkey-Johnston and Reynolds, 1974; Olney et al., 1973a, 1973b; Tafelski, 1976; Lamperti and Blaha, 1976; Takasaki, 1978a; Okaniwa et al., 1979; Olney et al., 1980) and kittens (Shimada et al., 1975; Applebaum et al., 1981). Neonatal rodents are more sensitive than adult rodents to dicarboxylic amino acid-induced neuronal necrosis (Lemkey-Johnston and Reynolds, 1974). Since glutamate and aspartate are additive in producing the rodent lesion (Olney and Ho, 1970), quantities of both amino acids must be considered when evaluating risk.

The susceptibility of the infant primate to dicarboxylic amino acid-induced neuronal damage is controversial. Initial reports by Olney and colleagues (Olney and Sharpe, 1969; Olney et al., 1972) indicated that administration of large glutamate loads to infant nonhuman primates also produced hypothalamic neuronal necrosis. However, four other research groups have been unable to confirm these reports (Reynolds et al., 1971, 1976, 1980; Abraham et al., 1971, 1975; Newman et al., 1973; Stegink et al., 1975; Wen et al., 1973; Heywood and James, 1979), even when plasma glutamate and aspartate concentrations were grossly elevated. In general, these groups had no difficulty in producing glutamate-induced neuronal damage in rodents.

The conflicting nonhuman primate data have contributed to controversy over the safety of glutamate and aspartate present in oral and intravenous nutrition preparations. This concern is greatest when glutamate- and aspartate-containing preparations are administered to human infants.

In previous studies (Stegink et al., 1979b) we demonstrated that the human metabolizes glutamate more rapidly than mice or monkeys. Our animal data further indicate that infant mice and monkeys metabolize glutamate less rapidly than the adults of these species. On the basis of these data, Olney suggested (1981) that human infants also metabolize glutamate and aspartate less rapidly than adults. He suggested that infants would be subjected to greater risk from intake of products containing these amino acids. If true, this would be of potential significance for parenterally fed infants, since a considerable portion of orally administered glutamate and aspartate is metabolized by the intestinal mucosa (Stegink, 1976).

This question, whether dicarboxylic amino acids should be present in nutritional products fed young infants, led us to evaluate potential risks from these amino acids by methods that do not depend directly upon neuropathologic studies (Stegink et al., 1974; Daabees et al., 1982). The degree and extent of neuronal necrosis in rodents administered large amounts of glutamate and/or aspartate are dose related. Plasma glutamate plus aspartate levels, the degree of neuronal necrosis, and the numbers of animals affected increase with increasing dose (Olney, 1969; Olney and Ho, 1970; Lemkey-Johnston and Reynolds, 1974; Stegink et al., 1974; Daabees et al., 1982).

Over the past several years, our research group (Stegink et al., 1974; Stegink et al., 1979a; Daabees et al., 1982) and others (Takasaki et al., 1979; Ohara and Takasaki, 1979) have attempted to determine the threshold plasma glutamate plus aspartate concentration associated with neuronal necrosis in the infant rodent. These studies indicate that the highly sensitive neonatal rodent tolerates plasma glutamate plus aspartate concentrations up to 60 μmol/dl (approximately four times normal) without evidence of neuronal necrosis. Only when plasma glutamate plus aspartate concentrations exceed 60 to 70 μmol/dl is neuronal necrosis noted.

One way of evaluating potential risk to human infants ingesting nutritional products containing glutamate and aspartate is to measure plasma and erythrocyte amino acid concentrations when such preparations are given parenterally or enterally. If plasma concentrations of glutamate and aspartate are not increased above normal, little risk of dicarboxylic amino acid-induced neuronal necrosis would be expected.

We first examined this problem in orally fed infants. Plasma amino acid concentrations were determined in term and premature infants fed conventional formulas containing little free glutamate and aspartate, or formulas based on protein hydrolysates that contained large quantities of free glutamate and aspartate. Plasma glutamate and aspartate levels were within the normal ranges for both term and premature infants (Filer et al., 1977a, 1977b, 1979), indicating adequate metabolism of ingested free glutamate and aspartate.

During parenteral feeding, both the gut and liver are bypassed to some degree since amino acids are administered directly into the peripheral circulation. Thus, while glutamate and aspartate fed orally with meals may not elevate plasma concentrations, parenteral administration of these amino acids might dramatically increase plasma levels.

This question was first examined in normal, healthy adult volunteers given amino acid solutions (Stegink, 1977). Subjects were infused with one of two parenteral solutions (25% dextrose–5% protein as a hydrolysate or a mixture of amino acids). One group of subjects received nitrogen in the form of a casein hydrolysate preparation (Amigen, Baxter-Travenol, Morton Grove, IL) containing glutamate and aspartate. The other group of subjects was given a mixture of crystalline amino acids (Aminosyn, Abbott Laboratories, North Chicago, IL) free of glutamate and aspartate. The mean daily intake and plasma amino acid concentrations of glycine, glutamate and aspartate are shown in Table 8-4. Plasma glycine values remained within normal limits when adult subjects were infused with the protein-hydrolysate based preparation providing 18 mg glycine/kg body weight/day, but increased sharply when the glycine intake was increased to 228 mg/kg/day. However, no significant difference in plasma glutamate or aspartate concentrations were noted between the two groups despite the wide difference in glutamate intake. This indicated that infusion of glutamate and aspartate at this level (113 mg/kg/day glutamate; 27 mg/kg/day aspartate) had no significant effect on plasma concentrations of these amino acids.

Table 8-4
Plasma Amino Acid Levels in Normal Adult Subjects Fed Totally by Vein Using Parenteral Solutions With and Without Glutamate and Aspartate

	Solution Content (mg/kg/day)		Plasma Level (μmol/dl)	
Amino Acid	*Aminosyn*	*Amigen*	*Aminosyn*	*Amigen*
Glutamate	0	113	4 ± 2	5 ± 2
Aspartate	0	27	0.8 ± 0.4	0.9 ± 0.3
Glycine	228	18	55 ± 10	24 ± 8

Next, we determined whether parenterally administered glutamate and aspartate were metabolized as efficiently by infants as adults. Although Olney (1981) postulated that human infants would metabolize glutamate and aspartate less efficiently than adults, we had reported 10 years earlier plasma amino acid values for a series of young infants given 22.5% dextrose–2.5% protein hydrolysate-based solutions parenterally (Stegink and Baker, 1971). The nitrogen source for these infusions was either enzymatically digested casein or fibrin, and provided large amounts of glutamate and aspartate. The intakes and plasma concentrations of glycine, glutamate and aspartate of these infants are shown in Table 8-5. Plasma glutamate and aspartate concentrations remained within the normal limits seen in normal orally fed infants during infusion of both preparations. However, total plasma dicarboxylic amino acid concentrations (aspartate + glutamate) were higher when the casein hydrolysate-based regimen was infused. This regimen provided larger quantities of glutamate + aspartate (213 mg/kg/day) than the fibrin hydrolysate-based solution (85 mg/kg/day). Plasma glycine values were higher in response to the increased glycine content of the fibrin hydrolysate-based solution, and values were greater than those observed postprandially in orally fed infants. These data indicate that intravenously fed infants metabolize glutamate and aspartate efficiently at these levels of infusion. They also suggest that the level of glycine in fibrin hydrolysates may be too high.

Table 8-5
Mean (± SD) Plasma Glycine, Aspartate and Glutamate Concentrations in Infants Infused with Protein-Hydrolysate Based Parenteral Solutions

	Plasma Concentration (μmol/dl)		
Amino Acid	*Casein Hydrolysate**	*Fibrin Hydrolysate†*	*Normal, Orally Fed‡*
Glycine	24.3 ± 5.63	48.0 ± 13.0	33.7 ± 8.2
Glutamate	6.12 ± 2.64	4.37 ± 1.12	10.7 ± 3.6
Aspartate	1.06 ± 0.54	0.42 ± 0.21	2.60 ± 1.40

*Regimen provided 34 mg glycine, 173 mg glutamate and 40 mg aspartate/kg body weight/day.
†Regimen provided 253 mg glycine, 32 mg glutamate, 53 mg aspartate/kg per day.
‡Data of Filer et al. (1977).

The low-birth-weight infant fed parenterally might be representative of a population with decreased ability to metabolize dicarboxylic amino acids. Such infants are biochemically immature and are further compromised by a feeding technique that bypasses the gut. We recently reported (Filer et al., 1979) plasma amino acid concentrations in two low-birth-weight infants (1.4 and 1.5 kg) fed parenterally with a casein hydrolysate-based preparation providing 165 to 201 mg glutamate and 39 to 48 mg aspartate/kg body weight/day. Mean plasma glutamate levels in these infants ranged from 3.6 to 3.9 μmol/dl, while plasma aspartate concentrations ranged from 1.6 to 1.7 μmol/dl (Table 8-6). Both sets of values are well within the normal range seen in normal orally fed low-birth-weight infants. Thus, even premature infants adequately metabolize parenterally administered glutamate and aspartate.

Solutions of crystalline amino acids have replaced protein hydrolysate solutions as the nitrogen source of choice for parenterally fed infants. Most solutions of amino

Table 8-6
Plasma Glutamate and Aspartate Concentrations in Low-Birth-Weight Infants on Total Parenteral Nutrition

	Weight	Intake (mg/kg)		Plasma Concentrations (μmol/dl)	
Patient	(kg)	*GLU*	*ASP*	*Glutamate*	*Aspartate*
1	1.4	165	39	3.6	1.6
2	1.5	201	48	3.9	1.7
Normal Orally Fed Infants*				10.7 ± 3.6	2.6 ± 1.4

*Values from Filer et al., 1977.

acids in general use in the United States contain large quantities of glycine, and no glutamate and aspartate. Recently, a solution of amino acids containing large quantities of glutamate and aspartate, with lower levels of glycine, became available for study. We have used that solution to further test the effect of glutamate, aspartate and glycine composition upon plasma amino acids in a group of low-birth-weight infants using a cross-over study design.

We also wished to investigate the possible role of the erythrocyte in glutamate and aspartate transfer during parenteral infusion. Since amino acids may be transported by the erythrocyte to a greater extent than plasma under some circumstances (Elwyn, 1966; Aoki et al., 1972; Elwyn et al., 1972; Felig et al., 1973; Drews et al., 1977), both erythrocyte and plasma dicarboxylic amino acid levels should be measured concurrently. There is some evidence to suggest that erythrocyte levels of glutamate and aspartate in infants might be affected by infusion of solutions containing these amino acids. First, erythrocyte levels of glutamate are considerably higher in infants than in adults. Second, erythrocyte concentrations of glutamate and aspartate in both infants and adults are considerably higher than plasma concentrations. This contrasts with concentrations for other amino acids, which are present in approximately equal quantities in plasma and erythrocytes (Levy and Barkin, 1971). Third, the response of erythrocyte dicarboxylic amino acid concentrations to elevations of plasma concentrations of those amino acids also differs from that noted with other amino acids. An increased plasma concentration of most amino acids produces a rapid and proportional increase in erythrocyte concentration of that amino acid. However, erythrocyte glutamate concentrations in humans do not respond in the same fashion. Elevated plasma glutamate levels (produced by glutamate loading) do not affect erythrocyte levels in normal adult subjects (Baker et al., 1979).

The direct transport of erythrocyte amino acids to organs such as liver and brain has been suggested (Elwyn, 1966; Elwyn et al., 1972; Drewes et al., 1977). Thus, it is possible that differences between the rodent and primate in the extent of erythrocyte glutamate and aspartate transport might be a factor predisposing the rodent to dicarboxylic amino acid-induced neuronal necrosis. Bizzi et al. (1977) and Airoldi et al. (1979) reported that glutamate transport occurred equally in plasma and erythrocytes of neonatal rodents after a glutamate load. In adult humans by contrast, the erythrocyte does not participate in glutamate and aspartate transport after glutamate loading (Baker et al., 1979).

Eight infants with birth weights between 1.05 and 2.68 kg and gestational ages between 28 and 41 weeks were studied (Bell et al., 1982). All infants were fed parenterally with dextrose–amino acid solutions and lipid emulsion. Mean daily intakes (per kg body weight) were 80 kcal energy, 2 g lipid, 15 g dextrose and 2 g amino acids. All infants received a similar intake of minerals and vitamins.

Two different infusion regimens, differing only in amino acid composition, were studied. In Regimen I, Neopham (Cutter Laboratories, Berkeley, CA) was used as the amino acid source; Travasol (Baxter-Travenol, Morton Grove, IL) provided the amino acids in Regimen II. The amino acid composition of these two amino acid solutions is shown in Table 8-2. Regimen I provided a mean of 226 mg of glutamate, 130 mg of aspartate and 67 mg glycine per kg body weight per day. Regimen II provided no glutamate or aspartate and 414 mg glycine/kg body weight per day. Subjects were infused with each regimen for successive three-day periods in a cross-over design. Initial baseline observations were obtained while these infants were receiving intravenous dextrose alone.

Mean (± SD) plasma glutamate, aspartate and glycine concentrations are shown in Table 8-7. The mean plasma glutamate concentration was slightly, but significantly higher (8.69 ± 2.85 μmol/dl) during infusion of Regimen I, containing dicarboxylic amino acids, than during infusion of Regimen II (6.65 ± 1.98 μmol/dl), which did not contain glutamate and aspartate. However, the plasma glutamate levels observed were all within two standard deviations of the mean observed for orally fed low-birth-weight infants (10.7 ± 3.6 μmol/dl; mean ± SD) (Filer et al., 1977b). No significant differences in plasma aspartate concentrations were noted between infusion regimens ($p > 0.05$, paired t-test).

Table 8-7
Plasma Glutamate, Aspartate and Glycine Concentrations in Low-Birth-Weight Infants on Total Parenteral Nutrition

	Intake (mg/kg/day)			Plasma concentrations (μmol/dl)		
Solution	*GLY*	*ASP*	*GLU*	*Glycine*	*Aspartate*	*Glutamate*
Dextrose	0	0	0	26.7 ± 13.9	1.92 ± 0.43	4.98 ± 3.41
Neopham	67	130	226	29.0 ± 7.05	3.44 ± 0.97	8.69 ± 2.85
Travasol	414	0	0	66.0 ± 14.2	2.74 ± 1.68	6.65 ± 1.98
Normal, Orally Fed Infants				33.7 ± 8.2	2.6 ± 1.4	10.7 ± 3.6

Although dicarboxylic amino acid content had only a minimal effect on plasma concentrations, glycine concentrations strongly reflected the composition of infused amino acids. Plasma concentrations of glycine were significantly higher, well above normal limits, when infants were infused with Regimen II, containing large amounts of glycine.

Erythrocyte concentrations of glutamate, aspartate and glycine are given in Table 8-8. No significant differences in erythrocyte aspartate or glutamate concentrations were noted between infusion regimens. As expected, erythrocyte glycine levels reflected plasma concentrations. Erythrocyte concentrations of glycine were significantly higher when the infants were infused with Regimen II, containing high levels of glycine, than during infusion of Regimen I. Thus, both plasma and erythrocyte data indicate that low-birth-weight infants adequately metabolize the infused glutamate (226 mg/kg/day) and aspartate (130 mg/kg/day).

Table 8-8
Erythrocyte Glutamate, Aspartate and Glycine Concentrations in Low-Birth-Weight Infants on Total Parenteral Nutrition

	Plasma Concentrations (μmol/100 g)		
Solution	*Glutamate*	*Aspartate*	*Glycine*
Dextrose	43.4 ± 13.2	11.9 ± 6.08	47.5 ± 15.6
Neopham	60.8 ± 15.0	18.2 ± 8.54	61.1 ± 22.6
Travasol	52.6 ± 14.4	16.1 ± 7.53	96.3 ± 24.1

These new data (Bell et al., 1982), as well as our earlier data using protein-hydrolysate-based parenteral regimens (Stegink and Baker, 1971) and later work by other investigators (Anderson et al., 1974, 1977; Patel et al., 1973; Winters et al., 1977), demonstrate that the amino acid composition of the infused solution directly affects plasma levels of many amino acids, and indicate that each amino acid preparation produces a characteristic plasma amino acid pattern. Our data in parenterally fed infants are summarized in Figure 8-12. Mean peak plasma glycine levels respond rapidly to increased glycine infusion. The observed response agrees with that reported earlier by Winters et al. (1977). They reported a correlation coefficient of 0.83 for the "raw glycine dose response curve." Little effect of aspartate and glutamate infusion on plasma concentrations was noted for either of these amino acids at the quantities infused. This response also agrees with that observed by Winters et al. (1977).

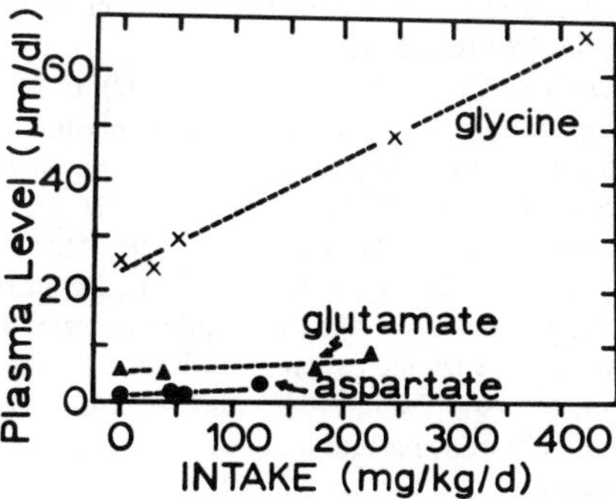

Figure 8-12 Mean peak plasma glycine (X), glutamate (▲) and aspartate (●) concentrations in young infants fed parenterally with various parenteral solutions of amino acids.

The data suggest that many of the currently used parenteral solutions could benefit from a decreased glycine content. Glutamate and aspartate are alternative sources of dispensable amino acid nitrogen.

REFERENCES

Abraham, R., Dougherty, W., Golberg, L., and Coulston, F. (1971): The response of the hypothalamus to high doses of monosodium glutamate in mice and monkeys. Cytochemistry and ultrastructural study of lysosomal changes. *Exp. Mol. Pathol.* 15:43–60.

Abraham, R., Swart, J., Golberg, L., and Coulston, F. (1975): Electron microscopic observations of hypothalami in neonatal rhesus monkeys (Macaca mulatta) after administration of monosodium-L-glutamate. *Exp. Mol. Pathol.* 23:203–213.

Adibi, S.A., Gray, S.J. and Menden, E. (1967): The kinetics of amino acid absorption and alteration of plasma composition of free amino acids after intestinal perfusion of amino acid mixtures. *Am. J. Clin. Nutr.* 20:24–33.

Airoldi, L., Bizzi, A., Salmona, M., Garattini, S. (1979): Attempts to establish the safety margin for neurotoxicity of monosodium glutamate. In: *Glutamic Acid: Advances in Biochemistry and Physiology* (eds: L.J. Filer, Jr., S. Garattini, M.R. Kare, W.A. Reynolds and R.J. Wurtman), pp. 321–331, Raven Press, New York.

Anantharaman, K. (1979): *In utero* and dietary administration of monosodium L-glutamate to mice: Reproductive performance and development in a multigeneration study. In: *Glutamic Acid: Advances in Biochemistry and Physiology,* (eds: L.J. Filer, Jr., S. Garattini, M.R. Kare, W.A. Reynolds and R.J. Wurtman), pp. 231–253, Raven Press, New York.

Anderson, G.H., Patel, D.G., and Jeejeebhoy, K.N. (1974): Design and evaluation by nitrogen balance and blood aminograms of an amino acid mixture for total parenteral nutrition of adults with gastrointestinal disease. *J. Clin. Invest.* 53:904–912.

Anderson, G.H., Bryan, H., Jeejeebhoy, K.N., and Corey, P. (1977): Dose-response relationships between amino acid intake and blood levels in newborn infants. *Am. J. Clin. Nutr.* 30:1110–1121.

Aoki, T.T., Brennen, M.F., Muller, W.A., Moore, F.D., and Cahill, G.F., Jr. (1972): Effect of insulin on muscle glutamate uptake. Whole blood versus plasma glutamate analysis. *J. Clin. Invest.* 51:2889–2894.

Applebaum, A.E., Daabees, T.T., Filer, L.J., Jr., and Stegink, L.D. (1981): Hypothalamic neuronal necrosis in neonatal cats administered pharmacologic doses of monosodium L-glutamate. *Society for Neuroscience,* Abstracts, 7:89.

Baker, G.L., Filer, L.J., Jr., and Stegink, L.D. (1979): Effect of carbohydrate on glutamate metabolism. *Fed. Proc.* 38:610 (abstract).

Bell, E.F., Filer, L.J., Jr., Wong, A. and Stegink, L.D. (1982): Effect of a parenteral nutrition regimen containing dicarboxylic amino acids upon plasma, erythrocyte and urinary amino acid concentrations of young infants. *Am. J. Clin. Nutr.* in press.

Bizzi, A., Veneroni, E., Salmona, M., and Garattini, S. (1977): Kinetics of monosodium glutamate in relation to its neurotoxicity. *Toxicol. Letters* 1:123–130.

Cox, W.M. Jr., Mueller, A.J., Elman, R., Albanese, A.A., Kemmerer, K.S., Bargon, R.W. and Holt, L.E., Jr. (1947): Nitrogen retention studies on rats, dogs and man. The effect of adding methionine to an enzymic casein hydrolysate. *J. Nutr.* 33:437–457.

Daabees, T.T., Finkelstein, M., Applebaum, A.E., and Stegink, L.D. (1982): Protective effect of carbohydrate or insulin on aspartate-induced neuronal necrosis in infant mice. *Fed. Proc.* 41:396 (abstract).

Dayhoff, (1978): *Atlas of Protein Sequence and Structure.* Volume 5, Suppl. 3, National Biomedical Research Foundation, Washington, D.C.

Doolittle, R.F. (1981): Similar amino acid sequences: Chance of common ancestry? *Science* 214:149–159.

Drewes, L.R., Conway, W.P., and Gilboe, D.D. (1977): Net amino acid transport between plasma and erythrocytes and perfused dog brain. *Am. J. Physiol.* 233:E320–325.

Elwyn, D.H. (1966): Distribution of amino acids between plasma and red blood cells in the dog. *Fed. Proc.* 25:854–861.

Elwyn, D.H., Launder, W.J., Parikh, H.C., and Wise, E.M., Jr. (1972): Roles of plasma and erythrocytes in interorgan transport of amino acids in dogs. *Am. J. Physiol.* 222: 1333–1342.

Felig P., Wahren, J., and Raf, L. (1973): Evidence of inter-organ amino-acid transport by blood cells in humans. *Proc. Nat. Acd. Sci. U.S.* 70:1775– 1779.

Filer, L.J., Jr., Baker, G.L., and Stegink, L.D. (1977a): Plasma aminograms in infants and adults fed an identical high protein meal. *Fed. Proc.* 36:1181 (abstract).

Filer, L.J., Jr., Stegink, L.D., and Chandramouli, B. (1977b): Effect of diet on plasma aminograms of low-birth-weight infants. *Am. J. Clin. Nutr.* 30:1036–1043.

Filer, L.J., Jr., Baker, G.L. and Stegink, L.D. (1979): Metabolism of free glutamate in clinical products fed infants. In: *Glutamic Acid: Advances in Biochemistry and Physiology* (eds: L.J. Filer, Jr., S. Garattini, M.R. Kare, W.A. Reynolds and R.J. Wurtman), pp. 353–362, Raven Press, New York.

Filler, R.M., Eraklis, A.J., Rubin, V.G., and Das, J.B. (1969): Long-term total parenteral nutrition in infants. *N. Engl. J. Med.* 281:589–595.

Gitler, C. (1964): Protein digestion and absorption in nonruminants. In: *Mammalian Protein Metabolism* (eds: H.N. Munro and J.B. Allison), Vol. I, pp. 35–69, Academic Press, New York.

Harper, A.E., Benevenga, N.J., and Wohlhueter, R.M. (1970): Effects of ingestion of disproportionate amounts of amino acids. *Physiol. Reviews* 50:428–558.

Heywood, R., and James, R.W. (1979): An attempt to induce neurotoxicity in an infant rhesus monkey with monosodium glutamate. *Toxicol. Letters* 4:285–286.

Jukes, T.H., Holmquist, R., and Moise, H. (1975): Amino acid composition of proteins: Selection against the genetic code. *Science* 189:50–51.

Lamperti A. and Blaha, G. (1976): The effects of neonatally-administered monosodium glutamate on the reproductive system of adult hamsters. *Biol. Reprod.* 14:362–369.

Lemkey-Johnston, N. and Reynolds, W.A. (1974): Nature and extent of brain lesions in mice related to ingestion of monosodium glutamate: A light and electron microscope study. *J. Neuropathol. Exptl. Neurol.* 33:74–97.

Levy, H.L. and Barkin, E. (1971): Comparison of amino acid concentrations between plasma and erythrocytes. Studies in normal human subjects and those with metabolic disorders. *J. Lab. Clin. Med.* 78:517–523.

Matthews, D.M. (1975): Intestinal absorption of peptides. *Physiol. Rev.* 55:537–608.

Neame, K.D. and Wiseman, G. (1957): The transamination of glutamic and aspartic acids during absorption by the small intestine of the dog *in vivo. J. Physiol.* 135:442–450.

Neame, K.D. and Wiseman, G. (1958): The alanine and oxo acid concentrations in mesenteric blood during the absorption of glutamic acid by the small intestine of the dog, cat, and rabbit *in vivo. J. Physiol.* 140:148–155.

Newman, A.J., Heywood, R., Plamer, A.K., Barry, D.H., Edwards, F.P., and Worden, A.N. (1973): The administration of monosodium L-glutamate to neonatal and pregnant monkeys. *Toxicology* 1:197–204.

Nixon, S.E. and Mawer, G.E. (1970a): The digestion and absorption of protein in man. 1. The site of absorption. *Br. J. Nutr.* 24:227–240.

Nixon, S.E. and Mawer, G.E. (1970b): The digestion and absorption of protein in man. 2. The form in which digested protein is absorbed. *Br. J. Nutr.* 24:241–258.

Nyhan, W. (1978): Nonketotic hyperglycinemia. In: *The Metabolic Basis of Inherited Disease.* (eds: J. Stanbury, J. Wyngaarden and D. Fredrickson), pp. 518–527, 4th Edition, McGraw-Hill, Inc., New York.

Ohara, Y. and Takasaki, Y. (1979): Relationship between plasma glutamate levels and hypothalamic lesions in rodents. *Toxicol. Letters* 4:499–505.

Okaniwa, A., Hori, M., Masuda, M., Takeshita, M., Hayashi, N., Wada, I., Doi, K., and Ohara, Y. (1979): Histopathological study on effects of potassium aspartate on the hypothalamus of rats. *J. Toxicol. Sci.* 4:31–46.

Olney, J.W. (1969): Brain lesions, obesity, and other disturbances in mice treated with monosodium glutamate. *Science* 164:719–721.

Olney, J.W. (1981): Excitatory neurotoxins as food additives: An evaluation of risk. *Neurotoxicol.* 2:163–192.

Olney, J.W. and Ho, O.L. (1970): Brain damage in infant mice following oral intake of glutamate, aspartate or cystine. *Nature* 227:609–611.

Olney, J.W., and Sharpe, L.G. (1969): Brain lesions in an infant rhesus monkey treated with monosodium glutamate. *Science* 166:386–388.

Olney, J.W., Sharpe, L.G., and Feigin, R.D. (1972): Glutamate-induced brain damage in infant primates. *J. Neuropathol. Exp. Neurol.* 31:464–488.

Olney, J.W., Ho, O.L., and Rhee, V. (1973a): Brain damaging potential of protein hydrolysates. *N. Engl. J. Med.* 289:391–395.

Olney, J.W., Rhee, V., and DeGubareff, T. (1973b): Neurotoxic effects of glutamate. *N. Engl. J. Med.* 289:1374–1375.

Olney, J.W., Labruyere, J., and DeGubareff, T. (1980): Brain damage in mice from voluntary ingestion of glutamate and aspartate. *Neurobehav. Toxicol.* 2:125–129.

Orr, M.L. and Watt, B.K. (1957): Amino acid content of foods. *Home Economics Research Report No. 4,* Household Economics Research Division, Institute of Home Economics, Agricultural Research Service, USDA, Washington, D.C.: Supt. of Documents, U.S. Government Printing Office, December.

Parsons, D.S. and Volman-Mitchell, H. (1974): The transamination of glutamate and aspartate during absorption in vitro of chicken, guinea pig and rat. *J. Physiol.* 239:677–694.

Patel, D.G., Anderson, G.H., and Jeejeebhoy, K.N. (1973): Amino acid adequacy of parenteral casein hydrolysate and oral cottage cheese in patients with gastrointestinal disease as measured by nitrogen balance and blood aminogram. *Gastroenterology* 65:427–437.

Ramaswamy, K. and Radhakrishnan, A.N. (1970): Labeling patterns using C^{14}-labelled glutamic acid, aspartic acid and alanine in transport studies with everted sacs of rat intestine. *Indian J. Biochem.* 7:50–54.

Reynolds, W.A., Lemkey-Johnston, N., Filer, L.J., Jr., and Pitkin, R.M. (1971): Monosodium glutamate: Absence of hypothalamic lesions after ingestion by newborn primates. *Science* 172:1342–1344.

Reynolds, W.A., Butler, V., Lemkey-Johnston, N. (1976): Hypothalamic morphology following ingestion of aspartame or MSG in the neonatal rodent and primate. A preliminary report. *J. Toxicol. Environ. Health* 2:471–480.

Reynolds, W.A., Lemkey-Johnston, N., and Stegink, L.D. (1979): Morphology of the fetal monkey hypothalamus after *in utero* exposure to monosodium glutamate. In: *Glutamic Acid: Advances in Biochemistry and Physiology,* (eds: L.J. Filer, Jr., S. Garattini, M.R. Kare, W.A. Reynolds, and R.J. Wurtman), pp. 217–229, Raven Press, New York.

Reynolds, W.A., Stegink, L.D., Filer, L.J., Jr., and Renn, E. (1980): Aspartame administration to the infant monkey: Hypothalamic morphology and plasma amino acid levels. *Anat. Rec.* 198:73–85.

Shimada, M., Wakamatsu, H., Tanaka, K., Nakao, H., and Kusunoki, T. (1975): Brain damage during the growth phase due to excessive administration of L-form amino acids. *Acta Pediatr. Jap.* 79:983–984.

Shohl, A.T., Butler, A.M., Blackfan, K.D., and McLachlan, E. (1939): Nitrogen metabolism during the oral and parenteral administration of the amino acids of hydrolyzed casein. *J. Pediat.* 15:469–475.

Silk, D.B.A., Marrs, T.C., Addison, J.M., Burston, D., Clark, M.L., and Matthews, D.M. (1973): Absorption of amino acids from an amino acid mixture stimulating casein and a tryptic hydrolysate of casein in man. *Clin. Sci. Mol. Med.* 45:715–719.

Stegink, L.D. (1976): Absorption, utilization and safety of aspartic acid. *J. Toxicol. Environ. Health* 2:215–242.

Stegink, L.D. (1977): Peptides in parenteral nutrition. In: *Clinical Nutrition Update—Amino Acids* (eds: H.L. Greene, M.A. Holliday, and H.N. Munro) pp. 192–198, Am. Med. Assoc., Chicago, IL.

Stegink, L.D. and Baker, G.L. (1971): Infusion of protein hydrolysates in the newborn infant. Plasma amino acid concentrations. *J. Pediat.* 78:595–602.

Stegink, L.D., Shepherd, J.A., Brummel, M.C., and Murray, L.M. (1974): Toxicity of protein hydrolysate solutions: Correlation of glutamate dose and neuronal necrosis to plasma amino acid levels in young mice. *Toxicology,* 2:285–299.

Stegink, L.D., Reynolds, W.A., Filer, L.J., Jr., Pitkin, R.M., Boaz, D.P., and Brummel, M.C. (1975): Monosodium glutamate metabolism in the neonatal monkey. *Am. J. Physiol.* 229:246–250.

Stegink, L.D., Filer, L.J., Jr., and Baker, G.L. (1977): Effect of aspartame and aspartate loading upon plasma and erythrocyte free amino acid levels in normal adult volunteers. *J. Nutr.* 107:1837–1845.

Stegink, L.D., Filer, L.J., Jr., Baker, G.L., Mueller, S.M. and M. Y-C Wu-Rideout (1979a): Factors affecting plasma glutamate levels in normal adult subjects. In: *Glutamic Acid: Advances in Biochemistry and Physiology,* (eds: L.J. Filer, Jr., S. Garattini, M.R. Kare, W.A. Reynolds, and R.J. Wurtman), pp. 333–351, Raven Press, New York.

Stegink, L.D., Reynolds, W.A., Filer, L.J., Jr., Baker, G.L., Daabees, T.T., and Pitkin, R.M. (1979b): Comparative metabolism of glutamate in the mouse, monkey, and man. In: *Glutamic Acid: Advances In Biochemistry and Physiology,* (eds: L.J. Filer, Jr., S. Garattini, M.R. Kare, W.A. Reynolds and R. J. Wurtman). pp. 85–102, Raven Press, New York.

Stegink, L.D., Baker, G.L. and Filer, L.J., Jr. (1982a): Plasma and erythrocyte concentrations of glutamate and aspartate in normal adults administered high doses of glutamate with meals. *Am. J. Clin. Nutr.* in press.

Stegink, L.D., Baker, G.L. and Filer, L.J., Jr. (1982b): Plasma and erythrocyte amino acid levels in normal adult subjects fed a high protein meal with and without added monosodium glutamate. *J. Nutr.* in press.

Takasaki, Y. (1978a): Studies on brain lesions by administration of monosodium L-glutamate to mice. I. Brain lesions in infant mice caused by administration of monosodium L-glutamate. *Toxicology* 9:293–305.

Takasaki, Y. (1978b): Studies on brain lesions by administration of monosodium L-glutamate to mice. II. Absence of brain damage following administration of monosodium L-glutamate in the diet. *Toxicology* 9:307–318.

Takasaki, Y., Matsuzawa, Y., Iwata, S., Ohara, Y., Yonetani, S., and Ichimura, M. (1979): Toxicological studies of monosodium L-glutamate in rodents: Relationship between routes of administration and neurotoxicity. In: *Glutamic Acid: Advances In Biochemistry and Physiology,* (eds: L.J. Filer, Jr., S. Garattini, M.R. Kare, W.A. Reynolds and R.J. Wurtman), pp. 255–275, Raven Press, New York.

Tafelski, T.J. (1976): Effects of monosodium glutamate on the neuroendocrine axis of the hamster. *Anat. Rec.* 184:543–544.

Wada, Y., Tada, K., Takada, G., Omura, K., Yoshida, T., Kuniya, T., Aoyama, T., Kakui, T., and Harada, S. (1972): Hyperglycinemia associated with hyperammonemia: In vitro glycine cleavage in liver. *Pediatr. Res.* 6:622–625.

Wen, C., Hayes, K.C., and Gershoff, S.N. (1973): Effects of dietary supplementation of monosodium glutamate on infant monkeys, weanling rats and suckling mice. *Am. J. Clin. Nutr.* 26:803–813.

Wilmore, D.W. and Dudrick, S.J. (1968): Growth and development of an infant receiving all nutrients exclusively by vein. *J. Am. Med. Assoc.* 203:860–864.

Wilmore, D.W., Groff, D.B., Bishop, H.C. and Dudrick, S.J. (1969): I. Total parenteral nutrition in infants with catastrophic gastrointestinal anomalies. *J. Pediatr. Surg.* 4:181–189.

Windmueller, H.G. and Spaeth, A.E. (1975): Intestinal metabolism of glutamine and glutamate from the lumen as compared to glutamine from blood. *Arch. Biochem. Biophys.* 171:662–672.

Windmueller, H.G. and Spaeth, A.E. (1976): Metabolism of absorbed aspartate, asparagine and arginine by rat small intestine *in vivo. Arch. Biochem. Biophys.* 175:670–676.

Windmueller, H.G. and Spaeth, A.E. (1980): Respiratory fuels and nitrogen metabolism *in vivo* in small intestine of fed rats. Quantitative importance of glutamine, glutamate and aspartate. *J. Biol. Chem.* 255:107–112.

Winters, R.W., Heird, W.C., Dell, R.B. and Nicholson, J.F. (1977): Plasma amino acids in infants receiving parenteral nutrition. In: *Clinical Nutrition Update—Amino Acids* (eds: H.L. Greene, M.A. Holliday and H.N. Munro). pp. 147–154, Am. Med. Assoc., Chicago, IL.

9 *In Vivo* and *In Vitro* Branched-Chain Amino Acid Interactions

Michael M. Meguid
Hanspeter Schwarz
Dwight E. Matthews
Irene E. Karl
Vernon R. Young
Dennis M. Bier

Because leucine, isoleucine, and valine share the same enzyme systems, branched-chain amino acid transferase (EC 2.6.1.6) and branched-chain α-ketoacid dehydrogenase (EC 1.2.4.4) for their initial degradative steps, the branched-chain amino acids are commonly thought of as a group in terms of their roles in amino acid homeostasis. For example, as recently as 1970 a review stated that "nature has dealt with the three branched-chain amino acids as a group" (Harper et al., 1970). Thus, both *in vivo* and *in vitro* experimental protocols frequently test a single branched-chain amino acid and extrapolate results to the group as a whole (Haymond and Miles, 1982; Glass et al., 1981). Recently, however, unique roles of individual branched-chain amino acids have been presented. For example, leucine-specific effects in regulating muscle protein metabolism (Buse and Weigand, 1977; Tischler et al., 1982) and adipose tissue valine oxidation (Frick et al., 1981) have been emphasized. Lately, we have had the opportunity to study unique aspects of the *in vivo* and *in vitro* relationships between leucine and valine metabolism. The present manuscript summarizes this work.

VALINE AND LEUCINE INTERACTIONS IN MAN

Almost 20 years ago Swendseid et al. (1965) reported dramatic reductions in plasma valine and isoleucine following leucine ingestion in man but no effect of oral valine on plasma levels of the other two branched-chain amino acids. Similarly, Hambraeus et al. (1976) found that subjects fed leucine-deficient diets had pronounced elevations of plasma valine but observed no change in plasma leucine when individuals received valine-deficient diets. To investigate the dynamics of these effects, we chose to examine both leucine and valine kinetics under circumstances where intake of one amino acid was reduced from a surfeit to a deficient level. A total of 15 normal weight, young adult volunteers participated in five dietary protocols. In each study, subjects received a crystalline amino acid mixture, patterned after the amino acid composition of egg proteins, which furnished an N equivalent of 0.8 g protein/kg•day. The subject's total energy requirement, based on his prior calorie intake, was furnished as mixed carbohydrate and fat with appropriate vitamin and mineral supplementation (Young et al., 1973). The diets, consumed for six days prior to study, were identical in each protocol except for the intake of valine or leucine which was adjusted to two different levels for leucine and three different intakes for valine as described below. Total nitrogen intake, however, was kept isonitrogenous by replacement of the reduced branched-chain amino acid with added aspartic acid in appropriate amounts. On the morning of the seventh day, and while consuming hourly aliquots of their test diet (Motil et al., 1981a,b) each subject was infused with either L[1-^{13}C]leucine or with L-[1-^{13}C]valine to determine branched-chain amino acid flux and oxidation as previously described (Matthews, 1980).

Table 9-1 shows the postabsorptive plasma leucine, valine, glucose, and insulin concentrations at each branched-chain amino acid intake level. As dietary leucine intake decreased, plasma leucine and insulin declined as anticipated. Plasma valine, on the other hand, rose significantly on the low dietary leucine intake. When dietary valine consumption was reduced, plasma valine fell and there was a small but insignificant decline in plasma insulin levels. Plasma leucine levels, however, remained unchanged. Plasma glucagon values (not shown) demonstrated no consistent change with altered valine or leucine consumption.

Table 9-1
Postabsorptive Plasma Leucine, Valine, and Insulin Concentrations in Subjects Consuming Graded Levels of Leucine or Valine

Dietary Intake Level (mg/kg•d)	Plasma Concentration			
	Leucine (μM)	*Valine* (μM)	*Glucose* (mg/dl)	*Insulin* (μU/ml)
Leucine 80*	130 ± 9	272 ± 16	80 ± 2	20 ± 2
Leucine 4*	80 ± 8	1004 ± 70	78 ± 4	10 ± 2
Valine 70†	135 ± 6	280 ± 7	89 ± 5	12 ± 3
Valine 16†	120 ± 7	107 ± 7	73 ± 4	12 ± 2
Valine 4†	127 ± 13	120 ± 11	83 ± 4	9 ± 1

*Dietary valine intake = 70 mg/kg•d
†Dietary leucine intake = 80 mg/kg•d

Figure 9-1 shows the effect of altering leucine intake from sufficient to deficient on plasma leucine and valine flux. Consistent with our previous observations (Motil et al., 1981a), leucine turnover decreased when dietary leucine consumption declined. Valine flux, on the other hand, rose dramatically in the circumstance of insufficient dietary leucine intake. Amino acid oxidation was also altered (Figure 9-2).

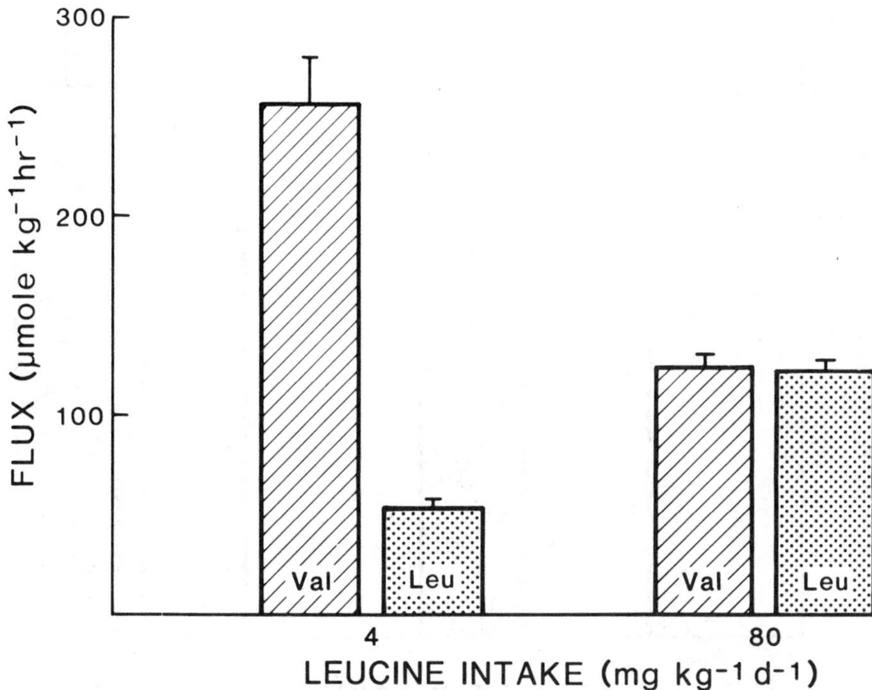

Figure 9-1 The effect of two different dietary leucine intake levels on the turnover of plasma leucine and valine.

Leucine oxidation declined, as expected, with reduced dietary leucine intake. However, despite the dramatic increase in valine turnover at lower dietary leucine consumption, the fraction of valine flux oxidized was reduced by 27%.

As observed for leucine flux and oxidation when dietary leucine intake was decreased, valine turnover (Figure 9-3) and oxidation (Figure 9-4) declined with reduced dietary valine intake. However, leucine turnover remained unchanged (Figure 9-3), and the fractional oxidation rate tended to increase (Figure 9-4), but not significantly so, as dietary valine consumption declined.

While it is tempting to explain these data in terms of specific leucine substrate effects on valine metabolism, such conclusions are not unequivocal in clinical studies where changes observed might be the result of secondary hormonal or other regulatory events consequent on altered dietary leucine consumption. For example, Clark et al. (1968) were unable to depress plasma valine in alloxan diabetic rats following ingestion of leucine. They interpreted these results as indicating that leucine-induced insulin release was the mediator of oral leucine's effect on plasma valine in nondiabetic animals. Similarly, whereas Hagenfeldt et al. (1980) suggested that the fall in plasma valine observed during a continuous 2.5-hour infusion of L-leucine (0.3 mmol/min) in man was independent of insulin action, peripheral plasma values rose from 17 to 22 microunits/ml, and it is conceivable that portal insulin levels rose even further. Thus, in order to determine whether the leucine-induced changes in valine metabolism we observed in our human subjects were a direct substrate-mediated effect, we undertook a series of correlative *in vitro* experiments in which the results of substrate alteration alone could be tested.

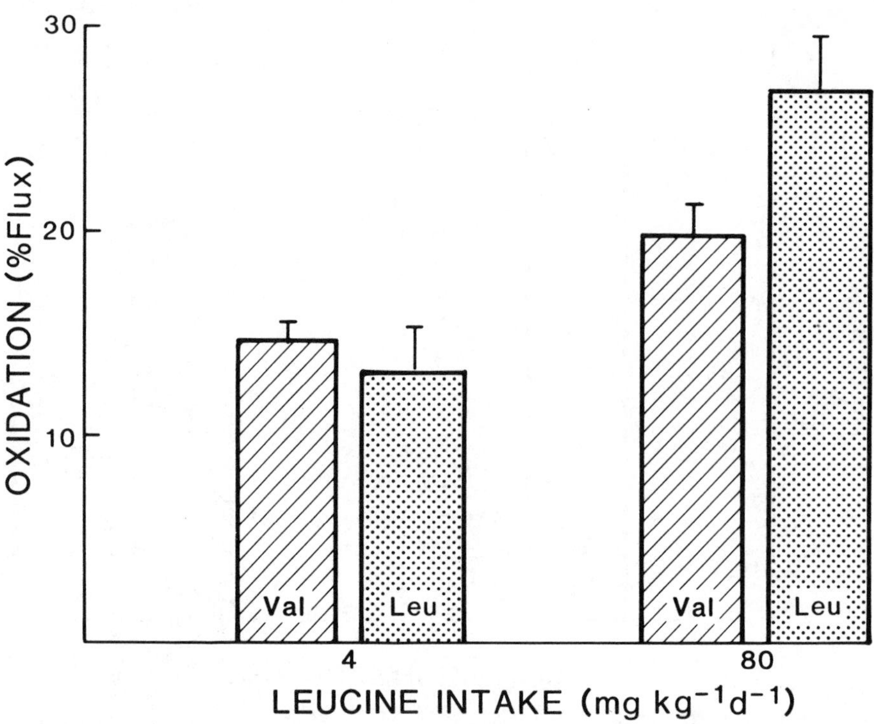

Figure 9-2 The effect of two different dietary leucine intake levels on the fractional oxidation of leucine and valine expressed as percent of the corresponding plasma flux.

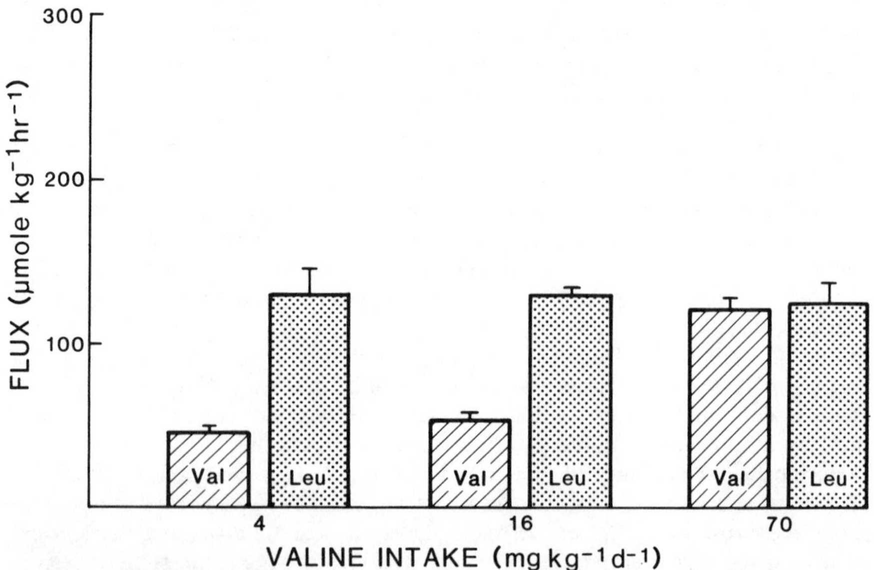

Figure 9-3 The effect of three different dietary valine intake levels on the turnover of plasma valine and leucine.

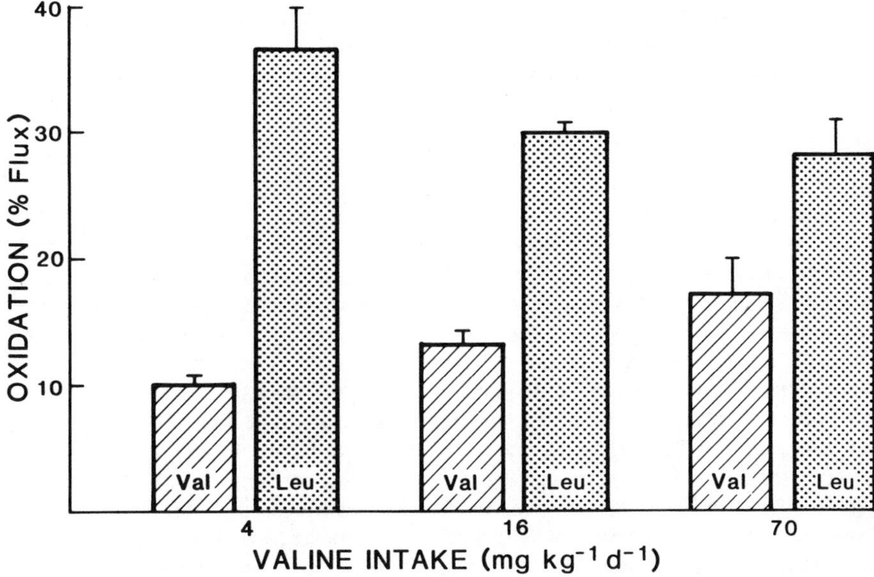

Figure 9-4 The effect of three different dietary valine intake levels on the fractional oxidation of valine and leucine expressed as percent of the corresponding plasma flux.

IN VITRO BRANCHED-CHAIN AMINO ACID INTERACTIONS

Intact epitrochlearis muscles were obtained as described (Garber et al., 1976) from 120 to 130 g male Sprague-Dawley rats kept for at least five days on an ad libitum Purina Lab Chow diet (22% crude protein). Single 20 to 30 mg muscles were incubated for two hours in Krebs-Henseleit buffer containing 5.5 mM glucose, 1 mM calcium chloride, 5 mM Hepes, and 0.15% dialyzed bovine serum albumin. Branched-chain amino acids were added in varying amounts (see below) either alone or in the presence of other amino acids at normal rat plasma concentrations.

Table 9-2 shows the effects of increasing incubation medium content of leucine or valine on muscle substrate release in the absence of other extracellular amino acids. As leucine concentration increased from zero to the supraphysiological range, muscle ketoisocaproate release increased, as anticipated, but there was a pronounced drop in ketoisovalerate release and a lesser, but still significant, decline in released valine. When extracellular valine content was modulated, however, there was essentially no effect on muscle leucine or ketoisocaproate release even though ketoisovalerate release increased dramatically. These effects were seen in the presence of all other amino acids as well.

The above data suggested that leucine was reducing the size of intracellular valine and ketoisovalerate pools. Leucine's role in accelerating muscle protein synthesis and ketoisocaproate's effect of attenuating muscle protein breakdown would have this result (Tischler et al., 1982). A similar effect, however, would occur if leucine accelerated muscle ketoisovalerate decarboxylation as recently described in adipose tissue (Frick et al., 1981) but not, to our knowledge, in muscle. Thus, we chose to investigate the latter process (Table 9-3). As in adipose tissue, leucine greatly enhanced valine decarboxylation. Valine, on the other hand, produced a slight decline in leucine degradation.

DISCUSSION

The above *in vivo* and *in vitro* data show remarkable similarities. As dietary leucine intake increased from deficient to surfeit, plasma valine (Table 9-1) and valine turnover decline (Figure 9-1), but the fraction of transported valine which is oxidized increases (Figure 9-2). Likewise, as medium extracellular leucine concentration increases, muscle valine and ketoisovalerate release decline (Table 9-2), and valine decarboxylation is accelerated (Table 9-3). On the other hand, when dietary valine intake increases from inadequate to excess, plasma leucine (Table 9-1) and leucine flux (Figure 9-3) are unaffected, but there is a slight decline in leucine oxidation (Figure 9-4). Similarly, when medium valine concentration was increased from zero to supranormal range, muscle leucine release was unchanged (Table 9-2) and a slight decrease in [1-^{14}C]leucine decarboxylation was observed (Table 9-3).

These results are consistent with previously reported observations in animals and man. As noted above, leucine's role in regulating muscle protein balance

Table 9-2
Effects of Leucine and Valine on Muscle Substrate Release

Addition (μM)	Substrate Released (nmol/min•g)			
	Leucine	*KIC*	*Valine*	*KIV*
Leucine				
0	–	0.3	2.6	0.5
200	–	1.5	2.3	0.2
1000	–	3.2	1.9	0.1
Valine				
0	4.2	0.4	–	0.3
200	4.4	0.3	–	1.9
1000	4.0	0.3	–	6.7

Table 9-3
Effects of Leucine and Valine on Each Other's Decarboxylation in Muscle

Additions (μM)			$^{14}CO_2$ Released (nmol/min•g)
Leucine	+	[1 – ^{14}C] Valine	
0		200	0.3
200		200	0.9
1000		200	1.3
Valine	+	[1 – ^{14}C] Leucine	
0		200	1.3
200		200	1.1
1000		200	1.0

(Tischler et al., 1982) can contribute to decreased intracellular availability of valine and consequently of ketoisovalerate. And, Hutson et al. (1978) also showed that hindlimb release of valine and ketoisovalerate were reduced as perfusate leucine concentration was increased from 100 to 500 mM. As also noted above, Frick et al. (1981) reported that adipose tissue valine oxidation doubled by addition of 200 to 500 μM leucine to the incubation buffer and that leucine, but not valine, accelerated isoleucine oxidation as well. Furthermore, Waymack et al. (1980) showed that ketoisovalerate perfusion of rat hearts "regularly resulted" in somewhat less activation of the branched-chain α-ketoacid dehydrogenase than did the other branched-chain α-ketoacids. These authors also showed that ketoisocaproate was about ten times more effective than ketoisovalerate in prevention of pyruvate-mediated inactivation of the branched-chain α-ketoacid dehydrogenase. While the reasons for these effects are not yet completely understood, recent observations on the kinase–phosphase-mediated phosphorylation–dephosphorylation interconversion of the branched-chain α-ketoacid dehydrogenase between its inactive and active forms, respectively, offer some insight. (Randle et al., 1981; Hughes and Halestrap, 1981). Ketoisocaproate is a potent inhibitor of phosphorylation and, consequently, prevents inactivation of the enzyme complex (Randle et al., 1981; Lau et al., 1981), whereas ketoisovalerate is fifteenfold less effective in this regard (Lau et al., 1981). Goodman and Frick (1981) have also concluded that ketoisocaproate inhibits the protein kinase which converts the branched-chain α-ketoacid dehydrogenase to its ineffective phosphorylated form, while Odessey (personal communication) has evidence that ketoisovalerate has little effect on this kinase.

CONCLUSION

The above results help explain leucine's reported *in vivo* effects on plasma valine levels (Swendseid et al., 1965; Hambraeus et al., 1976). Thus, while hormonal effects were not controlled in these studies, and while insulin is a regulator of branched-chain α-ketoacid dehydrogenase (Frick and Goodman, 1980), the above data demonstrate that direct substrate effects alone can explain the observed *in vivo* responses. Furthermore, the divergent actions of leucine and valine both in muscle and in the intact organism reaffirm both the need to consider each branched-chain amino acid as functionally unique and the potential hazards of extrapolating information obtained with a single index branched-chain amino acid to the group as a whole.

REFERENCES

Buse, M.G. and Weigand, D.A. (1977): Studies concerning the specificity of the effect of leucine on the turnover of protein in muscles of control and diabetic rats. *Biochim. et Biophys. Acta* 475:81–89.

Clark, A.J., Yamada, C., Swendseid, M.E. (1968): Effect of L-leucine on amino acid levels in plasma and tissue of normal and diabetic rats. *Am. J. Physiol.* 215:1324–1328.

Frick, G.P. and Goodman, H.M. (1980) Insulin regulation of branched chain α-keto acid dehydrogenase in adipose tissue. *J. Biol. Chem.* 255:6186–6192.

Frick, G.P., Tai, L-R., Blinder, L., and Goodman, H.M. (1981): L-leucine activates branched chain α-keto acid dehydrogenase in rat adipose tissue. *J. Biol. Chem.* 256:2618–2620.

Garber, A.J., Karl, I.E., and Kipnis, D.M. (1976): Alanine and glutamine release from skeletal muscle. I. Glycolysis and amino acid release. *J. Biol. Chem.* 251:826.

Glass, A.R., Bongiovanni, R., Smith, C.E., and Boehm, T.M. (1981): Normal valine disposal in obese subjects with impaired glucose disposal: Evidence for selective insulin resistance. *Metabolism* 30:578–582.

Goodman, H.M. and Frick, G.P. (1981): Metabolism of branched chain amino acids in adipose tissue. In: *Metabolism and Clinical Implications of Branched Chain Amino and Ketoacids* (eds: M. Walser and J.R. Williamson) p. 167, Elsevier/North Holland, New York.

Hagenfeldt, L., Eriksson, S., and Wahren, J. (1980): Influence of leucine on arterial concentrations and regional exchange of amino acids in healthy subjects. *Clin. Sci.* 59:173–181.

Hambraeus, L., Bilmazes, C., Dippel, C., Scrimshaw, N., Young, V.R. (1976): Regulatory role of dietary leucine on plasma branched chain amino acid levels in young men. *J. Nutr.* 106:230–240.

Harper, A.E., Benvenga, N.J., Wohlhueter, R.M. (1970): Effects of ingestion of disproportionate amounts of amino acids. *Physiol. Rev.* 50:523–558.

Haymond, M.W. and Miles, J.M. (1982): Branched chain amino acids as a major source of alanine nitrogen in man. *Diabetes* 31:86–89.

Hughes, W.A. and Halestrap, A.P. (1981): The regulation of branched-chain 2-oxoacid dehydrogenase of liver, kidney and heart by phosphorylation. *Biochem. J.* 196:459.

Hutson, S.M., Cree, T.C., and Harper, A.E. (1978): Regulation of leucine and α-ketoisocaproate metabolism in skeletal muscle. *J. Biol. Chem.* 253:8126–8133.

Lau, K.S., Fatania, H.R., and Randle, P.J. (1981): Inactivation of rat liver and kidney branched-chain 2-oxoacid dehydrogenase complex by adenosine triphosphate. *FEBS Lett.* 126:66.

Matthews, D.E., Motil, K.J., Rohrbaugh, D.K., Burke, J.F., Young, V.R., and Bier, D.M. (1980): Measurement of leucine metabolism in man from a primed, continuous infusion of L-[1-^{13}C]leucine. *Am. J. Physiol.* 238:E473–E479.

Motil, K.J., Bier, D.M., Matthews, D.E., Burke, J.F., and Young, V.R. (1981b): Whole body leucine and lysine metabolism studied with [l-^{13}C]leucine and [α-^{15}N]lysine: response in healthy young men given excess energy intake. *Metabolism* 30:783–791.

Motil, K.J., Matthews, D.E., Bier, D.M., Burke, J.F., Munro, H. M., and Young, V.R. (1981a): Whole-body leucine and lysine metabolism: response to dietary protein intake in young men. *Am. J. Physiol.* 240:E712–E721.

Randle, P.J., Lau, K.S., and Parker, P.J. (1981): Regulation of branched chain 2-oxoacid dehydrogenase complex. In: *Metabolism and Clinical Implications of Branched Chain Amino and Ketoacids* (eds: M. Walser and J.R. Williamson), p. 13, Elsevier/North Holland, New York.

Swendseid, M.E., Villalobos, J., Figueroa, W.S., Drenick, E.J. (1965): The effect of test doses of leucine, isoleucine or valine on plasma amino acid levels. The unique effect of leucine. *Am J. Clin. Nutr.* 17:317–321.

Tischler, M.E., Desautels, M., and Goldberg, A.L. (1982): Does leucine, leucyl-tRNA, or some metabolite of leucine regulate protein synthesis and degradation in skeletal and cardiac muscle? *J. Biol. Chem.* 257:1613–1621.

Waymack, P.P., DeBuysere, M.S., and Olson, M.S. (1980): Studies on the activation and inactivation of the branched chain α-keto acid dehydrogenase in the perfused rat heart. *J. Biol. Chem.* 255:9773–9781.

Young, V.R., Taylor, Y.S.M., Rand, W.M., and Scrimshaw, N.S. (1973): Protein requirements of man: efficiency of egg protein utilization at maintenance and submaintenance levels in young men. *J. Nutr.* 103:1164.

Interrelationship Between Phenylalanine and Tyrosine Metabolism in the Postabsorptive Rat

Lyle L. Moldawer, Isao Kawamura, Bruce R. Bistrian, and George L. Blackburn

L-tyrosine is a nutritionally dispensable amino acid (Meister, 1965). Its *de novo* synthesis represents the initial step in the oxidative pathway of phenylalanine. Estimates from man and laboratory animals have suggested that at least 90% to 95% of L-phenylalanine is catabolized through L-tyrosine, with the remainder via the urinary excretion of phenylpyruvate and its metabolites (Moss and Schoenheimer, 1940; Scriver and Rosenberg, 1973). Based upon this common pathway, plasma tyrosine appearance in a postabsorptive animal can be attributed to its *de novo* synthesis and release from protein breakdown. Because a component of tyrosine flux is an intermediate step in the oxidation of phenylalanine, a greater fraction of tyrosine appearance would be catabolized than anticipated with an indispensable amino acid. Based upon this model, the proportion of phenylalanine appearance that is ultimately oxidized would also be considerably less than with other indispensable amino acids since a major fate of L-tyrosine is not oxidation but incorporation into whole body protein.

The purpose of the present study was to estimate the quantitative importance of phenylalanine metabolism with respect to plasma tyrosine kinetics. Using a six-hour continuous infusion of either L-(U-^{14}C)-phenylalanine or L-(U-^{14}C)-tyrosine and L-(2,3-^{3}H)-phenylalanine, plasma phenylalanine and tyrosine appearance and oxidation, as well as phenylalanine conversion to plasma tyrosine were evaluated.

MATERIALS AND METHODS

Eighteen male, well-nourished rats (NEDH/kx strain) with an initial body weight of 90 to 120 g were studied following an overnight fast. Between 0800 and 1000 hours, the rats were restrained by gently wrapping in cloth and a 26 g catheter was inserted into the lateral tail vein. For the next six hours, the animals were infused with 2.3 to 2.4 ml/hr of physiologic saline containing 6 μCi of either L-(1-^{14}C)-leucine (n = 5), L-(U-^{14}C)-phenylalanine (n = 6), or L-(U-^{14}C)-tyrosine and L-(2,3-^{3}H)-phenylalanine (n = 7) (New England Nuclear Laboratories, Boston, MA). At hourly intervals, expired carbon dioxide was trapped in scintillation vials containing 200 μmols of hyamine hydroxide. Total carbon dioxide production was measured twice during the last two hours over 15-minute intervals, as previously described (Kawamura et al., 1982).

At the end of the six-hour infusion, the rats were sacrificed by decapitation. Plasma-free leucine-specific radioactivity was determined by using an automated amino acid analyzer (Moldawer et al., 1980). Quantitation of plasma phenylalanine-specific radioactivity was performed with the technique of Garlick and McNurlan (1981). ^{14}C-Tyrosine-specific radioactivity was determined according to Garlick and Marshall (1973). In rats infused with both L-(U-^{14}C)-tyrosine and

L-(2,3-^{3}H)-phenylalanine, ^{3}H-phenylalanine and ^{14}C- and ^{3}H-tyrosine-specific radioactivities were measured simultaneously. Because the isolation and extraction procedure for tyrosine (Garlick et al., 1973) is also specific for phenylalanine, ^{3}H-tyrosine-specific radioactivity was derived from the total tritium radioactivity, L-tyramine, and B-phenethylamine concentrations, and ^{3}H-phenylalanine-specific radioactivity.

Rates of amino acid flux and ^{14}C-amino acid oxidation were subsequently estimated from the dilution of tracer in the plasma compartment and its appearance in expired breath (Kawamura et al., 1982; Moldawer et al., 1980; Waterlow, 1982). The retention of metabolically generated ^{14}C-carbon dioxide was 24 ± 6% (S.D., n = 10; Moldawer, L.L., unpublished observations).

The percentage of total phenylalanine flux converted to plasma tyrosine was obtained from the equation:

$$\% \text{ converted} = (Q_t \cdot S_{p\ max.}/I) \cdot 100$$

where Q_t is the ^{14}C-tyrosine flux, in μmol/hr, $S_{p\ max.}$ is the ^{3}H-tyrosine-specific radioactivity, in d.p.m./μmol, and I is the infusion rate of L-(2,3-^{3}H)-phenylalanine, in d.p.m./hr. The percentage of phenylalanine flux converted to tyrosine was then multiplied by the plasma phenylalanine flux to obtain total conversion rates (μmols/hr).

RESULTS AND DISCUSSION

Plasma amino acid appearance and oxidation were investigated in three groups of well-nourished rats following an overnight fast. Since phenylalanine and leucine are nutritionally indispensable amino acids, their rates of plasma appearance in the postabsorptive state can be attributed solely to their release from protein breakdown. Plasma phenylalanine and leucine appearance paralleled their relative abundance in whole body protein (Table 1), suggesting that the endogenous flux of an indispensable amino acid can reflect the turnover of whole body protein when dietary protein is not administered.

Conversely, plasma tyrosine appearance was significantly greater than expected from its composition in whole body protein, and this apparent increase was due, in part, to its *de novo* synthesis via phenylalanine hydroxylation (Table 2). Under these conditions, the use of tyrosine or any other dispensable amino acid to quantitate whole body protein kinetics would give overestimates of protein breakdown, since a

Table 1
Relationship Between Plasma Appearance and Body Composition

	Protein Composition*		Amino Acid Flux	
	μmol/g protein	*Molar ratio*	*μmol/hr*	*Molar ratio*
Leucine	480	1.00	68.9 ± 3.0	1.00
Phenylalanine	260	0.54	43.7 ± 9.1	0.63
Tyrosine	176	0.37	42.1 ± 4.6	0.61

*Data obtained from Block, R.J., Weiss, K.W. (1956): *Amino Acid Handbook,* p. 292. Springfield, Ill., C.C. Thomas and Co.

Table 2
Individual Components of Plasma Tyrosine Kinetics

	Total Tyrosine	Due to Phenylalanine	Due to Endogenous Tyrosine
Appearance (μmol/hr)	42.1	9.1 ± 1.3 (21%)*	33.0 (79%)
Oxidation (μmol/hr)	10.3	5.6 ± 1.1 (54%)†	4.7 (46%)

*Derived from the conversion of L-(2,3-^{3}H)-phenylalanine to ^{3}H-tyrosine; see Materials and Methods section. (%) Refers to the percent of total tyrosine.
†Obtained from the plasma ^{14}C-specific radioactivity and the appearance of ^{14}C-carbon dioxide, during a continuous infusion of L-(U-^{14}C)-phenylalanine.

Table 3
Plasma Kinetics

	Appearance (μmol/hr)	Complete Oxidation*	Percentage of Flux Oxidized*
Leucine (L-(1-^{14}C))	68.9 ± 3.0	18.7 ± 2.2	27.1 ± 2.1
Phenylalanine (L-(U-^{14}C))	43.7 ± 9.1	5.6 ± 1.1	12.2 ± 1.4
Tyrosine (L-(U-^{14}C))	42.1 ± 4.6	10.3 ± 0.8	24.4 ± 2.2

*Assuming that 26% of metabolically generated carbonate does not appear as expired carbon dioxide.

component of tyrosine appearance is independent of protein synthesis and degradation. Considerations of this type could explain the considerably higher whole body protein dynamics reported by James et al. (1976) and Desai et al. (1981) with isotopic tyrosine when compared to leucine or lysine.

The appearance of ^{3}H-tyrosine in the plasma during a continuous infusion of L-(2,3-^{3}H)-phenylalanine was used to quantitate phenylalanine conversion to plasma tyrosine. In the postabsorptive rat, 9.1 μmol/hr of phenylalanine were converted to plasma tyrosine which represented 21% of total plasma tyrosine appearance (Table 2). This finding is in good agreement with the 16% contribution previously calculated by James et al. (1976).

An inherent assumption to the use of kinetic models for estimating whole body amino acid kinetics is that tyrosine derived from protein degradation, dietary intake, and phenylalanine hydroxylation enter a well-mixed homogenous free tyrosine pool. Theoretically, the 9.1 μmol/hr of plasma phenylalanine converted to plasma tyrosine would be further degraded at rates comparable to tyrosine released from protein degradation.

Table 3 summarizes tyrosine and phenylalanine oxidation. Based on the L-(U-^{14}C)-phenylalanine infusion and the appearance of ^{14}C-carbon dioxide, after adjusting for the retention of labeled carbonate, 5.3 μmol/hr of plasma phenylalanine were oxidized. Assuming that tyrosine and phenylalanine are degraded through a common pathway (2), then 54% of the 10.3 μmol/hr of plasma tyrosine oxidized was derived originally from plasma phenylalanine. However, if the 9.1 μmol/hr of phenylalanine converted to tyrosine had been catabolized in proportions similar to total plasma tyrosine flux, only 2.2 μmol/hr should have been oxidized entirely to carbon dioxide.

One possible conclusion is that tyrosine derived from phenylalanine is preferentially oxidized. Similarly, the disproportionate increase in apparent oxidation of tyrosine arising from phenylalanine hydroxylation may reflect a failure of tyrosine to equilibrate between the site of hydroxylation (presumably the hepatocyte) and the plasma compartment. Therefore, tyrosine generated from phenylalanine hydroxylation that is degraded further without first equilibrating with the plasma compartment will be measured as ^{14}C-phenylalanine oxidation but not as plasma appearance of ^{3}H-tyrosine during a ^{3}H-phenylalanine infusion. Although whole body amino acid kinetic studies based upon plasma enrichments are underestimates of absolute rates (see Jackson and Golden, 1982 for review), the potential to underestimate plasma appearance is considerably greater when the *de novo* synthesis of an amino acid occurs in a tissue where it may undergo further catabolism.

The findings suggest that in the postabsorptive animal, phenylalanine metabolism plays a principal role in the plasma appearance of tyrosine. These studies clearly demonstrate the dynamic interaction between tyrosine and phenylalanine metabolism *in vivo,* and emphasize the importance in considering the kinetics of both amino acids, concurrently.

ACKNOWLEDGMENT

Supported in part by grants GM-22691, GM-24206, and GM-24401, awarded by the National Institutes of General Medical Sciences and RR-05591, awarded by the Research Resources Division of the National Institutes of Health, DHHS. The authors gratefully acknowledge the assistance of Ajinomoto U.S.A., Inc.

REFERENCES

Desai, S.P., Moldawer, L.L., Bistrian, B.R., Blackburn, G.L., Bothe, A. Jr., Schulte, R.D. (1981): Amino acid and protein metabolism in humans using L-(U-^{14}C)-tyrosine and L-(l-^{14}C)-leucine. *Develop. Biochem.* 18:307–312.

Garlick, P.J., Millward, D.J., James, W.P.T. (1973): The diurnal response of muscle and liver protein synthesis in vivo in meal-fed rats. *Biochem. J.* 136:935–945.

Jackson, A.A., Golden, M.H.N. (1982), Interrelationships of amino acid pools and protein turnover. In *Nitrogen Metabolism in Man,* (eds: J.C. Waterlow and J.M.L. Stephen), Englewood, N.J., Applied Science Publishers.

James, W.P.T., Garlick, P.J., Sender, P.M., Waterlow, J.C. (1976): Studies of protein and amino acid metabolism in normal man with L-(U-^{14}C)-tyrosine. *Clin. Sci.* 53:277–288.

Kawamura, I., Moldawer, L.L., Keenan, R.A., Batist, G., Bothe, A. Jr., Bistrian, B.R., Blackburn, G.L. (1982): Altered amino acid kinetics in rats with progressive tumor growth. *Cancer Res.* 42:824–830.

McNurlan, M.A., Garlick, P.J. (1981): Protein synthesis in liver and small intestine in protein deprivation and diabetes. *Am. J. Physiol.* 241:E238–245.

Meister, A. (1965): *Biochemistry of the Amino Acids,* 2nd Edition. New York, Academic Press.

Moldawer, L.L., O'Keefe, S.J.D., Bothe, A. Jr., Bistrian, B.R., Blackburn, G.L. (1980): In vivo demonstration of the nitrogen-sparing mechanisms for glucose and amino acids in the injured rat. *Metabolism* 29:173–180.

Moss, A.R., Schoenheimer, R. (1940): Conversion of phenylalanine to tyrosine in the normal rat. *J. Biol. Chem.* 135:415–429.
Scriver, C.R., Rosenberg, L.E. (1973): *Amino Acid Metabolism and Its Disorders.* Philadelphia, W.B. Saunders and Co.
Waterlow, J.C. (1982): Methods of measuring protein turnover. In *Nitrogen Metabolism in Man* (eds: J.C. Waterlow and J.M.L. Stephen), Englewood, N.J., Applied Science Publishers, Inc.

Relationship of Plasma Leucine and α-Ketoisocaproate ^{13}C Enrichment During a L-[l-^{13}C] Leucine Infusion in Man

D.E. Matthews, H.P. Schwarz, R.D. Young, K.J. Motil, V.R. Young, and D.M. Bier

The branched-chain amino acids (BCAAs), leucine, valine, and isoleucine, play a prominent role in muscle amino acid metabolism. In contrast to the other dietary-indispensable amino acids that are oxidized principally in liver, the BCAAs are metabolized primarily in extrahepatic tissues such as muscle (Adibi, 1976; Harper and Zapalowski, 1981). The first two key steps in BCAA oxidation are common for all three BCAAs: (1) reversible transamination, e.g., leucine transamination to α-ketoisocaproate (KIC), and (2) decarboxylation of the carbonyl-carbon, e.g., KIC conversion to a CO_2 and an isovaleryl-CoA. In liver, transamination is thought to be rate limiting, but in muscle BCAA transamination is rapid and decarboxylation may be limiting (Harper and Zapalowski, 1981; Ichihara et al., 1981; Matthews et al., 1981). Peripheral tissues, such as muscle, can form and release into systemic circulation KIC for extraction and further oxidation by other tissues such as liver. Thus, the plasma KIC should reflect its precursor's history: the integrated release of intracellular KIC from the major tissues which transaminate leucine. This scheme is illustrated in Figure 1.

When a labeled amino acid is infused intravenously, the amino acid enrichment is higher in the extracellular plasma compartment than intracellularly because the label is infused directly into the extracellular space, while unlabeled amino acid from protein breakdown enters directly into the intracellular compartment. Of course, the ratio of enrichment between intracellular and extracellular compartments will depend upon the rate of tissue protein turnover; i.e., liver with a higher rate of proteolysis would be expected to produce lower intracellular enrichments than muscle (Waterlow et al., 1978). Although other workers have studied intracellular and extracellular free amino acid enrichments in animals (Waterlow et al., 1978), knowledge is more limited for the human because the equivalent tissue biopsy samples cannot be readily obtained.

Whole body leucine kinetics have been determined in man by a short, continuous infusion of L-(1-^{14}C)- or L-(1-^{13}C)leucine under a variety of metabolic conditions (Waterlow et al., 1978; Golden and Waterlow, 1977; Matthews et al., 1980; Motil et al., 1981a,b). Although this approach requires precursor ^{13}C enrichment for calculation of rates of flux, oxidation, or incorporation into protein via protein synthesis (Waterlow et al., 1978; Golden and Waterlow, 1977; Matthews et al., 1980), it

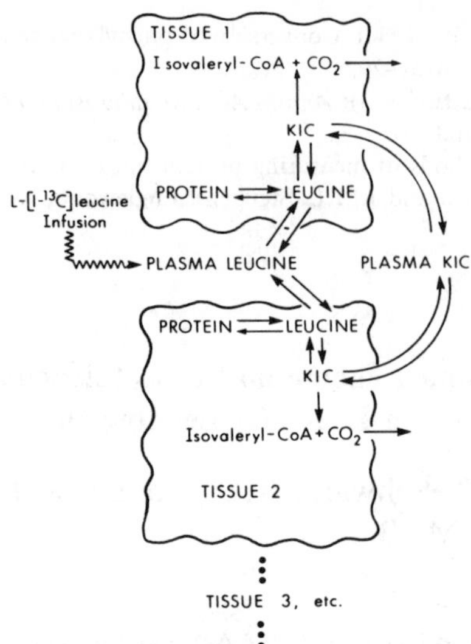

Figure 1 Multi-tissue model of whole body leucine metabolism. The model illustrates that plasma leucine is taken up and released by numerous tissues in the body. The KIC is formed from transamination of intracellular leucine and also released into the systemic circulation. At steady state during an infusion of L-(1-^{13}C)leucine intracellular KIC ^{13}C enrichment will match intracellular leucine ^{13}C enrichment for those tissues that release KIC into plasma, because intracellular leucine is the only net KIC producer source. Thus, plasma KIC ^{13}C enrichment should equal intracellular leucine ^{13}C enrichment integrated over the major KIC-exporting tissues.

is unclear whether the precursor is taken from the free intracellular leucine pool or, in large part, extracted directly from the extracellular free leucine pool (McKee et al., 1978; Schneible et al., 1981). The magnitude of uncertainty in the calculations will be bounded by the plasma leucine ^{13}C enrichment on the one hand, and the intracellular free leucine ^{13}C enrichment on the other. Using plasma (1-^{13}C)KIC enrichment as an index of the latter, we can address the question: what is the magnitude of the difference between plasma leucine and KIC ^{13}C enrichment in man, and is this difference affected by metabolic changes?

METHODS

Subjects, Diet, and Infusion Protocol

Young, healthy, normal weight for height, male adults were studied at the Massachusetts Institute of Technology (MIT) Clinical Research Center. Written consent was obtained from each subject in accordance with the protocols approved by the MIT Committee on the Use of Humans as Experimental Subjects and the Policy and Executive Committees of the MIT Clinical Research Center. Subjects were maintained for 5- to 7-day periods on whole-egg protein diets supplemented with vitamins, minerals, and trace elements as previously described (Motil et al., 1981a,b); the energy intake of each subject's diet was always maintained at each subject's normal level (ca. 47 kcal $kg^{-1}d^{-1}$). The protein content of the diet was reduced sequentially between dietary periods from a normal, generous protein intake (1.5 g $kg^{-1}d^{-1}$) to deficient protein intake (0.1 or 0.0 g $kg^{-1}d^{-1}$). At the end of each dietary period, subjects were given a primed, continuous infusion of L-(1-^{13}C)leucine. Two sets of infusion studies were conducted on different occasions with different L-(1-^{13}C)leucine infusion and dietary protocols. In the first set, subjects (group A) received L-(1-^{13}C)leucine infusions at three levels of protein intake: 1.5 (generous), 0.6 (maintenance), and 0.1 (deficient) g-protein $kg^{-1}d^{-1}$. Leucine kinetic data for these infusions have already been reported (Motil et al., 1981a,b). In the second infusion series, subjects (group B) received L-(1-^{13}C)leucine infusions at four levels of protein intake: 1.5, 0.6, 0.3, 0.0 g $kg^{-1}d^{-1}$.

At the end of each dietary period, each subject was given a primed, continuous infusion of L-(1-^{13}C)leucine via an antecubital vein. For group A subjects, blood was sampled from a contralateral antecubital vein. For group B subjects, blood was sampled from an ipsilateral superficial dorsal hand vein, while the hand was warmed in a heated-hand-box (autoregulated 68°C internal termperature) to obtain "arterialized" venous blood samples (Abumrad et al., 1981). Group A subjects were given a primed (1.9 μmol kg^{-1}) continuous infusion (2.3 μmol $kg^{-1}h^{-1}$) of L-(1-^{13}C)leucine for four hours; group B subjects were given a primed (4.2 μmol kg^{-1}) continuous infusion (4.8 μmol $kg^{-1}h^{-1}$) of L-(1-^{13}C)leucine for 3.5 hours. (Different L-(1-^{13}C)leucine primed and infusion doses were used for group A and B infusions because of different initial designs for each study.)

Two types of infusion protocols were used for both group A and B subjects: some subjects were infused in the postabsorptive state at 8 AM after fasting overnight for 12 hours; other subjects were infused in the fed state starting at 1 PM. The latter subjects received one twelfth of their daily food intake per hour during the infusion by combining their noon and evening meals into six aliquots, which were administered hourly beginning at noon, one hour prior to the start of the isotope infusion (Motil et al., 1981a,b).

Analytical Methods

Free amino acids were isolated from plasma and (1-^{13}C)leucine enrichments were measured by methane CI-GCMS and selected ion monitoring of the $[MH]^+$ and $[MH+1]^+$ ions (m/z = 216 and 217) as previously described (Matthews et al., 1979, 1980). Branched-chain α-keto acids were isolated from plasma and derivatized as the trimethylsilyl-quinoxalinol derivatives as previously reported (Schwarz et al., 1980). Plasma (1-^{13}C)KIC enrichments were determined by selected ion monitoring CI-GCMS of the $[MH]^+$ and $[MH+1]^+$ ions (m/z = 275 and 276) in the same fashion used for determining plasma (1-^{13}C)leucine enrichment (Matthews et al., 1979).

RESULTS

Figure 2 shows the measured plasma (1-^{13}C)KIC and (1-^{13}C)leucine enrichment ratios for plasma samples taken from study A L-(1-^{13}C)leucine infusion studies at three different levels of dietary protein intake. Select plasma samples obtained at isotopic steady state (three to four hours after start of the primed L-(1-^{13}C)leucine infusion) were measured, depending upon availability of plasma remaining from these former studies (Motil et al., 1981a,b). Typically, the plasma (1-^{13}C)leucine enrichment varied from 1.5 to 2.5 mol% excess over the range of dietary conditions used (Motil et al., 1981a,b). Because of the range of leucine ^{13}C enrichments between infusions, Figure 2 data are expressed directly as the ^{13}C enrichment ratio of plasma (1-^{13}C)KIC/(1-^{13}C)leucine. The ratio of KIC to leucine ^{13}C remained remarkably constant near 79%, both over a wide range of protein intakes and between the postabsorptive and fed states. Furthermore, there was no significant difference or correlation between either protein intake or the postabsorptive and fed states (two-way mixed-mode analysis of variance).

In study B, six subjects were infused over four levels of protein intake (Figure 3). The plasma (1-^{13}C)leucine ranged from 3 to 6 mol% excess across the dietary conditions used, and the enrichment ratio of plasma KIC/leucine ^{13}C enrichment ratio remained relatively constant (mean $\pm$ SE = 75 $\pm$ 1%). However, small significant differences in the KIC/leucine ^{13}C enrichment ratio were found between group B postabsorptively infused and fed infused individuals and between dietary protein intake levels ($p < 0.05$, two-way analysis of variance with replication). The variance between individuals was large enough, though, that no significant differences were found between the venous (Figure 2) and arterialized-venous plasma (Figure 3) KIC/leucine ^{13}C enrichment data.

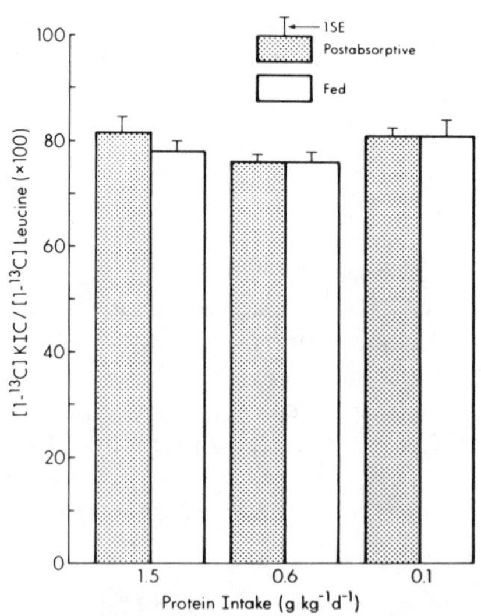

Figure 2 Plasma enrichment ratio of (1-^{13}C)KIC/(1-^{13}C)leucine for venous blood samples taken during a primed L-(1-^{13}C)leucine infusion. The enrichment ratio data are for study A. Between one and eight plasma samples per infusion per subject were taken at isotopic plateau. The number of subjects studied at each dietary intake level were 4, 10, and 4 at 1.5, 0.6, and 0.1 g-protein kg^{-1}d^{-1}, respectively.

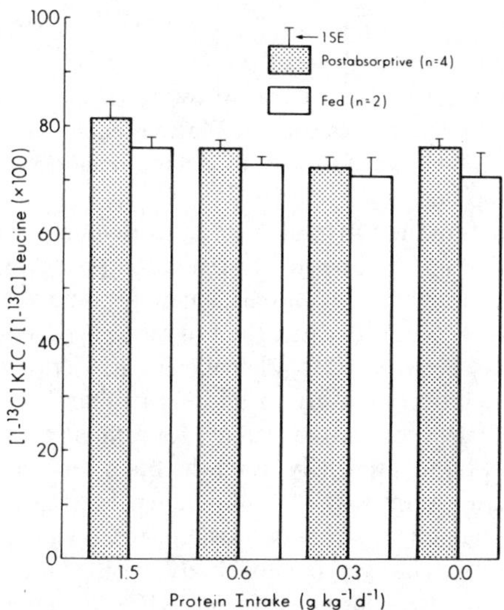

Figure 3 Plasma enrichment ratio of (1-^{13}C)KIC/(1-^{13}C)leucine for "arterialized" venous blood samples taken during a primed L-(1-^{13}C)leucine infusion. The enrichment ratio data are for study B. Four plasma samples, taken at isotopic plateau, were measured per infusion study and subject. The same four subjects were infused in the postabsorptive state, and the same two subjects were infused in the fed state at all four levels of dietary intake.

DISCUSSION

Because intracellular leucine is the precursor for plasma KIC (Adibi, 1976; Harper and Zapalowski, 1981), plasma KIC should reflect its former intracellular leucine environment. Therefore, plasma (1-^{13}C)KIC enrichment can be used to measure intracellular (1-^{13}C)leucine enrichment indirectly during a primed, continuous infusion of L-(1-^{13}C)leucine without the need for muscle biopsy specimens. We have measured the ratio of plasma KIC to leucine ^{13}C enrichment for subjects infused with L-(1-^{13}C)leucine over a wide range of protein intakes, from generous to deficient, and in both the postabsorptive and fed states. The KIC/leucine ^{13}C enrichment ratio was found to be remarkably constant (71% to 82%) over this extreme range of conditions (Figures 2 and 3). There was no significant correlation of KIC/leucine ^{13}C with protein intake or postabsorptive versus fed in the Figure 2 data, but there were small significant differences between protein intake levels and postabsorptive versus fed in the Figure 3 data. The latter represents the more detailed and defined study, but even here the magnitudes of the differences are remarkably minor: the largest difference in KIC/leucine ^{13}C enrichment ratio (81.7 − 71.0 = 10.7%) is small compared to the extreme dietary and protein intake differences (postabsorptive and 1.5 g kg^{-1}d^{-1} protein intake versus fed and 0.0 g kg^{-1}d^{-1} intake). The average value for the ratio between plasma (1-^{13}C)KIC and (1-^{13}C)leucine for the combined group A and group B mean data is 77 ± 1% (mean ± SE).

The intracellular (1-^{13}C)leucine enrichment, reflected by plasma (1-^{13}C)KIC enrichment, is expected to be lower than the corresponding plasma (1-^{13}C)leucine enrichment because of the preferential release of unlabeled leucine from protein breakdown into the intracellular milieu (Figure 1). Thus, the ^{13}C enrichment ratio of plasma KIC to leucine of 77% indicates that the inflow of plasma leucine into cells comprises 77% of the intracellular leucine inflow, with the remaining 23% coming from leucine release via protein breakdown. Plasma leucine inflow into cells would be, therefore, 77/23 = 3.4 times faster than leucine release via protein breakdown for the integrated whole body.

The above data define the range of isotopic enrichment that could be used to calculate whole body rates of leucine flux or oxidation (Waterlow et al., 1978; Matthews et al., 1980) from a high precursor enrichment (plasma (1-^{13}C)leucine) to a low enrichment (plasma (1-^{13}C)KIC). Because the full range between the two estimates is only 20% (the difference between plasma leucine and KIC enrichments) and because the true precursor enrichment is likely to be intermediate between the two values (Waterlow et al., 1978), the range of uncertainty for estimation of whole body amino acid kinetics is not that large, especially when the other assumptions of the method are considered. More importantly, the ^{13}C enrichment ratio between plasma leucine and KIC was found to remain remarkably constant over a wide range of dietary conditions. Thus, comparative changes in whole body leucine kinetics would still be the same regardless of whether plasma leucine, KIC, or intermediate value ^{13}C enrichments were used for the calculations.

ACKNOWLEDGMENT

The authors thank C. Bilmazes, L.L. Su-Chu, and B.J. Thielan for technical assistance. This work was supported in part by NIH grants AM25994, RR954, AM15856, RR88, the National Livestock and Meat Board, and the Schweizerischer Nationalfonds grant 83.748.079.

REFERENCES

Abumrad, N.N., Rabin, D., Diamond, M.P., and Lacy, W.W. (1981): Use of a heated superficial hand vein as an alternative site for the measurement of amino acid concentrations and for the study of glucose and alanine kinetics in man. *Metabolism* 30:936–940.

Adibi, S.A. (1976): Metabolism of branched-chain amino acids in altered nutrition. *Metabolism* 25:1287–1302.

Golden, M.H.N. and Waterlow, J.C. (1977): Total protein synthesis in elderly people: a comparison of results with (^{15}N)glycine and (^{14}C)leucine. *Clin. Sci. Mol. Med.* 53:277–288.

Harper, A.E., and Zapalowski, C. (1981): Interorgan relationships in the metabolism of the branched-chain amino and α-ketoacids. In *Metabolism and Clinical Implications of Branched Chain Amino and Ketoacids* (eds: M. Walser and J.R. Williamson), pp. 195–203, Elsevier/North-Holland, New York.

Ichihara, A., Noda, C., and Tanaka, K. (1981): Oxidation of branched chain amino acids with special reference to their transaminase. In *Metabolism and Clinical Implications of Branched Chain Amino and Ketoacids* (eds: M. Walser and J.R. Williamson), pp. 227–231, Elsevier/North-Holland, New York.

Matthews, D.E., Ben-Galim, E., and Bier, D.M. (1979): Determination of stable isotope enrichment in individual amino acids by chemical ionization mass spectrometry. *Anal. Chem.* 51:80–84.

Matthews, D.E., Bier, D.M., Rennie, M.J., Edwards, R.H.T., Halliday, D., Millward, D.J., and Clugston, G.A. (1981): Regulation of leucine metabolism in man: a stable isotope study. *Science* 214:1129–1131.

Matthews, D.E., Motil, K.J., Rohrbaugh, D.K., Burke, J.F., Young, V.R., and Bier, D.M. (1980): Measurement of leucine metabolism in man from a primed, continous infusion of L-(1-^{13}C)leucine. *Am. J. Physiol.* 238:E473–E479.

McKee, E.E., Cheung, J.Y., Rannels, D.E., and Morgan, H.E. (1978): Measurement of the rate of protein synthesis and compartmentation of heart phenylalanine. *J. Biol. Chem.* 253:1030–1040.

Motil, K.J., Bier, D.M., Matthews, D.E., Burke, J.F., and Young, V.R. (1981b): Whole body leucine and lysine metabolism: response in healthy young men given excess energy intake. *Metabolism* 30:783–791.

Motil, K.J., Matthews, D.E., Bier, D.M., Burke, J.F., Munro, H.N., and Young, V.R. (1981a): Whole-body leucine and lysine metabolism: response to dietary protein intake in young men. *Am. J. Physiol.* 240:E712–E721.

Schneible, P.A., Airhart, J., and Low, R.B. (1981): Differential compartmentation of leucine for oxidation and for protein synthesis in cultured skeletal muscle. *J. Biol. Chem.* 256:4888–4894.

Schwarz, H.P., Karl, I.E., and Bier, D.M. (1980): The α-keto acids of branched-chain amino acids: simplified derivatization for physiological samples and complete separation as quinoxalinols by packed column gas chromatography. *Anal. Biochem.* 108:360–366.

Waterlow, J.C., Garlick, P.J., and Millward, D.J. (1978): *Protein Turnover in Mammalian Tissues and in the Whole Body*. Elsevier/North-Holland, Amsterdam.

SECTION IV
Amino Acid–Organ Interrelationships

LIVER

10 Role of Amino Acid Availability in the Regulation of Liver Protein Synthesis

Leonard S. Jefferson
Kathryn E. Flaim

There has been considerable interest in the possible role of amino acid supply in the regulation of liver protein synthesis (Munro et al., 1975). However, the exact nature of such a role has been a controversial point. Furthermore, the mechanism(s) responsible for mediating effects of amino acid supply on liver protein synthesis is as yet unresolved. *In vivo,* the liver is exposed to wide fluctuations in amino acid supply and attempts have been made to describe the effects of such changes using the isolated perfused liver as a model system in which more precise control of amino acid concentrations is possible. Studies with perfused rat liver have demonstrated that maximum rates of protein synthesis are maintained only if amino acids are provided at concentrations higher than those present in normal rat plasma (Jefferson and Korner, 1969). However, this finding has been challenged by other studies. Whereas a limited ability of amino acids to stimulate liver protein synthesis has been observed by some investigators (Woodside and Mortimore, 1972), others have been unable to improve synthesis rates by providing higher than normal amino acid concentrations (Tavill et al., 1973; Peavy and Hansen, 1976).

It has been difficult to resolve conflicts among these reports because of variations in experimental technique. Determination of protein synthesis is complicated by several factors including difficulties inherent in separating actions of amino acids on protein synthesis from actions on protein degradation. If precursor-specific activity is not rigorously controlled, an increase in protein degradation can alter precursor-specific activity to give the appearance of a decrease in protein synthesis. The study of liver protein synthesis is further complicated by the fact that there are two categories of liver proteins, secretory and nonsecretory proteins. Determinations of protein synthesis made over short intervals indicate total liver protein synthesis, while measurements made over long intervals primarily represent nonsecretory protein synthesis.

Although measurements of protein synthesis which rely on incorporation of radioactively labeled precursors have produced inconsistent results, other approaches have indicated that protein synthesis in liver is indeed regulated by amino acid supply. Studies of polyribosome profiles on sucrose density gradients have shown a reduced state of ribosomal aggregation in livers perfused with a medium deficient in amino acids (Jefferson and Korner, 1969; Van Den Borre and Webb, 1972; McGown et al., 1973). This led to the proposal that inhibition of peptide-chain initiation is responsible for reduced protein synthesis occurring in livers perfused with amino acid-deficient medium (Jefferson and Korner, 1969).

Similar effects of amino acid deficiency on protein synthesis and polysomal aggregation have been shown to occur in a number of cell types (Eliasson et al., 1967; Lee et al., 1971; Vaughan et al., 1971; van Venrooij et al., 1972; Christman, 1973; Pain and Henshaw, 1975). In these studies a block in peptide-chain initiation is also indicated by the occurrence of polysomal disaggregation in cells made deficient in one or more amino acids. Although the nature of the defect in initiation is unknown, it does not appear to result from a loss of mRNA since reversal is rapid and is not prevented by actinomycin D (Eliasson et al., 1967; Lee et al., 1971; Vaughan et al., 1971; Christman, 1973).

We have investigated the effects of amino acid supply on protein synthesis in the perfused rat liver with the intent of resolving some of the controversy in the literature and providing insight into the underlying mechanisms (Flaim et al., 1982a and b). In our studies, livers have been perfused with a nonrecirculating medium to strictly control the perfusate amino acid concentrations, and the specific activity of the labeled precursor amino acid has been rigidly maintained by expansion of the intracellular amino acid pool to minimize dilution of specific activity by amino acids released during proteolysis. Additionally, rates of total protein (nonsecreted plus secreted) synthesis and the relative rate of synthesis of one secretory protein, albumin, have been determined in perfusions of varying durations to ensure that an effect of amino acids would not be missed due to the selection of an inappropriate time interval. We have investigated the mechanism of the impairment in protein synthesis occurring in livers perfused with a medium deficient in amino acids by determining if polysomal disaggregation is due to reduced availability of translatable mRNA or to reduced joining of initiation factors to form initiation complexes.

RESULTS AND DISCUSSION

The response of liver protein synthesis to variations in amino acid supply was tested using a continuous labeling technique in livers perfused for 30 minutes with a nonrecirculating medium consisting of Krebs-Henseleit bicarbonate buffer, pH 7.4, containing 10 mM glucose, 3% bovine serum albumin, 25% washed bovine erythrocytes, 5 mM [^{3}H]leucine (3.3 x 10^6 dpm/μmol) and other amino acids at 0, 1, 2, 5 or 10 times normal rat arterial plasma concentrations (Figure 10-1) (Tolman et al., 1973). [^{3}H]Leucine incorporation was determined in trichloroacetic acid precipitates of frozen liver powder and rates of protein synthesis were calculated using the leucine-specific activity, leucine content of liver protein, 9.6% (Peters, 1975), and protein content of liver, 200 mg/g (Flaim et al., 1982a).

Increasing perfusate amino acid concentrations up to five times those found in normal rat plasma stimulated protein synthesis above the rate measured when no amino acids were provided. The synthesis rate with either five or ten times plasma amino acid concentrations was twice the rate found in livers in the amino acid-deprived condition. This represents a synthesis rate of about 0.6 g protein per day which is similar to the *in vivo* rate reported by McNurlan et al. (1979). The addition of ten times plasma concentrations of amino acids was chosen for amino acid supplementation in subsequent experiments in which maximal synthesis rates were desired.

These results confirmed the earlier findings of Jefferson and Korner (1969). The failure of some investigations to substantiate these effects may reside in mistaken assumptions about the specific activity of the labeled amino acid precursor pool or in differences in the duration of experiments. The rates of protein synthesis presented in Figure 10-1 were calculated from the specific activity of extracellular [^{3}H]leucine assuming that in the presence of 5 mM leucine (approximately 25 times normal plasma levels) the specific activity of tRNA-bound leucine would be the same as that of the extracellular amino acid. That this was a valid assumption is illustrated in

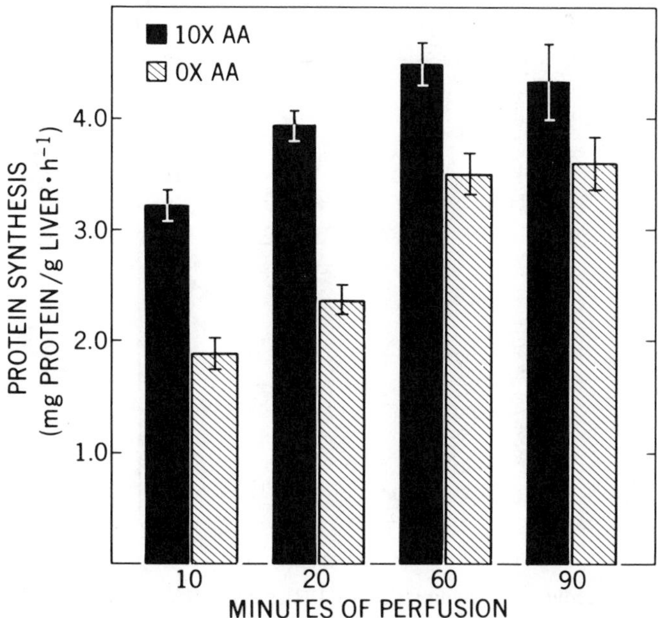

Figure 10-1 Rates of protein synthesis in perfused rat liver in response to varying perfusate amino acid concentrations. Synthesis rate with either five or ten times normal plasma amino acid concentrations was twice the rate measured when no amino acids were present. Values are means ± S.E.M.

Figure 10-2. In these experiments, rates of equilibration of the specific activities of tRNA-bound leucine were determined after a 15-minute preperfusion with a nonrecirculating medium consisting of Krebs-Henseleit bicarbonate buffer, pH 7.4, containing 10 mM glucose, 3% bovine serum albumin, 25% washed bovine erythrocytes, 5 mM leucine and other amino acids at zero or ten times normal rat arterial plasma concentrations (Panel A) (Tolman et al., 1973). After 15 minutes, livers were exposed to the same medium containing [^{3}H]leucine (3.3×10^6 dpm/μmol) and at intervals in frozen liquid nitrogen. The specific activities of [^{3}H]leucine in acid-soluble material in perfusate and in phenol-extracted leucyl-tRNA^{Leu} were determined (Flaim et al., 1982a). tRNA-bound leucine-specific activities were identical in perfusions containing zero or ten times normal plasma amino acid concentrations. Rates of equilibration were compared with the rate of incorporation of [^{3}H]leucine into total liver protein with the amino acid supplemented medium (Panel B). With leucine present at 5 mM concentrations, tRNA-bound leucine-specific activities in livers perfused with either amino acid-deficient or amino acid-supplemented medium were equal to the perfusate leucine-specific activity after two minutes. This two-minute equilibration period was associated with a delay of similar duration in the establishment of linear incorporation of [^{3}H]leucine into protein. Thus, the specific activity of perfusate leucine provides a good estimate of actual precursor specific activity. Synthesis rates measured over ten-minute intervals are slightly underestimated when calculated on the basis of perfusate-specific activity due to the two-minute equilibration period.

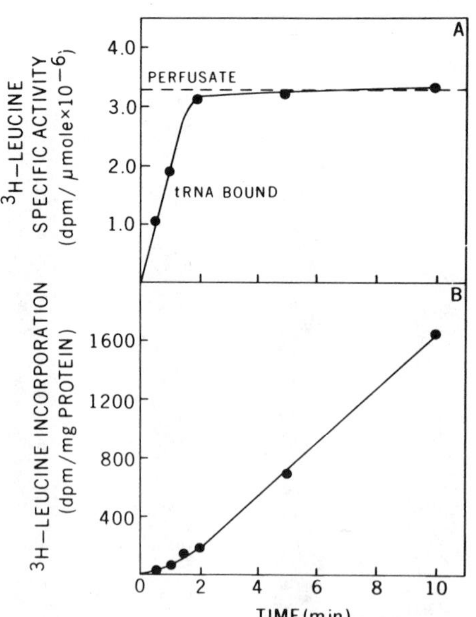

Figure 10-2 Time course of equilibration of [^{3}H]leucyl-tRNA^{Leu} specific activity and of [^{3}H]leucine incorporation into protein. See text for details. Panel A: tRNA-bound leucine-specific activities with zero or ten times normal amino acid concentrations. Perfusate leucine specific activity is indicated by the dashed line. Panel B: leucine incorporation into acid precipitable material in livers perfused with ten times plasma amino acid concentrations is shown. Values are means of two to four determinations.

We next examined the possibility that the influence of perfusate amino acid supply on liver protein synthesis may change with the duration of perfusion. A ten-minute pulse labeling interval was used to determine total protein synthesis (secreted plus nonsecreted) since radioactivity incorporated into secretory proteins would not be lost from the liver in less than 15 minutes (Feldhoff et al., 1977). As illustrated in Figure 10-3, after short preperfusions, five or 15 minutes, rates of synthesis obtained with amino acid-deficient and with amino acid-supplemented medium differed markedly. Synthesis rates increased with time of perfusion under both amino acid conditions. However, in the amino acid-deficient condition, synthesis rates increased more dramatically, such that after an 85 min preperfusion protein synthesis in livers receiving an amino acid-supplemented medium was only marginally higher than in the deficient condition. In many previous studies the perfusion medium was allowed to recirculate, thus permitting the amino acid concentrations to vary with time, which might account for the inability of higher than normal levels of amino acids to stimulate protein synthesis in those studies (Woodside and Mortimore, 1972; Tavill et al., 1973; Peavy and Hansen, 1976). Additionally, the fact that protein synthesis was assessed after perfusion periods in excess of one hour (Woodside and Mortimore, 1972; Peavy and Hanse, 1976) would, according to our findings, reduce the possibility of detecting an effect of exogenous amino acid concentrations on protein synthesis. In fact, Woodside and Mortimore (1972) were able to measure stimulation of protein synthesis by provision of excess amino acids in livers perfused for less than 30 minutes; however, this effect vanished with increased duration of perfusion.

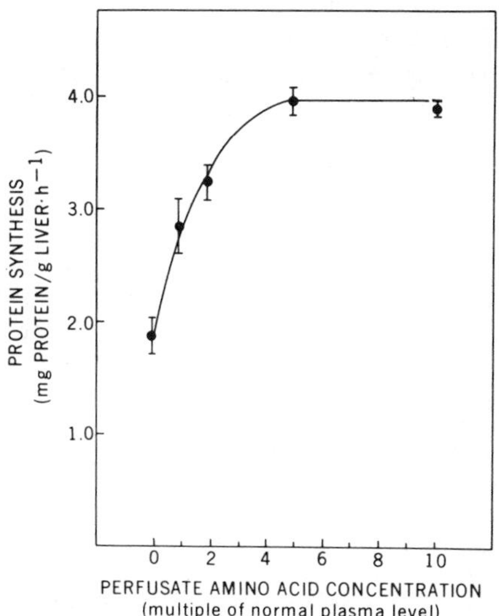

Figure 10-3 Time course of effects of amino acid-supplemented and amino acid-deficient media on rates of total protein synthesis in perfused rat liver. Livers were preperfused for 5, 15, 55, or 85 minutes with the standard medium containing 5 mM nonradioactive leucine and either no other amino acids (0X AA) or ten times plasma concentrations of other amino acids (10X AA). Livers were then labeled with [^{3}H]leucine (3.3×10^6 dpm/μmol) for ten minutes and were excised for determination of incorporation of radioactivity into acid precipitable material. Rates of protein synthesis were calculated for 10 (5–15), 20 (15–25), 60 (55–65) and 90 (85–95) minutes of perfusion. Values are means ± S.E.M.

The possibility that amino acid supply might have a selective effect on secretory protein synthesis was investigated by assessing the synthesis of albumin, the major secretory protein produced by the liver (Peters, 1975). The relative rate of albumin synthesis did not vary with perfusate amino acid concentrations or with duration of perfusion (Flaim et al., 1982a) and, therefore, the synthesis of secretory proteins is probably subject to regulation by amino acid supply in a manner similar to total liver proteins.

The recovery of protein synthesis during perfusion could be due to an accumulation of intracellular amino acids derived from internal sources. Such an accumulation could result from the spontaneous rise in proteolysis which occurs within 30 minutes of the start of perfusion with an amino acid-deficient medium (Woodside and Mortimore, 1972). To examine this possibility, we studied the effects of inhibitors of protein breakdown on the ability of the protein synthetic process to recover from inhibition in perfusions with amino acid-deficient medium. Both insulin (Mortimore and Mondon, 1970) and glutamine (Schworer and Mortimore, 1979) have been shown to suppress the rise in proteolysis which occurs in perfused livers. When insulin (500 μU/ml) or ten times normal plasma concentrations of glutamine were included in the amino acid-deficient medium, rates of synthesis after 25 minutes were low and were not increased in perfusions of 95-minutes duration (Figure 10-4). Thus, these data suggest that a rise in proteolysis is essential for the recovery of the protein synthetic process which has been limited by a lack of amino acids.

A possible source of the defect in protein synthesis in livers perfused with an amino acid-deficient medium is the extent of aminoacylation of tRNA. The effect of dietary tryptophan deficiency in rats to inhibit liver protein synthesis (Munro et al., 1975) has been attributed to a reduced charging of $tRNA^{Trp}$(Allen et al., 1969). Furthermore, experiments designed to alter charging of tRNA by using competitive in-

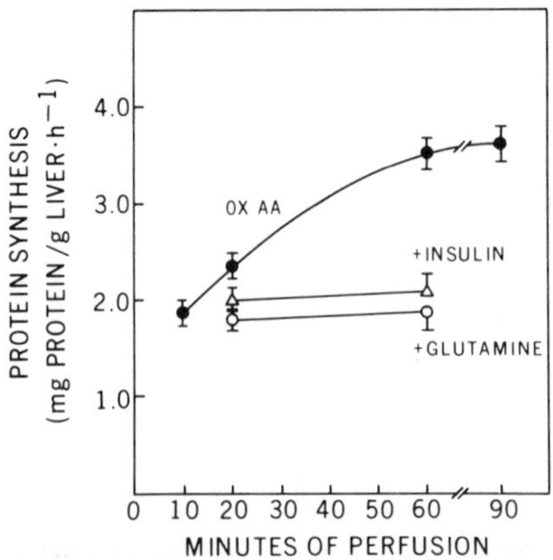

Figure 10-4 Effects of inhibitors of proteolysis on rates of protein synthesis in rat liver perfused with amino acid-deficient medium. Livers were perfused in a nonrecirculating manner with the standard medium containing 5 mM leucine and a) no other amino acids (0X AA, data from Figure 10-3); b) ten times normal rat plasma concentrations of glutamine; or c) 500 mU/ml of insulin. Rates of protein synthesis were determined from the rate of incorporation of [^{3}H]leucine into total protein during a ten-minute pulse labeling interval encompassing the indicated time points as described in Figure 10-3.

hibitors of aminoacylation of tRNA or mutant cell lines that have high Kms for tRNA synthetases have provided evidence in support of a role for tRNA in the regulation of protein synthesis (Vaughan and Hansen, 1973; Warrington et al., 1977; Lofgren and Thompson, 1979; Scornik et al., 1980).

We investigated this possibility by quantitating individual tRNA-bound amino acids in unperfused livers and livers perfused for 20 minutes with an amino acid-deficient or supplemented medium. The quantities of amino acids bound to tRNA for each of 16 amino acids are shown in Figure 10-5. In all cases, the quantities of tRNA-bound amino acids were virtually unchanged from the unperfused condition by perfusion with either an amino acid-deficient or supplemented medium at a time

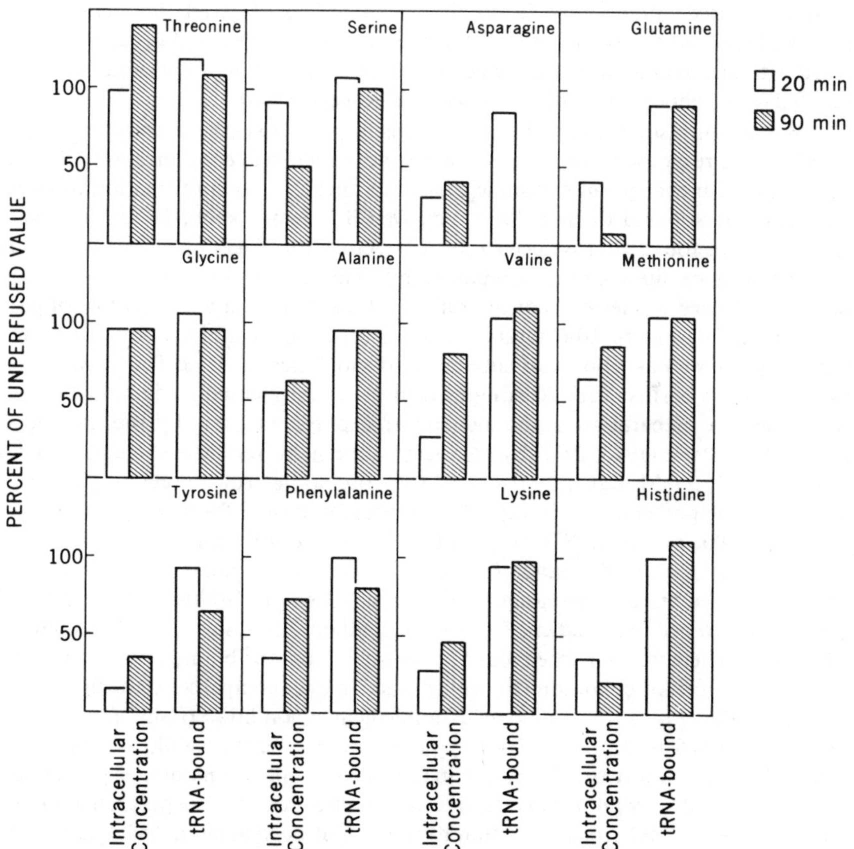

Figure 10-5 Effects of perfusion with amino acid deficient medium on quantities of intracellular and tRNA bound amino acids in rat liver. Livers were perfused for 20 or 90 minutes with the standard medium with no added amino acids other than 5 mM leucine. Following perfusion livers were excised, rapidly frozen, and intracellular amino acids were extracted with sulfosalicylic acid (Flaim et al., 1982a). Livers from three rats were pooled for extraction of tRNA-bound amino acids with phenol (Flaim et al., 1982a). Values for 16 amino acids are expressed as percentages of values obtained from unperfused liver tissue. Values were not obtained for asparagine bound to tRNA after 90 minutes of perfusion. All values are means of three to five determinations.

when rates of protein synthesis were maximally divergent in the two perfusion conditions. Similar amino acid values were obtained when aminoacyl-tRNA was extracted from livers perfused for 90 minutes with amino acid-deficient medium. The total amount of tRNA-bound amino acids averaged 32.5 nmol per g liver. Based on an average total RNA content of liver of 7.5 mg of RNA per g and assuming tRNA to have an average molecular weight of 25,000, the amount of tRNA which was aminoacylated represented 11% of the total liver RNA. This value is in good agreement with estimated values for the total tRNA content of liver (Munro, 1970), suggesting that tRNA was fully charged under all conditions examined. Therefore, neither a change in the charging levels of total tRNA nor a change in the amount of a specific amino acid bound to tRNA appears to be the basis for alterations in protein synthesis associated with amino acid supply. A similar lack of correlation between protein synthesis and the extent of tRNA charging has been reported in rat hearts perfused with different amino acid concentrations (Morgan et al., 1981) and in livers of rats fed a protein-deficient diet (Shenoy and Rogers, 1978).

We next investigated whether alterations in protein synthesis occurring in perfused liver in response to variations in perfusate amino acid concentrations could be correlated with changes in ribosome cycle intermediates. In confirmation of earlier reports (Jefferson and Korner, 1969; Van Den Borre and Webb, 1972; McGown et al., 1973), we found that reduced rates of synthesis in livers perfused with amino acid-deficient medium were accompanied by reduced rates of peptide-chain initiation as evidenced by elevated concentrations of ribosomal subunits and loss of polysomal material. Figure 10-6 illustrates the profiles of membrane-bound and free polysomes as well as ribosomal subunits and monomers isolated from unperfused liver and livers perfused for 20 minutes with the supplemented medium or the deficient medium. Separation of bound and free polysomes was by the method of Ramsey and Steele (1976; 1977) by homogenization in buffer (50 mM Hepes, pH 7.4, 250 mM KC1, 5 mM $MgCl_2$, and 250 mM sucrose) as described previously (Flaim et al., 1982b). Supernatants were centrifuged through linear 20% to 47% sucrose gradients at 41,000 rpm in an SW 41 rotor for 110 minutes for separation of polysomes (Panels b, d, f, h) or for seven hours for separation of nonpolysomal material, ribosomal subunits and monomers (Panels a, c, e, g). Gradients were pumped through a flow cell in a gradient fractionator and optical absorbance at 254 nm was monitored. There was a marked loss of polysomes from the bound population in the amino acid-deprived condition (Panel f, dashed line) as compared to the unperfused condition (Panel b) or the amino acid-supplemented condition (Panel f, solid line). The loss of RNA from the bound polysomes in the deficient condition was accompanied not only by a twofold increase in the free subunit and monomer populations (Panel g), but also by an increase in the RNA content of the free polysome population (Flaim et al., 1982b). In addition to the loss of polysomal material, a decrease occurred in the average size of bound polysomes from approximately 15 to 17 ribosomes per mRNA molecule in the unperfused and amino acid-supplemented conditions to approximately 10 to 11 ribosomes per mRNA molecule in the amino acid-deprived condition.

The loss of polysomal material did not appear to result from mRNA degradation for two reasons. First, the polysome profiles did not show a major increase in small polysomal material which would be expected if mRNA degradation had occurred. Second, after 90 minutes of perfusion with amino acid-deficient medium, subunit levels were reduced suggesting a movement of ribosomes back into

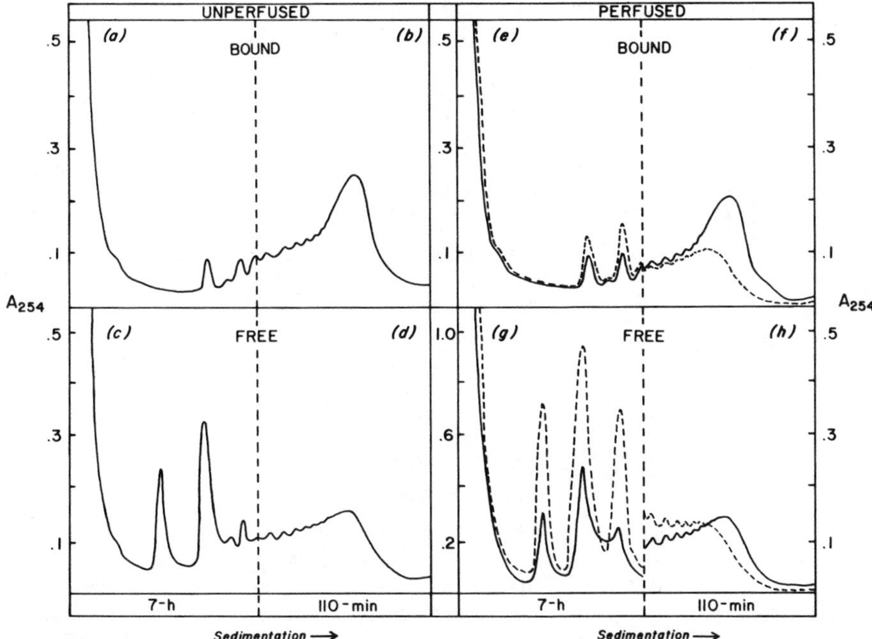

Figure 10-6 Effect of medium amino acid concentrations on distribution of ribosomal subunits and polysomes in perfused rat liver. Unperfused livers (Panels a–d), and livers perfused for 20 minutes (Panels e–h) with either the amino acid-deficient (0X, dashed line) or amino acid-supplemented (10X, solid line) medium. See text for details. Due to the recovery of large quantities of ribosomal subunits in the amino acid deprived condition, the A_{254} scale on Panel g is 1.0 as compared to 0.5 units on the other panels.

polysomes (Flaim et al., 1982b). Because this evidence is indirect, the reversibility of polysomal disaggregation was specifically examined. Livers were perfused with amino acid-deficient medium for 15 minutes to allow disaggregation to occur; perfusion was then continued with amino acid-supplemented medium for 5, 10, 15 or 20 minutes. Following perfusion, livers were homogenized in buffer (50 mM Hepes, pH 7.4, 250 mM KC1, 5 mM $MgCl_2$, and 250 mM sucrose) as described previously (Flaim et al., 1982b). Supernatants were centrifuged through 20% to 47% linear sucrose gradients for 110 minutes or seven hours for separation of ribosomal subunits and monomers (Panel a) and polysomes (Panel b) as described above. Optical absorbance at 254 nm was monitored. As seen in Figure 10-7, free ribosomal particles (Panel a) were able to move back into polysomes (Panel b) and this reversibility of disaggregation followed a time course such that after five minutes of resupplementation very little change had occurred (data not shown) and, after 20 minutes, profiles were nearly like those obtained from livers receiving the supplemented medium for the entire perfusion. Protein synthesis determined during ten minutes of supplementation following 15 minutes of deprivation also indicated a reversal of the inhibition (data not shown). Thus, as was the case with amino acid deficiency in several types of cultured cells (Eliasson et al., 1967; Vaughan et al., 1971; Lee et al., 1971; van Venrooij et al., 1972; Christman, 1973; Pain and Henshaw, 1975), reintroduction of amino acids to the medium induced reaggregation of liver polysomes.

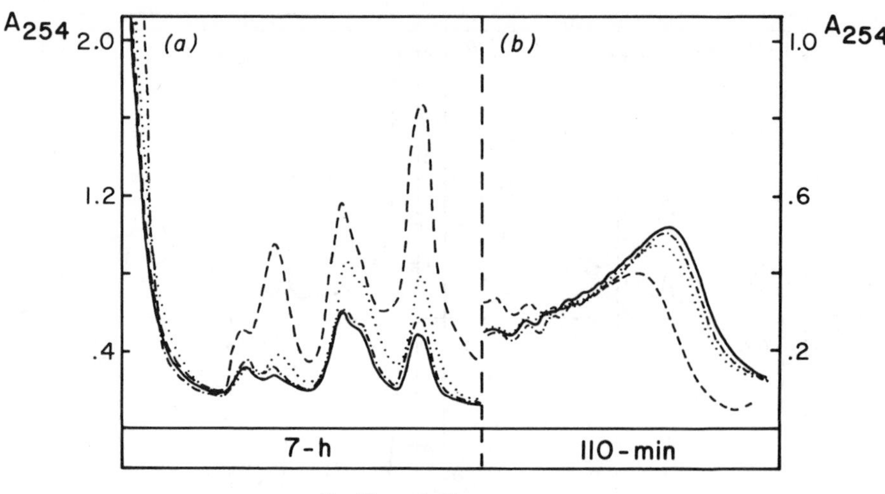

Figure 10-7 Reversibility of polysomal disaggregation induced by perfusion with amino acid deficient medium. Livers were perfused with the amino acid-deficient (0X, dashed line) or the amino acid-supplemented (10X, solid line) medium for 25 minutes, or livers were preperfused for 15 minutes with the amino acid-deficient medium followed by perfusion with the amino acid-supplemented medium for 10 minutes (dashed line) or 20 minutes (dash-dot line). Panel a: Ribosomal subunits and monomers. Panel b: Polysomes.

An inhibition of peptide-chain initiation resulting in a loss of polysomes could be due to a sequestering of mRNA such that there would be less available for initiation. An inhibition of initiation of this nature has been described in livers of starved rats. In those studies a significant sequestration of albumin mRNA as mRNP occurred with starvation and this effect was reversible by amino acid refeeding (Yap et al., 1978a and b). Under such circumstances, however, a decrease in polysome size would not be expected unless there was mRNA degradation or a selective sequestration of certain large species of mRNA. We examined the possibility of sequestration of mRNAs in an untranslatable pool by determining the distribution of a specific liver mRNA, that of albumin. Albumin is the major secretory protein synthesized by the liver and its synthesis responds to amino acid deficiency as does synthesis of total protein (Flaim et al., 1982a).

When the distribution of albumin mRNA in membrane-bound and free supernatant fractions as well as in bound and free polysomal fractions and free nonpolysomal fractions isolated on sucrose density gradients was determined, we obtained the results summarized in Figure 10-8. Livers were perfused for 20 minutes with the amino acid-supplemented (10X, 20 min) or amino acid-deficient (0X, 20 min) medium, or livers were perfused for 15 minutes with amino acid-deficient medium followed by perfusion for 20 minutes with amino acid-supplemented medium (0X, 15 min + 10X, 20 min). Separation of bound and free polysomes and nonpolysomal material, ribosomal subunits and monomers, from polysomes was achieved by the method of Ramsey and Steel (1976; 1977) as described above. Fractions containing membrane bound and free polysomes and the lighter free nonpolysomal material including ribosomal subunits, monomers and free mRNA were collected and total RNA was extracted with guanidine hydrochloride (Chirgwin et al., 1979; Flaim et al.,

1982b). Hybridization of extracted total RNA with albumin cDNA was performed (Tse et al., 1978) and $R_0t\frac{1}{2}$ values (R_0t in mol•s•l^{-1} at 50% hybridization) and albumin mRNA contents were determined (Liao et al., 1980; Flaim et al., 1982b). The albumin mRNA content of each fraction was determined by comparison of $R_0t\frac{1}{2}$ values to $R_0t\frac{1}{2}$ for pure albumin mRNA and from values for RNA contents of each fraction. The albumin mRNA content of each fraction was then expressed as a percentage of the total ablumin mRNA recovered from all fractions. In livers perfused with the supplemented medium, 91% of albumin mRNA was recovered in bound polysomes. The albumin mRNA in the free fraction was distributed almost equally between the polysomal pool and the nonpolysomal pool. Upon perfusion of liver with the amino acid-deficient medium, there was a loss of total polysomal RNA and a loss of half of the RNA in the bound polysome fraction. By comparison, 80% of the albumin mRNA was found in the bound fraction, resulting in a relative enrichment of albumin mRNA in bound polysomes in the amino acid-deficient condition. The free albumin mRNA was again distributed almost equally between the nonpolysomal and the polysomal pools. Contents of total RNA and albumin mRNA were decreased in the nonpolysomal fraction and increased in the polysomal fractions when perfusion with the supplemented medium followed induction of polysomal disaggregation with the deficient medium. Taken together, these results do not point to any significant sequestration of mRNA in a nontranslatable pool. Even though the albumin mRNA content of the free nonpolysomal fraction in the amino acid-deprived condition was twofold higher than in the amino acid-supplemented condition, this only represented 10% of the total albumin mRNA. If sequestration of mRNA, as RNP particles occurred with amino acid-deficient perfusion, an enrichment of mRNA with respect to ribosomes would be expected in the nonpolysomal fraction. This was not the case; albumin mRNA appeared in the nonpolysomal fraction in proportion to the increase in ribosomes. Furthermore, there was only a small loss of albumin mRNA from polysomes.

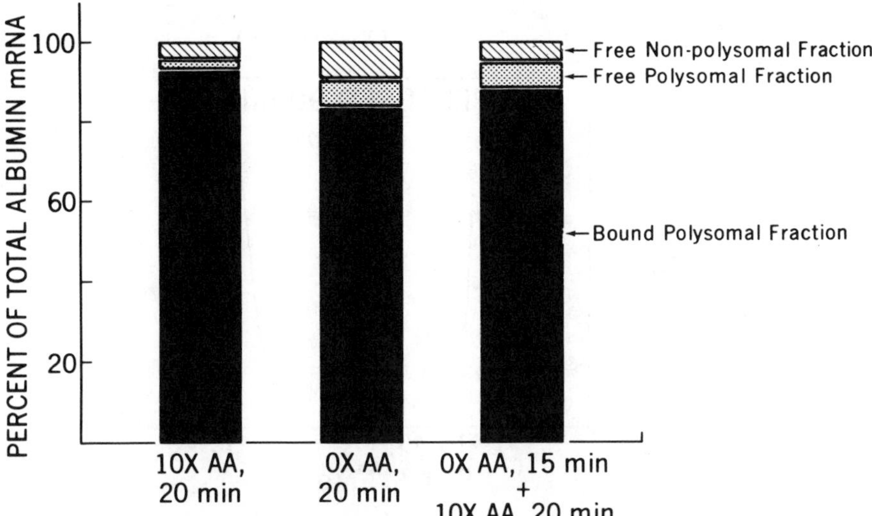

Figure 10-8 Effect of medium amino acid concentrations on albumin mRNA distribution in membrane-bound and free polysome fractions in perfused rat liver. See text for details.

An inhibition of peptide-chain initiation may also have its origin in reduced ability of one or more of the initiation factors to join with the ribosomal subunits and met-tRNA$_f^{Met}$ to form initiation complexes. We investigated this possibility by applying techniques that have proven useful for the study of initiation in Erlich ascites tumor cells (Pain and Henshaw, 1975; Henshaw, 1979). In ascites cells deprived of the essential amino acid lysine, an inhibition of peptide-chain initiation occurred such that ribosomes were released from polysomes (Pain and Henshaw, 1975). Additionally, the profiles of 40S subunits on CsCl density gradients were altered as compared to the profiles from fully supplemented cells (Pain and Henshaw, 1975). The response of the liver to amino acid deprivation appeared to be analogous to that of ascites cells. After 20 minutes of perfusion with the deficient or supplemented amino acid medium, the livers, along with unperfused livers, were homogenized in buffer (20mM triethanolamine, pH 7.4, 25 mM KC1, 2 mM Mg acetate, 0.5 mM dithiothreitol, 0.1 mM EDTA, and 250 mM sucrose) for separation of 40S ribosomal subunits on CsC1 gradient according to the method of Henshaw (1979) as described

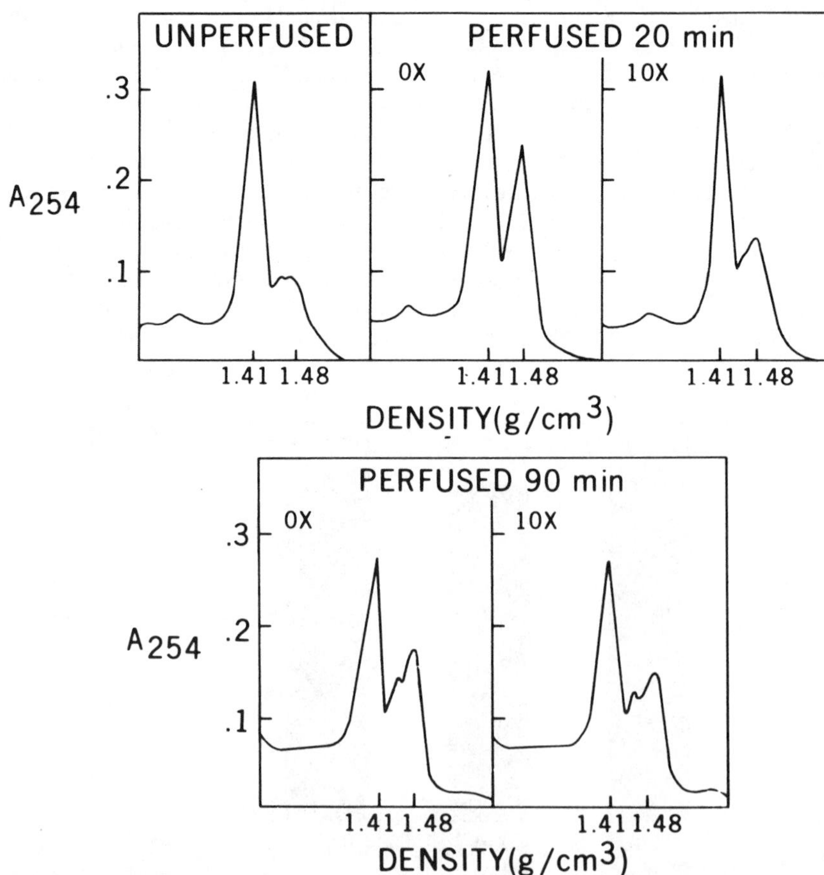

Figure 10-9 Effects of medium amino acid concentrations on the density of 40S ribosomal subunits in perfused rat liver. See text for details. Livers were perfused for 20 or 90 minutes with the amino acid-deficient (0X) or amino acid-supplemented medium (10X).

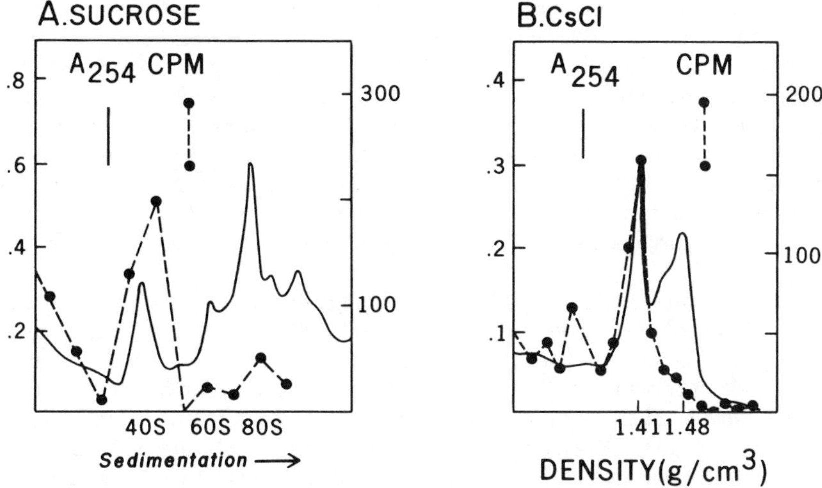

Figure 10-10 [35S]Methionine binding to 40S ribosomal subunits *in vivo*. See text for details. Absorbance at 254 nm (solid lines), radioactivity (dashed lines).

previously (Flaim et al., 1982b). Subunits of 40S isolated from other ribosomal particles on sucrose density gradients were centrifuged through CsCl of density 1.51 g/cm³ for 16 hours at 33,000 rpm in an SW41 rotor. Gradients were pumped through a flow cell and absorbance at 452 nm was monitored. Profiles of 40S subunits on CsCl density gradients resembled the profiles of 40S subunits obtained from unperfused liver with the exception that the species with a higher density, 1.48 g/cm³, showed a slight relative increase (Figure 10-9). When livers were perfused with the amino acid-deficient medium, however, the proportion of subunits existing in the 1.48 g/cm³ form was dramatically increased. After 90 minutes of perfusion, the profiles from the amino acid-deprived and amino acid-supplemented conditions were virtually identical. This correlated with the finding of similar synthesis rates in these conditions after a perfusion period of this duration. In ascites cells, density changes in the 40S subunits represented loss or addition of proteins (Pain and Henshaw, 1975). That these proteins were initiation factors was suggested by the finding of [35S] methionine bound as the 40S initiation complex to the lower density species of the 40S subunit (Smith and Henshaw, 1975). In our studies, [35S]Methionine (1.0 mCi) was infused into the hepatic portal vein of an anesthetized rat over an interval of 5 minutes (Figure 10-10). The liver was removed, homogenized as above, and 40S ribosomal subunits were resolved on sucrose density gradients (Panel A) and CsCl density gradients (Panel B). Absorbance at 254 nm was monitored, fractions were collected, and radioactivity associated with RNA was determined. The radioactivity was localized almost exclusively on the 40S subunit peak on sucrose density gradients. Upon further separation of subunits on CsCl density gradients, the radioactivity was associated only with the low density, 1.41 g/cm³, species of the 40S subunit. To determine the effect of perfusate amino acid concentration on [35S]methionine binding to 40S subunits, [35S]methionine was infused for two minutes in livers preperfused for 20 minutes with amino acid-deficient or supplemented medium. When livers were perfused with the supplemented medium, there were twice as many counts bound per unit RNA in the 40S fraction as compared to the binding when livers received no added amino acids. The intracellular methionine-specific activity in the supplemented condition was tenfold lower than in the deficient condition, undoubtedly as a result of greater competition for transport sites across the cell membrane. Thus, the difference in radioactivity bound in the two conditions would be even greater if intracellular-specific activities had been equal. These results indicated that formation of the 40S initiation complex in liver was inhibited by amino acid deprivation. Pain and Henshaw (1975) demonstrated a similar reduction in the binding of methionine to 40S particles in ascites cells deprived of lysine.

In summary, perfusion of liver with amino acid-deficient medium resulted in reduced rates of protein synthesis as compared to rates in livers receiving amino acid-supplemented medium. The lower synthesis rates were the result of an inhibition of peptide-chain initiation which caused polysomal disaggregation but did not correlate with limited availability of mRNA either due to degradation or sequestration. Examination of the relative amounts of different species of 40S ribosomal subunits and of [^{35}S]methionine binding to 40S subunits indicated reduced joining of initiation factors and met-tRNA$_f^{Met}$ to the 40S subunit. Thus, peptide-chain initiation appeared to be limited by a decreased formation of the 40S initiation complex in acute amino acid deficiency. The mechanism by which amino acid deficiency affects initiation complex formation remains to be described; however, potential regulatory sites for formation of the complex have been described in other systems (Austin and Clemens, 1980). Deficiency of a single or several amino acids may affect one of these regulatory steps. Possibilities include, activation of an eIF-2α kinase, inhibition of an eIF-2α phosphatase, decreased availability of tRNA$_f^{Met}$, inhibition of the synthetase which is specific for tRNA$_f^{Met}$, or decreased activity or availability of accessory factors which act to stabilize the association of eIF-2α with methionyl-tRNA$_f^{Met}$.

REFERENCES

Allen, R.E., Raines, P.L., and Regen, D.M. (1969): Regulatory significance of transfer RNA charging levels. Measurement of charging levels in livers of chow-fed rats, fasting rats, and rats fed balanced or imbalanced mixtures of amino acids. *Biochim. Biophys. Acta* 190:323–336.

Austin, S.A., and Clemens, M.J. (1980): Control of the initiation of protein synthesis in mammalian cells. *FEBS Lett.* 110:1–7.

Chirgwin, J.M., Przybyla, A.E., MacDonald, R.J., and Rutter, W.J. (1979): Isolation of biologically active ribonucleic acid from sources enriched in ribonuclease. *Biochemistry* 18:5294–5299.

Christman, J.K. (1973); Effects of elevated potassium level and amino acid deprivation on polysomal distribution and rate of protein synthesis in L cells. *Biochim. Biophys. Acta* 294:138–152.

Eliasson, E., Bauer, G.E., and Hultin, T. (1967): Reversible degradation of polyribosomes in Chang cells cultured in a glutamine-deficient medium. *J. Cell Biol.* 33:287–297.

Feldhoff, R.C., Taylor, J.M., and Jefferson, L.S. (1977): Synthesis and secretion of rat albumin *in vivo,* in perfused liver, and in isolated hepatocytes: Effects of hypophysectomy and growth hormone treatment. *J. Biol. Chem.* 252:3611–3616.

Flaim, K.E., Peavy, D.E., and Jefferson, L.S. (1982a): The role of amino acids in the regulation of protein synthesis in perfused rat liver. I. Reduction in rates of synthesis resulting from amino acid deprivation and recovery during flow-through perfusion. *J. Biol. Chem.* 257:2932–2938.

Flaim, K.E., Liao, W.S.L., Peavy, D.E., Taylor, J.M., and Jefferson, L.S. (1982b): The role of amino acids in the regulation of protein synthesis in perfused rat liver. II. Effects of amino acid deficiency on peptide-chain initiation, polysomal aggregation and distribution of albumin mRNA. *J. Biol. Chem.* 257:2939–2946.

Henshaw, E.C. (1979): CsC1 equilibrium density gradient analysis of native ribosomal subunits (and ribosomes). *Methods Enzmol.* 59:410–421.

Jefferson, L.S., and Korner, A. (1969): Influence of amino acid supply on ribosomes and protein synthesis of perfused rat liver. *Biochem. J.* 111:703–712.

Lee, S.Y., Krsmanovic, V., and Brawerman, G. (1971): Initiation of polysome formation in mouse sarcoma 180 ascites cells. Utilization of cytoplasmic messenger ribonucleic acid. *Biochemistry* 10:895–900.

Liao, W.S.L., Conn, A.R., and Taylor, J.M. (1980): Changes in rat alpha 1-fetoprotein and albumin mRNA levels during fetal and neonatal development. *J. Biol. Chem.* 255:10036–10039.

Lofgren, D.J., and Thompson, L.H. (1979): Relationship between histidyl-tRNA level and protein synthesis rate in wild-type and mutant Chinese hamster ovary cells. *J. Cell. Physiol.* 99:303–312.

McGown, E., Richardson, A.G., Henderson, L.M., and Swan, P.B. (1973): Effect of amino acids on ribosome aggregation and protein synthesis in perfused rat liver. *J. Nutr.* 103: 109–116.

McNurlan, M.A., Tomkins, A.M., and Garlick, P.J. (1979): The effect of starvation on the rate of protein synthesis in rat liver and small intestine. *Biochem. J.* 178:373–379.

Morgan, H.E., Chua, B.H., Boyd, T.A., and Jefferson, L.S. (1981): Branched-chain amino acids and the regulation of protein turnover in heart and skeletal muscle. In: *Developments in Biochemistry* (eds: M. Walser and J.R. Williamson), Vol. 18, pp. 217–226, Elsevier, New York.

Mortimore, G.E., and Mondon, C.E. (1970): Inhibition by insulin of valine turnover in liver. *J. Biol. Chem.* 245:2375–2383.

Munro, H.N. (1970): A general survey of mechanisms regulating protein metabolism in mammals. In: *Mammalian Protein Metabolism* (ed: H.N. Munro), Vol. IV, pp. 3–130, Academic Press, New York.

Munro, H.N., Hubert, C., and Baliga, B.S. (1975): Regulation of protein synthesis in relation to amino acid supply—a review. In: *Alcohol and Abnormal Protein Biosynthesis: Biochemical and Clinical* (eds: M.A. Rothschild, M. Oratz, and S.S. Schreiber), pp. 33–66, Pergamon Press, New York.

Pain, V.M., and Henshaw, E.C. (1975): Initiation of protein synthesis in Ehrlich ascites tumour cells. Evidence for physiological variation in the association of methionyl-$tRNA_f$ with native 40-S ribosomal subunits *in vivo*. *Eur. J. biochem.* 57:335–342.

Peavy, D.E., and Hansen, R.J. (1976): Lack of effect of amino acid concentration on protein synthesis in the perfused rat liver. *Biochem. J.* 160:797–801.

Peters, T. (1975): Serum albumin. In: *The Plasma Proteins* (ed: F.W. Putnam), Vol. 1, pp. 133–181, Academic Press, New York.

Ramsey, J.C., and Steele, W.J. (1976): A procedure for the quantitative recovery of homogeneous populations of undegraded free and bound polysomes from rat liver. *Biochemistry* 15:1704–1712.

Ramsey, J.C., and Steele, W.J. (1977): Differences in size, structure and function of free and membrane-bound polyribosomes of rat liver. Evidence for a single class of membrane-bound polyribosomes. *Biochem. J.* 168:1–8.

Schworer, C.M., and Mortimore, G.E. (1979): Glucagon-induced autophagy and proteolysis in rat liver: Mediation by selective deprivation of intracellular amino acids. *Proc. Natl. Acad. Sci., USA* 76:3169–3173.

Scornik, O.A., Ledbetter, M.L.S., and Malter, J.S. (1980): Role of amino-acylation of histidyl-tRNA in the regulation of protein degradation in Chinese hamster ovary cells. *J. Biol. Chem.* 225:6322–6329.

Shenoy, S.T., and Rogers, Q.R. (1978): Effects of dietary amino acids on transfer ribonucleic acid charging levels in rat liver. *J. Nutr.* 108:1412–1421.

Smith, K.E., and Henshaw, E.C. (1975): Binding of met-$tRNA_f$ to native and derived 40S ribosomal subunits. *Biochemistry* 14:1060–1067.

Tavill, A.S., East, A.G., Black, E.G., Nadkarni, D., and Hoffenberg, R. (1973): Regulatory factors in the synthesis of plasma proteins by the isolated perfused rat liver. In: *Protein Turnover,* Ciba Foundation Symposium 9, pp. 155–171, Elsevier, Amsterdam.

Tolman, E.L., Schworer, C.M., and Jefferson, L.S. (1973): Effects of hypophysectomy on amino acid metabolism and gluconeogenesis in the perfused rat liver. *J. Biol. Chem.* 248: 4552–4560.

Tse, T.P.H., Morris, H.P., and Taylor, J.M. (1978): Molecular basis of reduced albumin synthesis in Morris hepatoma 7777. *Biochemistry* 17:3121–3128.

Van Den Borre, M., and Webb, T.E. (1972): Perfusate composition and stability of polyribosomes in perfused liver. *Life Sci.* 11:347–354.

van Venrooij, W.J.W., Henshaw, E.C., and Hirsch, C.A. (1972): Effects on polyribosomal distribution and rate of protein synthesis in cultured mammalian cells. *Biochim. Biophys. Acta.* 259:127–137.

Vaughan, M.H., Pawlowski, P., and Frochhammer, J. (1971): Regulation of protein synthesis initiation in HeLa cells deprived of single essential amino acids. *Proc. Natl. Acad. Sci., USA* 68:2057–2061.

Vaughan, M.H., and Hansen, B.S. (1973): Control of initiation of protein synthesis in human cells. *J. Biol. Chem.* 248:7087–7096.

Warrington, R.C., Wratten, N., and Hechtman, R. (1977): L-Histidinol inhibits specifically and reversibly protein and ribosomal RNA synthesis in mouse L cells. *J. Biol. Chem.* 252:5251–5257.

Woodside, K.H., and Mortimore, G.E. (1972): Suppression of protein turnover by amino acids in the perfused rate liver. *J. Biol. Chem.* 247:6474–6481.

Yap, S.H., Strair, R.K., and Shafritz, D.A. (1978a): Identification of albumin mRNPs in the cytosol of fasting rat liver and influence of tryptophan or a mixture of amino acids. *Biochem. Biophys. Res. Commun.* 83:427–433.

Yap, S.H., Strair, R.K., and Shafritz, D.A. (1978b): Effect of a short term fast on the distribution of cytoplasmic albumin messenger ribonucleic acid in rat liver. *J. Biol. Chem.* 253:4944–4950.

11 Amino Acid Metabolism as Studied in the Isolated Hepatocyte

Khursheed N. Jeejeebhoy

A variety of nutrients flow through the liver with each meal. This flux in nutrient flow has numerous effects including a significant influence on protein synthesis and catabolism, as well as amino acid catabolism (Elwyn, 1970). *In vivo*, the effects of amino acids on protein metabolism *per se* cannot be dissociated from those of insulin secreted in response to the ingestion of a meal. Thus, in order to understand mechanisms, it is desirable to use a model in which effects of substrate and hormone can be controlled independently. The isolated hepatocyte in maintenance culture is one such model and has provided valuable insight into the way by which amino acids may influence hepatocyte protein catabolism and the way the hepatocyte metabolizes amino acids.

In this paper two aspects of amino acid–hepatocyte interaction will be presented: the effect of amino acids on protein synthesis and catabolism; and metabolism of amino acids by the fasted and fed hepatocyte and the influence of insulin.

EFFECT OF AMINO ACIDS ON PROTEIN SYNTHESIS AND CATABOLISM

Kirsch et al. (1969) noted that albumin synthesis in the isolated perfused liver was depressed by depriving this organ of amino acids (see also the chapter by Jefferson and Flaim). This depression could be corrected simply by adding branched-chain amino acids alone to the the fluid perfusing the liver. Thus, it was demonstrated that branched-chain amino acids may have a special role in promoting protein synthesis in the liver. Later, during *in vivo* studies, we showed that increasing plasma leucine concentration increased the synthesis of two liver-made plasma proteins, albumin and fibrinogen. Thus, it is clear that specific amino acids may have profound effects on liver protein synthesis.

Recently, Seglen et al. (1980a) found that freshly isolated hepatocytes in suspension are in a catabolic state as demonstrated by a net outward flux of amino acids into the incubation medium. Prior to isolation of the hepatocytes, they labeled hepatocyte protein with ^{14}C-valine and then followed the flux of free ^{14}C-valine from the isolated hepatocyte during incubation. Since valine is neither synthesized nor catabolized by the hepatocyte, the demonstration of a net outward flux of ^{14}C-valine from prelabeled hepatocyte protein must indicate protein catabolism. When hepatocytes were incubated in an amino acid-free medium, a rapid net outward flux of free valine was observed. However, addition of an amino acid mixture to the medium reduced the net outward flux of valine and, by inference, reduced protein catabolism. Maximal inhibition of amino acid catabolism by hepatocytes occurred when the content of amino acids in the medium was 10 to 12 times greater than that in normal plasma. When the inhibitory effect of amino acids was studied further, it became clear that six amino acids (leucine, phenylalanine, tyrosine, tryptophan, histidine and methionine) were responsible for 70% of this inhibitory effect. Experiments involving withdrawal of amino acids from the mixture showed that the removal of leucine alone diminished the inhibitory effect by 50%, whereas other amino acids had to be removed in pairs for the effect to become significant.

The anticatabolic effect of amino acids added to the medium was found to be due to an inhibition of the lysosomal pathway of protein degradation. Thus propylamine, an inhibitor of protein degradation by the lysosomal pathway, was as effective as a combination of leucine and asparagine in inhibiting protein catabolism. Furthermore, when propylamine had been added to the medium, further addition of these aforementioned amino acids did not enhance the inhibition of protein catabolism beyond that seen with propylamine alone.

PROTEIN SYNTHESIS

Addition of amino acids to culture media clearly stimulates incorporation of ^{14}C-valine into hepatocyte protein (Seglen et al., 1980b). Alanine is particularly effective. The stimulatory effect of alanine on protein synthesis is inhibited by amino oxyacetate (which blocks transamination) and is stimulated by pyruvate, suggesting that the function of amino acids in promoting protein synthesis may be related to their ability to be transaminated and thus provide energy substrate precursors.

EFFECT OF THE NUTRITIONAL STATE OF THE HEPATOCYTE AND INSULIN ON AMINO ACID AND PROTEIN METABOLISM

Hepatocytes from Fasted Donors

Hepatocytes from fasted animals, derived from a milieu of low insulin, have a net uptake from the media of only aspartate, phenylalanine and histidine. Such hepatocytes demonstrate a net transfer of alanine and branched-chain amino acids to the media. The transfer of alanine is clearly due to endogenous transamination from pyruvate as there is no alanine in the medium. The output of branched-chain amino acids, which are not synthesized or catabolized by the liver, indicates net proteolysis.

Net nitrogen balance is markedly negative in hepatocytes derived from fasted donors indicating that catabolism exceeds synthesis. The presence of rapid catabolism is supported also by observation of the release of ^{14}C-valine from prelabeled hepatocytes suggesting that about half of the hepatocyte protein is catabolized by 48 hours. Although there is concurrent protein synthesis, as demonstrated by the uptake of ^{3}H-valine into hepatocyte protein, an analysis of the specific activity of intracellular and medium valine suggests that catabolism exceeds synthesis by about 20% (unpublished results).

The addition of insulin to maintain physiological levels in the medium results in a significant net uptake of a variety of amino acids. This process could be due to either increased net protein catabolism increasing uptake or to better inward transport of amino acids. Both processes seem to occur. It has been noted that the net loss of branched-chain amino acids almost ceases after six hours of incubation with insulin. Further, since ^{14}C-valine loss from prelabeled cells (reflecting hepatocyte protein catabolism) is not affected by insulin, uptake of amino acids must increase. Increased uptake is supported by observations of a 30% increase in incorporation of ^{3}H-valine into hepatocyte protein. In addition, transamination is decreased since the output of alanine is markedly reduced after 12 hours of incubation. Yet the net amino acid uptake is not necessarily associated with their use in protein synthesis. For example, the enhanced inward flux of glycine is associated with an outward flux of serine—a product of glycine metabolism—to an extent that suggests that most of the glycine taken up may be converted to serine.

With the addition of insulin to the medium, the net negative nitrogen balance was changed to zero. Seglen (1980b), in contrast to our studies, did not find insulin improved protein synthesis over catabolism to an extent greater than that observed with amino acids alone. However, his studies were carried out for the period of an hour. In our studies the effect of insulin required at least six hours and became significant only after 24 hours of incubation.

Hepatocytes Derived from Fed Donors

When hepatocytes were derived from fed animals the fluxes of amino acids were quite different from those derived from fasted animals comparable to that seen in insulin-treated "fasted" hepatocytes. These hepatocytes had a net inward flux of aspartate, glutamate, glycine, cystine, methionine, and phenylalanine. Similarly, there was a net outward flux of threonine, serine, alanine, ornithine, lysine, and the branched-chain amino acids. Despite this enhanced rate of amino acid exchange in control hepatocytes from fed animals, protein synthesis and catabolism, as judged by the uptake and release of radiolabeled valine, were the same as in those from fasted animals. Thus, there was a dissociation of amino acid flux and protein synthesis. Addition of insulin to hepatocytes from fed donors had little effect on the flux of amino acids, but did significantly increase synthesis as judged by the intake and incorporation of ^{3}H-valine into protein and reduced output of ^{3}H-valine from prelabeled protein. Transamination, as judged by alanine output, continued despite the addition of insulin.

Data from the uptake and output of radiolabeled valine suggests that insulin increases net protein synthesis over catabolism. This concept is supported by the observation that net negative nitrogen balance was reduced by the addition of insulin, although the balance remained negative.

DISCUSSION

The isolated hepatocyte is normally in a net catabolic state as evidenced by a negative nitrogen balance and net outward flux of the branched-chain amino acids and alanine in excess of net inward flux of other amino acids. Observations of the output of ^{14}C-valine from prelabeled ^{14}C-hepatocyte protein confirms this impression. When hepatocytes are incubated in an amino acid-free medium, the output of ^{14}C-valine from prelabeled hepatocyte protein is 5% per hour. Thus, in 16 hours half of the cell protein is catabolized, but the net negative balance would be less, because there is simultaneous resynthesis not measured by the method. The use of an amino acid mixture enriched to about ten times normal plasma concentration reduces catabolism to 2% per hour. The amino acids most capable of this effect are leucine and asparagine. The addition of free amino acids alone will inhibit degradation to a rate of 2% per hour and over 48 hours this rate will result in catabolism of 96% of the protein. In a suspension culture with an enriched amino acid medium, our studies, using ^{3}H-valine, indicate a catabolic rate of 1% per hour, or 50% over 48 hours, which is less than that seen by Seglen et al. (1980a) with amino acids alone.

The addition of insulin to the medium reduced the rate of catabolism, as judged by the output of ^{3}H-valine from prelabeled hepatocyte protein, and significantly increased the incorporation of ^{3}H-valine into hepatocyte protein as well as reducing transamination. This effect of insulin was most pronounced after a delay of about 12 to 24 hours suggesting mediation through a process which may depend on transcription of messenger for protein synthesis. With reduced catabolism, the net fluxes of the branched-chain amino acids and of alanine reached equilibrium and became zero.

The effect of insulin was especially obvious in hepatocytes from depleted (fasted) animals coming from an endogenous environment of low insulin. These hepatocytes had a net inward flux of only three amino acids. The addition of a small amount of insulin increased inward flux dramatically. It could be argued that the enhanced inward flux was due to reduced catabolism and enhanced protein synthesis. However, data from isolated hepatocytes from fed donors does not support the contention that enhanced uptake of amino acids and increased net protein synthesis over catabolism are cause and effect. Hepatocytes from fed donors showed a net inward flux of a variety of amino acids, but had a comparable degree of negative nitrogen balance due to a net outward flux of the branched-chain amino acids and alanine. In addition, the uptake and release of radiolabeled valine were comparable to those seen in the control hepatocytes from fasted donors. Thus, enhanced exchange of amino acids occurred in hepatocytes from fed donors without better net protein synthesis over catabolism.

Insulin failed to suppress net outward flow of alanine and the branched-chain amino acids from the fed hepatocyte, but did reduce catabolism as seen by a reduced output of ^{3}H-valine from prelabeled hepatocyte protein, and increased uptake of ^{3}H-valine into hepatocyte protein. Thus, again, increased synthesis of protein and reduced catabolism was observed. The synthesis of hepatocyte protein in hepatocytes from both fasted and fed donors was not comparatively different in both controls and insulin-treated cells. Yet, the pattern of amino acid flux was quite different prior to insulin treatment. Thus, it appears that insulin may be important in the net inward flow of a variety of amino acids.

In conclusion, it appears that amino acids are utilized by the hepatocyte and in turn alter protein synthesis in different ways depending upon the prior nutritional state of the hepatocyte and the presence of insulin. In depleted hepatocytes, insulin suppresses net protein catabolism and transamination. In contrast, hepatocytes from fed animals continue to break down protein and to transaminate despite the presence of insulin which does, however, stimulate synthesis in both depleted and repleted states.

REFERENCES

Elwyn, D.H. (1970): The role of the liver in regulation of amino acid and protein metabolism. In: *Mammalian Protein Metabolism* (ed: H.N. Munro). Vol. 4, pp. 523–557. Academic Press, New York.

Kirsch, R.E., Saunders, S.J., Frith, L., Wicht, S., Kelman, L. and Brock, J.F. (1969): Plasma acid concentration and regulation of albumin synthesis. *Am. J. Clin. Nutr.* 22:1559–1562.

Seglen, O., Gordon, P.B. and Poli, A. (1980a): Amino acid inhibition of the autophagic/lysosomal pathway of protein degradation in isolated rat hepatocytes. *Biochim. Biophys. Acta* 630:103–118.

Seglen, O., Solheim, A.E., Grinde, B., Gordon, P.B., Schwartze, E., Gjessing, R. and Poli, A. (1980b): Amino acid control of protein synthesis and degradation in isolated rat hepatocytes. *Ann. N.Y. Acad. Sci.* 349:1–17.

The Effect of High Doses of Leucine on Protein Synthesis in Rat Tissues

Margaret A. McNurlan, Edward B. Fern, and Peter J. Garlick

There have been reports that leucine or branched-chain amino acid administration can spare nitrogen in the whole animal, and that leucine added to the medium of incubated or perfused muscle *in vitro* can stimulate protein synthesis. We have, therefore, investigated whether raising the concentration of leucine in the whole animal results in a stimulation of protein synthesis in tissues of the rat. Animals were injected with 100 μmol/100 g body weight of leucine and rates of protein synthesis were measured in skeletal muscle, cardiac muscle, smooth muscle of the small intestine (serosa), liver and intestinal mucosa by injection of a flooding dose of (^{3}H)phenylalanine.

METHODS

Animals

Forty male rats weighing approximately 135 g were fed a standard pelleted diet (23% crude protein) up to the morning of the experiment (fed groups), or starved for two days (starved groups). They were injected intravenously with either 150 μmol per 100 g (^{3}H)phenylalanine (control group) or 150 μmol (^{3}H) phenylalanine plus 100 μmol unlabeled leucine (leucine group) and incorporation of label was measured during the following ten minutes. A further 20 rats weighing approximately 113 g were given a protein-free, powdered diet for nine days before injection with (^{3}H)phenylalanine or (^{3}H)phenylalanine plus leucine, and incorporation of label was again measured after ten minutes. In another group of 20 rats, starved for two days as above, 100 μmol/100g unlabeled leucine or saline were injected intraperitoneally one hour before intravenous injection of (^{3}H)phenylalanine. Incorporation of label was again measured over ten minutes.

Measurement of Protein Synthesis

The rate of protein synthesis in tissues was estimated from the incorporation of label into protein ten minutes after the intravenous injection of a large dose of (^{3}H)phenylalanine. With this technique, the intracellular and extracellular pools of free amino acid are flooded and achieve nearly the same specific radioactivity (Henshaw et al., 1971; McNurlan et al., 1979). Problems of precursor compartmentation are therefore minimized, and the specific radioactivity at the site of protein synthesis is taken to be the same as that in the tissue homogenate.

Rats were immobilized and injected via a lateral tail vein with 150 μmol/100 g body weight (4^3H)phenylalanine (approximately 25 μCi). After either two minutes or ten minutes, animals were killed by decapitation and tissues (gastrocnemius muscle, heart, liver and jejunum) were rapidly removed and chilled in ice water. The jejunal mucosa and serosa were separated by scraping with a microscope slide. Tissues were homogenized in 2% perchloric acid and the supernatant was used for measurement of the specific activity of free phenylalanine. The precipitate was washed and hydrolyzed in HCl for measurement of the specific activity of protein-bound phenylalanine. Specific activities of free and bound phenylalanine were measured by enzymic conversion to β-phenylethylamine, followed by solvent extraction. Separate aliquots were counted and assayed for β-phenylethylamine by a fluorometric technique.

Fractional rates of protein synthesis (^{k}S; ie the % of the tissue protein renewed per day) were calculated from the following formula:

$$^{k}S = \frac{S_B \times 100}{S_A \times t}$$

where t is the period of incorporation, in days, and S_B is the specific activity of phenylalanine in protein of rats killed at ten minutes. S_A is the mean specific radioactivity of free phenylalanine during the period zero to ten minutes and is calculated from the measured values in rats killed at two minutes and ten minutes, on the assumption that the fall in specific activity is linear (McNurlan et al., 1979). Full details of the method have been described by Garlick et al. (1980).

RESULTS AND DISCUSSION

Rates of protein synthesis in fed rats are given in Table 1. Increasing the concentration of leucine (to about 1 mM) during the ten minute period of incorporation of label did not influence the rate of synthesis in any of the five tissues studied. In case synthesis was already maximal in fed rats, and hence not susceptible to further stimulation by leucine, the experiment was repeated in two-day starved and nine-day protein-deprived rats (Table 1). The free leucine concentration in the plasma of the protein-deprived rats was very low compared with that in both the fed and the starved animals, but insulin concentrations were low with both starvation and protein deprivation (McNurlan et al., 1982). Although these treatments resulted in synthesis rates that were much lower than in fed rats in all tissues, there was again no effect of leucine injection. In addition, to see whether a longer period of exposure to leucine was effective, two-day starved rats were given intraperitoneal injections of leucine one hour before the measurement of protein synthesis. However, this did not influence the rate obtained in any tissue.

These results contrast with the stimulation of protein synthesis observed in the presence of high concentrations of leucine in incubated skeletal muscle (e.g., Fulks et al., 1976; Buse and Reid, 1976) and in perfused skeletal and cardiac muscle (Li and Jefferson, 1978; Chua et al., 1979). This suggests that there is no direct link between these effects observed *in vitro* and the observation by some (e.g., Sherwin, 1978; Sakamoto et al., 1981), but not by others (e.g., Mitch et al., 1981) that administration of leucine *in vivo* can spare body nitrogen.

Table 1
Rates of Protein Synthesis (% per Day) in Tissues of Control and Leucine Injected Rats

	Experiment 1		Experiment 2		Experiment 3		Experiment 4	
	Control	*Leucine*	*Control*	*Leucine*	*Control*	*Leucine*	*Control*	*Leucine*
Gastrocnemius	16.9 ± 0.6	18.6 ± 0.9	5.8 ± 0.3	5.8 ± 0.6	4.1 ± 0.6	3.5 ± 0.3	4.5 ± 0.4	5.0 ± 0.3
Heart	19.6 ± 0.8	20.1 ± 0.7	11.9 ± 0.7	10.7 ± 0.9	10.3 ± 0.2	10.6 ± 0.4	12.2 ± 2.0	10.1 ± 1.3
Gut Serosa	52.1 ± 2.0	56.5 ± 2.8	31.4 ± 1.2	31.2 ± 1.2	–	–	34.6 ± 1.8	35.5 ± 2.1
Gut Mucosa	123 ± 4	117 ± 3	92.0 ± 3.2	101 ± 4	94.9 ± 6.0	99.7 ± 1.6	93.9 ± 2.1	88.8 ± 4.1
Liver	86.3 ± 5.6	82.1 ± 2.6	71.8 ± 2.9	73.6 ± 2.1	69.4 ± 4.3	68.6 ± 1.1	66.0 ± 2.5	67.0 ± 2.3

Experiment 1: Fed rats. Experiments 2 and 4: Two-day starved rats. Experiment 3: Nine-day protein-deprived rats. In experiments 1, 2 and 3 the leucine (100 μmol/100 g body weight) was given with the labeled phenylalanine and incorporation measured during the next ten minutes. In experiment 4 the leucine was injected one hour before the labeled phenylalanine.

REFERENCES

Buse, M.G., and Reid, S.S. (1975): Leucine: a possible regulator of protein turnover in muscle. *J. Clin. Invest.* 56:1250–61.
Chua, B., Siehl, D.L. and Morgan, H.E. (1979): Effect of leucine and metabolites of branched chain amino acids on protein turnover in heart. *J. Biol. Chem.* 254:8358–62.
Fulks, R.H., Li, J.B. and Goldberg, A.L. (1975): Effects of insulin, glucose and amino acids on protein turnover in rat diaphragms. *J. Biol. Chem.* 250:290–8.
Garlick, P.J., McNurlan, M.A. and Preedy, V.R. (1980): A rapid and convenient technique for measuring the rate of protein synthesis in tissues by injection of (^{3}H)phenylalanine. *Biochem. J.* 192:719–23.
Henshaw, E.C., Hirsch, C.A., Morton, B.E. and Hiatt, H.H. (1971): Control of protein synthesis in mammalian tissues through changes in ribosome activity, *J. Biol. Chem.* 246:436–46.
Li, J.B. and Jefferson, L.S. (1978): Influence of amino acid availability on protein turnover in perfused skeletal muscle. *Biochim. Biphys. Acta.* 544:351–9.
McNurlan, M.A., Tomkins, A.M. and Garlick, P.J. (1979): The effect of starvation on the rate of protein synthesis in rat liver and small intestine. *Biochem. J.* 178:373–9.
McNurlan, M.A., Tomkins, A.M. and Garlick, P.J. (1982): Failure of leucine to stimulate protein synthesis *in vivo. Biochem. J.* in press.
Mitch, W.E., Walser, M. and Sapir, D.G. (1981): Nitrogen sparing induced by leucine compared with that induced by its keto analogue, α-ketoisocaproate, in fasting obese man. *J. Clin. Invest.* 67:553–62.
Sakamoto, A., Moldawer, L.L., Bothe, A., Bistrian, B.R. and Blackburn, G.L. (1980): Nitrogen sparing mechanism of branched chain amino acid administration in acute experimental pancreatitis. Proc. 2nd European Congress of Parenteral and Enteral Nutrition, Newcastle-upon-Tyne, UK.
Sherwin, R.S. (1978): Effect of starvation on the turnover and metabolic response to leucine. *J. Clin. Invest.* 61:1471–81.

A Possible Role for the Muscle in the Regulation of Oxidation of Branched-Chain Amino Acid in the Liver

Harbhajan S. Paul and Siamak A. Adibi

The catabolism of three branched-chain amino acids (BCAA) leucine, isoleucine, and valine is initiated by the BCAA transaminase resulting in the formation of corresponding branched-chain α-keto acids (BCKA). In the subsequent reaction, the BCKA are oxidatively decarboxylated by the mitochondrial BCKA dehydrogenase (Meister, 1965). This enzyme plays an important role in the catabolism of BCAA by irreversibly committing these amino acids to the oxidative pathway. The activity of BCKA dehydrogenase is regulated by dietary and metabolic factors (Paul and Adibi, 1978a,b, 1980; Hutson et al., 1980). Recent investigations have shown that this enzyme is regulated by conversion from an inactive phosphorylated form to an active dephosphorylated form (Parker and Randle, 1980; Odessey, 1980a,b, Paul and Adibi, 1982). Furthermore, it has been shown that nutritional and hormonal factors affect this interconversion (Paul and Adibi, 1982).

Although it is well established that BCKA dehydrogenase is distributed in a variety of tissues, it is not yet known whether there are tissue factors which affect the activity of BCKA dehydrogenase in the mitochondria of the same or different tissues. The present studies were designed to investigate this possibility.

RESULTS

Effect of Muscle Fraction on BCKA Dehydrogenase Activity

As shown in Figure 1, addition of postmitochondrial fraction of gastrocnemius muscle increased the activity of BCKA dehyrogenase in liver mitochondria. The activity of this enzyme continued to increase with increasing amounts of muscle fraction for up to 1.0 mg protein. No further increase in the activity of BCKA dehydrogenase was observed when the amount of muscle fraction was increased to 2.0 mg protein, suggesting that the effect of this fraction was a saturable phenomenon (Figure 1). In contrast to liver mitochondria, the activity of BCKA dehydrogenase in gastrocnemius muscle mitochondria was not increased by the addition of the muscle fraction (Figure 1). Muscle fraction alone lacked any BCKA dehydrogenase activity. Our further studies revealed that, in addition to the gastrocnemius muscle, this factor was also present in other skeletal muscles such as soleus, vastus lateralis, and diaphragm. This factor was also found in low concentration in the heart muscle but was not found in the smooth muscle of uterus.

To investigate whether muscle factor has any effect on BCKA dehydrogenase in other tissues besides liver, we examined the effect of this factor on BCKA dehydrogenase activity in kidney, heart, and brain mitochondria. In kidney mitochondria, muscle factor at lower concentrations (0.25 to 0.50 mg protein) significantly inhibited the activity of BCKA dehydrogenase (Figure 2). However, when the amount of muscle factor was increased (1 to 3 mg protein), this inhibition was reversed (Figure 2). Muscle factor also inhibited the activity of BCKA dehydrogenase in heart mitochondria (Figure 2). However, unlike with kidney mitochondria, higher amounts of muscle factor (1 to 3 mg protein) failed to reverse the inhibition of BCKA dehydrogenase in heart mitochondria (Figure 2). Muscle factor had no significant effect on the BCKA dehydrogenase activity in brain mitochondria (Figure 2).

Effect of Other Tissue Fractions on BCKA Dehydrogenase

To determine whether fractions from tissues other than muscle can also affect the activity of BCKA dehydrogenase, we examined the effect of plasma and of postmitochondrial fraction of liver and kidney on the BCKA dehydrogenase activity in liver mitochondria. As shown in Figure 3, both liver and kidney fractions alone contained low BCKA dehydrogenase activities. Addition of these fractions to liver mitochondria did not result in any increment in the BCKA dehydrogenase activity (Figure 3). The enzyme activity observed by the combination of mitochondria and the tissue fractions was the sum of the activities observed individually by these components (Figure 3.)

In contrast to the liver and kidney fractions, addition of plasma greatly increased the BCKA dehydrogenase activity in liver mitochondria (Figure 4). The protein con-

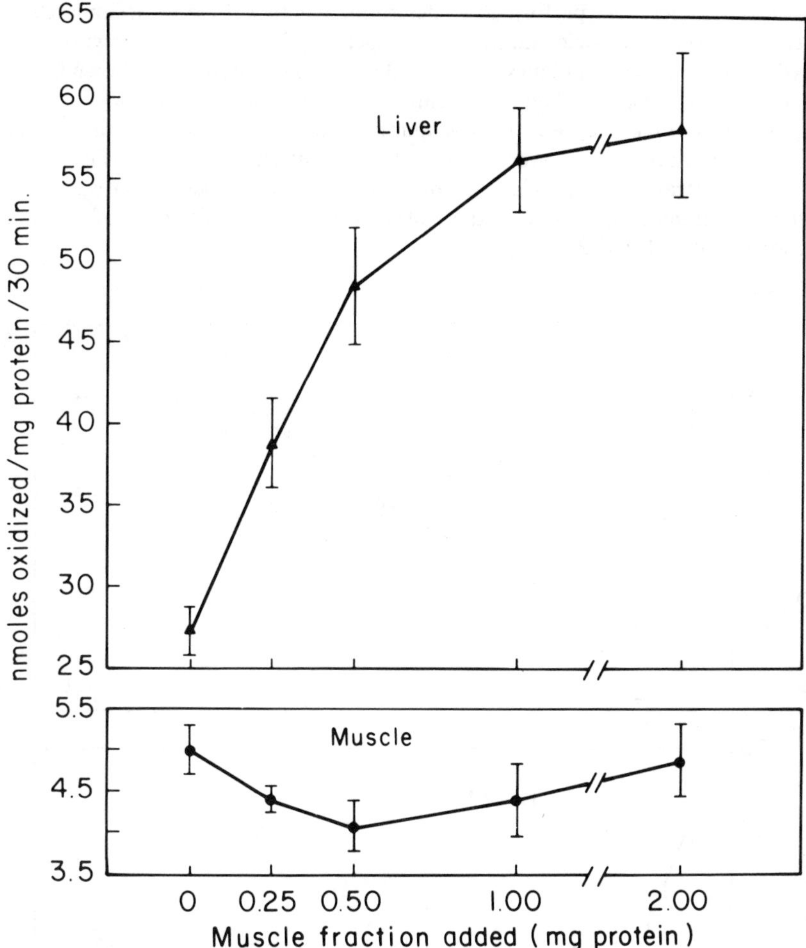

Figure 1 Effect of muscle fraction in BCKA dehydrogenase in liver and gastrocnemius muscle mitochondria. The activity of BCKA dehydrogenase was determined by measuring the rate of $^{14}CO_2$ production from α-keto [1-^{14}C] isocaproate incubated with mitochondria at 30°C for 30 minutes. Each point represents the mean ± S.E. of five to six rats.

tent of plasma did not appear responsible for the stimulatory effect of plasma. This was evident by the fact that when a comparable amount of protein, as bovine serum albumin, was added, the activity of BCKA dehydrogenase was not enhanced but actually decreased (Figure 4).

Similarities Between the Effects of Muscle and the Plasma Factors

Among the tissue fractions examined, only the muscle fraction and plasma increased the BCKA dehydrogenase activity in liver mitochondria (Figures 1 and 4).

Therefore, studies were performed to determine whether there were similarities between the effects of muscle and the plasma factors. The effect of plasma on BCKA dehydrogenase activity in kidney, heart, and muscle mitochondria is shown in Figure 5. Addition of plasma had no significant effect on the activity of BCKA dehydrogenase in kidney and muscle mitochondria, but inhibited this activity in heart mitochondria when lower concentrations of plasma were used (Figure 5). At higher concentrations of plasma this inhibition in heart mitochondria was reversed (Figure 5). In general, these effects of plasma were similar to those of the muscle fraction (Figures 1 and 2).

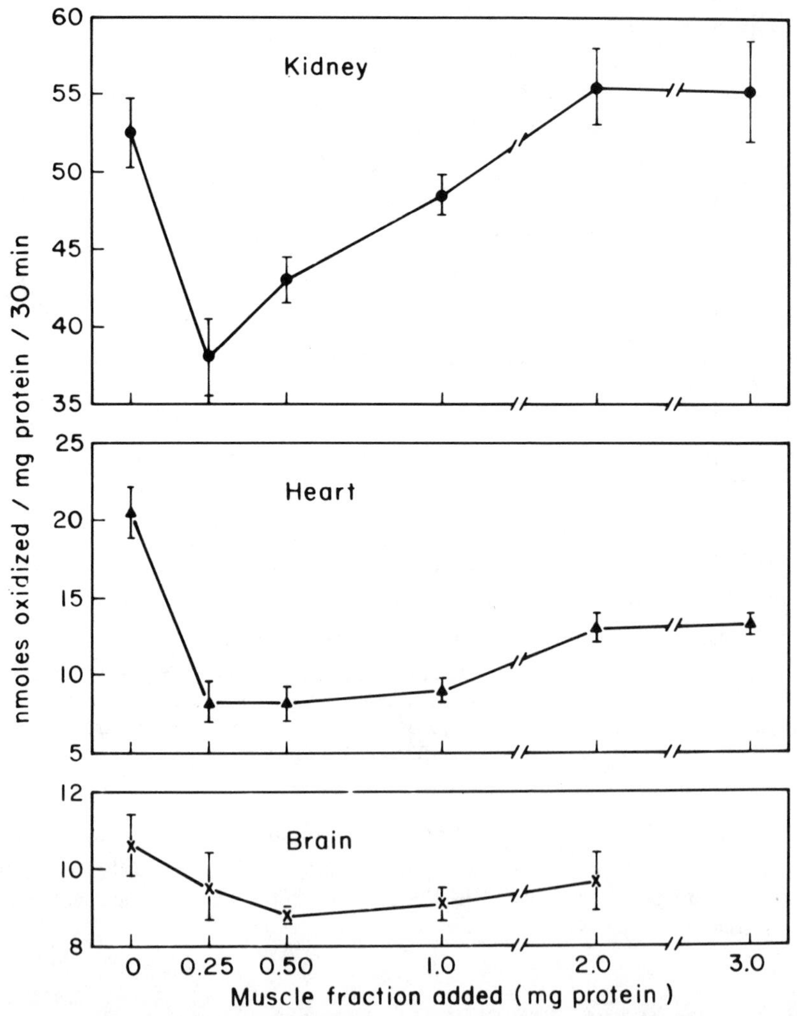

Figure 2 Effect of muscle fraction on BCKA dehydrogenase in kidney, heart, and brain mitochondria. All conditions were the same as described in Figure 1 with the exception that mitochondria from kidney, heart, and brain were used. Each point represents the mean ± S.E. of four rats.

In our further studies, we investigated the subcellular distribution and properties of the muscle factor. These studies revealed that this factor is present in the cytosolic fraction, is nondialyzable, is heat labile, and is a protein. The evidence for protein was based on the fact that muscle factor lost its activity after trypsin digestion.

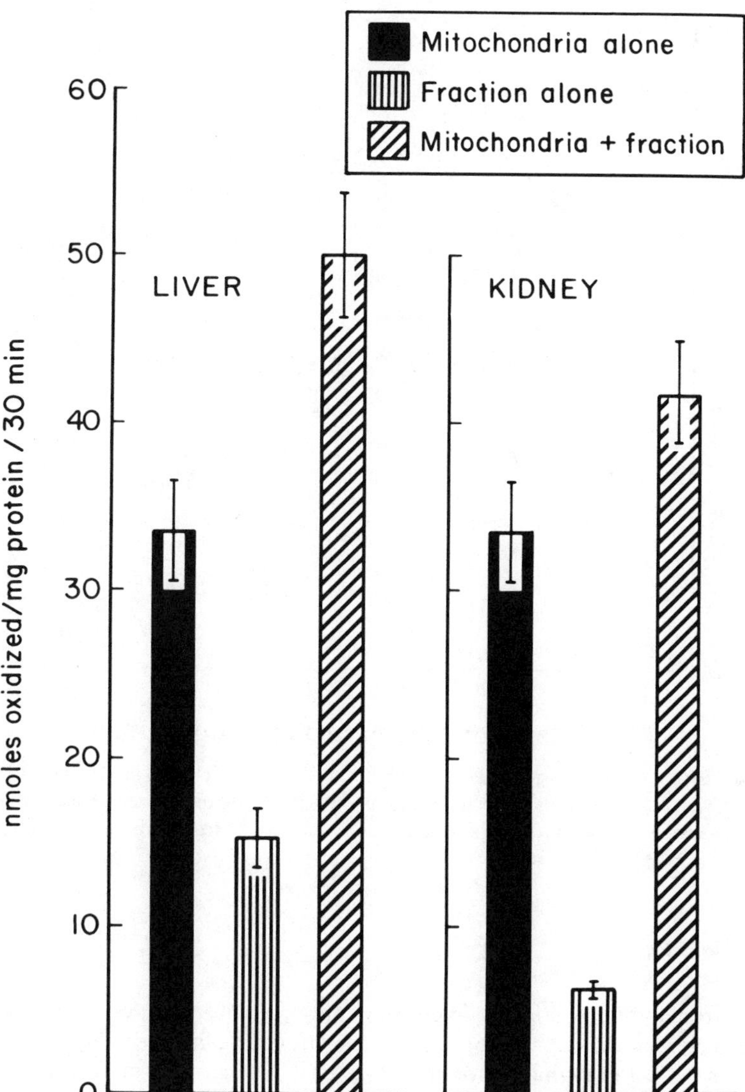

Figure 3 Effect of liver and kidney fractions on BCKA dehydrogenase in liver mitochondria. The activity of BCKA dehydrogenase in liver mitochondria was determined as described in Figure 1. Each bar represents the mean ± S.E. of five rats.

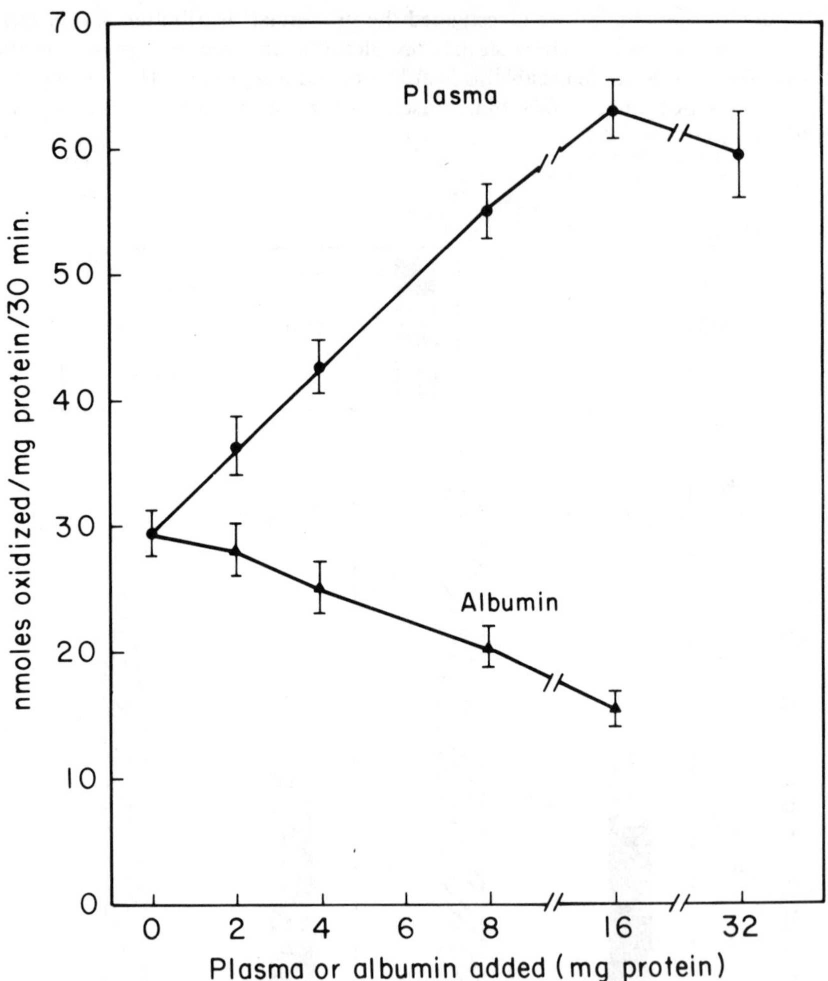

Figure 4 Effect of rat plasma and bovine serum albumin on BCKA dehydrogenase in liver mitochondria. All conditions were the same as described Figure 1 with the exception that varied amounts of rat plasma or bovine serum albumin were added. Each point represents the mean ± S.E. of four to six rats.

DISCUSSION

The results of the present studies show that a soluble fraction of the skeletal muscle increases the activity of BCKA dehydrogenase in liver (Figure 1). The stimulatory effect of muscle factor appears to be unique for liver mitochondria since no such effect is observed with mitochondria from skeletal muscle, kidney, heart, or brain (Figure 2). In fact, the muscle factor inhibits the activity of BCKA dehydrogenase in mitochondria from some tissues (Figure 2). Several lines of evidence suggest that this muscle factor is not one of the previously known factors

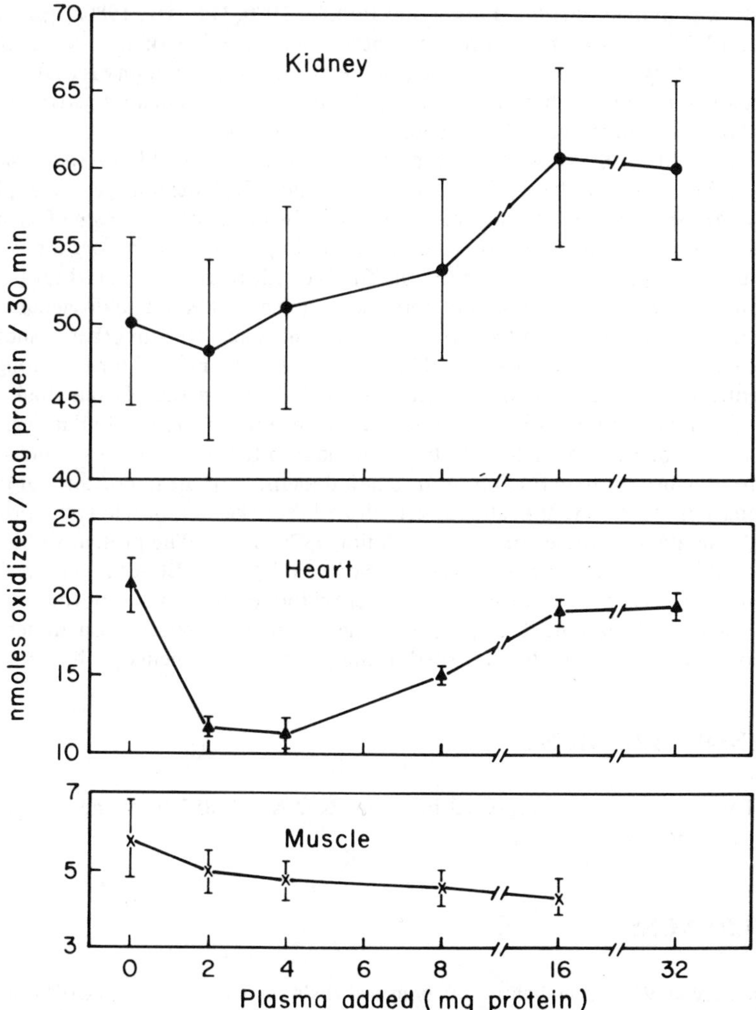

Figure 5 Effect of plasma on BCKA dehydrogenase in kidney, heart, and muscle mitochondria. All conditions were the same as described in Figure 2, with the exception that varied amounts of rat plasma were added. Each point represents the mean ± S.E. of four to six rats.

that increase the BCKA dehydrogenase activity. The previously known factors include metabolites such as carnitine (Paul and Adibi, 1978b) and substrates such as leucine and α-ketoisocaproate (Frick et al., 1981). Based on the physical properties such as being nondialyzable and heat labile, the muscle factor does not appear to be the same as previously known factors.

Recent investigations have shown activation of BCKA dehydrogenase by dephosphorylation of the enzyme protein (Parker and Randle, 1980; Odessey, 1980a,b; Paul and Adibi, 1982). Therefore, it is possible that the effect of muscle factor could be due to the presence of phosphatase in the muscle fraction. However, the activation of BCKA dehydrogenase by dephosphorylation has been observed in all tissues examined thus far (Parker and Randle, 1980; Odessey, 1980a,b; Paul and Adibi, 1982), whereas in the present experiments the effect of muscle factor was observed only with liver mitochondria (Figure 1). Another possibility is that the muscle factor is not a phosphatase but acts to stimulate the phosphatase activity in liver mitochondria. These possibilities require further investigation.

The results of the present experiments also show that, in addition to the skeletal muscle, there is a stimulatory factor for the hepatic BCKA dehydrogenase in plasma (Figure 4). Several lines of evidence suggest that the origin of the plasma factor may be the skeletal muscle. First, two metabolically important visceral organs, such as liver and kidney, lack this factor (Figure 3). Second, there are similarities between the effects of muscle and plasma factors. Both increase BCKA dehydrogenase activity in the liver (Figures 1 and 4), while they have no such effect in other tissues such as skeletal muscle, kidney, brain, and heart (Figures 1, 2, and 5). Third, although the concentration of the stimulatory factor is much lower in the plasma than in the skeletal muscle, both factors at saturating concentrations produce similar degrees of increases in the activity of BCKA dehydrogenase in the liver (Figures 1 and 4).

In conclusion, these findings bring a new dimension to the importance of muscle in oxidation of BCAA. It is already established that skeletal muscle is the principal site of oxidation of these amino acids (Adibi, 1976, 1980). The present results raise the possibility of another role for the muscle in oxidation of BCAA, namely, the activation of BCKA dehydrogenase in the liver by the release of a factor (protein) into the systemic circulation. This possibility needs further investigation under more physiological conditions than pursued in the present experiments.

ACKNOWLEDGMENT

These studies were supported by Grant No. AM 15855 from the National Institutes of Health.

REFERENCES

Adibi, S.A. (1976): Metabolism of branched-chain amino acids in altered nutrition. *Metabolism* 25:1287–1302.

Adibi, S.A. (1980): Roles of branched-chain amino acids in metabolic regulation. *J. Lab. Clin. Med.* 95:475–484.

Frick, G.P., Tai, L.R., Blinder, L., and Goodman, H.M. (1981): L-leucine activates branched-chain α-keto acid dehydrogenase in rat adipose tissue. *J. Biol. Chem.* 256:2618–2620.

Hutson, S.M., Zapalowski, C., Cree, T.C., and Harper, A.E. (1980): Regulation of leucine and α-ketoisocaproic acid metabolism in skeletal muscle. Effects of starvation and insulin. *J. Biol. Chem.* 255:2418–2426.

Meister, A. (1965): *Biochemistry of the Amino Acids,* 2nd ed. vol 2, pp 729–756, Academic Press, New York.

Odessey, R. (1980a): Reversible ATP-induced inactivation of branched-chain 2-oxoacid dehydrogenase. *Biochem. J.* 192:155–163.

Odessey, R. (1980b): Direct evidence for the inactivation of branched-chain oxo-acid dehydrogenase by enzyme phosphorylation. *FEBS Lett.* 121:306–308.

Parker, P.J., and Randle, P.J. (1980): Active and inactive forms of branched-chain 2-oxoacid dehydrogenase complex in rat heart and skeletal muscle. *FEBS Lett.* 112:186–190.

Paul, H.S., and Adibi, S.A. (1978a): Leucine oxidation in diabetes and starvation: Effect of ketone bodies on branched-chain amino acid oxidation in vitro. *Metabolism* 27:185–200.
Paul, H.S., and Adibi, S.A. (1978b): Effect of carnitine on branched-chain amino acid oxidation by liver and skeletal muscle. *Am. J. Physiol.* 234:E494–E499.
Paul, H.S., and Adibi, S.A. (1980): Leucine oxidation and protein turnover in clofibrate-induced muscle protein degradation in rats. *J. Clin. Invest.* 65:1285–1293.
Paul, H.S., and Adibi, S.A. (1982): Role of ATP in the regulation of branched-chain α-keto acid dehydrogenase activity in liver and muscle mitochondria of fed, fasted, and diabetic rats. *J. Biol. Chem.* 257:4875–4881.

12 Factors Affecting Protein Balance in Skeletal Muscle in Normal and Pathological States

Alfred L. Goldberg

Protein balance in skeletal muscle is of fundamental importance in the control of muscle size and also in overall energy homeostasis of the organism (Goldberg et al., 1980). For example, in fasting the mobilization of amino acids stored in muscle protein helps provide the organism with essential precursors for hepatic or renal gluconeogenesis and with substrates that can be directly oxidized for energy (Goldberg and Chang, 1978). Thus, protein breakdown in skeletal muscle should be viewed as an initial rate-limiting step in gluconeogenesis.

This chapter will review recent findings from our laboratory concerning the regulation of protein breakdown in muscle. Although I shall focus on the control of protein catabolism, it should be emphasized that skeletal muscle is also very active in amino acid metabolism (Goldberg and Chang, 1978; Felig, 1975; Ruderman, 1975). When net protein breakdown occurs in muscle, this tissue does not release all amino acids directly. The branched-chain amino acids are extensively oxidized within skeletal and cardiac muscle, and the amino groups are released in the form of alanine or glutamine, which are synthesized *de novo* in this tissue (Goldberg and Chang, 1978; Chang and Goldberg, 1978a,b). The latter amino acids are released in much larger amounts and the branched-chain amino acids in much lower amounts than would be expected from the composition of muscle protein (Felig, 1975; Ruderman, 1975). It is, therefore, important in analyzing protein balance in muscle to distinguish the breakdown and synthesis of amino acids from the synthesis and breakdown of muscle protein. Although these processes are distinct, important interrelationships exist between the regulation of protein and amino acid metabolism in skeletal muscle, as discussed below.

MEASUREMENT OF PROTEIN TURNOVER

A major factor limiting progress in this area has been various technical problems involved in measuring overall degradative rates of proteins (Goldberg and Dice, 1974). Such *in vivo* measurements are subject to a number of potential artifacts and have frequently engendered appreciable controversy. Our laboratory has employed simple *in vitro* techniques to analyze rates of protein degradation and synthesis under carefully controlled conditions. These studies employed certain thin rat muscles that can be maintained *in vitro* for many hours in a good physiological state, the diaphragm, red soleus muscle, or pale extensor digitorum longus (Goldberg et al., 1975a). The advantages of these methods have been discussed in detail elsewhere (Goldberg and Dice, 1974; Fulks et al., 1975; Li and Goldberg, 1976; Tischler et al., 1982).

Rates of protein synthesis in the incubated muscles are determined by measuring rates of incorporation of [^{14}C]tyrosine or [^{14}C]phenylalanine into muscle protein, after correcting for intracellular-specific activity. Rates of protein degradation are measured by following the net release of tyrosine from cell protein (Fulks et al., 1975). Tyrosine was chosen for such studies because sensitive fluorometric assays for tyrosine exist and because this amino acid is neither synthesized nor catabolized by muscle. Consequently, its production by isolated muscles must reflect net protein breakdown. This consideration is an important one that has been often overlooked; for example, many investigators have incorrectly equated protein breakdown with the release from muscle of alanine and glutamine which are synthesized *de novo* in large amounts by muscle (Goldberg and Chang, 1978).

Absolute rates of protein degradation can be determined by measuring net tyrosine release in the presence of cycloheximide, an inhibitor of protein synthesis. Alternatively, absolute rates of protein catabolism can be calculated from simultaneous measurements on the same muscle of net protein balance and rates of protein synthesis (Tischler et al., 1982). Thus, if the net generation of tyrosine from cell protein is added to the rate of tyrosine incorporation into proteins, the sum equals the absolute rate of tyrosine production by proteolysis.

AGENTS AFFECTING PROTEIN BALANCE IN ISOLATED MUSCLES

A number of factors known to be important for the growth of skeletal muscle have been shown with such techniques to alter the overall rates of protein degradation as well as protein synthesis in skeletal muscles incubated *in vitro,* although similar findings seem also to apply to cardiac muscle (Rannels et al., 1977). When rat muscles are incubated in unsupplemented Krebs-Ringer bicarbonate buffer, protein catabolism exceeds synthesis by severalfold (Fulks et al., 1975; Li and Goldberg,

1976). Because of the net protein breakdown, these muscles show a net release of amino acids into the medium and thus resemble skeletal muscle *in vivo* during a short fast. Various factors may be added to the incubation buffer to improve overall protein balance (Table 12-1).

Table 12-1
Factors Affecting Protein Turnover in Skeletal Muscle

	Protein Synthesis	Protein Degradation
Glucose	—	↓
Fatty Acids	—	—
Ketone Bodies	—	—
Insulin	↑	↓
Plasma Amino Acids	↑	↓
Leucine	↑	↓
α Keto-isocaproate	—	↓
Other Amino Acids	—	—
Arachidonic Acid		↑
Prostaglandin E_2	—	↑
Prostaglandin $F_{2\alpha}$	↑	—

1. *Insulin* is probably the most important physiological factor regulating overall protein balance in skeletal muscle (Cahill et al., 1972). The rise in insulin levels after meals stimulates the net uptake of amino acids by skeletal muscle and their incorporation into protein. The fall in insulin in the fasting organism signals a net release of amino acids from muscle (Cahill et al., 1972; Felig, 1975; Ruderman, 1975; Mortimore and Neely, 1975). In muscle and other tissues, insulin not only stimulates protein synthesis but also inhibits protein degradation (Goldberg, 1979; Rannels et al., 1975; Rannels et al., 1977; Fulks et al., 1975; Li and Goldberg, 1975; Mortimore, 1982) apparently by an effect on lysosomal function (Mortimore, 1982). These two hormonal actions have complementary effects in producing a net accumulation of tissue protein. These effects on protein synthesis and degradation can be demonstrated in the absence of exogenous glucose or amino acids and thus are not secondary to insulin's well-known ability to stimulate nutrient transport (Fulks et al., 1975).

2. *Glucose* by itself also inhibits protein degradation but does not affect overall protein synthesis (Fulks et al., 1975). The effects of insulin and glucose in general, appear additive in improving overall protein balance in muscle. By contrast, free fatty acids or ketone bodies at physiological levels do not affect protein synthesis or degradation in skeletal muscle (Fulks et al., 1975; Tischler et al., 1982), even though these compounds are an excellent source of energy for this tissue.

3. The addition of *plasma amino acids* to the incubation medium retards protein breakdown further and stimulates protein synthesis, but most of the amino acids found in plasma are not necessary for such effects. Studies in our laboratory (Fulks et al., 1975; Goldberg and Tischler, 1981) and by others in skeletal (Buse and Reid, 1975; Buse and Wiegand, 1977; Li and Jefferson, 1978) or cardiac muscle (Rannels et al., 1975; Rannels et al., 1977) have shown that *leucine* by itself promotes protein synthesis and inhibits protein breakdown (Table 12-2). No other plasma amino acid

can influence protein turnover in these preparations. The presence of leucine in the medium seems to stimulate the production of both soluble and myofibrillar proteins as also occurs upon exposure to insulin (Buse and Wiegand, 1977. See Table 12-3).

Leucine also is the only amino acid that can provide significant energy for muscle (Goldberg and Chang, 1978; Chang and Goldberg, 1978a,b) and in fasting, leucine, like fatty acids or ketone bodies, serves as an alternative substrate to glucose (Goldberg and Chang, 1978; Chang and Goldberg, 1978a,b). Such effects of leucine on protein turnover in muscle are obtained at concentrations of leucine (0.1 to 0.5 mM) found *in vivo* (Table 12-2). Thus, normal variations in the blood levels of leucine may regulate protein balance in muscle *in vivo*. Furthermore, intravenous administration of branched-chain amino acids, or leucine by itself, appears to be of therapeutic value in reducing the marked protein catabolism occurring in surgical patients (Williamson and Walzer, 1981). In our *in vitro* studies (Tischler et al., 1982), leucine also was found to progressively inhibit proteolysis at the high concentrations (0.3 to 1.0 mM) probably found in plasma of patients receiving amino acid mixtures intravenously or as dietary supplements.

Table 12-2
Comparison of Effects of Varied Concentrations of Leucine on Protein Synthesis and Degradation

	Protein Synthesis		Protein Degradation	
Leucine	*Absolute Increase*	*Stimulation*	*Absolute Decrease*	*Inhibition*
(mM)	(nmol/mg tissue/2h)	(percent)	(nmol/mg tissue/2h)	(percent)
0.1 (6)	+ 0.009 ± .002	10 ± 2[a]	− 0.005 ± .005	0
0.2 (6)	+ 0.016 ± .002	19 ± 2[b]	− 0.029 ± .005	6 ± 1[a]
0.25 (7)	ND		− 0.080 ± .016	15 ± 3[a]
0.5 (20)	+ 0.033 ± .004	42 ± 5[b]	− 0.171 ± .011	26 ± 2[b]

[a]$p < 0.005$; [b]$p < 0.001$
Data taken from Tischler et al., 1982.

Table 12-3
Effect of Branched-Chain Amino Acids on Synthesis of Soluble and Myofibrillar Proteins in Rat Diaphragm

		Tyrosine Incorporation (nmol tyr/h)		
		Control	*Leucine (0.5 mM)*	*% Stimulation*
Exp. I	Soluble	0.0450 ± .005	0.061 ± .006	36*
	Myofibrillar	0.081 ± .007	0.102 ± 0.006	26*
	Total	0.126 ± .009	0.163 ± 0.009	29*
Exp. II	Soluble	0.56 ± .005	0.70 ± .004	25
	Myofibrillar	0.65 ± .007	0.84 ± .006	29*
	Total	.121 ± .009	0.154 ± .008	27*
(6 animals)			*p < .05	

Protein synthesis was measured as described by Fulks et al. (1975), and soluble and myofibrillar proteins fractionated as described previously (Goldberg, 1969).

4. All these factors together still do not prevent net protein catabolism in the isolated muscles. Unlike muscles *in vivo,* these isolated tissues do not perform work, and it has long been recognized that disuse or denervation leads to muscle atrophy. Earlier studies *in vivo* and *in vitro* indicate that this process is primarily a consequence of an enhancement of protein breakdown (Goldberg, 1969; Goldspink, 1977). Several years ago, we obtained evidence that *repeated contractions in vitro* induced by electrical stimulation or *passive stretch* can retard protein breakdown by 15% to 25% in the isolated soleus or diaphragm (Goldberg et al., 1975; Goldberg et al., 1974). Under these same conditions, protein synthesis does not change in the muscles. When incubated muscles are provided with insulin, glucose, and amino acids and are maintained under some degree of tension, they are in a state of neutral or positive nitrogen balance.

This ability of contractile activity to retard protein breakdown probably is an important factor contributing to work-induced hypertrophy of muscle as well as disuse atrophy (Goldberg, 1980). These findings with passive tension of muscle are also of particular practical interest because of the evidence from several laboratories that passive tension of muscle may by itself induce compensatory hypertrophy (Goldberg et al., 1975a). In addition, these effects may contribute to certain beneficial results obtained by physical therapy. However, the cellular mechanisms by which passive or active tension may influence rates of proteolysis are completely unclear.

MECHANISMS OF LEUCINE'S EFFECTS ON PROTEIN SYNTHESIS AND BREAKDOWN

To investigate whether leucine in regulatory effects required leucine degradation, these studies have utilized a competitive inhibitor of leucine transamination, cycloserine. At low concentrations, this agent inhibits leucine oxidation in a reversible manner (Goldberg and Tischler, 1981; Tischler et al., 1982). In muscles incubated with cycloserine, the addition of leucine stimulated protein synthesis just as in the absence of this agent. However, this inhibitor completely prevented the reduction in protein breakdown in skeletal or atrial muscle by leucine. In other words, this agent dissociated the two anabolic effects of leucine; the inhibition of protein breakdown seems to require leucine catabolism, while the enhancement of synthesis does not (Goldberg and Tischler, 1981; Tischler et al., 1982). In additional experiments varying concentrations of leucine were added in the presence of cycloserine. By this approach, it was possible to show that the rates of leucine breakdown correlated closely with the ability of leucine to inhibit protein breakdown.

Further support for these conclusions came from incubating muscles with the keto acid derivative of leucine. As predicted, leucine's inhibitory effects on protein breakdown could be mimicked with α-ketoisocaproic acid, but unlike leucine, the keto acid derivative did not increase protein synthesis. It is noteworthy that in human patients, α-ketoisocaproate can improve protein balance (Walzer and Williamson, 1981). In fact, Mitch and coworkers (1981) have presented evidence that this agent is even more effective than leucine in improving nitrogen balance in humans with renal failure (perhaps because it is transported more rapidly across cells than leucine itself) (Odessey and Goldberg, 1979).

Additional studies attempted to clarify how extracellular leucine may stimulate protein synthesis. Specifically, we tested whether intracellular leucine itself might enhance protein synthesis or whether the supply of leucyl tRNA levels might be the rate-limiting factor for muscle protein synthesis. We, therefore, studied the kinetic properties of leucyl tRNA synthetase from muscle as well as liver and bacteria (Tischler et al., 1981) or muscle (Tischler et al., 1981). In each case, leucyl tRNA synthetase showed a Km of 6 μM or less, which is fiftyfold less than the apparent intracellular concentration in muscles, even in leucine-free medium. Consequently, under all physiological conditions, leucyl tRNA must be fully charged. In addition, formation of leucyl tRNA showed similar Kms as synthesis of phenylalanine tRNA even though phenylalanine has no regulatory influence on protein turnover in muscle.

Thus, the supply of leucyl tRNA should not vary with the changes in the extracellular levels of leucine between 0.1 and 0.5 mM or with parallel changes in the intracellular leucine concentrations (which are slightly higher than extracellular). To summarize, intracellular concentrations of this amino acid far exceed the levels required to fully charge leucyl tRNA, and the ability of leucine to control protein synthesis seems to depend directly on its intracellular concentration rather than on leucyl tRNA or any other known leucine metabolite.

PROSTAGLANDINS AND THE CONTROL OF PROTEIN BREAKDOWN

In a variety of pathological states, including fever, sepsis, traumatic injury, and cachexia, there is a marked negative nitrogen balance and a severe loss of body protein (Cuthbertson and Tilstone, 1969; Beisel et al., 1972; Garlick et al., 1980; Crane et al., 1977). A number of these studies have indicated that overall rates of protein breakdown increase in patients following traumatic injury, and it is generally presumed that these effects are occurring in skeletal muscle. We, therefore, undertook studies to attempt to identify the intracellular factors that may be responsible for this accelerated breakdown of muscle protein. Evidence has been obtained (Rodemann and Goldberg, 1982) that one important factor promoting protein breakdown in muscle is prostaglandin E_2, and that this agent triggers the excessive proteolysis in various pathological states (Rodemann et al., 1982; Rodemann and Goldberg, 1982; Baracos et al., 1982).

It is now well established that prostaglandins participate in a variety of pathological processes, including inflammatory responses, hemostasis, and fever. However, there have been no prior studies published concerning a possible role of prostaglandins, prostacyclins, or thromboxanes in the regulation of protein breakdown. In order to examine these possibilities, we have incubated rat skeletal and cardiac muscles with arachidonic acid or a number of its metabolites and also investigated whether prostaglandins were produced by the isolated rat muscles.

When the red soleus, pale extensor digitorum longus, diaphragm, or atrial muscles were incubated *in vitro* with arachidonic acid (10^{-6} to 10^{-7}M), rates of protein degradation increased by 20% to 40%. This increase in proteolysis was seen within 40 minutes after arachidonic acid addition (which was the shortest time studied). Arachidonate caused an acceleration of protein breakdown even when protein synthesis was inhibited; thus, this effect does not require the production of new proteases or regulatory proteins. Net protein breakdown increased in all muscles examined, although the overall rate of protein synthesis remained unchanged. (In one muscle, the dark soleus, protein synthesis also increased after addition of arachidonic acid, but this effect did not compensate for the greater increase in protein breakdown. The basis for this exceptional behavior of the soleus remains unclear.)

To clarify which of the various metabolites of arachidonate may be responsible for this effect, the muscles were incubated with aspirin, indomethacin, or meclofenamate. These compounds inhibit the cyclooxygenase necessary for prostaglandin and prostacyclin production from arachidonate. All three dramatically reduced the stimulation of protein breakdown by arachidonate (Table 12-4). (In addition, in the soleus they prevented the accompanying acceleration of protein synthesis.) By contrast, the cyclooxygenase inhibitors did not affect the basal rate of protein breakdown seen in control muscles.

These results suggest a specific role for prostaglandin in the acceleration of protein turnover. Accordingly, the product of the cyclooxygenase, PGH_2, mimicked the actions of arachidonic acid in stimulating proteolysis in the incubated muscles. Various metabolites of arachidonate (and of PGH_2) were also studied. Of the various compounds tested, only PGE_2 significantly stimulated the rate of protein degradation. This agent, caused net protein balance to become more negative by 20% to 40%, but it did not alter overall rates of protein synthesis. On the other hand, $PGE_{2\alpha}$ caused a reproducible stimulation of protein synthesis in both pale and dark muscles without affecting proteolysis.

These observations together strongly suggest that PGE_2 mediates the effects of arachidonate on protein breakdown. (Rodemann and Goldberg, 1982). Furthermore, the incubated muscles were found to synthesize and release into the medium, large amounts of PGE_2 and PGF_2, as shown by radioimmunoassay. The addition of arachidonate to the medium caused a five- to sixfold increase in the release of PGE_2 and a threefold increase of $PGF_{2\alpha}$. Indomethacin prevented these effects, just as it reduced the arachidonate effect on proteolysis (Table 12-4).

Table 12-4
Effect of Various Inhibitors of Cyclooxygenase on Protein Degradation in the Absence and Presence of Arachidonic Acid in Rat Diaphragm

Arachidonic Acid (5×10^{-6}M)	Inhibitor	Protein Degradation (nmol tyr/mg muscle/2 h)	% Change	p
None		0.509 ± 0.015		
+		0.678 ± 0.043	+33	<0.05
+	Aspirin	0.548 ± 0.023		N.S.
+	Indomethacin	0.527 ± 0.020		N.S.
None		0.499 ± 0.031		
+		0.633 ± 0.038	+41	<0.05
+	Indomethacin	0.525 ± 0.026		N.S.
+	Meclofenamate	0.538 ± 0.051		N.S.
None		0.604 ± 0.040		
None	Aspirin	0.620 ± 0.041		N.S.
None	Indomethacin	0.628 ± 0.033		N.S.
None	Meclofenamate	0.615 ± 0.032		N.S.

Data taken from Rodemann et al., 1982.

Further studies were undertaken to verify how prostaglandins may be activating protein breakdown in this tissue. It is now well established that mammalian cells contain multiple pathways for protein degradation, which may serve distinct physiological functions (Goldberg et al., 1980a; Etlinger and Goldberg, 1977; Mortimore, 1982). The lysosome has long been assumed to be the major, and perhaps the only site, for protein breakdown in mammalian cells (Mortimore, 1982). This organelle contains a high concentration of proteolytic enzymes, and is responsible for the degradation of many phagocytosed or pinocytosed proteins. It also plays an important role in the digestion of cellular proteins. In various physiological conditions, where overall protein breakdown increases (e.g., in the absence of insulin or amino acids), the intralysosomal proteolysis seems to rise through increased formation of autophagic vacuoles. The detailed mechanisms are unclear (Mortimore, 1982), but there is now strong evidence that areas of the cytoplasm are enclosed in vacuoles which then fuse with lysosomes.

In addition, mammalian and bacterial cells contain a soluble nonlysosomal degradative pathway that requires ATP (Etlinger and Goldberg, 1977). This cytoplasmic process seems responsible for the rapid elimination of abnormal proteins, as may arise by mutation or biosynthetic errors, as well as many short-lived proteins. In addition, mammalian mitochondria contain within them a similar system for degradation of intramitochondrial proteins (Desautels and Goldberg, 1982). Finally, in the cytoplasm of mammalian cells there exists an intriguing Ca^{2+}-requiring alkaline protease whose function remains unclear. To decide whether the prostaglandins may be activating the lysosomal apparatus, we incubated muscles with arachidonate or PGE_2, as well as specific inhibitors of lysosomal thiol proteases, leupeptin and Ep-475. These agents can enter muscle cells and inhibit in the intact tissue, cathepsin B and probably cathepsin H and L (Libby and Goldberg, 1978; Hanada et al., 1978). These inhibitors, however, do not affect the nonlysosomal ATP-dependent pathway, and therefore have proven very useful for dissecting the roles of these two systems (Hopgood et al., 1974; Libby and Goldberg, 1978; Seglen et al., 1979; Rodemann and Goldberg, 1982). These inhibitors also are of appreciable interest as possible tools for the treatment of excessive protein breakdown (e.g., in muscular dystrophy) (Stracher et al., 1978; Libby and Goldberg, 1978, 1980).

The stimulation of protein degradation by arachidonate and by PGE_2 could be inhibited almost completely with either leupeptin and Ep-475. Thus, somehow the prostaglandins appear to activate intralysosomal proteolysis, although the precise mechanisms by which they do so remain unclear. Most likely, PGE_2 in some way promotes autophagic vacuole formation which appears to be the rate-limiting step for protein catabolism (Mortimore, 1982), but the cellular mechanisms for such alterations in lysosomal function are an important subject for future research. It is well established that certain prostaglandins (especially PGE_1) can increase cyclic AMP levels in several cell systems, but such effects appear unrelated to the present findings. In our experience, dibutyryl cyclic AMP, catecholamines, or PGE_1 do not consistently alter rates of protein degradation or protein synthesis.

Another important question for future research is whether arachidonate or PGE_2 have similar effects on proteolysis in other tissues. Thus far, we have failed to show such effects of prostaglandins in cultured hamster fibroblasts or in rat hepatocytes.

SIGNIFICANCE

Although the mechanisms by which PGE_2 activates proteolysis are unknown, we have recently obtained extensive evidence that this compound plays an important role in triggering the acceleration of proteolysis in various pathological states. Thanks to the efforts of Drs. Rodemann, Baracos, and Waxman we have been able to demonstrate that PGE_2 is in large part responsible for the accelerated muscle proteolysis induced by Ca^{2+}-ionophores (Rodemann and Goldberg, 1982), by experimental fever in rats (Rodemann et al., in preparation) and by leukocyte pyrogen (Baracos et al., 1982). In fact, our recent findings, now in the course of publication, strongly suggest that leukocyte pyrogen (DiNarello and Wolff, 1978), the polypeptide that acts on the hypothalamus to induce the febrile state, also acts directly on muscle to stimulate prostaglandin release and proteolysis. In addition to their scientific interest, such observations are of appreciable clinical relevance. For example, they provide a strong new rationale for the use of the cyclooxygenase inhibitors to reduce negative nitrogen balance in human patients, suffering from burns, sepsis or fever.

ACKNOWLEDGMENTS

The author is grateful to Maureen Rush for her expert assistance in preparation of this manuscript. These studies have been supported by grants from the National Institute of Neurological Disease and Stroke and the Muscular Dystrophy Association of America. The conclusions presented here have been all made possible through the diligent efforts of my colleagues, Dr. Peter Rodemann, Dr. Vicky Baracos, Dr. Lloyd Waxman, and Dr. Marc Tischler, as well as the capable assistance of Timothy Meixsell and Shirley Li.

REFERENCES

Baracos, V., Rodemann, H.P., DiNarello, C. and Goldberg, A.L. (1982): Submitted for publication.

Beisel, W.R., Sawyer, W.D., and Ryll, W.D. (1972): Metabolic effects of intracellular infections in man. *Ann. Intern. Med.* 67:744–779.

Buse, M.G. and Reid, S.S. (1975): Leucine: a possible regulation of protein turnover in muscle. *J. Clin. Invest.* 56:1250–1261.

Buse, M.G. and Weigand, D.A. (1977): Studies concerning the specificity of the effects of leucine on the turnover of proteins in muscles of control and diabetic rats. *Biochim. Biophys. Acta* 475:81–89.

Cahill, G.F., Aoki, T.T., Marliss, E.B. (1972): In *Handbook of Physiology-Endocrinology* (eds: R.O. Greep and E.B. Astwood), Vol. 1, pp. 563–577, Am. Physiol. Soc., Washington, D.C.

Chang, T.W. and Goldberg, A.L. (1978A): The metabolic fats of amino acids and the formation of glutamine in skeletal muscle. *J. Biol. Chem.* 253:3685–3693.

Chang, T.W. and Goldberg, A.L. (1978B): Leucine inhibits oxidation of glucose and pyruvate in skeletal muscles during fasting. *J. Biol. Chem.* 253:3696–3701.

Crane, C.W., Picou, D., Smith, R., and Waterlow, J.C. (1977): Protein turnover in patients before and after elective orthopaedic operations. *Br. J. Surg.* 64:129–133.

Cuthbertson, D., and Tilstone, W.J. (1969): Metabolism during the postinjury period. *Adv. Clin. Chem.* 12:1-55.

Desautels, M. and Goldberg, A.L. (1982): Liver Mitochondria contain an ATP-dependent, vanadate-sensitive pathway for the degradation of proteins. *Proc. Nat. Acad. Sci.* USA, 79:1869-1873.

DiNarello, C.A., and Wolff, S.M. (1978): Pathogenesis of fever in man. *N. Eng. J. Med.* 298: 607-612.

Etlinger, J.D. and Goldberg, A.L. (1977): A soluable ATP-dependent proteolytic system responsible for the degradation of abnormal proteins in reticulocytes. *Proc. Nat. Acad. Sci.* 74:54-58.

Felig, P. (1975): Amino acid metabolism in man. *Ann. Rev. Biochem.* 44:933-954.

Frick, G.P. and Goodman, H.M. (1981): In *Metabolism and Clinical Implications of Branched Chain Amino and Ketoacids* (eds: M. Walser and J.R. Williamson), Vol. 18, p. 73, Elsevier/North Holland, New York.

Fulks, R., Li, J.B., and Goldberg, A.L. (1975): Effects of insulin, glucose, and amino acids on protein turnover in rat diaphragm. *J. Biol. Chem.* 250:290-298.

Garlick, P.J., McNurlan, M.A., Fern, E.B., Tomkins, A.H., and Waterlow, J.C. (1980): Stimulation of protein synthesis and breakdown by vaccination. *Br. Med. J.* 281: 263-265.

Goldberg, A.L. (1969): Protein turnover in skeletal muscle. *J. Biol. Chem.* 244:3223-3229.

Goldberg, A.L. (1979): Influence of insulin and contractile activity on muscle size and protein balance. *Diabetes,* 28(1):18-24.

Goldberg, A.L. and Chang, T.W. (1978): Regulation and significance of amino acid metabolism in skeletal muscle. *Fed. Proc.* 37:2301-2307.

Goldberg, A.L. and Dice, J.F. (1974): Intracellular protein degradation in mammalian and bacterial cells. *Ann. Rev. Biochem.* 43:835-869.

Goldberg, A.L. and Tischler, M.E. (1981): In *Metabolism and Clinical Implications of Branched Chain Amino and Ketoacids* (eds: J.H. Williamson and M. Walser), pp. 205-216, Elsevier/North Holland, New York.

Goldberg, A.L., Jablecki, C.N. and Li, J.B. (1974): Effects of use and disuse of amino acid transport and protein turnover in muscle. *Ann. N.Y. Acad. Sci.* 228:190-201.

Goldberg, A.L., Etlinger, J.J., Goldspink, D.F., Jablecki, C. (1975): Mechanism of work-induced hypertrophy of skeletal muscle. *Med. Sci. Sports* 7:185-198.

Goldberg, A.L., Martel, S.B. and Kushmerick, M.J. (1975B): *In vitro* preparations of the diaphragm and other skeletal muscles. *Methods Enzymol.* 39:82-93.

Goldberg, A.L. (1980): In *Plasticity of Muscle* (ed: D. Pette), pp. 470-492, W. de Gruyter, New York.

Goldberg, A.L., Strnad, N. and Swamy, K.H.S. (1980a): In *Protein Degradation in Health and Disease,* pp. 227-251, CIBA Symposium, Excerpta Medica, Amsterdam, Oxford, New York.

Goldberg, A.L., Tischler, M., DeMartino, G. and Griffin, G. (1980b): Hormonal regulation of protein degradation and synthesis in skeletal muscle. *Fed. Proc.* 39:31-36.

Hanada, K., Tamai, M., Yamagashi, M., Ohmura, S., Sawada, J., and Tanaka, I. (1978): *Agric. Biol. Chem.* 42:523-528.

Hopgood, M.F., Clark, M.G., Ballard, F.J.: Inhibition of protein degradation in isolated rat hepatocytes. *Biochem. J.* (1977):164:399-407.

Libby, P., Bursztajn, S. and Goldberg, A.L. (1980): Degradation of the acetylcholine receptor in cultured muscle cells: selective inhibitors and the fate of undergraded receptors. *Cell* 19:481-491.

Libby, P. and Goldberg, A.L. (1978): Leupeptin: a proteinase inhibitor decreases protein degradation in normal and diseased muscles. *Science* 199:534-536.

Libby, P. and Goldberg, A.L. (1976): Effects of Chymostatin and other proteinase inhibitors on protein breakdown and proteolytic activities in muscle. *Biochem. J.* 188:213-220.

Li, J.B. and Goldberg, A.L. (1976): Effects of food deprivation on protein synthesis and degradation in rat skeletal muscles. *Am. J. Physiol.* 231:441–448.

Li, J.B. and Jefferson, L.S. (1978): Influence of amino acid availability on protein turnover in perfused skeletal muscle. *Biochim. Biophys. Acta.* 544:351–359.

Mitch, W.E., M. Walser, and D.G. Sapir (1981): In *Metabolism and Clinical Implications of Branched Chain Amino and Ketoacids* (eds: M. Walser and J. R. Williamson), Vol. 18, pp. 349–354, Elsevier/North Holland, New York.

Mortimore, G. (1982): Mechanisms of cellular protein catabolism. *Nutrit. Rev.* 40:1–12.

Neff, N.T., DeMartino, G.N. and Goldberg, A.L. (1979): The effect of protease inhibitors and decreased temperature on the degradation of different classes of proteins in cultured hepatocytes. *J. Cell Physiol.* 101:439–457.

Odessey, R. and Goldberg, A.L. (1979): Leucine degradation in cell free extracts of skeletal muscle. *Biochem. J.* 178:475–489.

Rannels, D.E., Kao, R., Morgan, H.E. (1975): Effect of insulin on protein turnover in heart muscles. *J. Biol. Chem.* 250:1694–1701.

Rannels, D.E., McKee, E.E., Morgan, H.E. (1977): In *Biochemical Actions of Hormones* (ed: G. Litwack), pp. 135–195, Academic Press, New York.

Rodemann, H.P. and Goldberg, A.L. (1982): Arachidonic acid, prostaglandin E_2 and F_2 influence rates of protein turnover in skeletal and cardiac muscle. *J. Biol. Chem.* 257: 1632–1638.

Rodemann, H.P., Waxman, L., and Goldberg, A.L. (1982): *J. Biol. Chem.* in press.

Ruderman, N.B. (1975): Muscle amino acid metabolism and gluconeogenesis. *Ann. Rev. Med.* 26:245–258.

Seglen, P.O., Grinde, B., and Solheim, A.E. (1979): Inhibition of the lysosomal pathway of protein degradation in isolated rat hepatocytes by ammonia, methylamine, choroquine and leupeptin. *Eur. J. Biochem.* 95:215–225.

Stracher, A., McGowan, E.B. and Shafiq, S.A. (1978): Muscular dystrophy: Inhibition of degeneration *in vivo* with protease inhibitors. *Science* 200:50–51.

Tischler, M.E., Desautels, M. and Goldberg, A.L. (1982): Does leucine, leucyl-tRNA, or some metabolite of leucine regulate protein synthesis and degradation in skeletal and cardiac muscle? *J. Biol. Chem.* 257:1613–1621.

Tischler, M.E. and Goldberg, A.L. (1980): Amino acid degradation and effect of leucine on pyruvate oxidation in rat atrial muscle. *Am. J. Physiol.* 238:E480–E486.

Williamson, J.H. and M. Walser (eds.) (1981): *Metabolism and Clinical Implications of Branched Chain Amino and Ketoacids.* Elsevier/North Holland, New York.

Is the Liver or the Periphery Limiting for Hepatic Utilization of Amino Acids in Cancer-Induced Malnutrition?

Lars Ekman and Kent G. Lundholm

A characteristic finding in patients suffering from cancer, trauma or infection is loss of body proteins, especially from skeletal muscles. In contrast, the liver seems to be protected from the overall body N catabolism in cancer disease and may even remain in nitrogen balance in spite of tumor growth. In this situation there is, generally, an increased gluconeogenesis. Muscle amino acids may, therefore, play an important role in supplying the liver and the tumor with nitrogen and energy-yielding precursors. It has been suggested that an elevated gluconeogenesis may not reflect an actual increased need for glucose, but rather that this process may function as an alternative excretory pathway for the disposal of surplus amino acids originating from protein breakdown in peripheral tissues (Stein, 1978). It is controversial as to whether peripheral mobilization or hepatic utilization of amino acids is the limiting step in negative nitrogen balance.

The aim of this study was to evaluate this question.

MATERIAL AND METHODS

Nongrowing sarcoma-bearing C57/BL6J mice were used as the tumor-bearing animal model. We have used this experimental model extensively to study tumor-host metabolism (Lundholm et al., 1978; Lundholm et al., 1980a,b; Lundholm et al., 1981; Karlberg et al., 1981, Lundholm et al., 1979). A description of the measurement of energy expenditure has been reported (Schersten et al., 1979) as well as measurements of food intake, pair-feeding experiments, urinary excretion of nitrogen, urea and potassium, nitrogen balance and body composition (Lundholm et al., 1980a). The rate and capacity of gluconeogenesis have been estimated both *in vitro* and *in vivo* (Lundholm et al., 1980a). The incorporation of [U-^{14}C]lactate and [U-^{14}C]glycerol into glucose were measured in relation to different substrate levels of lactate and glycerol in incubated liver slices from tumor-bearing mice compared with ad-libitum fed controls. The incorporation rate of [U-^{14}C]alanine into glucose was measured both *in vitro* and *in vivo*. Urea synthesis was measured *in vivo* as the cumulative excretion of urea over the entire period of tumor growth. The *in vitro* synthesis of urea was measured in incubated liver slices, in the presence of 20 amino acids at high concentrations (Lundholm et al., 1980a). The protein imbalance of skeletal muscles was estimated from the net loss of nitrogen in the extensor digitorum longus and quadriceps muscles (Svaninger et al., 1982). Hepatic protein synthesis was measured *in vivo* and *in vitro* using incubated liver slices, isolated mouse liver cells, a cell-free system, and by determination of the activities of RNA polymerases I, II and III (Lundholm et al., 1979; Ternell and Lundholm, 1981). Hepatic protein synthesis *in vivo* was calculated by dividing the area of the specific activity time curve for [^{14}C]arginyl-tRNA by the area of the specific activity time curve for [^{14}C]arginine in acid-precipitable proteins (method to be published). Total hepatic RNA content was measured according to Munro and Fleck (1966). The total hepatic pool of free amino acids was quantified after homogenization of liver and precipitation with perchloric acid. Amino acids were quantified in an automatic amino acid analyzer. Oxygen uptake by isolated liver cells was measured by means of an oxygen electrode.

RESULTS

The tumor-bearing animals (carcass plus tumor) were in negative energy balance but in overall positive nitrogen balance due to the growth of the tumor (Figure 1). However, the carcass was in negative nitrogen balance. Pair-fed controls maintained their body composition, which shows that the anorexia itself was not a sufficient condition to induce negative energy and nitrogen balance. Pair-fed mice conserved energy by reducing the metabolic rate and protein turnover, while the corresponding adaptation in the tumor-bearing animals was insufficient to achieve energy and nitrogen balance. Nitrogen was lost from the skeletal muscles primarily due to reduced synthesis, while total degradation of protein in skeletal muscles was unchanged. The gluconeogenesis rate was increased, as measured both *in vivo* and *in vitro* (Figure 2). Lactate and glycerol were quantitatively the most important precursors for gluconeogenesis. The hepatic protein synthesis was elevated by around 30% to 40% compared with that of freely fed controls (Figure 3). The increased protein synthesis appears to be due to an increased hepatic RNA content. All the above changes of liver metabolism in tumor-host livers were concomitant with a pronounced reduction

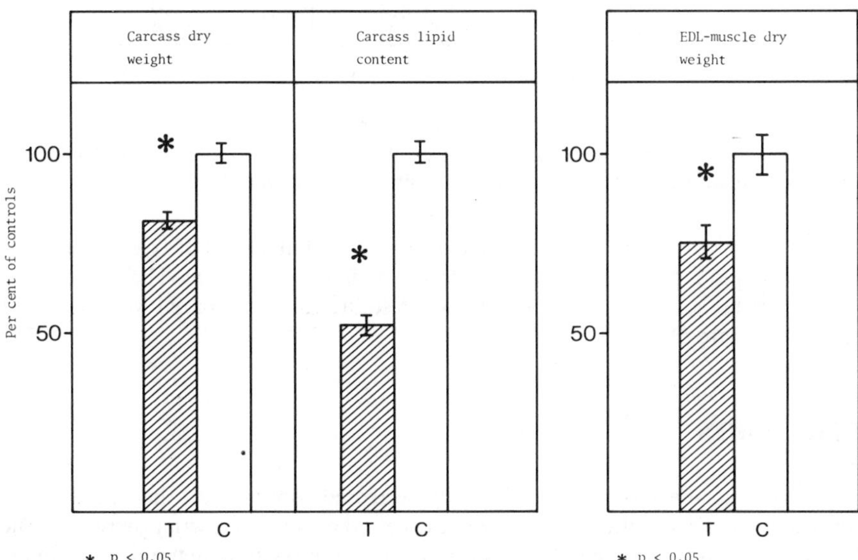

Figure 1 Dry weight in carcass and EDL muscles and carcass lipid content in tumor-bearing mice (T) compared with freely fed (C) controls.

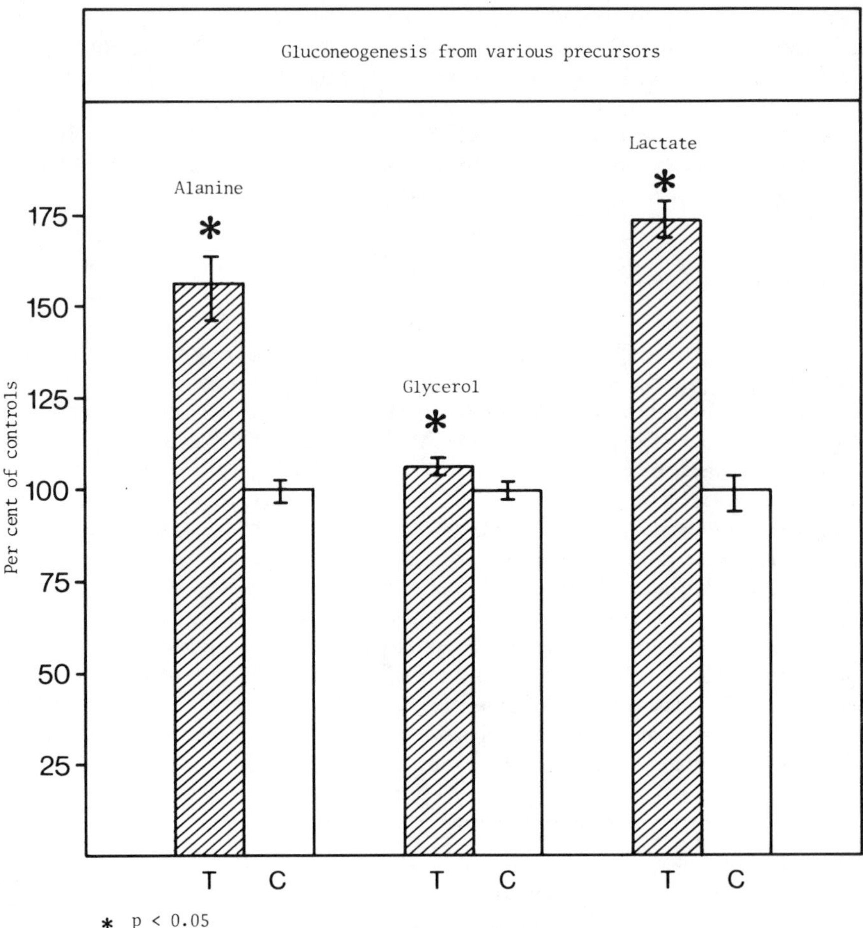

Figure 2 Gluconeogenesis from alanine, glycerol and lactate measured in incubated liver slices from tumor-bearing mice (T) compared with freely fed controls (C).

in urea synthesis (Figure 4), an increase of the intracellular pool of free amino acids (Figure 5), and a decreased oxygen consumption in the liver tissue. The intracellular pool of amino acids in skeletal muscles was also increased compared with freely fed controls (Figure 5).

DISCUSSION

The tumor-bearing mice in this study decreased continuously their food intake toward about 50% of the initial value as the period of tumor growth progressed. The loss of body lipids provided the energy for the tumor growth, as determined from the pair-feeding experiments. The nitrogen, which was necessary for the proliferation of the tumor, was made available by a net breakdown of skeletal muscles (Lundholm,

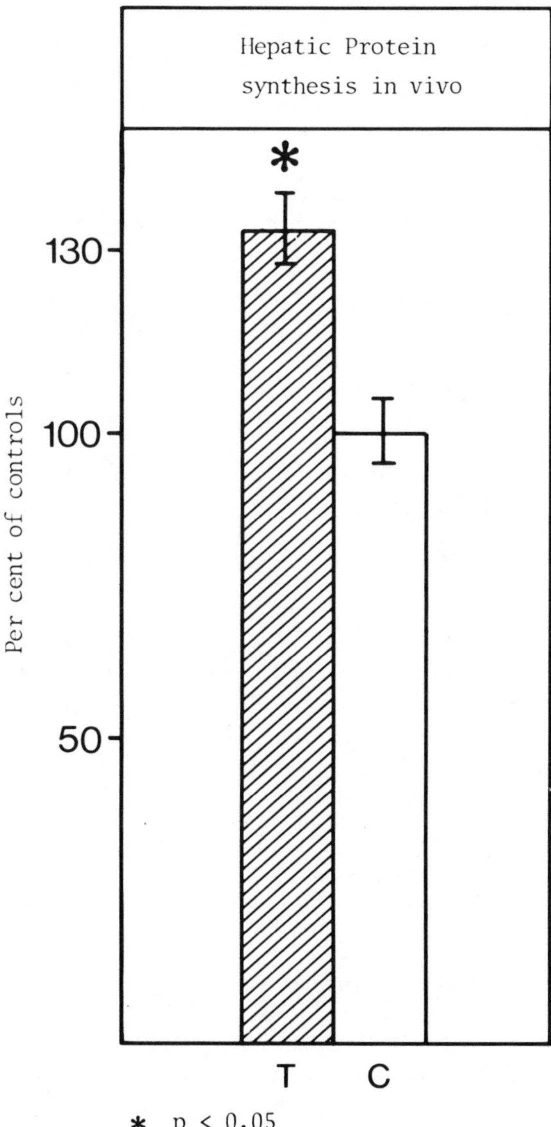

Figure 3 Hepatic protein synthesis *in vivo* in tumor bearing mice (T), compared with that of freely fed controls (C). Hepatic protein synthesis was measured as described in "Material and Methods".

et al., 1980a). Muscle protein turnover accounts for a significant proportion of whole body protein turnover. Therefore, any reduction in muscle turnover is a suitable way to save energy and to channel amino acids toward protein synthesis and gluconeogenesis elsewhere. This was probably an induced adaptation to make energy available for use elsewhere and so compensating for diminished availability of energy due to decreased food intake. Some authors have favored the view that net

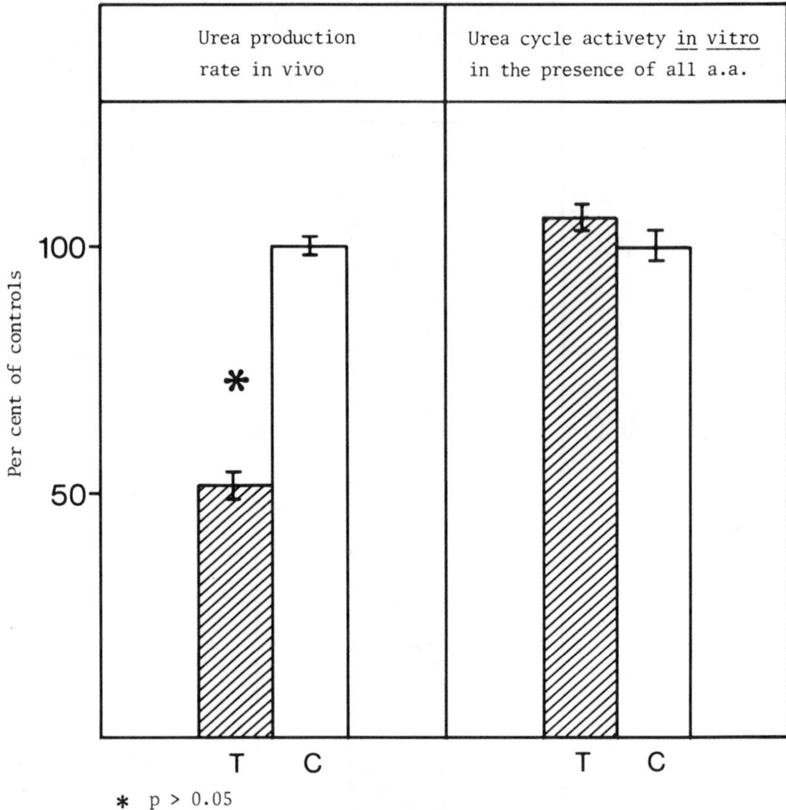

Figure 4 Urea production rate *in vivo* and *in vitro* in tumor-bearing mice(T) compared with that of freely fed controls (C). Urea production rate *in vivo* was measured as the cumulative excretion of urea along the tumor growth. Urea cycle activity *in vitro* was measured as urea synthesis in the presence of high concentrations of all amino acids.

breakdown of muscles is aimed at supplying amino acids for gluconeogenesis in conditions of negative nitrogen and energy balance. Another hypothesis may be that the liver or other central organ lacks certain amino acids for protein synthesis or as metabolic precursors for the intermediary metabolism. Whatever the explanation may be, our results suggest that incoming amino acids from the periphery are not randomly distributed intracellularly. This is supported by the finding that the free hepatic pool of amino acids was expanded concomitantly with increased protein synthesis, increased gluconeogenesis and decreased urea synthesis. It appears that nitrogen from amino acids can escape the urea cycle enzymes under certain conditions. The urea cycle enzymes *per se* were not the limiting factor for decreased urea synthesis in our study, since urea enzymes did function normally *in vitro*. Moreover, we have also found kinetic evidence of nonrandom distribution of amino acids in these tumor-bearing animals using isotopes (Karlberg et al., 1982).

The discrepancy between decreased urea production and increased gluconeogenesis from alanine may be that the total oxidation rate of amino acids was decreased, contributing less amino nitrogen for urea synthesis. This was supported

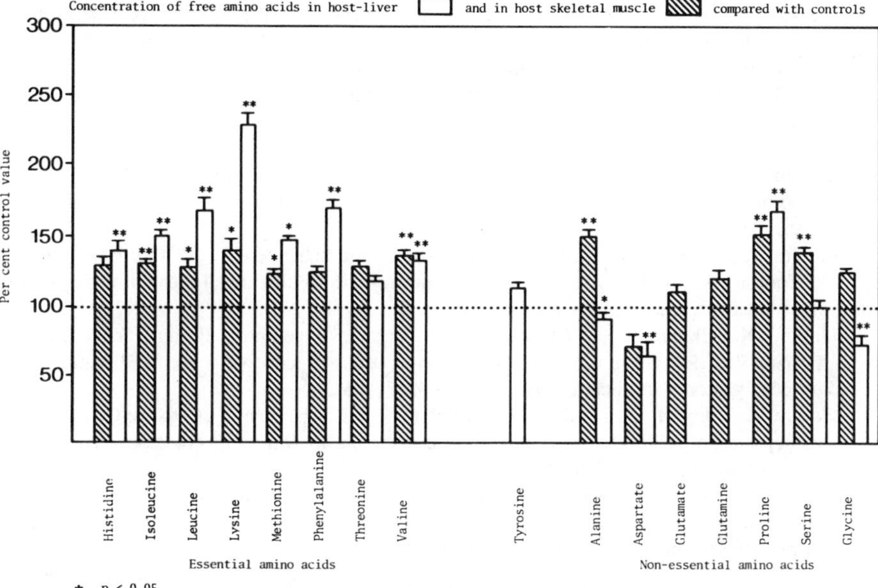

Figure 5 Concentration of free amino acids in host liver and in host skeletal muscle tissue compared with that of freely fed controls. Concentration of amino acids in tissues from control animals was set to 100%.

by our finding that the sarcoma-bearing mice had a decreased oxidation of amino acids measured *in vivo* (unpublished results).

The finding that the free pool of amino acids was increased in the liver and skeletal muscles from tumor-bearing mice means that the inflow of amino acids exceeded the outflow. The outflow pathway consists of protein synthesis and amino acid catabolism including hepatic and renal gluconeogenesis. These results suggest that the rate of net breakdown of skeletal muscles is not well controlled, since it appears to exceed the need of amino acids as metabolic precursors. Our results are at variance with those reported by Wu and Bauer (1960), who reported a decreased amount of free amino acids in skeletal muscle tissue from growing tumor-bearing rats. However, growing animals represent a condition necessitating a positive nitrogen balance. Therefore, growing animals do not provide an appropriate model for studies of wasting of skeletal muscles. An increased free pool of amino acids has recently been demonstrated in muscle biopsies from cancer patients (Wu and Bauer, 1960).

In summary, our results indicate that net breakdown of peripheral tissues is not the limiting step for the hepatic utilization of amino acids in cancer-induced malnutrition.

REFERENCES

Karlberg, I., Ekman, L., Edström, S., Scherstén, T. and Lundholm, K. (1982): Reutilization of amino acid carbons in relation to albumin turnover in non-growing mice with sarcoma. *Cancer Res;* accepted for publication.

Karlberg, I., Edström, S., Ekman, L., Johansson, S., Scherstén, T. and Lundholm, K. (1981): Metabolic host reaction in response to the proliferation of nonmalignant cells versus malignant cells *in vivo*. *Cancer Res.* 41:4154–4161.

Larsson, J., Baum, A., Symreng, T., Wetterfors, J. and Liljedahl S-O. (1981): Muscle amino acid pattern in gastrointestinal cancer. Espen. Third European Congress on Parenteral and Enteral Nutrition, Maastricht, The Netherlands.

Lundholm, K., Edström, S., Ekman, L., Karlberg, I., Bylund, A-C. and Scherstén, T. (1979): A comparative study of the influence of malignant tumor on host metabolism in mice and man. *Cancer* 42:453–461.

Lundholm, K., Edström, S., Karlberg, I., Ekman, L. and Scherstén, T. (1980a): Relationship of food intake, body composition, and tumor growth to host metabolism in nongrowing mice with sarcoma. *Cancer Res* 40:2516–2522.

Lundholm, K., Ekman, L., Edström, S., Karlberg, I., Jagenburg, R. and Scherstén, T. (1979): Protein synthesis in liver tissue under the influence of a methylcholanthrene-induced sarcoma in mice. *Cancer Res.* 39:4657–4661.

Lundholm, K., Ekman, L., Karlberg, I., Edström, S. and Scherstén, T. (1980b): Comparison of hepatic cathepsin D activity in response to tumor growth and to caloric restriction in mice. *Cancer Res.* 40:1680–1685.

Lundholm, K., Ekman, L., Karlberg, I., Edström, S. and Scherstén, T (1981): Evaluation of anorexia as the cause of altered protein synthesis in skeletal muscles from nongrowing mice with sarcoma. *Cancer Res.* 41:1989–1996.

Munro, H.N. and Fleck, A.A. (1966): Determination of nucleic acids. *Methods Biochem. Anal.* 14:113–176.

Scherstén, T., Lundholm, K., Edén, E., Edström, S., Ekman, L., Karlberg, I. and Warnold, I. (1979): Energy metabolism in cancer. *Acta Chir. Scand.* 498:130–136.

Stein, T.P. (1978): Cachexia, gluconeogenesis and progressive weight loss in cancer patients. *J. Theor. Biol.* 73:51–59.

Svaninger, G., Ekman, L., Ternell, M. and Lundholm, K. (1982): Is wastage of skeletal muscles in cancer cachexia associated with increased degradation? *Eur. Soc. Clin. Invest., Luxembourg.*

Ternell, M. and Lundholm, K. (1981): DNA dependent RNA synthesis in tumor-host liver. Espen. Third European Congress on Parenteral and Enteral Nutrition, Maastricht, The Netherlands.

Wu, C. & Bauer, J.M. (1960): A study of free amino acids and of glutamine synthesis in tumor-bearing rats. *Cancer Res.* 20:848–857.

BRAIN

13 Implications of Parenteral and Enteral Amino Acid Mixtures in Brain Function

Richard J. Wurtman

The brain is a part of the body: When food consumption or peripheral metabolic events alter plasma levels of key nutrients, the brain's composition is as likely to be affected as any other organ, and perhaps more so (Wurtman and Wurtman, 1977, 1979; Wurtman, Hefti and Melamed, 1980; Wurtman, 1982). A blood-brain barrier does indeed exist, and does control the flux of chemicals between blood and brain (Pardridge, 1977); however, perhaps contrary to earlier views, for many compounds this barrier can act not to keep them out of the brain but to facilitate their entry. The small number of highly lipid-soluble chemicals in the bloodstream (like the hormones melatonin or progesterone, or many drugs) pass right through the capillary endothelia that comprise the blood-brain barrier. In contrast, the ability of water-soluble molecules to enter or leave the brain is contingent on the existence within the endothelial cells of specific macromolecules ("transport systems") that recognize and bind them, then carry them between the cells' "brain" and "blood" surfaces. Nine such transport systems have been identified; this means that at least nine circulating compounds (e.g., choline; thyroxine) or families of compounds (e.g., large neutral amino acids [LNAA]; hexoses) can traverse the barrier in one direction or the other. The kinetic properties and cellular localizations of these macromolecules determine the rates and directions of transport; for example, glutamate—which is synthesized in large excess within brain tissue—is poorly transported from blood to brain (and its rate of influx is independent of plasma glutamate concentrations), but very well transported from brain to blood at a rate that increases when brain glutamate levels are elevated. In general, the "transport systems" are unable to transport their ligand against a concentration gradient; rather, they facilitate the ligand's diffusion along the gradient.

A major implication of the existence of these transport systems is that each time blood levels of some of their ligands change (for example, after eating) brain levels may also change, *passively,* with important functional consequences. The best-characterized blood constituents whose levels affect brain composition are certain nutrients (tryptophan; tyrosine; choline), all reviewed recently in the references cited above, which are also precursors of central and peripheral neurotransmitters (serotonin; the catecholamines dopamine, norepinephrine, and epinephrine; acetylcholine). When brain levels of these nutrients increase after their administration, or after the consumption of meals of appropriate composition, the synthesis of their neurotransmitter products can also rapidly rise, with important functional consequences. However, it seems equally likely that changes in plasma levels of additional, less well-explored nutrients or metabolites (for example, adenosine; basic amino acids) will also be found in future studies to be important for brain function.

Until proved otherwise, it is prudent to assume that every nutrient present in or absent from a meal or a synthetic mixture may, under appropriate conditions, influence neuronal function, and thereby affect any of the myriad processes controlled by the brain (for example, alertness; cognition; the control of cardiovascular function; respiration; hormone secretion; pain sensitivity). Situations in which such inclusions or omissions seem most likely to become clinically manifest are those involving parenteral or enteral mixtures, both because by bypassing some or all gastrointestinal buffering mechanisms these cause the greatest changes in plasma composition and because these products tend to be administered to the sickest patients, who can least afford to deny their neurons the precursors needed to sustain optimal neurotransmitter synthesis. One thus views with concern the fact that all commercially available parenteral mixtures contain little or no choline, and either lack tyrosine entirely or contain quantities of it that are disproportionately small when compared with their contents of other LNAA, which complete with circulating tyrosine for uptake into the brain. Similarly, severe metabolic diseases—like uncontrolled diabetes or liver failure—in which plasma levels of neurotransmitter precursors are pathologically elevated or depressed independent of food consumption, may cause severe and even life threatening changes in brain function by disturbing the synthesis of precursor-dependent neurotransmitters. However, it is important to recognize that relatively small, meal-induced changes in plasma levels of particular nutrients may *normally* participate in physiological control mechanisms, for example, those through which the brain decides when and for what to be hungry, or when to be sleepy. Moreover, the deliberate administration of individual nutrients or groups of nutrients, as though they were drugs, can have significant therapeutic effects in diseases in which the release of one or another neurotransmitter happens to be inadequate.

MECHANISMS COUPLING FOOD CONSUMPTION TO NEUROTRANSMITTER SYNTHESIS

Similar sequences of metabolic events mediate the effects of particular foods or nutrients on the synthesis of serotonin, the catecholamines, and acetylcholine.

First, consumption of food or administration of the nutrient causes its plasma levels to rise, either absolutely or in relation to those of the other nutrients that compete with it for blood-brain barrier transport. Hence, consumption of lecithin (phosphatidylcholine) elevates plasma choline levels; consumption of a carbohydrate-rich, protein-poor meal lowers plasma levels of the other LNAA, which compete with tryptophan for blood-brain barrier transport without lowering typtophan itself, thereby increasing the *plasma tryptophan ratio;* consumption of a protein-rich meal can increase plasma tyrosine levels more than those of other LNAA, thereby elevating the *plasma tyrosine ratio.* The tryptophan and tyrosine ratios can, of course, be selectively elevated by administering the pure amino acids; if this treatment is combined with carbohydrate administration, the resulting decrease in plasma LNAA enhances the rises in the tryptophan and tyrosine ratios and thereby potentiates their effect on the brain. Plasma levels of amino acids and of choline apparently are not regulated by classical "feedback loops"; instead they reflect at any instant the composition of the food that is then being digested. Thus, plasma concentrations of tryptophan, tyrosine, or choline can undergo as much as threefold daily ratios, or can exhibit no diurnal changes at all, depending solely on what the subject has chosen to eat on that particular day.

Next, the change in plasma choline, or in the plasma tryptophan or tyrosine ratios, causes a parallel change in the extent to which the blood-brain barrier transport system for choline or for LNAA happens to be saturated. The kinetic characteristics of these transport systems are such that they normally are highly *un*-saturated with their ligands; hence a rise in, for example, the tryptophan/LNAA ratio will increase the proportion of transport molecules occupied with tryptophan, and thus accelerate tryptophan's entry into the brain. Once the precursor's concentration in the brain's extracellular fluid has increased, its levels within individual brain cells, neurons and glia, apparently change in parallel. At present there is no evidence that the uptake of any of the precursors into neurons using it for neurotransmitter synthesis is at all different from its uptake into any other brain cell. It is certainly possible that the functional properties of the blood-brain barrier transport systems for LNAA or choline differ among individuals, especially those suffering from diseases such as liver disease, as discussed by Dr. Hawkins (p. 239), or uncontrolled diabetes, which has been shown (McCall et al., 1982) to diminish blood-brain barrier glucose uptake.

Next, the increase in the precursor's intraneuronal concentration causes a parallel change in the substrate saturation of the enzyme (tryptophan hydroxylase; tyrosine hydroxylase; choline acetyltransferase) that initiates its conversion to its neurotransmitter product. This relationship obtains because of the kinetic properties of these enzymes: they have relatively poor affinities for their precursor substrates and are thus highly susceptible to changes in substrate concentration. None of the three enzymes is subject to significant end-product inhibition *in vivo.* The increase in, for example, neuronal serotonin concentration that follows tryptophan administration does not cause the inhibition of tryptophan hydroxylase. This allows the enzyme to continue to respond to changes in its substrate's availability.

Apparently serotonin's synthesis can always be enhanced by giving people or animals tryptophan or a carbohydrate meal. In contrast, the synthesis of the catecholamines or of acetylcholine within particular neurons may or may not be enhanced at any particular time by providing more tyrosine or choline. The determining factor seems to be the frequency with which the neuron happens to be firing at that time: Rapidly firing neurons are very responsive to changes in tyrosine or choline levels; slowly firing or quiescent neurons are largely unresponsive. The mechanism by which a high-firing frequency causes tyrosine hydroxylase to become tyrosine-responsive seems to involve a short-lived phosphorylation of the enzyme protein; this causes the protein to exhibit a vastly increased affinity for its cofactor, tetrahydrobiopterin, making it more dependent on tyrosine levels. The biochemical mechanism that couples the firing frequency of cholinergic neurons to their choline responsiveness awaits exploration. Thus, for example, the administration of tyrosine to the otherwise untreated rat has little or no effect on dopamine release within its corpus striatum (assessed by measuring striatal levels of the dopamine metabolites homovanillic acid or dihydroxyphenylacetic acid); however, tyrosine markedly enhances dopamine's release following any of a variety of treatments known to accelerate nigrostriatal firing (e.g., administration of drugs that deplete presynaptic dopamine or block postsynaptic dopamine receptors; production of lesions that destroy some of the neurons). This dependence on firing frequency probably explains why so few cholinergic or catecholaminergic side effects follow the administration of lecithin or tyrosine. As soon as most "normal" CNS neurons are "forced" (by giving them more choline or tyrosine) to release more acetylcholine or dopamine, the brain compensates by making these neurons fire less frequently; this renders them less responsive to the additional precursor. It also explains how a given dose of tyrosine can lower blood pressure in hypertensive animals, raise it in hemorrhagic shock, and fail to affect it in normotensive animals or people. The amino acid selectively amplifies the neurotransmitter output from rapidly firing brain-stem noradrenergic neurons in the first situation, from sympathetic nerves and the adrenal medulla in the shocked animals, and from neither group in the normotensives. Serotoninergic neurons, whose output always is affected by tryptophan availability and plasma amino acid pattern, thus serve as "sensors" of peripheral metabolic state, normally informing the rest of the brain about what is currently being digested. In contrast, in catecholaminergic and cholinergic neurons, the ability to respond to changes in precursor availability provides them with a means of *amplifying* their neurotransmission. The utility to the brain of having "sensors" is apparent and can readily be illustrated by experiments on appetite control which show that an increase in serotonin release, as occurs after carbohydrate consumption, tryptophan administration, or drugs like fenfluramine, *decreases* the proportion of carbohydrate that the animal or human chooses to consume in its next meal. However, the utility to the animal of allowing plasma composition to "amplify" catecholaminergic or cholinergic neurotransmission remains a mystery. Although it provides the physician with additional chemicals for treating neuronal disorders, one wonders why the evolutionary process chose to build it into the brain.

IMPLICATIONS FOR AMINO ACID FORMULATIONS OF THE PRECURSOR CONTROL OF NEUROTRANSMITTER SYNTHESIS

As proposed earlier in this chapter, it must be assumed that any preparation, administered by any route, that contains one or more amino acids (or which includes compounds like carbohydrates that modify plasma amino acid levels) can affect brain composition and neuronal function. In trying to determine whether such alterations are likely to be significant to the patient's health, an obvious first task is to characterize them in detail, and to calculate the changes that are generated in the plasma tryptophan and tyrosine ratios. All things being equal, preparations that increase or decrease these ratios will cause parallel changes in brain tryptophan and tyrosine levels, and can thereby affect serotonin and catecholamine synthesis (i.e., in catecholaminergic neurons that happen to be firing frequently). Circulating tyrosine levels can also be expected to affect catecholamine production in sympathetic nerves and the adrenal medulla, just as plasma choline levels can affect acetylcholine release both from central and peripheral cholinergic neurons. It goes without saying that enteral and parenteral preparations should be formulated so as to keep plasma tryptophan and tyrosine ratios, and plasma choline levels, within their normal physiological ranges, unless there is a good therapeutic reason for doing otherwise.

If a disease process has caused major distortions of the tyrosine or tryptophan ratios (or has markedly altered plasma choline levels), and if that disease is associated with aberrations in any of the myriad processes controlled by the brain, the investigator should at least consider the possibility that the plasma disturbance is etiologic in the neuronal malfunction. He can explore whether treatments designed to correct that plasma imbalance also help the patient. One's expectations shouldn't be too high. As discussed above, it is possible, and even likely, that abnormalities in other plasma constituents (e.g. glucose), including some whose brain effects have not yet been studied, also are involved in the neuronal disturbances.

In characterizing the disturbances in plasma composition associated with metabolic disease, or the plasma responses to amino acid mixtures, the investigator should not fall into the intellectual trap of lumping together all of the aromatic amino acids for purposes of calculating ratios, just as one often lumps together the branched-chain amino acids. Phenylalanine is *not* a substitute for tyrosine as far as catecholaminergic neurons are concerned. It both blocks tyrosine's passage across the blood-brain barrier and directly inhibits the enzyme, tyrosine hydroxylase, that converts tyrosine to the catechols.

The brain's responses to plasma amino acids constitute both an opportunity and a nuisance to the clinician. They probably underlie the severe neuronal disturbances associated with certain metabolic diseases, and they allow amino acid mixtures formulated without the brain in mind to produce neurologic side effects. Clearly, anyone who treats patients whose diseases involve amino acids, etiologically or therapeutically, must be aware of the effects of plasma constituents on the brain. However, in at least one case—the responses of serotoninergic neurons to carbohydrate consumption—these effects constitute a perfectly normal mechanism for allowing the brain to sense peripheral metabolic state, and make decisions according to the information it receives. Moreover, individual amino acids like tyrosine or tryptophan, given alone or with insulin-releasing carbohydrates, may become useful "drugs" for treating clinical states in which more or less catecholamine or serotonin somewhere in the body would be helpful to the patient. The growing list of situations in which this approach is being tested includes appetite disturbances (especially carbohydrate-craving associated with obesity), insomnia, various neurologic disorders, depression, the propensity towards ventricular arrhythmias, and hyper- or hypotension. As always with the body, complexity generates opportunity.

REFERENCES

McCall, A.L., Millington, W.R., Temple, S. and Wurtman, R.J.: Metabolic fuel and amino acid transport into the brain in experimental diabetes mellitus. (submitted to) *Proc. Nat. Acad. Sci.*

Pardridge, W. (1977): Regulation of amino acid availability to the brain, in: *Nutrition and the Brain* (eds: R.J. Wurtman and J.J. Wurtman) Vol. 1, pp. 141–204, Raven Press, New York.

Wurtman, R.J. and Wurtman, J.J. (1977): *Nutrition and the Brain,* Vols. I & II, Raven Press, New York.

Wurtman, R.J. and Wurtman, J.J. (1979): *Nutrition and the Brain,* Vols. III, IV & V, Raven Press, New York.

Wurtman, R.J., Hefti, F. and Melamed, E. (1980): Precursor control of neurotransmitter synthesis. *Pharmacological Reviews* 32:315–335.

Wurtman, R.J. (1982): Nutrients that modify brain function. *Scientific American* 246:50–59.

14 Amino Acids and the Regulation of Quantitative and Qualitative Aspects of Food Intake

G. Harvey Anderson
N. Theresa Glanville
Edmund T. S. Li

Control of food intake and the correlated regulation of body energy balance has been studied for many years, and the literature on the subject contains many theories on the mechanisms involved. Although a complete understanding of the control mechanisms is still lacking, it is generally accepted that these controls result in the regulation of energy balance. It follows, then, that the animal's response to the energy producing macronutrients, particularly glucose and fat, would be examined rigorously in attempts to define control mechanisms. Receiving less attention as a possible component of control mechanisms has been protein, or amino acids.

A role for amino acids from the diet and for the free amino acid pools of blood and tissues in control mechanisms regulating food intake is suggested by several lines of evidence. First, high protein diets suppress food intake in both man and experimental animals, suggesting specific signals arise from this constituent of food (Harper et al., 1970). Second, protein consumption is a regulated aspect of food intake in experimental animals and possibly man (Anderson, 1979) emphasizing that underlying control mechanisms based on amino acids must be present. Third, the synthesis of serotonin and of the catecholamines, which are the central nervous system neurotransmitters most implicated in feeding behavior, is partially regulated by the availability of their dietary amino acid precursors, tyrosine and tryptophan, respectively (Wurtman and Fernstrom, 1976). This relationship suggests that diet, by its effect on plasma amino acids and brain uptake of these amino acids, can directly influence brain neurotransmitter synthesis and brain response to diet. Finally, dietary amino acids cause release of a number of hormones including insulin and cholecystokinin. The actions of these hormones may serve to enhance or modulate the direct impact of dietary amino acids on tissue uptake of amino acids, as is the case for insulin; or may serve as a more direct messenger to the brain's food intake regulating center, such as is the case for cholecystokinin (Smith and Gibbs, 1981).

In the following, each of the lines of evidence for a role of amino acids in control mechanisms regulating food intake is considered in detail.

HIGH PROTEIN AND AMINO ACID DIETS AND FOOD INTAKE

Studies of the effect of the protein and amino acid component of food on food intake of experimental animals have led the way in showing that amino acids are involved in the regulation of food intake. In general, when protein concentration is 40% or greater in diets fed to rats, long-term food intake is depressed (Harper et al., 1970; Anderson, 1979) depending to some extent on the protein type (Musten et al., 1974), the age of the rats (Anderson, 1979), and possibly other dietary components such as the mineral content (Li and Anderson, 1982). Similarly, feeding imbalanced amino acid diets, or diets with excessive quantities of single amino acids depress appetite (Harper et al., 1970). Although this research has shown a role for amino acids in feeding behavior, the impression gained is that they are only important when extremes of diet composition are fed. The importance of dietary amino acids to normal food intake regulation may be more relevant than is apparent from this earlier work.

High protein diets also affect food consumption in man. Although this possible aspect of dietary control as received surprisingly little direct investigation, studies have shown both long-term and short-term effects of protein on appetite. Artificial diets containing less than 13% protein by weight were reported to leave people always hungry, whereas diets low in carbohydrate or fat, but high in protein, were satiating (Fryer et al., 1955). An indication that the protein content of breakfast can have an influence throughout the day comes from the observation that adolescent girls consumed 10% to 15% less daily food energy when breakfasts were given containing similar energy content (600 kcal) but containing 24 g rather than 9 g protein (Ohlson and Hart, 1965). Protein content of a meal was found to have an effect on the next meal in the studies of Booth et al. (1970). They fed volunteers a high and low protein meal, 40% and 6% of calories, respectively. Food consumption within the meal was not different. The amount of food eaten in a subsequent meal (20% protein) four hours later, however, by the subjects fed the high protein meal was 30% less than that of the subjects fed the low protein meal. More immediate responses to protein have also been suggested (Quaade et al., 1981). Subjects asked to consume a protein supplement 30 minutes before ad lib meals lost as much weight as subjects who were advised to follow a 1000 kcal energy restricted diet and take an appetite suppressant (Quaade et al., 1981). Presumably, the subjects voluntarily ate less food in each meal taken after the protein drink, although this was not documented.

Two reports have appeared indicating a role for individual amino acids, or groups of amino acids, in regulating short-term aspects of normal feeding behavior such as meal size and food selection in man. A mixture of four amino acids (phenylalanine 3 g; valine 2 g; methionine 2 g; tryptophan 1 g), taken a half-hour before a midday meal, reduced food intake by 22.5% in subjects whose weight was greater than 5% above the ideal, whereas it had no effect in normal subjects (Butler et al., 1981). Furthermore, when tryptophan alone was administered after lunch, subjects reduced their intake of carbohydrate-containing snacks between the midday and evening meal (Wurtman et al., 1981). Taken together these findings demonstrate the potent appetite-suppressing effect of protein in man and suggest that some amino acids may be more important than others in mediating this response.

REGULATION OF PROTEIN INTAKE

A second line of evidence that indirectly supports a role for amino acids in food intake is offered by the recent literature on the animals' ability to self-select for nutrients. The ability of rats and experimental animals to select for nutrients was studied vigorously in the first half of this century. However, due to incomplete knowledge of nutrient requirements, the animals studied were often nutrient deficient (Lát, 1967). For example, early attempts to study macronutrient selection involved placing in the animal's cage sources of fat, protein and carbohydrate, but either no vitamins and minerals or incomplete mixtures were made available. With time, the rats became deficient in essential nutrients, which in turn interfered with selection patterns (Gershoff, 1977).

The concept of protein selection is not new and the rat's ability to possibly regulate this component of its diet was stated first by Osborne and Mendel (1918). It re-emerged in the late 1960s with the report that rats fed liquid forms of fat, carbohydrate and protein would maintain their intake of protein even if the protein source was diluted (Rozin, 1968). Our first contribution was to put the concept of protein regulation on firmer ground (Musten et al., 1974). In these studies, young rats were simultaneously presented with a protein-containing and a protein-free diet or else two diets differing only in protein concentration. Except for protein and carbohydrate, both diets were complete and contained identical nutrient-to-energy ratios. For a wide range of dietary choices, rats regulated their protein intake at a constant proportion of the dietary energy consumed, and this regulation was almost as precise as the regulation of total energy intake (Musten et al., 1974). Although most of our initial studies were based on two- or four-week experiments, the ability of the rat to regulate protein intake is apparent *within the first day* that the dietary choices are fed, and occurs on a meal-to-meal basis (Johnson et al., 1979).

A protein intake regulatory mechanism may also exist in man. Whenever the diet is adequate, man consumes 14% to 16% of the dietary calories as protein, even though food varies in protein concentration from zero to 96%, and the quantity of fat and carbohydrate calories vary markedly (FAO/WHO, 1973). More direct evidence comes from a recent study of the dietary patterns of monozygotic versus dizygotic twins. Dietary records obtained on each of twin pairs raised in separate home environments, showed that dietary protein concentration selected by identical twin pairs was similar. The diets of dizygotic twins who were raised in different home environments were quite dissimilar, suggesting that a primitive, genetically determined control mechanism may underlie protein intake by man (Wade et al., 1981).

Protein intake regulation appears to be separate from energy intake regulation, although it is reasonable to assume that both mechanisms interact to determine food intake (Anderson, 1979). For example, strategies which increase the animal's energy requirement such as cold exposure (Musten et al., 1974) or increased activity (Collier et al., 1969) result in the animal making a selective adjustment in energy intake while maintaining a constant intake of protein. Similarly, when given choices of high and low protein diets, both ventromedial hypothalamus-lesioned rats and Zucker rats exhibited a selective drive to overeat total energy but maintained relative control over protein intake (Anderson et al., 1979; Kanarak et al., 1981). Conversely, protein consumption may be manipulated while energy intake is unaffected. The quantity of protein consumed in relation to total dietary calories is characteristic of the protein fed, but the animal's usual intake can be altered by the addition of certain amino acids to the protein. For example, adding lysine to gluten (Ashley and Anderson, 1975), or tryptophan to casein (Woodger et al., 1979) or zein (Ashley and Anderson, 1975) causes the rat to select a lower proportion of dietary calories as protein, but not necessarily to change the total energy consumed.

AMINO ACIDS IN THE REGULATION OF PROTEIN AND ENERGY INTAKE

The involvement of the central nervous system in the mechanisms by which amino acids elicit feeding responses provides a third line of evidence for a role of amino acids in food intake regulation. Although, the exact mechanisms are unknown, at least three possibilities exist. First, food ingestion results in a change in concentration and turnover of body-free amino acid pools. Possibly brain uptake of many amino acids, or of single amino acids, has a direct affect on brain function through presently unidentified mechanisms such as altered brain protein synthesis. Second, it is possible that the primary mechanism involves amino acids that are neurotransmitters or neurotransmitter precursors in the brain, and this allows the feeding centers to receive information about the diet and state of peripheral metabolism (Anderson, 1979). Finally, it is possible that any of these changes are secondary to hormone responses directed by food ingestion and the primary effect is the release of hormones such as cholecystokinin, which have an appetite-suppressing effect (Gibbs et al., 1973).

Plasma Amino Acids and Food Intake

The significance of general changes in plasma-free amino acid pools to feeding control remains unknown. The aminostatic hypothesis recognized that high protein diets or high concentrations of amino acids infused intravenously caused satiety in man (Mellinkoff, 1956). Subsequent studies in animals showed that appetite suppression caused by feeding a single high protein diet or imbalanced diet was associated with large shifts in the plasma amino acid (Harper et al., 1970) and brain amino acid patterns (Peng et al., 1972). Harper and his associates have contributed greatly to describing the animals' feeding response to diets containing disproportionate amounts of amino acids. They have presented arguments in favor of the brain responding to the most limiting amino acid in a deficient or imbalanced amino acid diet, rather than the amino acids in excess or ammonia, although the mechanism for this response is not clear at present (Rogers and Leung, 1977; Tews et al., 1980).

Similarly, little headway has been made toward describing the mechanism for the suppression of food intake by a high protein diet. In this situation the plasma branched-chain amino acids are particularly elevated (Johnson and Anderson, 1982), suggesting that they may be playing a role in the animal's feeding response (Anderson et al., 1968), either directly due to their elevation in brain-free amino acid pools or indirectly by blocking brain uptake of other large neutral amino acids including tryptophan and histidine (Tews et al., 1978).

In a review on the subject, Rogers and Leung (1977) stated that "there appears to be a broad range of dietary protein levels above the minimum requirements, but not excessively high, and a wide range of disproportionality possible among the dietary amino acids, which within reasonable ranges a normal animal may tolerate the excess, deficiency or disproportionality with little or no effect on food intake." This statement, however, applies to rats given no dietary choice and appears to underestimate the role amino acids may play in regulating normal feeding behaviors, which in addition to quantitative aspects of food intake include food (nutrient) selection and meal feeding patterns.

As pointed out earlier, our studies of food intake regulation have emphasized the use of the self-selecting animal (Anderson, 1979). This approach is based on the simple rationale that in both man and experimental animals there are physiological control mechanisms, based on peripheral and central amino acid metabolism, which lead to the regulation of both quantitative and qualitative aspects of food intake.

On examining plasma amino acid patterns in self-selecting rats we found certain unique relationships with protein and energy intake (Anderson, 1979). First, we observed an inverse relationship between the quantity of protein the rat selected (expressed as a proportion of total energy) and the plasma concentration of tryptophan (TRP) relative to other large neutral amino acids (NAA), namely, leucine, isoleucine, valine, phenylalanine and tyrosine (Ashley and Anderson, 1975). We also found that the plasma tyrosine-to-phenylalanine ratio (TYR/PHE), and to the lesser extent the TYR/NAA ratio, correlated with long-term energy consumption in the weanling rat (Anderson and Ashley, 1977). More recently we have reported that such an association between the quantitative and qualitative aspects of food exists in man (Anderson and Blendis, 1981).

Since our first report (Ashley and Anderson, 1975), other studies have substantiated the view that selected protein intake is correlated with the plasma TRP/NAA ratio. Reeves and O'Dell (1981) found that the morning TRP/NAA ratio in rats is inversely related to previous chronic self-selected dietary protein concentration, and similar data have been reported for mice (Chee et al., 1981a,b.) Although Peters and Rogers (1981) concluded that food selection and daily protein intake of self-selecting rats is unrelated to the morning plasma TRP/NAA ratio, a further analysis of the data reported suggests a reinterpretation is required. Reanalysis of their data shows a statistically significant negative correlation between the plasma TRP/NAA ratio and either protein intake expressed in grams or as a concentration in the food selected for seven of the eight diet groups fed casein (Figure 14-1). Because the majority of these diets were the same as those used by Ashley and Anderson (1975), their results provide strong support for the original observation. The plasma TRP/NAA ratio of their eighth group was high (0.20), but this may be explained by the fact that tryptophan was added in equal quantities (2 g/100 g) to both diets. Due to mechanisms described in the following, the relatively high protein intake selected by the rats, despite this high plasma ratio, may be expected.

The specific relationships between amino acid ratios and protein and energy intakes strongly support the contention that amino acids play a role in food intake regulation. The motivation for us to seek and find these relationships of plasma amino acid ratios to food intake was based on two new concepts. First, Wurtman and Fernstrom (1976) had shown that the regulation of the synthesis of certain neu-

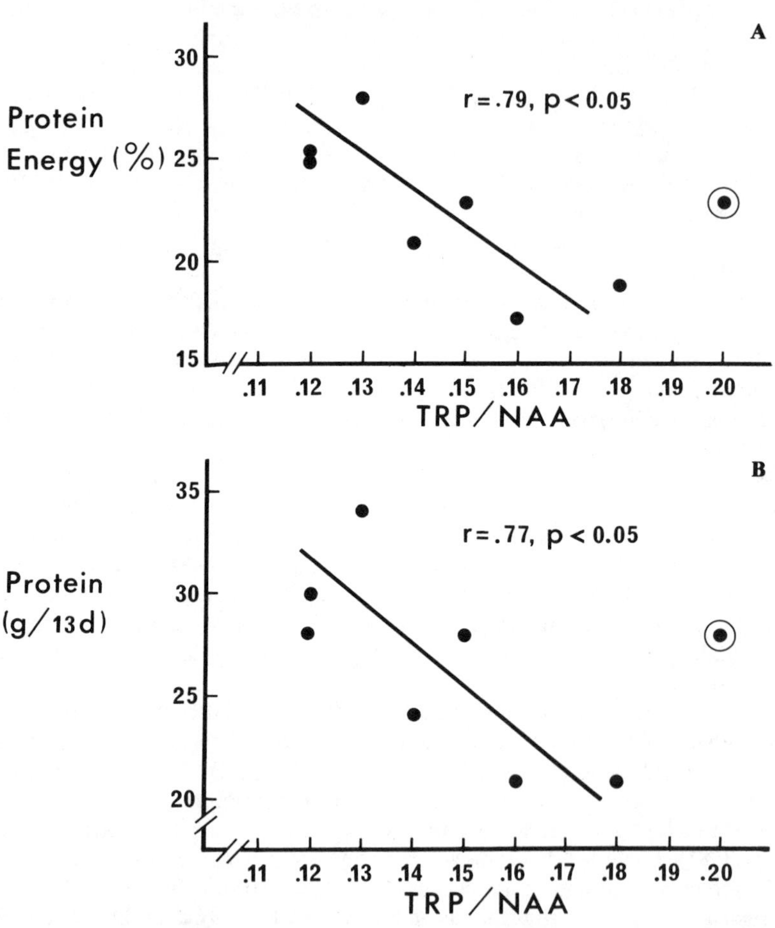

Figure 14-1 The relationship between the morning plasma TRP/NAA amino acid ratio and prior protein intake, expressed either as protein-energy % (A), or as protein intake in grams per 13 days (B), for seven groups (x) of weanling rats fed casein diets for 13 days. Each diet group was fed a choice of 15% and 55% casein diets to which various amino acid additions were made. Although protein intake selected by the groups varied and correlated with the plasma TRP/NAA ratio, energy intakes and growth rates of all groups were similar. The final diet group (⊙) was provided the choice of 15% and 55% casein to which a high level of tryptophan (2 g/100 g diet) was added to both diets. This figure and the data shown are adapted from Table 1 of Peters and Harper (1981). NAA = phenylalanine, tyrosine, leucine, isoleucine and valine.

rotransmitters, namely serotonin (5-HT) and the catecholamines (CA), was under partial precursor control. Second, these two neurotransmitter systems were giving rise to the monoamine hypothesis for the control of feeding behavior (Blundell, 1980). It seemed possible that shifts in plasma amino acid patterns of significance to the central nervous system control of feeding behavior might be those that influenced the activity of these specific neuronal systems.

Precursor Control of Neurotransmitter Synthesis

The synthesis of serotonin and the catecholamines, under certain circumstances, is partially controlled by the availability of their amino acid precursors in the diet and the blood (Wurtman and Fernstrom, 1976). Tryptophan, because it cannot be synthesized within the body, appears in the blood as a result of protein ingestion and body protein breakdown. Along with tyrosine, it is transported across the blood-brain barrier via an amino acid uptake system specific for large neutral amino acids (NAA) including phenylalanine, tyrosine, valine, isoleucine and leucine (Pardridge, 1977). Tryptophan administration alone will raise the concentration of plasma and brain tryptophan and serotonin. Due to its competition for brain uptake with other NAA at the blood-brain barrier, however, the effect of food ingestion on brain serotonin is not simply related to its tryptophan content. Protein ingestion, which causes the plasma concentration of branched-chain amino acids to rise more quickly than tryptophan results in a decreased ratio of plasma TRP to NAA and, therefore, leads to decreased brain TRP uptake. Conversely, CHO ingestion results in an increase in the concentration of plasma tryptophan relative to other NAA (Wurtman and Fernstrom, 1976). This is due to the CHO-induced insulin release which results in the increased uptake of all amino acids into tissues, with the least effect on tryptophan because of its binding to plasma albumin (McMenamy and Oncley, 1978).

Catecholamine synthesis and turnover is also influenced by tyrosine availability under certain conditions (Wurtman et al., 1981). The relationship between diet composition and brain tyrosine fluctuations is less clear than that for tryptophan. Single meals of both CHO and protein increase brain tyrosine levels, with protein having the greater effect (Fernstrom and Faller, 1978). Furthermore, a comparison between long-term and short-term feeding studies indicates that while the short-term effect of a high protein meal is to increase brain tyrosine and norepinephrine (NE) turnover, chronic high protein feeding decreases brain TYR levels (Anderson, unpublished data).

Monoamines and the Control of Feeding Behavior

At the present time there is considerable evidence for a role of the catecholamines, dopamine and norepinephrine, and of serotonin in the regulation of feeding behavior (Blundell and Rogers, 1980). While the manipulation of these systems gives rise to changes in feeding behavior, a specific description of their involvement in control mechanisms is not possible (Blundell, 1980). Nevertheless, it is possible to suggest that the synthesis of these neurotransmitters and their influence on food consumption is controlled in part by the nature of the food eaten.

Diet, Plasma Amino Acids and Monoamine Control of Feeding Behavior

A current working conceptualization of the relationships among quantitative and qualitative aspects of food intake, plasma amino acid ratios, and catecholamine and serotonin control of feeding behavior can be described (Figure 14-2).

In the animal allowed to select for macronutrients, shifts in the plasma TRP/NAA ratio caused by either protein or carbohydrate may be read out in the serotonergic system which in turn controls aspects of the animal's appetite for protein (Anderson, 1979) or carbohydrate (Wurtman and Wurtman, 1979), or the proportion of protein relative to carbohydrate, as well as total food intake (Blundell, 1980). In contrast, shifts in plasma tyrosine, brought about by many factors, including food selected and possibly in tune with the total food energy consumed (Anderson and Ashley, 1979), may influence catecholamine synthesis and subsequent regulation of energy balance. One needs to recognize that this is a simplistic description constructed on correlative associations. Testing this conceptualization of the feedback of serotonin and the catecholamines on the qualitative and quantitative aspects, respectively, of food intake regulation has proven difficult. Nevertheless, considerable evidence has emerged to support a view of serotonergic neurons in the regulation of the qualitative aspects of food selection.

A relatively clear picture of serotonin involvement in food selection can be constructed from studies of short-term (meal) feeding responses after manipulation of the serotonergic system. Animals given a choice of diets after administration of serotonergic agonists, reduce total food mainly from carbohydrate but not protein (Wurtman and Wurtman, 1978; Wurtman and Wurtman, 1979), suggesting that serotonin stimulation creates a relative preference for protein. Fenfluramine administered to nonobese humans also exerts a preferential decrease in carbohydrate consumption in a test meal (Blundell and Rogers, 1980) and the frequency of carbohydrate snacking following a meal (Wurtman et al., 1981), while tryptophan alone has a modest effect in reducing carbohydrate snacking in some obese human subjects (Wurtman et al., 1981). Presumably, this is also by a mechanism of increased serotonergic activity. Because carbohydrate consumption increases brain serotonin

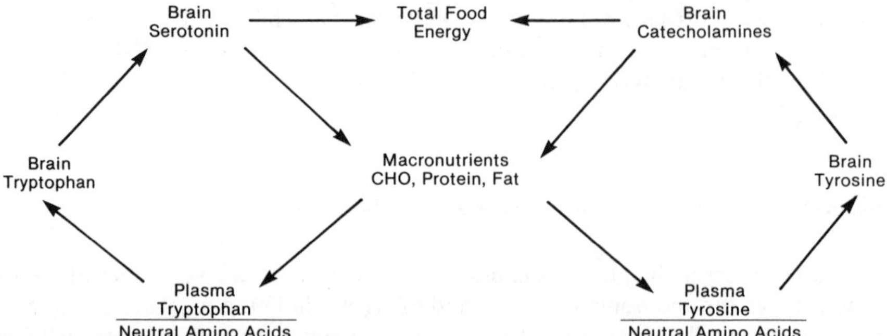

Figure 14-2 A proposed relationship among plasma amino acids, brain neurotransmitters, and quantitative and qualitative aspects of food intake in animals allowed to select from diets varying in macronutrients (protein, carbohydrate and fat composition). Modified from Anderson (1979).

content, it seems reasonable to expect that increases of brain serotonin by alternate means would reduce the animal's preference for carbohydrate, and possibly enhance a relative preference for protein. Conversely, approaches designed to reduce serotonergic transmission should result in the rat preferring carbohydrate as a compensatory mechanism for increasing serotonergic transmission. Hence, the reduced protein enhanced carbohydrate selection over several days following drug-induced lesions (p-chlorophenylanine and 5,7-dihydroxytryptamine) or surgical lesions of the serotonergic system (raphé nuclei) is consistent (Ashley et al., 1979). The only literature that does not fit with this general view that increased brain serotonergic activity results in relative protein preference or carbohydrate avoidance is a report of the decreased protein but increased carbohydrate selected by both normal and diabetic rats after the tryptophan content of the diets was increased (Woodger et al., 1979). It seems possible that this later observation is misleading. In this study the tryptophan content of the protein (casein) was enhanced prior to mixing the protein in the diets. Hence, the two diet choices offered the rats varied in tryptophan as well as protein content. Perhaps the rats decreased their intake of the high protein diet in favor of the high carbohydrate diet in an effort to decrease free tryptophan intake. In this way, the rats would reduce the impact of the high tryptophan diet on brain serotonin metabolism. Support for this conjecture is provided by the Peters and Harper data (1981) (Figure 14-1). The diet group not fitting the expected relationship between the plasma TRP/NAA ratio and protein selection was fed a choice of 15% and 55% casein, both diets contained 2 g/100 g of tryptophan. This means that the dietary TRP/NAA ratio was much higher in the 15% casein diet, possibly enhancing serotonergic transmission and hence a relative preference for the high casein diet with the lower TRP/NAA ratio.

There is less information on the effect of catecholamine manipulations on food selection. Clonidine, a drug which acts centrally to reduce noradrenergic tone, increases total food and protein intake of rats selecting from 45% and 5% protein diets (Mauron et al., 1980). Amphetamine, a central catecholinergic agonist, decreases total food intake, but has been reported to either decrease protein proportionately (Kanarak et al., 1981), or relatively more than total calories (Blundell and McArthur, 1979), while at the same time more selectively reducing fat intake (Kanarak et al., 1981). While it seems clear, based on pharmacological manipulations, that the catecholamines are involved in both the quantitative and qualitative aspects of food intake, there are no published reports demonstrating that diet-induced variations in tyrosine availability over normal ranges will alter nutrient selection or quantitative aspects of food intake.

The foregoing working conceptualization of neurotransmitters and feeding is undoubtedly oversimplified. A number of other neurotransmitter substances, such as gamma-amino-butyric acid and peptides, are currently recognized as influencing food intake (Morley, 1980). More directly relevant to the precursor hypothesis are the observations that the neurotransmitters, glycine and histamine, may also be under the influence of their precursors, threonine (Maher and Wurtman, 1980) and histidine (Schwartz et al., 1972), respectively. Therefore, it is relevant to note that threonine- and histidine-imbalanced diets result in reduced brain levels of these two amino acids and are associated with a marked depression of feeding (Harper et al., 1970; Rogers and Leung, 1977). Further evidence for histamine involvement in feeding is provided by studies showing that a brain histidine decarboxylase inhibitor decreases food and water intake (Menon et al., 1971). Because brain threonine and histidine uptakes are inhibited by large neutral amino acids (Tews et al., 1978), we cannot ignore the possibility that food composition influences brain histidine and threonine levels and by this route influences feeding behavior.

A broader view of the picture would rationally suggest that feeding is controlled by a balance of activities in several neurochemical systems. In addition to amino acids acting directly on the central nervous system, another possibility for their action resides in their effects in the gastrointestinal tract and resulting interactions with the monoamines.

BRAIN-GUT PEPTIDES, MONOAMINES AND THE CONTROL OF FOOD INTAKE

In any study of the mechanism of short-term feeding behavior, the possible involvement of the peptidergic system must be considered. Although many naturally occurring peptides elicit satiety upon intraperitoneal or intravenous injection (Smith and Gibbs, 1981), their mechanisms of action are basically unknown. Certainly, the discovery of gut hormones in the brain has significant physiological implications; however, the role of brain peptides in food intake regulation remains unclear. A general consensus is that while gut hormones possess mostly endocrine or paracrine actions peripherally, the small peptides present in the brain may act as neuromodulators (Krieger and Martin, 1981).

Ten gut peptides have been shown to inhibit feeding. These are cholecystokinin, bombesin, gastrin, secretin, glucagon, insulin, somatostatin, neurotensin, substance P, and pancreatic polypeptide (Smith and Gibbs, 1981). Of these ten, the peptide receiving the most investigation is cholecystokinin (CCK).

Fasting and feeding have been shown to alter central and peripheral CCK metabolism. For example, the number of CCK receptors increases in the hypothalamus of mice after fasting, suggesting a role for the receptor site in hunger and satiety (Saito et al., 1981). Although Straus and Yalow (1980) have reported a lower cortical immunoreactive CCK concentration in food-deprived mice, it would be premature to suggest that food ingestion directly affects brain peptide synthesis. On the other hand, peripheral hormonal response to food ingestion has been well documented. For example, human serum iCCK level increased from approximately 25 pg/ml to 16 ng/ml within 35 minutes of food ingestion (Harvey et al., 1973). Of particular interest here is the peripheral and central compartmentation of these small peptides. Certain regions of the brain, such as the pituitary, are outside the blood-brain barrier and may be susceptible to alterations in circulating peptide concentration. The contribution of peripheral peptides to the central pool is largely unresolved.

Although it is highly unlikely that amino acid precursors of these peptides influence their synthesis and release due to the genetic control involved, their presence and release is relevant to the possible role of amino acids in food intake regulation. This is in part due to the fact that amino acids trigger their release. For example, tryptophan and phenylalanine are strong stimulators of cholecystokinin release (Meyer and Grossman, 1972), which is in turn a particularly potent appetite suppressant (Gibbs et al., 1973). It may act either by altering gastrointestinal function (e.g., gut motility) or by interaction with several central neurotransmitter systems that are involved in food intake. The satiating effect of CCK depends on intact gastric vagal fibers (Smith et al., 1981), and impulses along these projections to the diencephalon may activate certain hypothalamic noradrenergic neurons (Myers and McCaleb, 1981). This mechanism might be responsible for the suppression of norepinephrine-induced feeding after intraperitoneal CCK injection (McCaleb and Myer, 1980). Taken together, these results suggest that CCK interacts functionally with the hypothalamic noradrenergic system to mediate changes in feeding behavior. CCK also interacts with the serotonergic system, because intraventricularly injected CCK alters brain serotonin turnover (Fekete et al., 1981). Conversely, tryptophan (200 mg/kg) injected intraperitoneally caused a decrease in hypothalamic CCK-like activity (Lamers et al., 1980), offering evidence that 5HT or CA precursor availability may influence this peptide's effect on food intake.

SUMMARY

In summary, amino acids would appear to have a unique potential to be part of food intake control mechanisms. They are substances which in some instances (the indispensable or essential amino acids) can only arise from the diet because they cannot be synthesized in the body. Their release from food proteins triggers the release of hormones that may be part of feeding control mechanisms, while at the same time the entry of dietary amino acids into free amino acid pools and into the brain allows them to play a possible direct neurotransmitter role or, in some instances, influence the formation of neurotransmitters. Furthermore, brain-free amino acid pools and brain neurotransmitter synthesis are influenced in a predictable manner by the carbohydrate and fat as well as the protein components of the diet. Thus, all the macrocomponents of food are able to provide information to the brain via free amino acids, which may participate in mechanisms regulating qualitative as well as quantitative (energy) aspects of food intake.

REFERENCES

Anderson, G.H. (1979): Control of protein and energy intake: role of plasma amino acids and brain neurotransmitters. *Can. J. Physiol. Pharmacol.* 57:1043–1057.

Anderson, G.H. and Ashley, D.V.M. (1977): Correlation of the plasma tyrosine to phenylalanine ratio with energy intake in self-selecting rats. *Life Sci.* 21:1227–1234.

Anderson, G.H. and Blendis, L.M. (1981): Plasma neutral amino acid ratios in normal man and in patients with hepatic encephalopathy: correlations with self-selected protein and energy consumption. *Am. J. Clin. Nutr.* 34:377–385.

Anderson, G.H., Leprohon, C., Chambers, J.H. and Coscina, D.V. (1979): Intact regulation of protein intake during the development of hypothalamic or genetic obesity in rats. *Physiol. Behav.* 22:777–780.

Anderson, H.L., Benevenga, N.J. and Harper, A.E. (1968): Associations among food intake and protein intake, serine dehydratase and plasma amino acids. *Am. J. Physiol.* 214: 1008–1013.

Ashley, D.V.M. and Anderson, G.H. (1975): Food intake regulation in the weanling rat: the effect of the most limiting essential amino acids of gluten, casein and zein on the self selection of protein and energy. *J. Nutr.* 105:1405–1411.

Ashley, D.V.M. and Anderson G.H. (1975): Correlation between the plasma tryptophan to neutral amino acid ratio and protein intake in the self-selecting rat. *J. Nutr.* 105: 1412–1421.

Ashley, D.V.M., Coscina, D.V. and Anderson, G.H. (1979): Selective decrease in protein intake following drug induced brain serotonin depletion. *Life Sci.* 24:973–984.

Blundell, J.E. (1980): Pharmacological adjustments of the mechanisms underlying feeding and obesity. In: *Obesity* (ed: A.J. Stunkard), pp. 182–207, W.B. Saunders, Toronto, Ontario.

Blundell, J.E. and McArthur, R.A. (1979): Investigation of food consumption using a dietary self-selection procedure: effects of pharmacological manipulation and feeding schedules. *Br. J. Pharmacol.* 67:436–438.

Blundell, J.E. and Rogers, P.J. (1980): Effects of anorexic drugs on food intake, food selection and preferences and hunger motivation and subjective experiences. *Appetite* 1:151–165.

Booth, D.A., Chase, A. and Campbell, A.T. (1970): Relative effectiveness of protein in the late stages of appetite suppression in man. *Physiol. Behav.* 5:1299–1302.

Butler, R.M., Davies, M., Gehling, N.J. and Grant, A.K. (1981): The effect of preloads of amino acids on short-term satiety. *Am. J. Clin. Nutr.* 34:2045–2047.

Chee, K.M., Romsos, D.R. and Bergen, H.G. (1981): Effect of dietary fat on protein intake regulation in young obese and lean mice. *J. Nutr.* 111:668–672.

Chee, K.M., Romsos, D.R., Bergen, W.G. and Leveille, G.A. (1981): Protein intake regulation and nitrogen retention in young obese (ob/ob) and lean mice. *J. Nutr.* 111:58–67.

Collier, G., Leshner, A.I. and Squibbs, R.L.(1969): Dietary self-selection in active and nonactive rats. *Physiol. Behav.* 4:79–82.

FAO/WHO (1973): Joint expert committee on energy and protein requirement. *World Health Organization Technical Report Series.* No. 522, Geneva.

Fekete, M., Kádár, T., Penke, B., Kovács, K. and Telegdy, G. (1981): Influence of cholecystokin in octapeptide sulphate ester on brain monoamine metabolism in rats. *J. Neural Transm.* 50:81–88.

Fernstrom, J.D. and Faller, D.V. (1978): Neutral amino acids in the brain: Changes in response to food ingestion. *J. Neurochem.* 30:1531–1538.

Fryer, J.H., Moore, N.S., Williams, H.H. and Young, C.M. (1955): A study of the interrelationships of the energy yielding nutrients, blood glucose levels and subjective appetite in man. *J. Lab. Clin. Med.* 45:684–696.

Gershoff, S.N. (1977): The role of vitamins and minerals in taste. In: *The Chemical Senses and Nutrition* (eds: M.R. Kare and O. Maller), pp. 201–212, Academic Press, New York.

Gibbs, J.R., Young, R.C. and Smith, G.P. (1973): Cholecystokinin decreases food intake in rats. *J. Comp. Physiol. Psychol.* 84:488–495.

Harper, A.E., Benevenga, N.J. and Wohlhueter, R.M. (1970): Effect of ingestion of disproportionate amounts of amino acids. *Physiol. Rev.* 50:428–558.

Harvey, R.F., Dowsett, L., Hartog, M. and Read, A.E. (1973): A radioimmunoassay for cholecystokinin-pancreozymin. *Lancet* 2:826–828.

Johnson, D.J. and Anderson, G.H. (1982): The prediction of plasma amino acid concentration from diet amino acid content. *Am. J. Physiol.* (in press).

Johnson, D.J., Li, E.T.S., Coscina, D.V. and Anderson, G.H. (1979): Different diurnal rhythms of protein and non-protein intake by rats. *Physiol. Behav.* 22:777–780.

Kanarak, R.B., Feldman, P.G. and Hanes, C. (1981): Pattern of dietary self-selection in VMH-lesioned rats. *Physiol. Behav.* 27:337–343.

Kanarak, R.B., Ho, L. and Meade, R.G. (1981): Sustained decrease in fat consumption produced by amphetamine in rats maintained on a dietary self-selection regime. *Pharmacol. Biochem. Behav.* 14:539–542.

Krieger, D.T. and Martin, J.B. (1981): Brain peptides. *N. Engl. J. Med.* 304:876–885.

Krieger, D.T. and Martin, J.B. (1981): Brain peptides. *N. Engl. J. Med.* 304:944–951.

Larners, C.B., Morley, J.E., Poitras, P., Sharp, B., Carlson, H.E., Hershman, J.M. and Walsh, J.H. (1980): Immunological and biological studies on cholecystokinin in rat brain. *Am. J. Physiol.* 239:E232–E235.

Lát, J. (1967): Self-selection of dietary components. In: *Handbook of Physiology,* Section 6, Vol. 1, Chapter 27, pp. 367–386. American Physiological Society, Washington, D.C.

Li, E.T.S., and Anderson, G.H. (1982): Dietary minerals modify the food intake suppressing effects of high casein diets fed to rats. *J. Nutr.* 112:April.

Maher, T.J. and Wurtman, R.J. (1980): L-Threonine administration increases glycine concentrations in the rat central nervous system. *Life Sci.* 26:1283–1286.

Mauron, C., Wurtman, J.J. and Wurtman, R.J. (1980): Clonidine increases food and protein consumption in rats. *Life Sci.* 27:781–791.

McCaleb, M.L. and Myers, R.D. (1980): Cholecystokinin acts on the hypothalamic 'noradrenergic system' involved in feeding. *Peptides* 1:47–49.

McMenamy, R.H. and Oncley, J.L. (1978): The specific binding of L-tryptophan to serum albumin. *J. Biol. Chem.* 233:1436–1447.

Mellinkoff, S.M., Frankland, M., Boyle, D., and Geipell, M. (1956): Relationship between serum amino acid concentration and fluctuations in appetite. *J. Appl. Physiol.* 8:535–538.

Menon, M.K., Clark, W.G. and Aures, D. (1971): Effect of thiazol-4-ylmethoxyamine, a new inhibitor of histamine biosynthesis on brain histamine, monoamine levels and behaviour. *Life Sci.* 10:1097–1109.

Meyer, J.H. and Grossman, M.I. (1972): Release of secretin and cholecystokinin. In: *Gastrointestinal Hormones* (ed: L. Demling), pp. 50–53, Georg Thieme Verlag, Stuttgart.

Morley, J.E. (1980): The neuroendocrine control of appetite: The role of the endogenous opiates, cholecystokinin, TRH, gamma-amino-butyric-acid and the diazepam receptors. *Life Sci.* 27:355–368.

Musten, B., Peace, D. and Anderson, G.H. (1974): Food intake regulation in the weanling rat: self-selection of protein and energy. *J. Nutr.* 104:563–572.

Myers, R.D. and McCaleb, M.L., (1981): Peripheral and intrahypothalamic cholecystokinin act on the noradrenergic 'feeding circuit' in the rat's diencephalon. *Neurosci.* 6:645–655.

Ohlson, M.A. and Hart, B.P. (1965): Influence of breakfast on total day's food intake. *J. Am. Diet. Assoc.* 47:282–286.

Osborne, T.B. and Mendel, L.B. (1918): The choice between adequate and inadequate diets, as made by rats. *J. Biol. Chem.* 35:19–27.

Pardridge, W.M. (1977): Regulation of amino acid availability to the brain. In: *Nutrition and the Brain.* (eds: R.J. Wurtman and J.J. Wurtman), Vol. 1, pp. 141–204, Raven Press, New York.

Peng, Y., Tews, J.K. and Harper, A.E. (1972): Amino acid imbalance, protein intake and changes in rat brain and plasma amino acids. *Am. J. Physiol.* 222:314–321.

Peters, J.C. and Harper, A.E. (1981): Protein and energy consumption, plasma amino acid ratios, and brain neurotransmitter concentrations. *Physiol. Behav.* 27:287–298.

Quaade, F., Hyldstrup, L. and Andersen, T. (1981): The Copenhagen PRODI project: preliminary results. *Int. J. Obesity* 5:263–266.

Reeves, P.G. and O'Dell, B.L. (1981): Short term zinc deficiency in the rat and self-selection of dietary protein level. *J. Nutr.* 111:375–383.

Rogers, Q.R. and Leung, P.M.B. (1977): The control of food intake: when and how are amino acids involved. In: *The Chemical Senses and Nutrition* (eds: M.B. Kare and O. Maller), pp. 213–248, Academic Press, New York.

Rozin, P. (1968): Are carbohydrate and protein intakes separately regulated? *J. Comp. Physiol. Psychol.* 65:23–29.

Saito, A., Williams, J.A. and Goldfine, I.D. (1981): Alterations in brain cholecystokinin receptors after fasting. *Nature* 289:599–600.

Schwartz, J.C., Lampart, C. and Rose, C. (1972): Histamine formation in rat brain in vivo: Effects of histidine loads. *J. Neurochem.* 19:801–810.

Smith, G.P. and Gibbs, J. (1981): Brain-gut peptides and the control of food intake. In: *Neurosecretion and Brain Peptides* (eds: J.B. Martin, S. Reichlin and K.L. Bick), pp. 389–395, Raven Press, New York.

Straus, E. and Yalow, R.S. (1980): Brain cholecystokinin in fasted and fed mice. *Life Sci.* 26: 969–970.

Tews, J.K., Good, S.S. and Harper, A.E. (1978): Transport of threonine and tryptophan by rat brain slices: relation to other amino acids at concentrations found in plasma. *J. Neurochem.* 31:581–589.

Tews, J.K., Kim, Y.L. and Harper, A.E. (1980): Induction of threonine imbalance by dispensable amino acids: relationships between tissue amino acids and diet in rats. *J. Nutr.* 110: 394–408.

Wade, J., Milner, J. and Krondl, M. (1981): Evidence for a physiological regulation of food selection and nutrient intake in twins. *Am. J. Clin. Nutr.* 34:143–147.

Woodger, T.L., Sirek, A. and Anderson, G.H. (1979): Diabetes, dietary tryptophan, and protein intake regulation in weanling rats. *Am. J. Physiol.* 236:R307–R311.

Wurtman, J.J. and Wurtman, R.J. (1978): Fenfluramine and fluoxetine spare protein consumption while suppressing caloric intake by rats. *Science.* 198:1178–1180.

Wurtman, J.J. and Wurtman, R.J. (1979): Drugs that enhance central serotonergic transmission diminish elective carbohydrate consumption by rats. *Life Sci.* 24:895–904.

Wurtman, J.J., Wurtman, R.J., Growden, J.H., Henry, P., Lipscomb, A. and Zeisel, S.H. (1981): Carbohydrate craving in obese people: suppression by treatments affecting serotoninergic transmission. *Int. J. Eating Disorders* 11:2–15.

Wurtman, R.J. and Fernstrom, J.D. (1976): Control of brain neurotransmitter synthesis by precursor availability and nutritional state. *Biochem. Pharmacol.* 25:1691–1696.

Wurtman, R.J., Hefti, F. and Melamed, E. (1981): Precursor control of neurotransmitter synthesis. *Pharmacol. Rev.* 32:315–335.

Communication

Alterations in Amino Acid Transport Across Blood-Brain Barrier in Rats Following Portacaval Shunting

Richard A. Hawkins, Anke M. Mans, and Julien F. Biebuyck

The brain requires a continuous and balanced supply of essential amino acids to sustain protein synthesis and for the formation of small polypeptides and certain neurotransmitters such as serotonin and the catecholamines. The availability of amino acids to cerebral cells is determined by the blood-brain barrier, which has many of the kinetic properties of a cell membrane. The entry of hydrophilic amino acids depends on specific transport carriers that mediate facilitated diffusion, a process that is equilibratory (not concentrative), sodium- and energy-independent (Betz et al., 1975; Pardridge, 1977), and stereospecific (Oldendorf, 1973). Because the amino acid transport activities of nerve and glial cell membranes are much greater (Bauman et al., 1974; Pardridge and Oldendorf, 1975; Parfitt and Graham-Smith, 1974), it has been inferred that transport across the blood-brain barrier is the rate-limiting step in the supply of amino acids to brain cells (Pardridge, 1977; Pardridge et al., 1975).

Studies of amino acid transport *in vivo* have shown that most amino acids could be assigned to one of three carriers: one for the acidic amino acids glutamate and aspartate; one for the basic amino acids arginine, ornithine, and lysine; and one for the neutral amino acids (Oldendorf and Szabo, 1976). The last system carries several large neutral amino acids at simiar rates, namely phenylalanine, tyrosine, tryptophan, valine, leucine, isoleucine, histidine, and threonine. Transport by this system appears to obey Michaelis-Menten saturation kinetics, with the affinity constant for each amino acid being similar to its plasma concentration (Pardridge and Oldendorf, 1975). Because of this, the rate of entry of any particular amino acid is strongly influenced by the presence of the other competing amino acids.

In addition to competition, the rate of influx of an amino acid may be affected by alterations in the carrier itself. The kinetic constants of the blood-brain barrier transport systems are subject to change in various conditions (Betz et al., 1976; Daniel et al., 1975; Mans et al., 1982; James et al., 1978). Because a close relationship exists between amino acid supply and metabolic demand (Pardridge, 1977) a change in blood-brain barrier permeability may be of importance in abnormal states.

The transport step becomes especially important in conditions where plasma amino acid concentrations are also altered, such as during hepatic failure and after portacaval shunting. During these conditions, both in man and experimental animals, characteristic decreases in plasma branched-chain amino acids are seen, together with increases in the aromatic amino acids phenylalanine, tyrosine, and unbound tryptophan (Bloxam and Curzon, 1978; James et al., 1976; Maddrey et al., 1976). It was suggested that the decreased branched-chain amino acids in the plasma lead to reduced competition for entry into brain of the aromatic amino acids, in particular tryptophan, and thus cause the brain amino acid and neurotransmitter changes characteristic of portacaval shunting (Munro et al., 1975; Soeters and

Fischer, 1976). These hypotheses were based on studies of amino acid transport in normal experimental animals (Fernstrom and Wurtman, 1972). It was tacitly assumed that the carrier mechanisms remained unchanged in abnormal conditions such as hepatic encephalopathy. However, it is now clear that there are specific alterations in the blood-brain barrier transport mechanisms during experimental hepatic failure. The kinetics of the neutral amino acid carrier are changed so as to increase influx of tryptophan and the other amino acids transported by this carrier into the brain, whereas transport of the basic amino acid arginine is decreased (James et al., 1978; Mans et al., 1979, 1982; Zanchin et al., 1979).

In most of the above-mentioned studies of transport across the blood-brain barrier, a technique first described by Oldendorf (1970) was used. This is a dual-label method in which the uptake of a substance from a defined medium is measured following a single pass through a portion of the capillary bed. The permeability of the test substance relative to that of a reference is expressed as the brain uptake index. This convenient method was not designed for determining influx rates of substrates as affected by all of the physiological factors, such as plasma amino acids and other consitituents, which may vary in different conditions. In addition, because the solution is injected into one of the carotid arteries, transport studies are limited to a portion of the ipsilateral cerebral hemisphere.

Because of the key role of the blood-brain barrier in cerebral metabolism, it is important to know what the actual rate of penetration of an amino acid is under physiological conditions, that is, in the presence of competitors, hormones, proteins, and other circulating blood constituents. Of even greater interest is the determination of the rate of influx into specific anatomical structures of the brain. With this information, it would be possible to determine whether changes were localized to specific areas or occurred throughout the whole brain. A detailed study of amino acid entry into brain may reveal areas of etiological significance to the encephalopathic process. In this study the influx of tryptophan, tyrosine, phenylalanine, leucine, and lysine was examined in rats with portacaval shunts, using quantitative autoradiography, which allows individual determinations of influx to be made in most cerebral structures (Hawkins et al., 1982).

METHODS

Rats

All rats used were Long-Evans males weighing 225–250 g. Normal rats, those with an end-to-side portacaval shunt, as well as sham-operated rats, were bought from Zivic-Miller Laboratories, Inc., Allison Park, PA. The protacaval shunt procedure was carried out according to a modification of the technique described by Lee and Fisher (1961). The rats were allowed free access to standard laboratory chow (RMH 3000, containing protein 22% minimum, fat 5% minimum, fiber 5% maximum), obtained from Agway, Inc., Syracuse, NY, and water until the morning of the experiment.

Measurement of Amino Acid Transport

Regional transport of amino acids across the blood-brain barrier was studied seven to eight weeks after the portacaval shunt operation. The procedure used was an autoradiographic adaptation of the method of Baños et al. (1973). Since it is explained in detail elsewhere (Hawkins et al., 1982), only a brief description will be given here. Anesthesia was induced with halothane in O_2 and cannulae were placed in the femoral artery, femoral vein, and the trachea. The rats were paralyzed with Tubocurarine (1.5 mg/kg) and artificially ventilated with N_2O:O_2(70:30, v/v) at a rate that maintained normal blood gas and pH values. Body temperature was maintained at 38°C with a homeothermic electric blanket. After a 45-minute period of stabilization, the transport experiment was carried out. Radiolabeled amino acid was infused through the femoral venous cannula for a period of 1.5 minutes (phenylalanine, tyrosine, leucine, and tryptophan), or four to six minutes (lysine).

The ^{14}C-labeled amino acid was made up in 0.154M NaCl solution (50 μCi/ml) except in the case of tryptophan, which was dissolved in plasma obtained from a normal rat just before the experiment. This was done to allow equilibration of [^{14}C]tryptophan with unlabeled tryptophan bound to plasma albumin before infusion. The rate of infusion was adjusted so that a rapid rise of isotope was obtained in the plasma followed by an approximately steady level for the duration of the experiment. Frequent blood samples were collected from the femoral artery during the experiment for determination of dpm/ml in plasma. The rat was then decapitated and an additional blood sample collected from the cervical wound for plasma amino acid analysis.

The brain was removed from the skull and prepared for quantitative autoradiography as previously described (Hawkins et al., 1979). The ^{14}C content in individual regions was obtained densitometrically by comparison with calibrated standards. A computer-driven scanning densitometer was used for a few representative rats from each group studied to provide more detailed images for regional comparison.

Calculations

The plasma clearance (μl•min^{-1}•g^{-1}) was calculated from the following equation:

$$\text{Clearance} \cong C_b{}^*\!\int_0^T C_p{}^*dt \qquad [1]$$

and influx (nmol•min^{-1}•g^{-1}) from:

$$\text{Influx} = C_b{}^*\!\int_0^T C_p{}^*/C_p dt \qquad [2]$$

where $C_b{}^*$ = tracer concentration of labeled substance in brain tissue (d.p.m./g); $C_p{}^*$ = tracer concentration of labeled substance in plasma (d.p.m./μl); t = experimental time (min); T = duration of experiment (min). $C_b{}^*$ was corrected for radioactivity in blood remaining in the brain tissue by subtracting a background value for each region:

$$\text{Background d.p.m.} = (\mu\text{l blood/g}) \times (\text{d.p.m.}/\mu\text{l blood}) \qquad [3]$$

A correction for the effect of blood flow on amino acid influx was not necessary in this study. The permeability of the blood-brain barrier to amino acids is relatively low; therefore, their entry into brain is not seriously affected by blood flow. For a more complete discussion of the various considerations, see Hawkins et al. (1982).

To calculate tryptophan influx, total plasma tryptophan concentrations were used. As described above, the [^{14}C]tryptophan was mixed with plasma before infusion to allow the specific activities of free and bound tryptophan to equilibrate. Thus movement of label into brain represented the total tryptophan entry irrespective of whether it was free or associated with albumin.

RESULTS

Physiological Parameters

Rats with portacaval shunts weighed 40% less than controls (control: 433 ± 61 [S.D.]g; portacaval shunt: 263 ± 33 g). This is in agreement with other studies showing that these rats gain little if any weight after the operation (Gjedde et al., 1978; Rossouw et al., 1978). The shunted rats appeared alert but had some hair loss and testicular atrophy, changes which have also been observed by others (Bircher, 1979). The blood pressure was significantly lower after portacaval shunting (107 ± 19 [S.D.] mm Hg) than in control rats (135 ± 12 mm Hg) although the values remained well within physiological limits for the autoregulation of cerebral blood flow (Hernandez et al., 1978). Arterial blood gases and pH were maintained close to normal values during the experimental period by adjustment of the rate of ventilation.

Integrity of the Blood-Brain Barrier

Before beginning the transport experiments, it was necessary to examine the integrity of the blood-brain barrier in all regions. This was done by infusing a relatively impermeable substance, [^{14}C] sucrose, in a separate group of rats. Since sucrose passes the blood-brain barrier at a very slow rate (Ohno et al., 1978), it can be considered to be restricted to cerebral vessels during the first 1.5 minutes unless the blood-brain barrier has been disrupted. Normal and shunted rats were infused with sucrose for a period of 1.5 minutes then decapitated and the brains removed for quantitative autoradiography. The small volume of sucrose distribution, which was interpreted as being due to the blood remaining in cerebral vessels, amounted to 7 μl in the globus pallidus to 21 μl in the pons. No differences were found between normal and portacaval shunted rats. This demonstrated that the physical integrity of the blood-brain barrier was retained in the rats with portacaval shunts.

Plasma Amino Acids

Changes were observed in the concentrations of many amino acids after portacaval shunting (Table 1), which are characteristic of this disorder (Bloxam and Curzon, 1978; Cummings et al., 1976a; James et al., 1976). Significant decreases were found in the branched-chain amino acids leucine, isoleucine, and valine, the basic amino acid lysine, and the neutral amino acid threonine. Increased concentrations of tyrosine, phenylalanine, histidine, and unbound tryptophan were found, as well as increases in a few nonessential amino acids, asparagine, alanine, glycine and glutamine. Cystine concentrations were decreased.

Brain Amino Acids

The content of some essential neutral and basic amino acids, as well as glutamine, was measured in whole brain of normal and shunted rats. Tryptophan, phenylalanine, tyrosine, methionine, histidine, and glutamine were increased (Table 2) whereas the other neutral amino acids were not significantly affected. Basic amino acid content (not shown) was generally decreased, although none of the individual amino acids showed a statistically significant changes.

Table 1
Plasma Amino Acids After Portacaval Shunting

Amino acid	Control (μM)	Portacaval shunt (μM)	%Difference
Large neutral			
Tryptophan, unbound	15 ± 3	21 ± 2	+ 40
Tryptophan, total	169 ± 10	145 ± 13	
Phenylalanine	64 ± 2	107 ± 4	+ 67
Tyrosine	54 ± 2	109 ± 4	+ 102
Methionine	55 ± 2	52 ± 3	
Histidine	74 ± 7	107 ± 10	+ 45
Leucine	183 ± 10	127 ± 5	− 31
Isoleucine	90 ± 4	63 ± 2	− 30
Valine	194 ± 7	134 ± 5	− 31
Threonine	201 ± 8	115 ± 5	− 43
Small Neutral			
Asparagine	42 ± 5	109 ± 11	+ 160
Serine	198 ± 6	205 ± 9	
Proline	177 ± 9	186 ± 10	
Glutamine	538 ± 22	779 ± 37	+ 45
Basic			
Ornithine	87 ± 7	109 ± 14	
Lysine	358 ± 11	303 ± 13	− 15
Arginine	173 ± 15	167 ± 17	
Acidic			
Glutamate	70 ± 5	75 ± 4	
Unassigned			
Alanine	369 ± 16	407 ± 19	
Glycine	248 ± 11	360 ± 16	+ 45
Taurine	137 ± 13	179 ± 20	
Cystine	69 ± 16	31 ± 6	− 55

Results are the means ± S.E.M. of 12 to 34 rats. The amino acids are grouped according to their blood-brain barrier transport mechanisms (Oldendorf and Szabo, 1976). Only percentage differences significant at the 5% level or less are shown.

Table 2
Amino Acid Concent of Brain from Normal Rats and Rats with Portacaval shunts

	Control	Shunt
Tryptophan	23 ± 2	70 ± 11
Phenylalanine	44 ± 5	179 ± 23
Tyrosine	50 ± 4	195 ± 16
Methionine	65 ± 5	92 ± 6
Histidine	105 ± 10	183 ± 15
Glutamine	5.97 ± 0.34	21.4 ± 1.6

All values are means (± S.E.M.) of five or six individual determinations. The data are expressed in nmol/g except glutamine, which is given in μmol/g. All values in the shunted group were significantly different from control of the 5% level.

Amino Acid Transport

The influx of all four neutral amino acids was increased substantially in almost every area examined; however, the different areas were not affected equally (Table 3). The hypothalamus, for example, was generally less affected whereas the fluxes into the reticular formation, hippocampus, and amygdala were much greater. This pattern was especially consistent with phenylalanine, tyrosine, and tryptophan. The influx of phenylalanine in different brain regions was significantly correlated with that of tryptophan, tyrosine and leucine, both in normal and shunted rats. This showed that the proportions between influx in different regions were similar for these amino acids. The increased rates of phenylalaine and tyrosine influx were caused in part by the increased circulating concentrations. On the other hand, the plasma concentrations of tryptophan and leucine were decreased (Table 1). The changes in the transport properties of the blood-brain barrier itself are better seen by using plasma clearance to describe the transport process (Table 4). The clearance values show that the transport mechanism was altered in favor of increased transport for all four neutral amino acids. The rate of tryptophan transport was enhanced to a greater degree (about 200%) and leucine to a lesser degree (about 30%) than was the transport of phenylalanine (about 80%) and tyrosine (about 70%). These findings are in close agreement with an earlier study by Zanchin et al. (1979), where the brain uptake index technique was used. They also found that the uptake of tryptophan was increased to a much greater extent than that of any of the other neutral amino acids examined.

The regional distribution of lysine transport was generally similar to that of the neutral amino acids. After portacaval shunting, the rate of lysine clearance was decreased by 50% to 88% (Table 4). Lysine influx was decreased even more as a result of reduced concentrations of plasma lysine (Tables 1 and 3). These results demonstrate the very specific changes in blood-brain barrier transport that occur in this condition. Furthermore, the decreased permeability to lysine supports the contention that the blood-brain barrier remains intact.

Figures 1A and B (see color illustrations) show phenylalanine clearance in a series of coronal sections from a control rat and a rat with a portacaval shunt, respectively, analyzed by a computer-driven scanning densitometer. Both the heterogeneity of the transport process among the different brain areas and the increases after portacaval shunting can be clearly seen.

Table 3

Influx of Neutral and Basic Amino Acids into Various Cerebral Structures

	INFLUX														
	Phenylalanine			Tyrosine			Tryptophan			Leucine			Lysine		
	Control	Shunt	%Diff	Control	Shunt	%Diff	Control	Shunt	%Diff	Control	Shunt	%Diff	Control	Shunt	%Diff
TELENCEPHALON															
Frontal cortex	8	24	+ 184	5	14	+ 180	4	12	+ 180	15	18		9	3	− 68
Cingulate gyrus	8	24	+ 203	4	13	+ 225	4	11	+ 212	14	18		9	2	− 73
Parietal cortex	8	22	+ 192	5	13	+ 160	4	11	+ 203	14	17	+ 21	8	3	− 61
Pyriform cortex	6	18	+ 200	3	10	+ 233	3	8	+ 167	11	14	+ 27	6	2	− 67
Insular cortex	7	22	+ 214	4	12	+ 200	4	11	+ 175	11	15	+ 39	9	3	− 67
Occipital cortex	7	22	+ 204	4	12	+ 200	4	11	+ 185	13	17	+ 33	8	4	− 56
Caudate nucleus	7	19	+ 185	3	11	+ 267	3	9	+ 206	11	14	+ 28	6	1	− 80
Globus pallidus	5	15	+ 174	3	8	+ 167	2	6	+ 175	9	11		4	1	− 77
Amygdala	7	19	+ 193	3	11	+ 267	3	10	+ 237	11	14	+ 23	7	2	− 72
Hippocampus –															
anterior	6	19	+ 225	3	11	+ 267	3	8	+ 225	10	14	+ 40	5	1	− 70
posterior	6	18	+ 210	3	11	+ 267	3	9	+ 225	10	14	+ 46	5	2	− 68
Lateral septal n.	7	18	+ 161	3	11	+ 267	3	9	+ 191	13	13		6	2	− 59
Corpus callosum	3	9	+ 200	2	7	+ 250	1	4		9	11		3	1	− 79
DIENCEPHALON															
Habenula	9	30	+ 233	5	15	+ 200	5	15	+ 200	18	21		12	3	− 75
Hypothalamus	8	18	+ 123	4	11	+ 175	4	8	+ 123	13	13		6	1	− 80
Thalamus –															
anterior	10	29	+ 199	5	14	+ 180	5	13	+ 146	17	20		11	2	− 80
ventral	8	24	+ 191	5	13	+ 160	5	12	+ 170	15	18	+ 18	9	2	− 82
medial	8	24	+ 195	5	14	+ 180	4	12	+ 182	15	18	+ 22	10	1	− 86
lateral	8	23	+ 191	5	12	+ 140	4	12	+ 192	14	16	+ 19	8	2	− 80
Internal capsule	3	9	+ 200	2	7	+ 250	1	4	+ 300	8	11	+ 29	3	1	− 72
MESENCEPHALON															
Substantia nigra	7	19	+ 164	3	10	+ 233	4	9	+ 119	14	14		6	1	− 82
Red nucleus	8	25	+ 224	5	13	+ 160	4	13	+ 221	16	19		9	1	− 91
Occulomotor complex	6	19	+ 198	5	14	+ 180	3	9	+ 252	19	19		11	1	− 89
Interpeduncular n.	11	29	+ 165	6	16	+ 167	5	16	+ 208	18	20		8	2	− 76
Reticular formation	6	19	+ 218	3	10	+ 233	3	9	+ 238	11	13		6	1	− 84
Superior colliculus	8	23	+ 192	5	14	+ 180	4	12	+ 181	15	18		10	3	− 67
Inferior colliculus	11	31	+ 170	7	18	+ 157	7	17	+ 130	21	23		14	3	− 81

Table 3 (continued)

	INFLUX														
	Phenylalanine			Tyrosine			Tryptophan			Leucine			Lysine		
	Control	Shunt	%Diff	Control	Shunt	%Diff	Control	Shunt	%Diff	Control	Shunt	%Diff	Control	Shunt	%Diff
METENCEPHALON															
Pons	9	23	+ 160	5	14	+ 180	6	14	+ 147	19	19		15	3	− 80
Cerebellar gray—															
molecular	7	20	+ 193	4	12	+ 200	3	10	+ 262	10	15	+ 39	7	2	− 78
granular	8	21	+ 167	5	13	+ 160	4	12	+ 209	16	19	+ 17	9	2	− 83
vermis	8	22	+ 166	5	14	+ 180	5	11	+ 147	19	18		10	2	− 81
Cerebellar white	4	10	+ 150	2	8	+ 300	1	4	+ 300	9	11	+ 25	5	1	− 82
Dentate nucleus	12	31	+ 158	6	16	+ 167	7	17	+ 143	20	20		13	2	− 85
MYELENCEPHALON															
Vestibular nucleus	12	33	+ 175	6	17	+ 183	7	19	+ 171	24	24		15	3	− 80
Cochlear nucleus	13	33	+ 153	6	17	+ 183	8	18	+ 125	25	24		13	3	− 77
Superior olive	12	35	+ 192	7	18	+ 157	8	21	+ 163	22	22		15	3	− 80
Inferior olive	10	30	+ 200	5	15	+ 200	5	16	+ 220	18	21		14	3	− 79
Reticular formation	7	19	+ 150	4	12	+ 200	3	9	+ 204	14	15		10	1	− 88

All values are means of six to ten rats expressed in $nmol \cdot min^{-1} \cdot g^{-1}$. Only percentage differences significant at the 5% level or less are given.

Table 4
Plasma Clearance of Neutral and Basic Amino Acids by Various Cerebral Structures

	CLEARANCE														
	Phenylalanine			Tyrosine			Tryptophan			Leucine			Lysine		
	Control	Shunt	%Diff	Control	Shunt	%Diff	Control	Shunt	%Diff	Control	Shunt	%Diff	Control	Shunt	%Diff
TELENCEPHALON															
Frontal cortex	127	229	+ 80	86	140	+ 63	23	70	+ 204	98	130	+ 33	26	10	− 63
Cingulate gyrus	120	230	+ 92	77	127	+ 65	20	67	+ 235	94	128	+ 36	26	8	− 70
Parietal cortex	117	214	+ 83	78	133	+ 70	20	68	+ 240	95	122	+ 28	24	10	− 56
Pyriform cortex	88	173	+ 97	55	101	+ 84	16	47	+ 194	69	96	+ 39	17	7	− 59
Insular cortex	113	215	+ 90	68	119	+ 74	22	64	+ 191	69	105	+ 52	24	11	− 96
Occipital cortex	112	215	+ 92	68	123	+ 81	21	66	+ 214	82	120	+ 46	23	11	− 51
Caudate nucleus	102	183	+ 79	59	104	+ 78	17	56	+ 229	70	101	+ 44	17	4	− 78
Globus pallidus	82	141	+ 72	42	77	+ 82	13	38	+ 192	58	75	+ 29	10	3	− 75
Amygdala	101	186	+ 84	56	109	+ 94	17	60	+ 253	72	99	+ 38	21	7	− 69
Hippocampus –															
anterior	88	118	+ 106	56	104	+ 86	14	50	+ 257	64	98	+ 53	13	5	− 66
posterior	90	175	+ 94	56	105	+ 88	15	51	+ 240	62	101	+ 63	15	6	− 63
Lateral septal n.	107	175	+ 64	59	105	+ 78	17	51	+ 200	79	93		16	8	− 54
Corpus callosum	51	89	+ 75	43	71	+ 66	8	25	+ 213	60	79	+ 32	8	2	− 75
DIENCEPHALON															
Habenula	140	286	+ 104	91	142	+ 56	28	87	+ 211	118	150	+ 27	35	9	− 74
Hypothalamus	121	170	+ 40	74	104	+ 41	21	49	+ 133	88	96		18	4	− 78
Thalamus –															
anterior nuclei	147	277	+ 88	89	141	+ 59	29	79	+ 172	109	141	+ 29	33	7	− 79
ventral nuclei	128	236	+ 84	83	130	+ 57	25	73	+ 192	98	128	+ 31	25	5	− 80
medial genicul.	126	236	+ 87	85	138	+ 62	24	72	+ 200	97	130	+ 34	29	4	− 85
lateral genicul.	120	220	+ 83	77	123	+ 59	22	70	+ 218	89	117	+ 31	22	5	− 78
Internal capsule	51	87	+ 71	41	70	+ 70	8	22	+ 175	54	74	+ 37	9	3	− 70
MESENCEPHALON															
Substantia nigra	112	185	+ 65	58	94	+ 61	23	54	+ 135	87	97		17	3	− 80
Red nucleus	118	239	+ 103	78	130	+ 67	23	80	+ 248	101	138	+ 37	26	3	− 90
Occulomotor complex	96	180	+ 88	87	138	+ 59	15	55	+ 267	107	138	+ 29	31	4	− 88
Interpeduncular n.	166	279	+ 68	103	155	+ 50	29	94	+ 224	114	145	+ 27	24	6	− 73
Reticular formation	89	177	+ 99	58	102	+ 75	14	51	+ 264	73	93	+ 27	17	3	− 82
Superior colliculus	120	220	+ 83	82	134	+ 63	24	74	+ 208	95	130	+ 37	27	10	− 63
Inferior colliculus	172	295	+ 72	112	179	+ 60	40	98	+ 145	136	166	+ 22	40	8	− 80

Table 4 (continued)

	CLEARANCE														
	Phenylalanine			Tyrosine			Tryptophan			Leucine			Lysine		
	Control	Shunt	%Diff	Control	Shunt	%Diff	Control	Shunt	%Diff	Control	Shunt	%Diff	Control	Shunt	%Diff
METENCEPHALON															
Pons	137	228	+ 66	89	138	+ 55	31	83	+ 168	121	137		42	9	− 77
Cerebellar gray—															
molecular	104	195	+ 88	65	122	+ 87	16	61	+ 281	66	107	+ 62	21	5	− 77
granular	119	198	+ 66	88	128	+ 45	22	73	+ 232	105	135	+ 29	25	5	− 80
vermis	128	212	+ 66	86	136	+ 58	25	67	+ 168	112	129		28	6	− 78
Cerebellar white	128	212	+ 66	41	74	+ 81	22	71	+ 223	58	81	+ 40	13	2	− 81
Dentate nucleus	176	296	+ 68	104	160	+ 54	43	101	+ 135	127	147		38	5	− 87
MYELENCEPHALON															
Vestibular nucleus	176	316	+ 80	110	170	+ 54	39	112	+ 187	153	173		44	7	− 84
Cochlear nucleus	200	314	+ 57	107	167	+ 57	43	106	+ 147	160	167		40	9	− 78
Superior olive	181	334	+ 85	115	178	+ 55	45	122	+ 171	143	161		41	9	− 79
Inferior olive	148	285	+ 93	93	152	+ 63	27	88	+ 226	118	152		39	9	− 77
Reticular formation	111	168	+ 51	65	116	+ 78	15	51	+ 240	90	108		30	4	− 86

All values are means of six to ten rats expressed in $\mu l \cdot min^{-1} \cdot g^{-1}$. Only percentage differences significant at the 5% level or less are given.

Figure 1 Computerized analysis of phenylalanine clearance (μl/min/g) in a control rat and a rat with a portacaval shunt. Autoradiographs of coronal sections from a control rat (numbers 1–7) and a shunted rat (numbers 9–15) were read with a computer-driven scanning densitometer (10,000 measurements/cm^2). The readings were converted to values of phenylalanine clearance and displayed by colors corresponding to discrete levels of transport. Please note that a different color key is used for each group. The sections are placed rostrally to caudally, as indicated by the numbers.

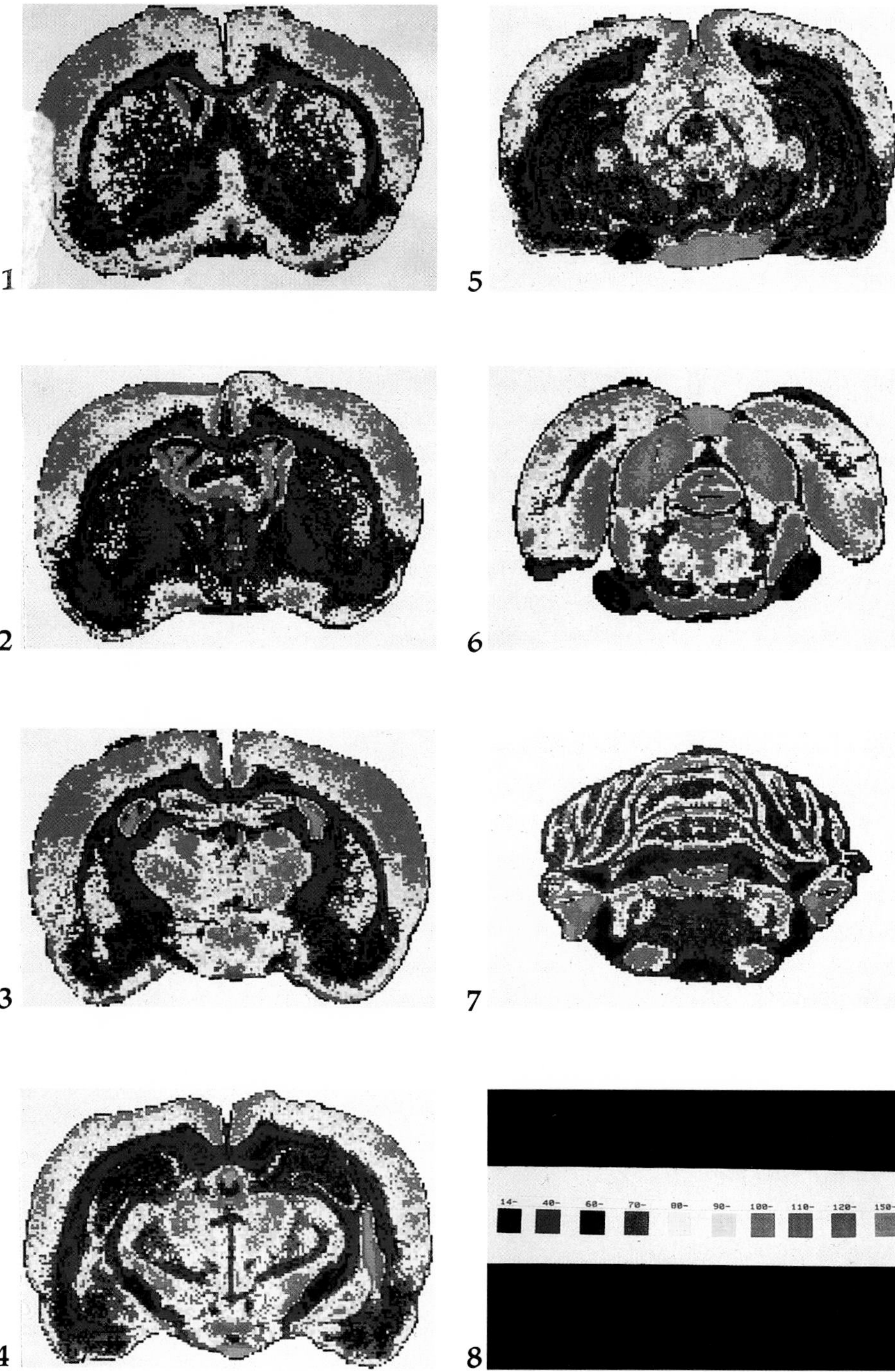
1
5
2
6
3
7
4
8
14-
40-
60-
70-
80-
90-
100-
110-
120-
150-

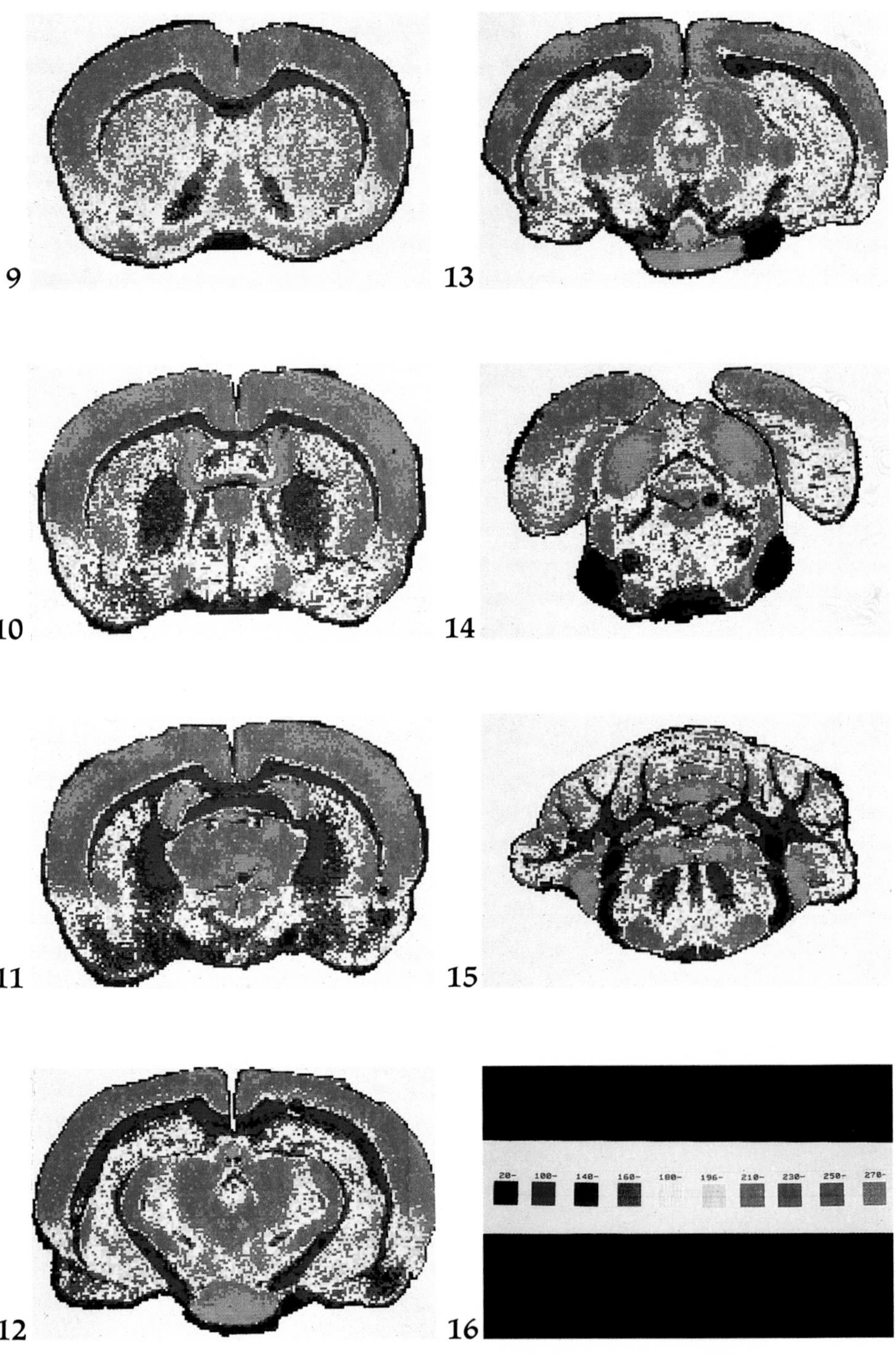

9
10
11
12
13
14
15
16
20-
100-
140-
160-
180-
196-
210-
230-
250-
270-

DISCUSSION

These studies are, we believe, the first applications of quantitative autoradiographic techniques to the determination of essential amino acid transport across the blood-brain barrier. The data demonstrate a marked heterogeneity in the rates of transport which can best be appreciated from Figure 1. It is interesting to consider what the cause of such different regional rates may be. The movement of molecules from plasma into brain must be related to the quantity of transport carriers available, which, in turn, is probably related to the capillary surface area. Although we know of no data concerning the density of transport carriers in capillaries from different portions of brain, the relative vascularity of cerebral structures was studied in detail by Craigie (1920). When his data for regional capillarity are compared to phenylalanine influx, there is a significant correlation (Hawkins et al., 1982). Therefore, it is probable that transport is at least partially related to vascularity and presumbably surface area. It does not necessarily follow that the density of transport carriers (number of carriers per unit area) is the same in the capillaries of all brain areas, but this possibility is not ruled out. Certainly an increase in transport carrier density is a likely possibility to explain the changes observed in rats with portacaval shunts, since capillaries isolated from such rats have increased transport rates (Cardelli-Cangiano et al., 1981).

The possibility of a physical breakdown of the blood-brain barrier after portacaval shunting must be considered when interpreting the data. In one study of acute hepatic failure, staining of the brain by trypan blue was observed, as well as increased penetration of some molecules that do not normally enter brain, such as insulin and L-glucose, indicating a loss of blood-brain barrier function (Livingstone et al., 1977). However, in that study a complete hepatectomy was performed which rapidly produced a severe condition with cerebral edema and histological changes such as vacuolation around the capillaries. Such changes have not been observed after a portacaval shunt operation (Cavanagh, 1974; Zamora et al., 1973). The changes in the rates of amino acid passage across the blood-brain barrier after portacaval shunting reported here were due to specific changes in the carrier mechanisms themselves and not to changes in the physical integrity of the blood-brain barrier. This was shown conclusively by the finding that the brain capillaries of shunted rats remained essentially impermeable to sucrose, a molecule that does not readily cross the blood-brain barrier unless damage has occurred. Furthermore, the permeability of the blood-brain barrier to lysine was decreased by about 70%. The results of other studies support this conclusion. Transport of glucose was unchanged by portacaval shunting (James et al., 1978) and the relative impermeability of the blood-brain barrier to ^{22}Na, [^{51}CR]EDTA, insulin, or tyramine was unaltered (James et al., 1978; Sarna et al., 1977).

The presence of vesicles transporting horseradish peroxidase has been observed within cerebral capillary endothelial cells in rats with portacaval shunts (Laursen and Westergaard, 1977). Conceivably, amino acids and other small molecules could be transported by such a mechanism in these rats. Dr. Robert Page examined the cortex of a few brains from shunted rats for the presence of vesicles and found none. However, even if present they could not have been a physiologically significant means of transport of the substrates tested, especially in view of the decrease in permeability to lysine and impermeability to sucrose.

It has been shown in normal rats that the main factors controlling the influx and thereby influencing the brain content of an amino acid are its plasma concentration and the concentrations of its competitors for the common transport system (Fernstrom and Faller, 1978; Gessa et al., 1974; Perez-Cruet et al., 1974). An additional factor must be taken into account in rats with portacaval shunts, namely the specific alterations in the carrier mechanisms. It is clear, therefore, that in the pathological condition included by a portacaval shunt, changes in the rate of influx cannot be predicted only on the basis of plasma amino acid concentrations. The changes in the rates of clearance suggest that the kinetic characteristics of the blood-brain barrier changed in such a way that the increase in transport was greater for tryptophan than for phenylalanine and tyrosine, which in turn were more affected than leucine. It is possible that more than one carrier mechanism exists for the neutral amino acids. Several studies have shown the presence of an apparently nonsaturable component of neutral amino acid transport (Brender et al., 1975; Etienne et al., 1976; Mans et al., 1979). Perhaps the separate components of the multicomponent system are affected differently by portacaval shunting.

The blood-brain barrier is in a strategic position to moderate brain metabolism. The influx of several substrates such as amino acids, ketone bodies, and glucose is not much in excess of cerebral requirements (Hawkins and Biebuyck, 1979; Lund-Anderson, 1979; Pardridge, 1977). There appears, therefore, to be a closely balanced relationship between the kinetic characteristics of the blood-brain barrier and brain metabolism. It is plausible that a disturbance in this normal relationship may be of etiologic significance for the cerebral dysfunction that occurs after portacaval shunting or during hepatic failure. The increased influx of tryptophan, phenylalanine, and tyrosine undoubtedly contributes to the high brain content of these amino acids found after portacaval shunting. (However, it must be borne in mind that the brain content of an amino acid reflects the processes of influx, as well as efflux, incorporation into and release from protein, metabolism to neurotransmitters, oxidative metabolism, etc.). Since brain monoamine metabolism may be dependent on precursor availability (Wurtman and Fernstrom, 1976), it has been suggested that the increased amounts of these amino acids can interfere with normal neurotransmitter metabolism and thus lead to disturbances of brain function (Cummings et al., 1976b; Curzon et al., 1975; Fischer and Baldessarini, 1971). If this is true, then it may be expected that some structures such as the hippocampus and reticular formation will be more severely affected, as they showed the greatest permeability changes.

The decreased influx of lysine and possibly arginine, both of which are essential basic amino acids transported by the same carrier, raises the possibility of interference with protein synthesis. In rats with portacaval shunts, the rate of influx for lysine is reduced to well below the estimated rate of protein synthesis (Mans et al., 1982) and under these circumstances availability of the precursor may become limiting. On the other hand, the brain content of lysine was not significantly altered. It is possible that protein turnover is decreased (both synthesis and degradation) or that lysine is very efficiently recycled. Studies of protein synthesis after portacaval shunting, as determined by the rate of label incorporation from various substrates, are inconclusive. The substrates used, acetate (Patel et al., 1972) and lysine (Wasterlain et al., 1978), have decreased influx rates after portacaval shunting. Therefore, it is not clear whether the decreased rate of label accumulation in these studies is an artifact of the altered transport or reflects decreased protein synthesis. Cremer et al., (1977) found that the incorporation of leucine into brain protein was the same in rats with portacaval shunts as in controls, suggesting that protein synthesis, at least from this amino acid, was unimpaired. Thus, the possibility of interference with brain protein synthesis after portacaval shunting remains to be clarified. Nonetheless, it is clear that the transport of essential amino acids is vital for normal brain metabolism and, therefore, any changes occurring after portacaval shunting are of major importance and may possibly have etiological significance in the development of encephalopathy.

ACKNOWLEDGMENT

This work was partially supported by the National Institute of Health grants NS 16737 and NS 16389.

REFERENCES

Baños, G., Daniel, P.M., Moorhouse, S.R., and Pratt, O.E. (1973): The influx of amino acids into the brain of the rat *in vivo:* the essential compared with some non-essential amino acids. *Proc. R. Soc. Lond.* (Biol.) 183:59–70.

Bauman, A., Bourgoin, S., Benda, P., Glowinski, J., and Hamon, M. (1974): Characteristics of tryptophan accumulation by glial cells. *Brain Res.* 66:253–263.

Betz, A.L., Gilboe, D.D., and Drewes, L.R. (1975): Kinetics of unidirectional leucine transport into brain: effects of isoleucine, valine, and anoxia. *Am. J. Physiol.* 228:895–900.

Betz, A.L., Gilboe, D.D., and Drewes, L.R. (1976): The characteristics of glucose transport across the blood brain barrier and its relation to cerebral glucose metabolism. *Adv. Exp. Biol. Med.* 69:133–149.

Bircher, J. (1979): The rat with portacaval shunt: An animal model with chronic hepatic failure. *Pharmac. Ther.* 5:219–222.

Bloxam, D.L., and Curzon, G. (1978): A study of proposed determinants of brain tryptophan concentration in rats after portacaval anastomosis or sham operation. *J. Neurochem.* 31: 1255–1263.

Brender, J., Andersen, P.E., and Rafaelsen, O.J. (1975): Blood-brain barrier transfer of D-glucose, L-leucine, and L-tryptophan in the rat. *Acta Physiol. Scand.* 93:490–499.

Cavanagh, J.B. (1974): Liver by-pass and the glia. *Res. Publ. Assoc. Res. Nerv. Ment. Dis.* 53: 13–38.

Cardelli-Cangiano, P., Cangiano, C., James, J.H., Jeppson, B., Brenner, W., and Fischer, J.E. (1981): Uptake of amino acids by brain microvessels isolated from rats after portacaval anastomosis. *J. Neurochem.* 36:627–632.

Craigie, E.H. (1920): On the relative vascularity of various parts of the central nervous system of the albino rat. *J. Comp. Neurol.* 31:429–464.

Cremer, J.E., Teal, H.M., Heath, D.F., and Cavanagh, J.B. (1977): The influence of portacaval anastomosis on the metabolism of labeled octanoate, butyrate and leucine in rat brain. *J. Neurochem.* 28:215–222.

Cummings, M.G., Soeters, P.B., James, J.H., Keane, J.M., and Fischer, J.E. (1967a): Regional brain indoleamine metabolism following chronic portacaval anastomosis in the rat. *J. Neurochem.* 27:501–509.

Cummings, M.G., James, H.J., Soeters, P.B., Keane, J.M., Foster, J., and Fischer, J.E. (1976b): Regional brain study of indoleamine metabolism in the rat in acute hepatic failure. *J. Neurochem.* 27:741–746.

Curzon, B., Kantameneni, B.D., Fernando, J.C., Woods, M.S., and Cavanagh, J.B. (1975):

Effects of chronic porto-caval anastomosis on brain tryptophan, tyrosine and 5-hydroxytryptamine. *J. Neurochem.* 24:1065–1070.

Daniel, P.M., Love, E.R., and Pratt, O.E. (1975): Hypothyroidism and amino acid entry into brain and muscle. *Lancet* 2:872.

Etienne, P., Young, S.N., and Sourkes, T.C. (1976): Inhibition by albumin of tryptophan uptake by rat brain. *Nature* (Lond.) 262:144–145.

Fernstrom, J.D., and Faller, D.V. (1978): Neutral amino acids in the brain: Changes in response to food ingestion. *J. Neurochem.* 30:1531–1538.

Fernstrom, J.D., and Wurtman, R.J. (1972): Brain serotonin content: Physiological regulation by plasma neutral amino acids. *Science* 78:414–416.

Fischer, J.E., and Baldessarini, R.J. (1971): False neurotransmitters and hepatic failure. *Lancet* ii:75–79.

Gessa, G.L., Biggio, G., Fadda, F., Gorsini, F.U., and Tagliamente, R. (1974): Effect of the oral administration of tryptophan-free amino acid mixtures on serum tryptophan, brain tryptophan and serotonin metabolism. *J. Neurochem.* 22:869–870.

Gjedde, A., Lockwood, A.H., Duffy, T.E., and Plum, F. (1978): Cerebral blood flow and metabolism in chronically hyperammonemic rats: Effect of an acute ammonia challenge. *Ann. Neurol.* 3:325–330.

Hawkins, R.A., and Biebuyck, J.F. (1979): Ketone bodies are selectively used by individual brain regions. *Science* 205:325–327.

Hawkins, R.A., Hass, W.K., and Ransohoff, J. (1979): Measurement of regional brain glucose utilization *in vivo* using [2-^{14}C] glucose. *Stroke* 10:690–703.

Hawkins, R.A., Mans, A.M., and Biebuyck, J.F. (1982): Amino acid supply to individual cerebral structures in awake and anesthetized rats. *Am. J. Physiol.* 242:E1–E11.

Hernandez, M.J., Brennan, R.W., Vannucci, R.C., and Bowman, G.S. (1978): Cerebral blood flow and oxygen consumption in the newborn dog. *Am. J. Physiol.* 234:R209–R215.

James, J.H., Hodgman, J.M., Funovics, J.M., Yoshimura, N., and Fischer, J.E. (1976): Brain tryptophan, plasma free tryptophan and distribution of plasma neutral amino acids. *Metabolism* 25:471–476.

James, J.H., Escourrou, J., and Fischer, J.E. (1978): Blood-brain neutral amino acid transport activity is increased after portacaval anastomosis. *Science* 200:1385–1397.

Laursen, H., and Westergaard, E. (1977): Enhanced permeability to horseradish peroxidase across cerebral vessels in the rat after portacaval anastomosis. *Neuropath. Appl. Neurobiol.* 3:29–43.

Lee, S.H., and Fisher, B. (1961): Portacaval shunt in the rat. *Surgery* 50:668–672.

Livingstone, A.S., Potvin, M., Goresky, C.A., Finlayson, M.H., and Hinchey, E.J. (1977): Changes in the blood-brain barrier in hepatic coma after hepatectomy in the rat. *Gastroenterology* 73:697–704.

Lund-Anderson, H. (1979): Transport of glucose from blood to brain. *Physiol. Rev.* 59:304–352.

Maddrey, W.C., Weber, F.L., Coulter, A.W., Chura, C.M., Chapanis, N.P., and Walser, M. (1976): Effects of keto analogues of essential amino acids in portal-systemic encephalopathy. *Gastroenterology* 71:190–195.

Mans, A.M., Biebuyck, J.F., Saunders, S.J., Kirsch, R.E., and Hawkins, R.A. (1979): Tryptophan transport across the blood-brain barrier during acute hepatic failure. *J. Neurochem.* 33:409–418.

Mans, A.M., Biebuyck, J.F., Shelly, K., and Hawkins, R.A. (1982): Regional blood-brain permeability to amino acids after portacaval anastomosis. *J. Neurochem.* 38:705–717.

Munro, H.N., Fernstrom, J.D., and Wurtman, R.J. (1975): Insulin, plasma amino acid imbalance and hepatic coma. *Lancet* i:722–724.

Ohno, K., Pettigrew, J.D., and Rapoport, S.I. (1978): Lower limits of cerebrovascular permeability to nonelectrolytes in the conscious rat. *Am. J. Physiol.* 235:H299–H307.

Oldendorf, W.H. (1970): Measurement of brain uptake of radiolabeled substances using a tritiated water internal standard. *Brain Res.* 24:382–376.

Oldendorf, W.H. (1973): Stereospecificity of blood-brain barrier permeability to amino acids. *Am. J. Physiol.* 224:967–979.

Oldendorf, W.H., and Szabo, J. (1976): Amino acid assignment to one of three blood-brain barrier amino acid carriers. *Am. J. Physiol.* 230:94–98.

Pardridge, W.M. (1977): Regulation of amino acid availability to the brain. In *Nutrition and the Brain* (eds: R.J. Wurtman and J.J. Wurtman), Vol. 1, pp. 141–204, Raven Press, New York.

Pardridge, W.M., Connor, J.D., and Crawford, I.L. (1975): Permeability changes in the brain barrier: causes and consequences. *CRC Crit. Rev. Toxicol.* 3:159–199, 1975.

Pardridge, W.M., and Oldendorf, W.H. (1975): Kinetic analysis of blood-brain barrier transport of amino acids. *Biochim. Biophys. Acta* 401:128–136.

Parfitt, A., and Graham-Smith, D.G. (1974): The transfer of tryptophan across the synaptosomal membrane. In: *Aromatic Amino Acids in the Brain* (Ciba Foundation Symp. 22), pp. 175–196, Associated Scientific Publishers, New York.

Patel, A.J., Balazs, R., Kyu, M.H., and Cavanagh, J.B. (1972): Effects of portacaval anastomosis on the metabolism of [1 – ^{14}C] acetate and on metabolic compartmentation in brain. *Biochem. J.* 127:85P.

Perez-Cruet, J., Chase, T.N., and Murphy, D.L. (1974): Dietary regulation of brain bryptophan metabolism by plasma ratio of free tryptophan and neutral amino acids in humans. *Nature* (Lond.) 248:693–695.

Rossouw, J.E., Labadario, D., Vinik, A.I., and DeVilliers, A.S. (1978): Liver glycogen after portacaval shunt in rats. *Metabolism* 27:1067–1073.

Sarna, G.S., Bradbury, M.W.B., and Cavanagh, J. (1977): Permeability of the blood-brain barrier after portacaval anastomosis in the rat. *Brain Res.* 138:550–555.

Soeters, P.B., and Fischer, J.E. (1976): Insulin, glucagon, amino acid imbalance and hepatic encephalopathy. *Lancet* ii:880–882.

Wasterlain, C.G., Lockwood, A.H., and Conn, M. (1978): Chronic inhibition of brain protein synthesis after portacaval shunting. A possible pathogenic mechanism in chronic hepatic encephalopathy in the rat. *Neurology* 28:233–238.

Wurtman, R.J., and Fernstrom, J.D. (1976): Control of brain neurotransmitter synthesis by precursor availability and nutritional state. *Biochem. Pharmacol.* 25:1691–1696.

Zamora, A.J., Cavanagh, J.B., and Kyu, M.H. (1973): Ultrastructural responses of the astrocytes to portacaval anastomosis in the rat. *J. Neurol. Sci.* 18:25–45.

Zanchin, G., Rigotti, P., Dussini, N., Vassanelli, P., and Battistin, L. (1979): Cerebral amino acid levels and uptake in rats after portacaval anastomosis: II. Regional studies *in vivo*. *J. Neurosci. Res.* 4:301–310.

GASTROINTESTINAL

15 Amino Acid and Peptide Absorption in Human Intestine: Implications for Enteral Nutrition

Siamak A. Adibi

Metabolically, the first step in protein nutrition is the breakdown of dietary protein to amino acids for delivery to portal circulation. Studies within the past decade have established that this process is accomplished in three sequential phases in the small intestine. The anatomical sites for these phases are: gut lumen; brush border membrane; and mucosal cytoplasm.

GUT LUMEN PHASE

In the initial phase dietary proteins are hydrolyzed to amino acids and oligopeptides in the gut lumen. This reaction is catalyzed principally by pancreatic proteolytic enzymes. The gastric proteolytic enzymes do not appear to play a major role in this regard, as suggested by the fact that there is increased fecal loss of nitrogen when pancreatic secretion is impaired, while it is hardly affected by the absence of gastric secretion (Adibi, 1976). Studies in our laboratory (Adibi and Mercer, 1973) as well as those by other investigators (Chung et al., 1979) have shown that the main product of protein hydrolysis in the gut lumen of human small intestine is oligopeptides. In both of these studies there was greater accumulation of oligopeptides than amino acids in the gut lumen after a well-balanced protein meal (Adibi and Mercer, 1973;

Chung et al., 1979). The greater accumulation in the gut lumen is not the result of the difference between absorption of peptides and amino acids since, as will be discussed later, peptides are actually absorbed at a greater rate than amino acids.

BRUSH BORDER MEMBRANE PHASE

As mentioned above, the end products of protein digestion in the gut lumen are mixtures of amino acids and oligopeptides. In the second phase of protein assimilation, the brush border membrane of intestinal mucosa clears these products from the gut lumen. This function is accomplished by the following components of the brush border membrane: 1) amino acid transport system, 2) peptide transport system, and 3) peptide hydrolase.

Amino Acid Transport System

Among the three components of the brush border membrane mentioned above, historically the amino acid system was the first to have its existence established. Studies completed during the 1950s clearly showed the presence of an active transport system for amino acids in animal intestine. Studies performed during the 1960s, including those in my laboratory, showed the presence of this system in human intestine. These experiments investigated various aspects of intestinal transport of amino acids, which include the following: heterogeneity, stereospecificity, affinity, ionic requirement, pH dependency, site of maximal transport, and response to nutritional and metabolic alteration.

Heterogeneity The absorption of neutral and basic amino acids is mediated by separate carrier systems. The most convincing evidence for this notion comes from observations of amino acid absorption in the intestine of patients with hereditary disorders of amino acid absorption (McCarthy et al., 1964; Thier et al., 1965; Shih et al., 1971). There are patients who have impaired intestinal absorption of neutral amino acids but can absorb the basic amino acids normally (Hartnup disease). The reverse of this is true in patients with cystinuria. Although several other transport systems for amino acids, such as imino and acidic amino acids, have been proposed, the evidence is not as strong as that for neutral and basic amino acids.

Stereospecificity The intestinal absorption of L-amino acids is much faster than the corresponding D-isomers (Gibson and Wiseman, 1951). In fact, D-amino acids may not be actively transported. However, there is uptake of D-amino acids by the carrier system for L-amino acids but at much reduced affinity.

Affinity The kinetic constants of absorption of amino acids are influenced by their affinity for the transport system. The molecular structure of the side chain of amino acids is a key factor in this regard. For example, amino acids with a long side chain appear to have a greater affinity than amino acids with a short side chain for the transport system (Adibi, 1969). The importance of affinity is evident from the selective rate of absorption of amino acids containing equivalent amounts of either eight essential or the 18 common dietary amino acids (Adibi and Gray, 1967; Adibi et al., 1967).

Ionic requirement The active transport of amino acids by preparations of intestine *in vitro* requires sodium (Rosenberg et al., 1965). However, *in vivo* absorption of amino acids does not appear to be affected by marked reduction in the luminal concentration of sodium (Adibi, 1970). An explanation for the difference between *in vitro* and *in vivo* transport may be that amino acid absorption *in vivo,* unlike *in vitro,* is usually downhill, and therefore does not require sodium as a driving force.

pH dependency Amino acid absorption in human intestine does not appear to be affected within a wide range of changes in intraluminal pH (Adibi et al., 1972). However, reduction of the intraluminal pH to a value between 4.5 and 3.0 reduces the amino acid absorption rate. This reduction appears to be principally the result of protonation of the amino acid molecule. This molecular alteration reduces the interaction of the amino acid with its carrier system, resulting in comparatively slow transport.

Site of maximal transport Studies in human intestine have shown that absorption of amino acids is most rapid in the upper jejunum (Adibi, 1969; Schedl et al., 1968). In contrast, most studies in animal intestine have shown that absorption is greatest in the distal half of the small intestine (Nathans et al., 1960).

Response to nutritional and hormonal alteration Several laboratories (Kershaw et al., 1960; Levin et al., 1965; Steiner and Gray, 1969) have reported that caloric restriction increases amino acid absorption in animal intestine, the opposite has been found in human intestine. Our studies of amino acid absorption in man *in vivo* (Adibi and Allen, 1970) and those of other investigators (Steiner et al., 1969) *in vitro* have shown that amino acid absorption is reduced by starvation. Our studies have also shown that the selectivity of amino acid absorption is maintained during a period of starvation. In other words, the sequence of amino acid absorption from an amino acid mixture is the same before and during fasting (Adibi and Allen, 1970). Although the effect of diabetes on intestinal absorption of amino acids in human intestine is not known there have been extensive studies of this problem in animal intestine. It appears that experimental diabetes increases the transport of both neutral and basic amino acids in rat intestine (Lal and Schedl, 1974).

Peptide Transport System

For a long time it was generally believed that amino acid absorption was the only mechanism for assimilation of the amino acid constituents of dietary proteins. At the time it was thought that dietary proteins had to be completely hydrolyzed to amino acids in the gut lumen, and furthermore that there was no significant absorption of peptides. The first notion was invalidated by the results of studies of protein digestion in the gut lumen (Adibi, 1976). The second notion became untenable in view of the results of two independent but parallel studies performed during the 1960s (Matthews and Adibi, 1976), which showed that there is large-scale absorption of dipeptides and tripeptides in human intestine (Adibi and co-workers) and in animal intestine (Matthews and co-workers). These studies led to the characterization of a common transport system for dipeptides and tripeptides, which appears to play an important if not predominant role in assimilation of the amino acid constituents of dietary proteins (Adibi and Kim, 1981). Although the peptide transport system has not been as extensively studied as the amino acid transport system, there is sufficient information to allow a comparison of the characteristics of the two systems.

Heterogeneity Initially, it was thought that there were several peptide transport systems, but the most recent data suggests that neutral, basic, and acidic dipeptides share a common mediated mechanism for transport (Adibi and Kim, 1981). Apparently, peptide uptake, unlike amino acid uptake, is indifferent to the net charge on the amino acid side chain.

Stereospecificity The peptide transport system, like the amino acid transport system, has a preference for peptides with amino acid residues in the L rather than the D form (Asatoor et al., 1973). This is suggested by the results of studies of jejunal absorption rates of dipeptides containing amino acids either in L or D form or a mixture of both forms (Asatoor et al., 1973). Absorption was greatest when both amino acids were in L form and smallest when both amino acids were in D form.

Affinity The key factor determining the affinity of dipeptides and tripeptides for the transport system appears to be the structure of the amino acid in the N-terminal position (Adibi and Morse, 1981). In this position an amino acid with a short side chain will confer a greater affinity than an amino acid with a long side chain.

Ionic requirement There have been conflicting reports regarding the sodium requirement for peptide transport *in vitro*. Generally, most results seem to indicate that peptide transport is not as strongly sodium-dependent as amino acid transport. In fact, recent studies using isolated brush border membrane vesicles of rat intestine have found no sodium dependency for peptide transport (Ganapathy and Leibach, 1982).

pH dependency Acidification of intraluminal pH results in a greater reduction in amino acid absorption from solutions of free amino acids than from equivalent peptide solutions (Fogel and Adibi, 1974). This greater effect appears to be related to greater protonation of amino acids when they are in free than in peptide form. Those amino groups involved in peptide bonds are no longer subject to the effect of acidic pH.

Site of maximal transport Investigators (Crampton et al., 1973) studying absorption of dipeptides and their corresponding amino acids along the length of the small intestine of rats found that dipeptide absorption was maximal in the proximal half of the intestine, whereas amino acid absorption was maximal in the distal half. Our studies in human intestine have shown that dipeptide absorption is greatest in the jejunum and smallest in the duodenum, with ileal absorption being between these two extremes (Adibi, 1971). An unexpected finding of this study was the observation that the ileum has a greater capacity for peptide hydrolysis than the jejunum and, therefore, hydrolysis plays a greater role in dipeptide disappearance in the ileum than in the jejunum (Adibi, 1971).

Response to nutritional and metabolic alterations Several studies have compared the effect of dietary restriction on peptide and amino acid absorption in animal intestine, but the results are conflicting. Some studies have shown that dietary restriction results in a greater reduction in amino acid than peptide transport (Lis et al., 1972a, b), while other studies have shown the opposite effect (Schedl et al., 1979). Experimental diabetes alters intestinal transport of amino acids, but has no effect on peptide transport in rat intestine (Schedl et al., 1978). Although there has not yet been extensive study of the effect of altered nutrition on peptide transport in human intestine, there is some evidence that the effect on peptide transport differs from that on amino acid transport. Jejuno-ileal bypass, which causes protein-calorie malnutrition, significantly reduces the absorption of amino acids but not that of dipeptides (Fogel et al., 1976).

Peptide Hydrolases

Recent studies have shown that the brush border membrane contains several different hydrolases (for review, see Adibi and Kim, 1981). These enzymes are designated as:

Aminooligopeptidases
Aminopeptidase A
Dipeptidase (I)
Dipeptidase (III)
Dipeptidyl Aminopeptidase (IV)

Among the above enzymes, aminooligopeptidases appear to be the predominant enzymes. Although the substrates for the membrane peptide hydrolases are peptides with two to eight amino acid residues, the hydrolytic activity against these peptides varies markedly. The activities, expressed as percent of the total cellular activity, are as follows:

Dipeptides	5% to 12%
Tripeptides	10% to 60%
Tetrapeptides	90%
Higher peptides	98%

These data show a remarkable coordination of labor between hydrolytic and transport systems for assimilation of peptides. The hydrolase activity is small against peptides that can be transported intact, but high against peptides that cannot be transported. Therefore, the chief function of brush border membrane enzymes appears to be hydrolysis of unabsorbable peptides to absorbable products (tripeptides, dipeptides, and amino acids).

MUCOSAL CYTOPLASMIC PHASE

The final phase of protein assimilation, which takes place in the cytoplasm of intestinal mucosa, is concerned with two events: completion of peptide hydrolysis and amino acid transport to portal circulation.

PEPTIDE HYDROLYSIS

Recently several studies have shown that the mucosal cytoplasm has several peptide hydrolases (for reveiw, see Adibi and Kim, 1981). These enzymes which are totally different from the ones in the brush border membrane are designated as:

Dipeptidase
Aminotripeptidase
Proline dipeptidase

The substrates for the above enzymes are peptides with two to four amino acid residues. The activities, expressed as percent of the total cellular activity, are as follows:

Dipeptides	80% to 95%
Tripeptides	30% to 60%
Tetrapeptides	Trace to 10%
Higher peptides	Nil

The above data show that the order of the activities of the cytoplasmic enzymes is the reverse of the order of the activities of brush border peptide hydrolases. Therefore, the cytoplasmic enzymes appear well specialized for completing the hydrolysis of absorbed peptides. In fact, because of substantial hydrolase activity against dipeptides and tripeptides, hardly any of the absorbed peptides accumulate in mucosal cells or reach portal circulation in intact form. Nevertheless, there is evidence that certain peptides may reach the portal vein in intact form (Adibi and Kim, 1981). A number of studies in our laboratory have shown that if peptides enter the systemic circulation, they are efficiently hydrolyzed to amino acids by extraintestinal tissues in the body (Adibi et al., 1977; Krzysik and Adibi, 1977; Krzysik and Adibi, 1979).

Amino Acid Transport to Portal Circulation

Amino acids produced as the result of intracellular hydrolysis of dipeptides and tripeptides, together with amino acids absorbed from the lumen, are transported to portal circulation via a special mechanism located in the basolateral membrane. Due to limited studies, characteristics of this mechanism are not yet well understood.

Advantages of Peptides over Amino Acids as Substrates for Enteral Nutrition

There is increasing recognition of the importance and use of enteral nutrition in patients who cannot either grow or maintain their body weight by oral intake of foodstuffs. A variety of formula diets have been made available for enteral nutrition. Among these diets, probably the elemental diet, Vivonex, has been most extensively used. The nitrogen source of this diet is provided entirely as free amino acids. Substitution of these amino acids with dipeptides, or even better with tripeptides, has the following advantages: 1) reduction or abolition of hypertonicity and 2) enhancement of amino acid absorption.

Hypertonicity Elemental diets are usually quite hypertonic. The maintenance of isotonicity is required by all living cells, including those of the gastrointestinal mucosa. If this physiological principle is violated by feeding hypertonic solutions, the gastrointestinal tract must make every effort to correct it. As might be expected, there are consequences to this adjustment. Although there is meager useful information on the effect of hypertonicity on the gastrointestinal tract, there is some evidence that the effect is deleterious. For example, it has been shown (Teichberg et al., 1978) that a single force-feeding of a hypertonic solution causes structural and functional damage to the rat jejunum.

Efficiency of absorption Our previous studies have shown that the rate of amino acid absorption is significantly greater from dipeptide and tripeptide solutions than from corresponding amino acid solutions (Adibi, 1971; Adibi et al., 1975). In fact, this difference in absorption is magnified in diseases of the small intestine such as celiac-sprue (Adibi et al., 1974). These observations have been confirmed by other investigators (Silk et al., 1974; Nutzenadel et al., 1981). Greater amino acid absorption from peptides appears to be due to the greater efficiency and stability of the peptide transport system than the amino acid transport system described above (Adibi and Soleimanpour, 1974). These observations have led to a change in the concept of the proper nitrogen source for elemental diets. Many formula diets no longer include crystalline amino acids but instead include protein hydrolysates as the nitrogen source. A protein hydrolysate is a heterogeneous mixture of peptides of different sizes and composition. The size and composition determines whether a peptide is a substrate for the peptide transport system. For example, peptides with bulky amino acids in the N-terminal position or greater than three amino acid residues have very little or no affinity for the uptake sites of the peptide transport system (Adibi et al., 1975; Adibi and Morse, 1977). Another problem with protein hydrolysates is the possibility of inhibition of the activity of mucosal peptide hydrolases by amino acids which are present in protein hydrolysates (Adibi and Kim, 1981). These problems could be resolved by using a crystalline mixture of dipeptides or tripeptides containing no free amino acids and having an appropriate amino acid in the N-terminal position. However, such a mixture is not currently commercially available. In its absence, protein hydrolysates seem to be superior to crystalline amino acids as the nitrogen source for enteral nutrition (Silk et al., 1973; Silk et al., 1979). In fact, other investigators (Smith et al., 1982) believe that feeding the crystalline amino acid diet may be potentially dangerous. These investigators were surprised to find that during enteral nutrition with a crystalline amino acid diet (High Nitrogen Vivonex) weight gain was primarily extracellular water and fat and the net retention of nitrogen was negligible. These observations led them to conduct a series of balance studies comparing the effect of High Nitrogen Vivonex with two other diets (Smith et al., 1982). One diet was solid food, the other was a protein hydrolysate diet. Despite similar intake of calories and nitrogen on each of the three diets, nitrogen retention was much greater with the protein hydrolysate diet (16 times) than with the crystalline amino acid diet. The solid diet was also far superior to the crystalline amino acid diet in this regard. During the feeding of High Nitrogen Vivonex, there were increases in the levels of urea-nitrogen in both the plasma and urine of these patients. The increases were reversed by the alternative diets. It thus appears that the reason for poor nitrogen retention with the High Nitrogen Vivonex is that the ingested nitrogen is converted to urea rather than to body proteins.

REFERENCES

Adibi, S.A. (1969): The influence of molecular structure of neutral amino acids on their absorption kinetics in the jejunum and ileum of human intestine in vivo. *Gastroenterology* 56:903–913.

Adibi, S.A. (1970): Leucine absorption rate and net movements of sodium and water in human jejunum. *J. Appl. Physiol.* 28:753–757.

Adibi, S.A. (1971): Intestinal transport of dipeptides in man: relative importance of hydrolysis and intact absorption. *J. Clin. Invest.* 50:2266–2275.

Adibi, S.A. (1976): Intestinal phase of protein assimilation. *Am. J. Clin. Nutr.* 29:205–215.

Adibi, S.A. and Allen, E.R. (1970): Impaired jejunal absorption rates of essential amino acids induced by either dietary caloric or protein deprivation in man. *Gastroenterology* 59:404–413.

Adibi, S.A., Fogel, M.R., and Agrawal, R.M. (1974): Comparison of free amino acid and dipeptide absorption in the jejunum of sprue patients. *Gastroenterology* 67:586–591.

Adibi, S.A. and Gray, S.J. (1967): Intestinal absorption of essential amino acids in man. *Gastroenterology* 52:837–845.

Adibi, S.A., Gray, S.J., and Menden, E. (1967): The kinetics of amino acid absorption and alteration of plasma composition of free amino acids after intestinal perfusion of amino acid mixtures. *Am. J. Clin. Nutr.* 20:24–33.

Adibi, S.A. and Kim, Y.S. (1981): Peptide absorption and hydrolysis. In: *Physiology of the Gastrointestinal Tract* (ed: L.R. Johnson), Vol. 2, pp. 1073–1095, Raven Press, New York.

Adibi, S.A., Krzysik, B.A. and Drash, A.L. (1977): Metabolism of intravenously administered dipeptides in rats: effects on amino acid pools, glucose concentration and insulin and glucagon secretion. *Clin. Sci. Molec. Med.* 52:193–204.

Adibi, S.A. and Mercer, D.W. (1973): Protein digestion in human intestine as reflected in luminal, mucosal, and plasma amino acid concentrations after meals. *J. Clin. Invest.* 52: 1586–1594.

Adibi, S.A. and Morse, E.L. (1977): The number of glycine residues which limits intact absorption of glycine oligopeptides in human jejunum. *J. Clin. Invest.* 60:1008–1016.

Adibi, S.A. and Morse, E.L. (1981): Rearranging the sequence of amino acid residues in a tripeptide to favor its intestinal transport or hydrolysis. *Gastroenterology* 80:1096.

Adibi, S.A., Morse, E.L., Masilamani, S.S. and Amin, P.M. (1975): Evidence for two different modes of tripeptide disappearance in human intestine: uptake by peptide carrier systems and hydrolysis by peptide hydrolases. *J. Clin. Invest.* 56:1355–1363.

Adibi, S.A., Ruiz, C., Glaser, P., and Fogel, M.R. (1972): Effect of intraluminal pH on absorption rates of leucine, water, and electrolytes in human jejunum. *Gastroenterology* 63:611–618.

Adibi, S.A. and Soleimanpour, M.R. (1974): Functional characterization of dipeptide transport system in human jejunum. *J. Clin. Invest.* 53:1368–1374.

Asatoor, A.M., Chadra, A., Milne, M.D., and Prosser, D.I. (1973): Intestinal absorption of stereoisomers of dipeptides in the rat. *Clin. Sci. Molec. Med.* 45:199–212.

Chung, Y.C., Kim, Y.S., Shadchehr, A., Garrido, A., MacGregor, I.L., and Sleisenger, M.H. (1979): Protein digestion and absorption in human small intestine. *Gastroenterology* 76: 1415–1421.

Crampton, R.F., Lis, M.T., and Matthews, D.M. (1973): Sites of maximal absorption and hydrolysis of two dipeptides by rat small intestine. *Clin. Sci.* 44:583–594.

Fogel, M.R. and Adibi, S.A. (1974): Assessment of the role of brush-border peptide hydrolases in luminal disappearance of dipeptides in man. *J. Lab. Clin. Med.* 84:327–333.

Fogel, M.R., Ravitch, M.M., and Adibi, S.A. (1976): Absorptive and digestive function of the jejunum after jejunoileal bypass for treatment of human obesity. *Gastroenterology* 71: 729–733.

Ganapathy, V., and Leibach, F.H. (1982): Peptide transport in intestinal and renal brush border membrane vesicles. *Life Sci.* 30:2137–2146.

Gibson, Q.H. and Wiseman, G. (1951): Selective absorption of stereoisomers of amino acids from loops of the small intestine of the rat. *Biochem. J.* 48:426–429.

Kershaw, T.G., Neame, K.D., and Wiseman, G. (1960): The effect of semistarvation on absorption by the rat small intestine in vitro and in vivo. *J. Physiol.* 152:182–190.

Krzysik, B.A. and Adibi, S.A. (1977): Cytoplasmic dipeptidase activities of kidney, ileum, jejunum, liver, muscle, and blood. *Am. J. Physiol.* 233:E450–E456.

Krzysik, B.A. and Adibi, S.A. (1979): Comparison of metabolism of glycine injected intravenously in free and dipeptide forms. *Metabolism* 28:1211–1217.

Lal, D., and Schedl, H.P. (1974): Intestinal adaptation in diabetes: amino acid absorption. *Am. J. Physiol.* 227:827–831.

Levin, R.J., Newey, H., and Smyth, D.H. (1965): The effects of adrenalectomy and fasting on intestinal function in the rat. *J. Physiol.* 177:58–73.

Lis, M.T., Crampton, R.F., and Matthews, D.M. (1972a): Effect of dietary changes on intestinal absorption of L-methionine and L-methionyl-L-methionine in the rat. *Br. J. Nutr.* 27:159–167.

Lis, M.T., Matthews, D.M., and Crampton, R.F. (1972b): Effects of dietary restriction and protein deprivation on intestinal absorption of protein digestion products in the rat. *Br. J. Nutr.* 28:443–446.

Matthews, D.M. and Adibi, S.A. (1976): Progress in gastroenterology: peptide absorption. *Gastroenterology* 71:151–161.

McCarthy, C.F., Borland, J.L., Lynch, H.J., Owen, E.E., and Tyor, M.P. (1964): Defective uptake of basic amino acids and L-cystine by intestinal mucosa of patients with cystinuria. *J. Clin. Invest.* 43:1518–1524.

Nathans, D., Tapley, D.F., and Ross, J.E. (1960): Intestinal transport of amino acids studied in vitro with L-[^{131}I]monoiodotyrosine. *Biochim. Biophys. Acta.* 41:264–271.

Nutzenadel, W., Fahr, K., and Lutz, P. (1981): Absorption of free and peptide-linked glycine and phenylalanine in children with active celiac disease. *Pediat. Res.* 15:309–312.

Rosenberg, I.H., Coleman, A.L., and Rosenberg, L.E. (1965): The role of sodium ion in the transport of amino acids by the intestine. *Biochim. Biophys. Acta.* 102:161–171.

Schedl, H.P., Burston, D., Taylor, E., and Matthews, D.M. (1979): Kinetics of uptake of an amino acid and a dipeptide into hamster jejunum and ileum: the effect of semistarvation and starvation. *Clin. Sci.* 56:487–492.

Schedl, H.P., Pierce, C.E., Rider, A., and Clifton, J.A. (1968): Absorption of L-methionine from the human small intestine. *J. Clin. Invest.* 47:417–425.

Schedl, H.P., Wenger, J., and Adibi, S.A. (1978): Diglycine absorption in streptozotocin diabetic rat. *Am. J. Physiol.* 235:E457–E460.

Shih, V.E., Bixby, E.M., Alpers, D.H., Bartsocas, C.S. and Thier, S.O. (1971): Studies of intestinal transport defect in Hartnup disease. *Gastroenterology* 61:445–453.

Silk, D.B.A., Chung, Y.C., Berger, K.L., Conley, K., Beigler, M., Sleisenger, M.H., Spiller, G.A., and Kim, Y.S. (1979): Comparison of oral feeding of peptide and amino acid meals to normal human subjects. *Gut* 20:291–299.

Silk, D.B.A., Kumar, P.J., Perrett, D., Clark, M.L., and Dawson, A.M. (1974): Amino acid and peptide absorption in patients with coeliac disease and dermatitis herpetiformis. *Gut* 15:1–8.

Silk, D.B.A., Marrs, T.C., Addison, J.M., Burston, D., Clark, M.L., and Matthews, D.M. (1973): Absorption of amino acids from an amino acid mixture simulating casein and a tryptic hydrolysate of casein in man. *Clin. Sci. Molec. Med.* 45:715–719.

Smith, J.L., Arteaga, C., and Heymsfield, S.B. (1982): Increased ureagenesis and impaired nitrogen use during infusion of a synthetic amino acid formula. *N. Engl. J. Med.* 306: 1013–1018.

Steiner, M., Farrish, G.C.M., and Gray, S.J. (1969): Intestinal uptake of valine in calorie and protein deprivation. *Am. J. Clin. Nutr.* 22:871–877.

Steiner, M., and Gray, S.J. (1969): Effect of starvation on intestinal amino acid absorption. *Am. J. Physiol.* 217:747–752.

Teichberg, S., Lifshitz, F., Pergolizzi, R., and Wapnir, R.A. (1978): Response of rat intestine to a hyperosmotic feeding. *Pediat. Res.* 12:720–725.

Their, S.O., Segal, S., Fox, M., Blair, A., and Rosenberg, L.E. (1965): Cystinuria: defective intestinal transport of dibasic amino acids and cystine. *J. Clin. Invest.* 44:442–448.

SECTION V
Clinical Aspects of Amino Acid Metabolism

GENERAL CONSIDERATIONS

16 An Evaluation of Techniques for Estimating Amino Acid Requirements in Hospitalized Patients

George L. Blackburn
Lyle L. Moldawer

Determining the requirements for total protein and individual amino acids in man poses a number of theoretical and technical problems which become even more complex in the hospitalized patient with injury or infection. The following chapters illustrate how new approaches and improved technology have greatly increased our present understanding of the amino acid needs of the hospitalized patient. This article will review selected methods currently available for investigating amino acid metabolism in the hospitalized patient and will emphasize the importance of stratifying patient populations based upon their nutritional status and degree of stress. The traditional approaches for estimating amino acid requirements such as the use of nitrogen balance, amino acid profiles, and arteriovenous differences of amino acid concentrations will be examined and then the more recent measurements of amino acid flux and oxidation using isotopically labeled amino acids will be presented. The subsequent chapters in this section will report on the use of these techniques in various clinical states and will examine more extensively the many variables affecting amino acid requirements, such as the degree of malnutrition and the presence of trauma, burns, cancer, or organ failure.

The primary difficulty encountered when estimating appropriate dietary protein or individual amino acid intakes is identification of a valid parameter(s) by which to measure requirements accurately. For the healthy individual, considerable controversy exists as to which criteria is best for assessing that the requirements for dietary indispensable amino acids and for total nitrogen have been met. Recent studies by Vernon Young and his colleagues at M.I.T., summarized in Chapter 2, have raised considerable concern regarding the accuracy of previous estimates in healthy man based solely on nitrogen balance measurements as well as the applicability of such techniques to the general problem of protein malnutrition which is prevalent in the critically ill (Bistrian et al., 1974, 1976). Unfortunately, investigation into the amino acid requirements of the critically ill has been less well defined. It might appear that the difficulties in estimating protein and amino acid requirements in the hospitalized individual are insurmountable, given the diversity of the patient population and disease process as well as the technical and ethical limits placed upon research conducted in hospitalized patients. However, as this symposium has clearly demonstrated, increased investigation into the metabolism of individual amino acids has greatly enhanced our capacity to develop and test new amino acid formulations. It is this concerted effort that will result in the development of appropriate amino acid solutions which will more effectively support the hospitalized patient.

GOALS OF AMINO ACID SUPPORT

The primary goal of amino acid nutrition in the hospitalized individual is to support protein synthesis, particularly in those tissues involved in host defense and recovery. This priority is a result of the need by the hospitalized patient for amino acids to maintain host defense (Alexander et al., 1980), prevent bacterial colonization and assure that the body's immunologic competence will function to reduce the likelihood of secondary bacterial infections (Sobrado et al., 1983). With the clinical use of amino acids, the metabolic pathways that determine the fate of each individual amino acid interact with the new hormone and nonprotein substrate milieu present in individual disease states. It is these interactions that result in the specific requirements for different amounts of individual amino acids important in the clinical treatment (Blackburn and Wolfe, 1981).

Amino acid requirements in previously well-nourished, unstressed adults can therefore only serve as a starting point for evaluating the needs of the ill and debilitated patient. Unlike the healthy state, injury and infection are associated with increased plasma amino acid appearance. (Table 16-1). Many investigators (Birkhahn et al., 1980; Wolfe et al., 1982b; Elia et al., 1980) have demonstrated an enhanced appearance of leucine in the plasma compartment after major injury or burns and similar findings have been reported for total α-amino nitrogen (Stein et al., 1977), 1982b; Kien et al., 1978b; Garlick et al., 1980b) in patients with various diseases. We have also reported increased tyrosine appearance during the catabolic phase of experimental injury in rats (Sakamoto et al., 1979) and in tumor-bearing animals (Kawamura et al., 1982). Contrary to many earlier studies (O'Keefe et al., 1974; Kien et al., 1978a; Crane et al., 1977; Moldawer et al., 1980), it also appears that after most severe forms of injury or in the presence of infection, the patient has increased rates of protein synthesis (Stein et al., 1982b) even when dietary protein is not administered. This phenomenon is in striking contrast to the reduced protein synthesis

Table 16-1
Summary of Earlier Studies Investigating Amino Acid Kinetics After Injury

Investigator	Species (Metabolic State)	Tracer	Changes in Amino Acid Appearance	Changes in Protein Synthesis
O'Keefe et al., 1974	Man (elective surgery)	L-(1-^{14}C)-leucine	none	reduced
Crane et al., 1977	Man (elective orthopedic surgery)	^{15}N-glycine	none	reduced
Long et al., 1977	Man (sepsis)	L-(a-^{15}N)-alanine	increased	increased
Kien et al., 1978a	Pediatrics (elective reconstructive surgery of the skin)	^{15}N-glycine	none	reduced
Kien et al., 1978b	Pediatrics (thermal injury)	^{15}N-glycine	increased	increased
Birkhahn et al., 1980	Man (multiple long bone fracture)	L-(1-^{14}C)-leucine	increased	increased
Elia et al., 1980	Man (emergency abdominal surgery)	Nonisotopic methodology	increased	ND*
O'Keefe et al., 1981	Man (fulminant hepatic failure)	L-(U-^{14}C)-tyrosine	increased	increased
Garlick et al., 1981	Man (postvaccination)	^{15}N-glycine	increased	increased
Stein et al., 1982	Man (multiple clinical disorders)	^{15}N-glycine	increased	increased

*ND = not determined

observed in the healthy individual deprived of dietary protein or an indispensable amino acid (Garlick, Millward, and James, 1973; Conway et al., 1980, Motil et al., 1981).

Limited consensus exists on the concept that mobilization of body protein and increases in protein synthesis in the injured or infected patient have a purposeful function; the few animal studies conducted to date (Moldawer et al., 1980; Stein et al., 1977; Augustine and Swick, 1980) suggest that increased synthesis is occurring predominantly in visceral tissues and may play a role in the synthesis of proteins necessary for host defense and recovery (Yang et al., 1981). Furthermore, in the malnourished animal, certain aspects of this protein metabolic response are lost and host defense and survival are impaired.

USE OF NITROGEN BALANCE STUDIES

For the patient being fed, there is a need to determine the effectiveness of a given nutritional regimen in promoting recovery and maintaining immunological function. These two factors have historically been related to the protein status of the patient and thus (Moore, 1959; Rhoades and Alexander, 1955) considerable effort has been directed toward reducing body protein losses, as measured by the urinary excretion of nitrogen, sulfur, and potassium (Moldawer, Bistrian, and Blackburn, 1981).

Unfortunately, nitrogen balance techniques or even the newer whole body methods which measure body protein content directly, such as neutron activation (Hill et al., 1978), total body potassium (Palombo et al., 1981), or exchangeable potassium (Shizgal et al., 1977) have serious methodologic limitations which restrict their usefulness for assessing the value of different amino acid-containing regimens. Whole body potassium or nitrogen analysis have analytical (Forbes et al., 1968) errors of approximately 3%, thus precluding their utility for short-term (less than one week) or acute studies. The techniques are of potential benefit, however, to evaluate differences in protein status in large populations (Forbes and Hursh, 1963) or in long-term studies (Palombo et al., 1981) where changes in body protein content exceed the analytical variability of the method. Neither these whole body measurements, nor nitrogen balance for that matter, can easily differentiate between body compartments so that they fail to provide information regarding the loss or accretion of protein by individual tissues. In an excellent review, W.P.T. James (1982) observed that the minimum quantities of dietary protein necessary to achieve nitrogen equilibrium in malnourished children result in subnormal synthetic rates of physiologically significant plasma proteins. Under such conditions, amino acid or protein intakes must be substantially increased to maximally promote albumin synthesis while less is necessary to achieve nitrogen equilibrium.

O'Keefe et al. (1981) have also demonstrated that crystalline amino acid infusions support albumin synthesis better than solutions containing amino acids, dextrose, and insulin, despite the fact that nitrogen balance is significantly better with added dextrose and insulin. Similar findings have been reported by Rosenoer et al. (1980) and Skillman et al. (1976).

Nitrogen balance measurements based on urinary nitrogen excretion are also difficult to conduct in the clinical setting. As previous investigators (Blackburn et al., 1973; Jeejeebhoy, 1976; Elwyn et al., 1979) have suggested, feeding regimens need to be continued for at least three days and preferably seven days to allow for equilibration of the rather large body urea pool. Elsewhere in this book, Dr. Elwyn more fully discusses the time limitations inherent in nitrogen balance studies. However, in a clinical situation, it is recognized that the status of the patient will rarely remain constant over any length of time; temporal factors must always be considered in the interpretation of the results. Furthermore, because of the relatively large free urea pool in the body, nitrogen excretion rates should be evaluated in the context of changes in blood urea nitrogen levels (Benotti and Blackburn, 1978).

Although nitrogen balance has its restrictions, this technique still remains the benchmark for assessment of the efficiency of a given amino acid regimen. There is a need, however, to expand upon nitrogen balance studies and evaluate both the mechanism of nitrogen sparing as well as the actual tissues involved.

AMINO ACID CONCENTRATIONS

Although plasma amino acid concentrations are altered from fasting or postprandial levels in a variety of metabolic states, interpretation of these changes is often difficult and misleading. Previous studies in healthy adults have emphasized the importance of a change in an individual amino acid concentration relative to the others in response to feeding. Plasma concentrations of an amino acid that is contained in the diet in the smallest amount relative to its requirement will generally show the greatest fall or smallest rise postprandially (Young et al., 1971). Conversely, plasma concentrations of an individual amino acid that is provided in the greatest excess of requirements (Young et al., 1972) or that the body cannot degrade efficiently is usually most elevated (Freund et al., 1979). Such observations have been the basis for the earlier evaluation of various amino acid formulations used in hospitalized patients and is the subject of Dr. C. Long's chapter.

Although disproportionate changes in plasma amino acid concentrations in response to parenteral or enteral feedings can serve as an indicator that the amino acid mixture has affected the capacity of the patient to metabolize amino acids, the difficulty arises with the subsequent interpretation of such observations.

A characteristic pattern of plasma amino acid concentrations has been described in the unfed, stressed patient (Wannemacher, 1977). Although changes in branched-chain amino acid concentrations appear to be quite variable after different forms of surgery or trauma, most investigators have reported no change or a slight increase in their levels (Clowes et al., 1980b; Shenkin et al., 1980). The concentration of some other indispensable amino acids such as phenylalanine and methionine also appear to increase (Wannemacher, 1977) whereas levels of the dispensable amino acids, glutamine and glycine, are generally decreased. Different patterns of plasma amino acid concentrations have been reported in thermal injury (Stinnett et al., 1982; Aulick and Wilmore, 1979) and cirrhosis (Fischer et al., 1975).

There are two questions which need to be addressed when evaluating plasma amino acid concentrations in respect to determining amino acid requirements. The first is simply one of understanding: Is the change in plasma concentration or pool size due to an alteration in the production and release of the amino acid or does it reflect, merely, a change in its clearance? This question is central to determination of amino acid requirements since a rise in concentration may imply either a relative failure of the body to clear amino acid sufficiently or an increased production or infusion rate. Although the differences appear subtle, they have important clinical implications. A reduced capacity by the body to metabolize an amino acid suggests that its intake should be decreased. The rationale to decrease the intake of an amino acid simply because endogenous appearance is increased is less convincing. Recent studies by Elia, Farrell, and Williamson (1980) have evaluated the mechanism by which plasma leucine concentrations rise in early starvation, uncontrolled diabetes, and severe injury. Their findings demonstrate that changes in plasma concentration cannot always be attributed to one explanation (Table 16-2). Unlike a short-term fast where the rise in plasma leucine concentrations was due to a reduced clearance of the amino acid, after severe injury the increase in plasma concentration was attributed solely to a more rapid appearance, presumably from protein breakdown. The increase in plasma leucine concentration observed in uncontrolled diabetes was due to both an increased appearance and reduced clearance.

Table 16-2
Mechanisms by Which Plasma Leucine Concentrations Increase in Different Physiologic Settings*

	Appearance or Production	Clearance
Short-term fast	unchanged	reduced
Surgical injury	increased	increased
Diabetes	increased	reduced

*Data from Elia, Farrell and Williamson (1980)

SIMILARITIES BETWEEN PLASMA AMINO ACID CONCENTRATIONS AND APPEARANCE

We recently completed a series of studies in rats subjected to a simple femur fracture that were infused with different hypocaloric feeding regimens (Moldawer et al., 1980). In this study, we attempted to determine if a correlation between plasma leucine concentrations and appearance (flux) existed. As observed in Figure 16-1, such a correlation was observed, suggesting that in this mildly stressed model the alterations in leucine pool size produced by nutritional means are primarily associated with changes in appearance rates and did not reflect a change in metabolic clearance.

In general, most investigators have concluded (Munro, 1974; Pain and Manchester, 1970; Waterlow, Garlick, and Millward, 1978) that due to the complexity of factors regulating amino acid pool sizes (plasma and intracellular concentrations), the significance of changes cannot be properly understood without some additional knowledge of rates of amino acid appearance and disappearance. Although changes in concentration may serve to alert the individual that some alterations in amino acid metabolism have occurred, they fail to provide information about what that change may be.

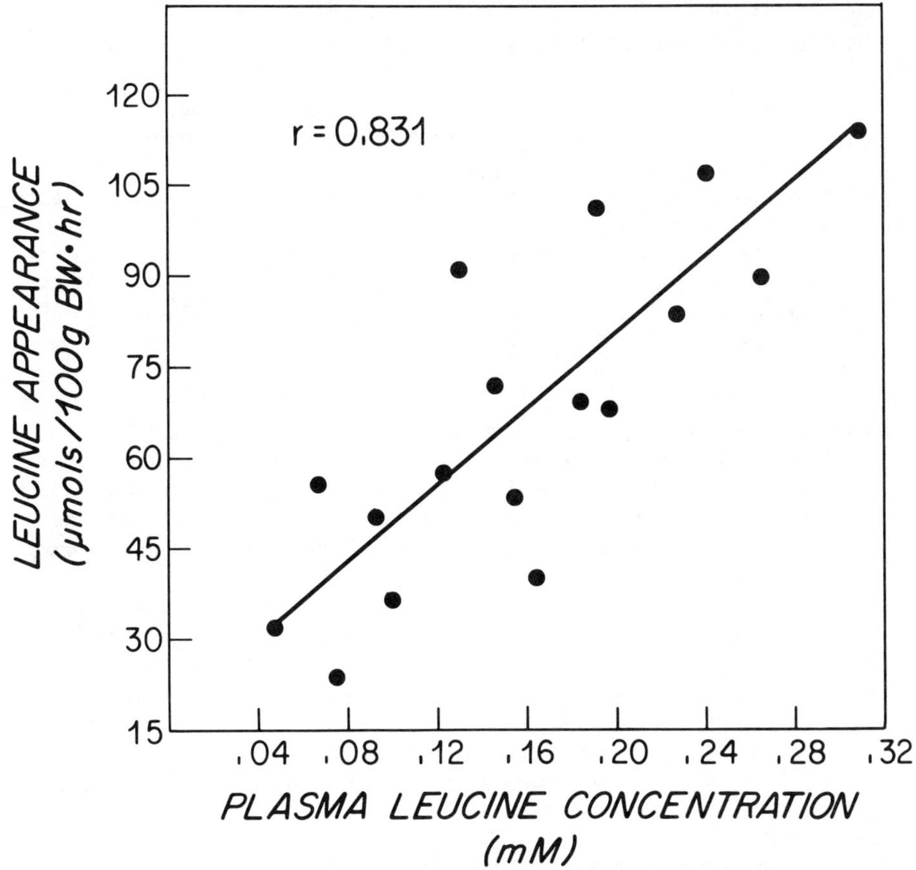

Figure 16-1 Correlation between plasma leucine concentration and appearance rate. Rats were subjected to a simple femur fracture and were infused with either crystalline amino acids, hypocaloric dextrose or physiologic saline. Rates of leucine disappearance were determined from a constant intravenous infusion of L-(1-^{14}C)-leucine. The regression line is significant at greater than 99% level of confidence.

The more important question about pool sizes and their significance when considering dietary amino acid requirements is whether amino acid concentrations in themselves regulate protein synthesis and degradation, rather than merely reflecting such changes. The question is key to studies evaluating amino acid requirements in the hospitalized patient since an affirmative answer would suggest that the goal for amino acid therapy in different disease states would be to devise an amino acid formulation that expands the free concentration of all amino acids, thereby stimulating protein synthesis. This subject has been extensively reviewed in healthy animals by others (Munro, 1974; Pain and Manchester, 1970; Waterlow, Garlick, and Millward, 1978; Jackson and Golden, 1982) and will only be discussed in the context of how it may apply to the injured patient.

BRANCHED-CHAIN AMINO ACID METABOLISM IN STRESSED, HOSPITALIZED PATIENTS

Of relevance to our laboratory has been the regulatory nature of dietary branched-chain amino acid administration in reducing protein catabolism after injury. We have suggested in earlier reports (Blackburn et al., 1979; Moldawer et al., 1981; Sakamoto et al., 1982) that by increasing branched-chain amino acid intake, we could offset the increased oxidation of these amino acids in injury and stimulate protein synthesis. However, Millward and Waterlow (Millward et al., 1976) have questioned the regulatory nature of branched-chain amino acids *in vivo,* based upon their observations that plasma and intracellular concentrations rise in starvation while synthesis rates in muscle decline. A more recent report by McNurlan, Fern, and Garlick (1982) has failed to show a stimulatory effect of infused leucine *in vivo* in healthy animals. Justifiably, one can criticize *in vitro* and perfusion studies that have shown increased muscle protein synthesis with elevated levels of branched-chain amino acids, because the changes in amino acid concentrations in such *in vitro* systems are generally much greater than seen under physiologic conditions (Goldberg and Chang, 1981). Furthermore, by using tissues removed from the body, the interaction between amino acid administration and hormone and substrate response is not investigated.

Desai et al. (1981, 1982) from this laboratory have recently evaluated *in vivo* the interaction between dietary administration of branched-chain amino acids and their effect on protein metabolism in surgically traumatized patients. Summarized in Table 16-3 are five patients who were studied prior to gastric bypass surgery while receiving crystalline amino acids and on postoperative days two through four while receiving only 85 to 100 g/day of isomolar branched-chain amino acids. L-(U-^{14}C)-tyrosine (5 uCi/hr for 10 hours) was infused to estimate the effect of such infusions

Table 16-3
Effect of Branched-Chain Amino Acid Administration on Postoperative Tyrosine Kinetics*

	Percentage of Tyrosine Flux Oxidized	
Patient ID	*Preoperative*†	*Postoperative*‡
GK	30.4% (0.68 mmol/hr)§	18.4% (0.46 mmol/hr)
MT	32.7% (1.08 mmol/hr)	19.4% (0.80 mmol/hr)
CD	18.5% (0.64 mmol/hr)	13.3% (0.21 mmol/hr)
EK	33.8% (0.57 mmol/hr)	22.5% (0.45 mmol/hr)
RK	19.4% (1.55 mmol/hr)	24.4% (1.73 mmol/hr)

*Unpublished data of Desai, S.P.
†while receiving 50 to 70 g/day crystalline amino acids (Travasol).
‡while receiving isonitrogenous quantities of isomolar branched-chain amino acids (approx. 85 g/day).
§total oxidation of plasma derived tyrosine.

on the behavior of another amino acid that was not contained in the diet. Plasma leucine, isoleucine, and valine concentrations were expectedly increased from 0.144, 0.097, and 0.220 μmols/ml to 0.988, 0.912, and 1.806 μmols/ml, respectively. Other indispensable amino acids declined slightly with only changes in methionine levels being statistically significant.

However, with this expansion of the plasma branched-chain amino acid pool, the proportion of free tyrosine in the body that was oxidized entirely to carbon dioxide declined in four of the five patients, suggesting that in these patients the administration of branched-chain amino acids and the expansion of the plasma branched-chain amino acid pool increased the efficiency with which tyrosine was incorporated into whole body protein. Of course, it cannot be concluded that these increases were attributed directly to a branched-chain amino acid stimulation of protein synthesis, since leucine in particular is insulinogenic, but similar findings have not been reported in rats given isonitrogenous quantities of L-alanine (Sakamoto et al., 1982; Freund, Yoshimura, and Fischer, 1980) which is equally insulinogenic (Freund, Yoshimura, and Fischer, 1980) *in vivo*.

As expected, the cost of this increased amino acid availability and incorporation into protein is a much higher proportion of the administered amino acids being oxidized. Numerous investigators (Waterlow, Garlick, and Millward, 1978; Jackson and Golden, 1982) have emphasized that the control of amino acid oxidation is more closely regulated than rates of protein synthesis or breakdown. Echenique et al. (1982) from this laboratory administered two crystalline amino acid solutions as part

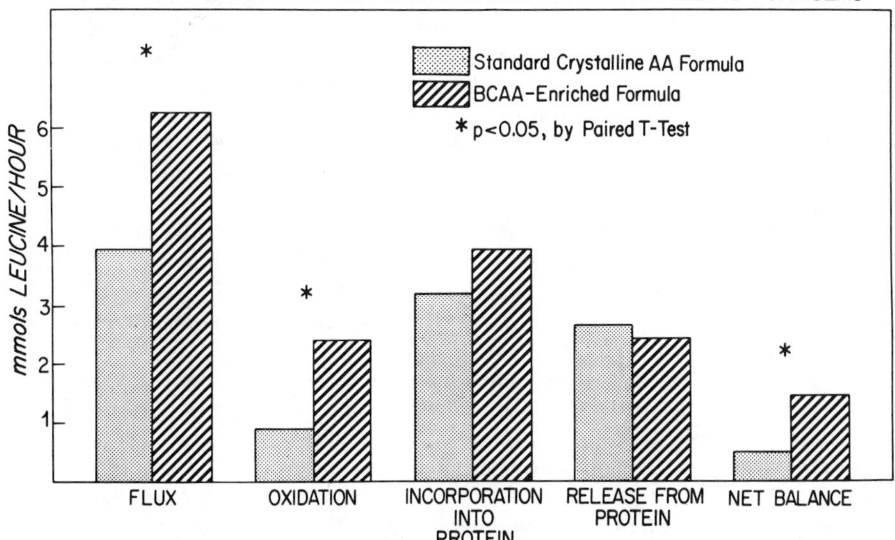

Figure 16-2 Whole body leucine kinetics in critically ill patients infused with either a standard crystalline amino acid formula or one enriched to 50% branched-chain amino acids. Five critically ill patients in the surgical intensive care unit were infused with 0.9 g/kg BW•day of either Travasol (crystalline amino acids) or a newer formula consisting of 50% branched-chain amino acids, sequentially. Rates of leucine oxidation, flux and net balance were significantly different between the two diets.

of a total parenteral nutrition regimen into five critically ill individuals and measured leucine oxidation rates with a continuous infusion of L-(1-^{14}C)-leucine. One solution contained 15% of the total amino acids as branched-chain amino acids, whereas the second contained 50% as branched-chain amino acids. Plasma branched-chain amino acid concentrations increased from 0.091 ± 0.011 to 0.165 ± 0.027 μmols/ml (leucine), 0.051 ± 0.008 to 0.134 ± 0.023 μmols/ml (isoleucine), and 0.197 ± 0.030 to 0.412 ± 0.086 μmols/ml (valine) with the 50% branched-chain amino acid administration. Furthermore, leucine oxidation (Figure 16-2) increased from 0.83 mmols/hr (21% of plasma appearance) to 2.39 mmols (38% of plasma appearance). Nevertheless, the patients were in improved net leucine balance, implying that rates of protein anabolism had also been increased.

Earlier studies by O'Keefe et al. (1981) showed that oxidation of leucine was also closely correlated to plasma concentration and availability (appearance).

The only conclusion that can be reached at the present time regarding the usefulness of plasma amino acid concentrations is that they can identify changes in amino acid metabolism. However, at present, they serve primarily to reflect whether changes have occurred, and until further studies are conducted, their role in interpreting amino acid dynamics is unclear.

ARTERIOVENOUS DIFFERENCES AND TISSUE DISPOSAL OF AMINO ACIDS

Amino acid concentrations are useful in the clinical setting because of their ease of analysis. However, information on the disposal of individual amino acids by organs or tissues have been difficult to obtain and as a result, there is a scarcity of such data. Those studies that have examined the disposal of an individual amino acid have done so generally in healthy animals following ingestion of a protein meal and have utilized a measurement of amino acid concentrations in arterial and venous samples either across a muscle, the splanchnic bed, liver or kidney. The need to invasively place catheters in the artery and vein limits the widespread applicability of this technique as does the necessity to obtain accurate measurements of blood flow. Although differences in amino acid concentrations between arterial and venous samples provides valuable information about the overall fate of amino acids, it cannot detail whether the disposal of amino acids is due to changes in protein breakdown or synthesis nor determine whether the uptake of an amino acid results in an oxidative or anabolic fate.

Clowes et al. (1980a) have estimated the net release of amino acids by skeletal muscle and the hepatic clearance in septic patients and in septic pigs receiving total parenteral nutrition (Lindberg and Clowes, 1981). Aulick and Wilmore (1979) have evaluated the release of amino acids from the leg in burned, postabsorptive individuals. Owen and Robinson (1963), Pozefesky et al. (1969, 1970), Aoki, Brennan, and Muller (1976), Wahren, Felig, and Hagenfeldt (1976), and Chiasson et al. (1977) have also reported the disposal of amino acids in man in response to various physiological states, including the effects of feeding, obesity, and diabetes. However, only recently have Abumrad et al. (1982) utilized this technique to evaluate the effect of intravenous amino acid intake on skeletal muscle metabolism. By measuring blood flow access to the forearm and arterial and venous amino acid concentrations in healthy young adults, Abumrad et al. (1982) noted that in the postabsorptive state, skeletal muscle was releasing approximately 300 nmols of total amino acids/100 g muscle•minute of which glutamine and alanine accounted for a major fraction (Table 16-4). Two hours after initiating an infusion of 17.5 g, complete amino acid/hour rates of total amino acid uptake by skeletal muscle were approximately 1200 nmols/100 g muscle•minute. The authors concluded that the skeletal muscle response to a complete amino acid infusion was similar to that following ingestion of a protein meal. Although it is apparent that a significant amount of the infused amino acids were extracted by skeletal muscle, the fate of those amino acids within the tissue was unclear. Whether such a technique will prove useful for estimating the requirements of individual amino acids is unknown, but the methodology is valuable in providing unique information about the individual organ response to different feeding regimens.

Table 16-4
Changes in Amino Acid Balance Across the Forearm of Healthy Young Adults Prior to and During an Amino Acid Infusion*

	Postabsorptive	Amino Acid Infusion
Arterial *Amino Acid,* mM	3.093 ± 0.088	6.613 ± 0.153‡
Disposal, nmol/100g muscle•minute	− 300 ± 97†	+ 1195 ± 209§
Arterial *Branched-Chain Amino Acid,* mM	0.369 ± 0.230	1.229 ± 0.047‡
Disposal, nmol/100g muscle•minute	− 31 ± 15	+ 513 ± 75§
Arterial *Ketoisocaproate,* mM	0.022 ± 0.006	0.026 ± 0.007
Disposal, nmol/100g muscle•minute	− 37 ± 9	− 32 ± 11
Arterial *Glutamine,* mM	0.614 ± 0.052	0.655 ± 0.052
Disposal, nmol/100g muscle•minute	− 144 ± 17	− 218 ± 42‡
Arterial *Alanine,* mM	0.290 ± 0.015	0.575 ± 0.034‡
Disposal, nmol/100g muscle•minute	− 116 ± 32	− 68 ± 23

*Data of Abumrad, et al. (1982).
†(−) signifies release, (+) signifies uptake.
‡p < 0.05, versus postabsorptive.
§p < 0.01, versus postabsorptive.

USE OF ISOTOPICALLY LABELED AMINO ACIDS

We have recently utilized an alternative approach for estimating amino acid needs of hospitalized patients. By continuously infusing either a ^{14}C-, ^{13}C-, ^{2}H-, ^{3}H-, or ^{15}N-labeled amino acid and measuring the enrichment in both the plasma compartment and an endproduct pool, rates of amino acid appearance and metabolic fate are determined. During the course of a constant intravenous infusion of labeled amino acid, the specific radioactivity in the plasma compartment will rise to "pseudo" plateau (Shipley and Clarke, 1964). At steady state enrichments, the appearance of amino acid can be derived from the dilution of tracer in the plasma compartment. As initially described by Waterlow and Stephens (1967), the whole body can be considered as a simplified two-pool system containing an exchangeable free amino acid pool that is measured by the plasma compartment (Figure 16-3) and a single protein pool.

In this model, amino acids enter the metabolic pool by either dietary intake, protein degradation, or *de novo* synthesis, and exit the pool via oxidation, incorporation into protein, or synthesis of nonprotein compounds. For most amino acids, the synthesis of nonprotein compounds can be considered quantitatively unimportant and disappearance from the plasma can be assumed to represent either amino acid oxidation or incorporation into protein. Similarly, use of a dietary indispensable amino acid as an isotopic tracer precludes *de novo* synthesis and rates of appearance can be assigned to either dietary intake or protein degradation.

The usefulness of this model has been equated to a measurement of oxygen consumption or energy expenditure, which necessarily represents the mean for many individual tissues. The benefits of the whole body measurements centers around their ability to provide an overall representation of protein metabolism rather than determining individual components.

However, with the opportunity to isolate selected tissue proteins, fractional rates of protein synthesis can also be determined. The fractional synthesis rate of albumin and other plasma proteins has frequently been determined with this technique (Waterlow and Stephens, 1967; Moldawer et al., 1980; O'Keefe et al., 1981a, 1981b; Clague et al., 1982). Halliday and McKeran (1975) as well as Stein et al. (1978, 1982a) have also used the technique to measure muscle protein and mixed tissue synthetic rates, respectively.

The assumption and limitations inherent to the stochastic model for measuring whole body protein kinetics and its usefulness for estimating amino acid requirements have been the subject of numerous excellent reviews (Shipley and Clarke, 1972: Waterlow, Garlick, and Millward, 1978; Waterlow and Stephens, 1982). However, its use in critically ill individuals has only been initiated in the past few years, and it is in the hospital setting that the value of this technique can be best seen.

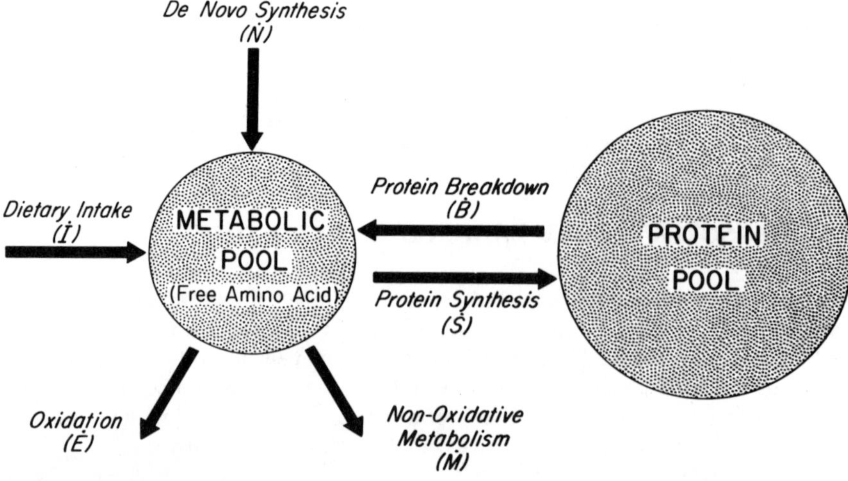

Figure 16-3 Two-pool model for estimating whole body amino acid metabolism.

USE OF ISOTOPICALLY LABELED AMINO ACIDS CAN REDUCE THE TIME PERIOD REQUIRED TO ESTIMATE REQUIREMENTS

Use of nitrogen excretion to evaluate a given diet requires a minimum of two days and crossover studies generally require a week. Since this period is usually too long to assure that the patient has remained clinically stable, we have used isotopic tracers to shorten the analytical period. Previous studies by Young and his colleagues (1981), Motil et al. (1981), Conway et al. (1980), Garlick et al. (1980a), and Clugston and Garlick (1982) have shown that in the healthy or obese young adult, isotopic steady states in the plasma and expired carbon dioxide can be achieved in a matter of hours with the infusion of most isotopic amino acids. We have recently demonstrated similar findings in hospitalized patients in the immediate postoperative period (O'Keefe et al., 1981). During a 20-hour continuous infusion of L-(1-^{14}C)-leucine, patients were infused for the first ten hours with only physiologic saline and isotopic steady states were reached within six to eight hours. Rates of leucine appearance and oxidation were subsequently determined during this baseline period and for the last ten hours the patients were then administered crystalline amino acids (85 g/day) with the ^{14}C-leucine.

As is evident in Figure 16-4, new isotopic steady states were achieved within six hours of changing the nutrient infusion and second estimates of amino acid oxidation and appearance could be determined. In this manner, the acute effects of an amino acid administration were elucidated in an immediately postoperative patient

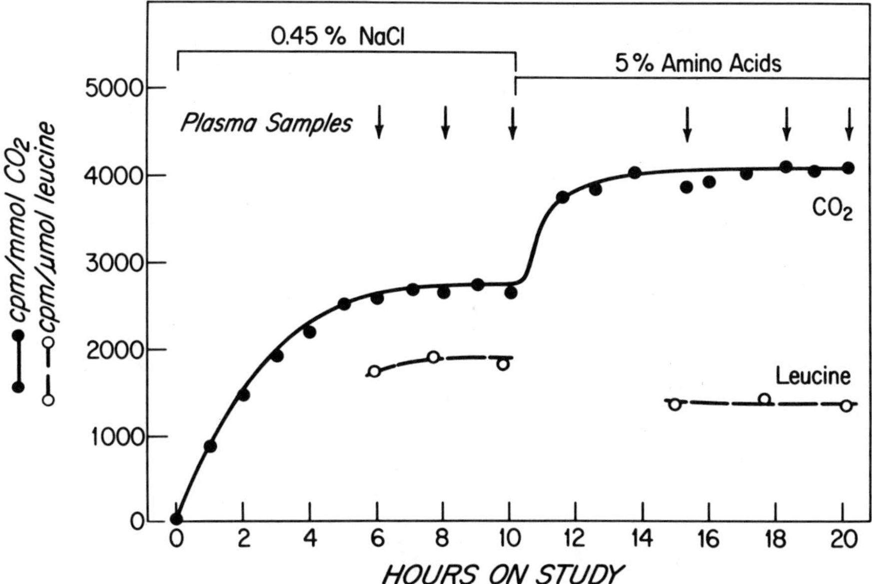

Figure 16-4 Attainment of plasma leucine and expired carbon dioxide specific radioactivities in an immediate postoperative patient. The patient received a 20-hour continuous infusion of L-(1-^{14}C)-leucine (5 μCi/hr). During the first ten hours, the patient received only physiologic saline and during the last ten hours, received 85 g/day of crystalline amino acids. Attainment of isotopic steady states was achieved within six hours of initiating the infusion or changing the composition of the diet.

where similar data on the effectiveness of a diet could not have been obtained by other techniques. The reliability of these results was subsequently confirmed by correlating leucine oxidation obtained over the ten hours with urinary nitrogen excretion over the following three days (r = 0.736).

We have recently completed similar studies (Echenique et al., 1982) in the intensive care unit with five stressed patients (as documented by increased urea production and amino acid appearance) receiving different crystalline amino acid formulas. In this setting, where clinical status is constantly changing and patient mortality is

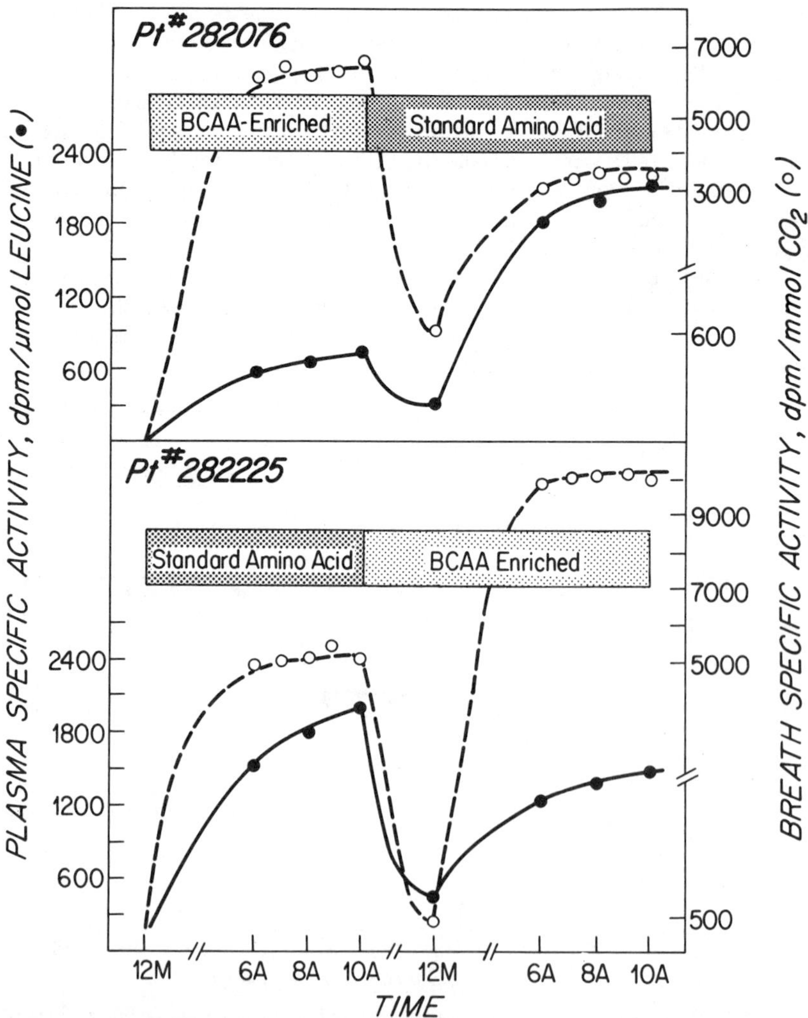

Figure 16-5 Attainment of plateau-specific radioactivities in two critically ill individuals infused with L-(1-^{14}C)-leucine. On two sequential days, patients were infused with either a standard crystalline amino acid formula or one enriched with branched-chain amino acids. Leucine kinetics were evaluated on each day and baseline enrichments were obtained prior to starting the second infusion.

high (80% of this population), administration of isotopic tracers permitted a rapid evaluation of amino acid utilization. Summarized in Figure 16-5 are results from two patients infused with L-(1-^{14}C)-leucine on two consecutive days. During one day, the patients were administered a standard crystalline amino acid formula at 0.9 g amino acid/kg•day, and on the other day were infused with an isonitrogenous formula which contained 50% branched-chain amino acids by weight. In this population, isotopic steady states in both the plasma compartment and expired carbon dioxide were also obtained within eight to ten hours. Although the quality of plateaus was clearly not as good as in the postoperative period (see Figure 16-4), the progressive increase in specific radioactivity was small compared to the differences due to dietary intake.

LIMITATIONS OF THE MODEL

Even though the use of isotopically labeled amino acids offers some distinct advantages over other techniques, such as the rapidity of measurement and the ability to obtain additional estimates of protein synthesis and breakdown, the reliability of the methodology is dependent to a great extent upon a thorough appreciation of its limitations. The theoretical justification for estimating rates of whole body protein synthesis and breakdown from the constant infusion of an isotopically labeled amino acid has been extensively described (Waterlow, Garlick, and Millward, 1978; Stein, 1982b) and is beyond the scope of this work. Nevertheless, the applicability of this technique to the hospitalized patient, particularly in regard to the derivation of whole body protein synthesis and breakdown rates, remains controversial.

As Waterlow has stated earlier (Waterlow, Garlick, and Millward, 1978), measurements of amino acid flux based upon plasma enrichments are only estimates of true rates and the reliability of these measurements depends in part upon the ability of the plasma pool to reflect intracellular enrichments. During a continuous infusion, it is assumed that the enrichment of plasma-free amino acid pool is in some fashion reflecting the specific radioactivity of the amino acid at its true site of oxidation and protein synthesis. Although such an assumption is not necessary to obtain an estimate of plasma amino acid appearance and ultimate fate, it is essential that such a constant ratio exist if extrapolating the flux or appearance of an amino acid to the total protein turnover rate is desired.

The effect of amino acid compartmentalization and reliance on the plasma compartment as an estimate of the true precursor specific radioactivity has not been evaluated extensively in the injured state. The potential for error has been demonstrated, however. For tyrosine, changes in the ratio of intracellular-to-plasma specific radioactivity have been reported in fasting and protein deficiency (Garlick, Millward, and James, 1973; Garlick et al., 1975), although similar findings have not been reported with a single amino acid deficiency (Harney, Swick, and Benevenega, 1976).

More important to this discussion is the observation of Sakamoto et al. (1982) from this laboratory who reported that compartmentalization of tyrosine in skeletal muscle was altered in rats suffering experimentally induced injury. As shown in Table 16-5, alterations of tyrosine compartmentalization were only observed in the most catabolic forms of injury, and the changes were consistent with a reduced efficiency of tyrosine recycling within the muscle cell.

Table 16-5
Effect of Increasingly Catabolic Forms of Experimental Injury on Whole Body Tyrosine Oxidation and Compartmentation in Skeletal Muscle

	Tyrosine Oxidation (μmol/100g BW•hr)	Plasma Tyrosine Specific Radioactivity† (d.p.m./μmol)	Intracellular‡ to Plasma Tyrosine Specific Radioactivity Ratio
Healthy, fasted	4.58 ± 0.33	40,561 ± 2,332	0.461 ± 0.057
Anesthesia only	4.71 ± 0.25	43,987 ± 3,578	0.453 ± 0.042
Experimental laparotomy	5.84 ± 0.57*	36,259 ± 2,749*	0.479 ± 0.087
Acute pancreatitis	7.42 ± 0.43*	33,600 ± 1,536*	0.700 ± 0.061*

Data of Sakamoto et al. (1982).
*$p < 0.05$ versus healthy fasted.
†Based upon the continuous infusion of L-(U-^{14}C)-tyrosine (1 μCi/hr).
‡'Acid-soluble' fraction.

Unfortunately, similar techniques are not readily available for measuring amino acid compartmentalization in humans nor is there consensus that the "acid-soluble" fraction of tissue is representative of the precursor pool for amino acid oxidation and protein synthesis (Wheatley, 1979). An alternative approach used by our group, Dr. Robert R. Wolfe at Harvard Medical School, Dr. Vernon Young at M.I.T., and Drs. Dwight Matthews and Dennis Bier at Washington University, is to determine the specific activity of an intracellular metabolite of the indispensable amino acid. If the isotopic amino acid is in equilibrium with the product and, in itself, is indispensable, then the specific radioactivity of the metabolite will reflect the specific radioactivity of the amino acid at its site of metabolism within the cell (Matthews et al., 1982). For those using carboxy-labeled leucine as an isotopic tracer, evaluation of L-ketoisocaproate (KIC) specific radioactivity offers the opportunity to evaluate an intracellular enrichment.

Figure 16-6 presents a theroretical model explaining why the specific activity of plasma KIC would be more representative of the specific activity of leucine at its site of oxidation. Plasma ^{14}C-leucine, from the continuous infusion of the tracer, is transported into the cell where it is assumed to mix freely with unlabeled leucine also derived from intracellular protein breakdown. The specific activity of leucine in the intracellular pool must theoretically have a specific radioactivity less than that of plasma to a degree dependent upon the rate of protein breakdown relative to the quantity of labeled amino acid entering from the plasma compartment (Waterlow, Garlick, and Millward, 1978). Because leucine and its ketoacid, L-ketoisocaproate are in equilibrium (Krebs and Lund, 1977; Matthews at al., 1981), the ketoisocaproate would attain the specific radioactivity of the intracellular leucine. Ketoisocaproate that is not oxidatively decarboxylated further but rather reenters the plasma compartment (Hutson, Cree and Harper, 1978) will have a specific radioactivity less than that of leucine in the plasma compartment and the decrease in enrichment would reflect the relative underestimate of leucine oxidation based upon plasma leucine enrichments. Recent studies (Matthews et al., 1982) have demonstrated that the underestimate in leucine oxidation based upon plasma leucine enrichments is about 20% in man and, more importantly, does not appear to be affected by dietary intake. Brehon Laurent, in collaboration with Vernon Young, completed a

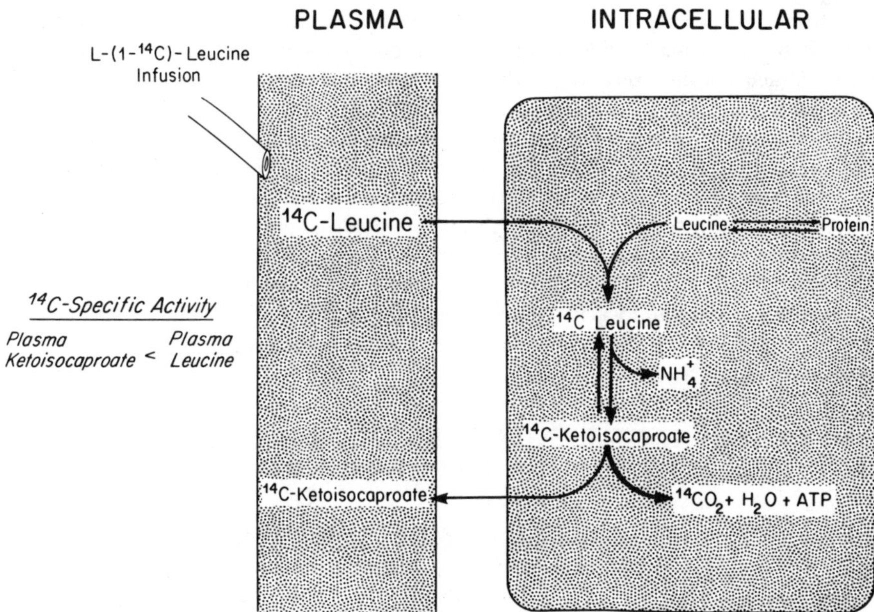

Figure 16-6 Theoretical model for the use of ketoisocaproate-specific radioactivity as a precursor for leucine oxidation. The reduction in plasma ketoisocaproate enrichment relative to leucine reflects the contribution of intracellular dilution and quantitates the relative underestimate in leucine oxidation based upon plasma leucine enrichments.

similar study in rats in this laboratory and observed that the ratio of ketoisocaproate to leucine-specific radioactivity was 0.7 and was also unaffected by prior dietary protein intake (Table 16-6). Interestingly, the specific activity of ketoisocaproate in the plasma was very similar to the specific activity of free leucine in the muscle "acid-soluble" fraction. This is consistent with the suggestion that muscle is a principal site of leucine deamination in the rat (Krebs and Lung, 1978).

Table 16-6
Relationship Between Plasma and Muscle Intracellular Leucine and Plasma Ketoisocaproate Specific Radioactivities in Rats Fed Different Levels of Casein*

Diet Composition	Plasma Leucine Specific Radioactivity, d.p.m/μmol†	Plasma Ketoisocaproate: Leucine Specific Radioactivity Ratio	Muscle 'Acid-Soluble' Leucine: Plasma Leucine Specific Radioactivity Ratio
2% Casein	50,574 ± 3,854[a]	0.719 ± 0.062	0.753 ± 0.060
5% Casein	32,457 ± 1,345[b]	0.758 ± 0.043	0.910 ± 0.113
20% Casein	20,524 ± 1,279[c]	0.749 ± 0.039	0.778 ± 0.036
40% Casein	20,254 ± 1,728[c]	0.688 ± 0.045	0.820 ± 0.041

*Unpublished data of Laurent, B. et al.
†Based upon a continuous infusion of L-(1-^{14}C)-leucine (1 μCi/hr).
[a,b,c]Values with different superscripts are significantly different, p 0.05.

Robert Wolfe and his colleagues (1982a) have recently investigated the relationship between plasma leucine and ketoisocaproate enrichments with an infusion of L-(1-^{13}C)-leucine in exercising individuals and in burned adults receiving total parenteral nutrition (Wolfe et al., 1982b). Surprisingly, the ratio of plasma ketoisocaproate to leucine-specific radioactivity significantly decreased from 0.8 both with exercise and injury. Such data is of importance because it implies that in some altered physiologic states greater proportions of free leucine derived from intracellular protein rather than from plasma are oxidized and that estimates of whole body leucine metabolism based on plasma enrichments will become substantially greater underestimates. Until more work can be evaluated, caution must be exercised when interpreting amino acid kinetics based on plasma enrichments in injured individuals, and efforts will have to continue to identify the proper precursor pool for protein synthesis.

AMINO ACID APPEARANCE AS AN ESTIMATE OF WHOLE BODY PROTEIN TURNOVER

An additional assumption that will require further validation is the extrapolation of individual amino acid kinetics to whole body protein turnover. Such a mathematical derivation requires that some knowledge of the body composition be known and the presumption that other amino acids are behaving in a similar manner. Although it is unrealistic to suggest that the kinetics of dispensable amino acids would be similar to indispensable amino acids, since a component of their appearance is independent of protein intake and degradation, the behavior of some indispensable and semi-indispensable amino acids appear similar when balanced amino acid or protein-containing diets are administered.

In a recently completed series of studies, Desai et al. (1982) evaluated the similarities between leucine and tyrosine kinetics in ten hospitalized adults, either postabsorptive or receiving complete crystalline amino acids or total parenteral nutrition (Table 16-7). On Day 1, the patients were infused for ten hours starting at midnight with 35 to 50 μCi of L-(1-^{14}C)-leucine. The following night at midnight an additional blood and breath sample was obtained for baseline radioactivity and the patients were infused with 30 to 50 μCi of L-(U-^{14}C)-tyrosine. Rates of leucine and tyrosine kinetics were subsequently determined based upon the dilution of tracer in the plasma compartment and appearance in expired carbon dioxide. As demon-

Table 16-7
Comparison between Leucine and Tyrosine Kinetics Obtained in Hospitalized Patients Sequentially*

	Leucine†	Tyrosine‡
Amino acid appearance, mmol/hr	5.60 ± 0.47	2.45 ± 0.24
Amino acid oxidation, mmol/hr	0.70 ± 0.11	0.29 ± 0.06
Amino acid incorporation into protein, mmol/hr	4.90 ± 0.41	2.16 ± 0.20

*Unpublished data of Desai, S.P.
†Obtained from a 10-hr continuous infusion of L-(1-^{14}C)-leucine (3 5o 5 μCi/hr).
‡Obtained from a 10-hr continuous infusion of L-(U-^{14}C)-tyrosine (3 to 5 μCi/hr).

strated in Table 16-7, rates of leucine and tyrosine appearance, incorporation into protein and oxidation were found to differ significantly with the two tracers. Although tyrosine kinetics were significantly less than leucine, the proportion of tyrosine and leucine flux that were oxidized and incorporated into protein were remarkably similar (Table 16-8). This was somewhat unexpected since approximately 15% to 20% of tyrosine appearance is due to the hydroxylation of phenylalinine (Clark and Bier, 1982; James, Garlick, and Sender, 1976; see also Moldawer et al., Section III), and for this reason, it would be expected that a greater proportion of tyrosine appearance would be oxidized than for an indispensable amino acid-like leucine. However, this has not been observed (James, Garlick, and Sender, 1976), and it appears that tyrosine derived from the hydroxylation of phenylalanine does not equilibrate freely with plasma tyrosine, but rather is oxidized preferentially. Motil et al. (1981) also reported similar changes in plasma leucine and lysine kinetics when healthy volunteers had the protein component of their diet varied.

Although the data suggests that in healthy or mildly stressed individuals either receiving no dietary intake or a balanced amino acid formula, tyrosine, leucine, and lysine kinetics behave in a similar fashion, it does not imply that the isotopic amino acids are interchangeable for estimating whole body dynamics under different physiologic states. In a recent report, O'Keefe et al. (1981b) used L-(U-^{14}C)-tyrosine to estimate whole body protein kinetics in patients with hepatic dysfunction and obtained reports which suggested that patients with fulminant hepatic failure were degrading protein at rates equal to 13 g/kg•day approximately four times that observed in healthy adults. Stein (see Section V) has also observed very high whole body protein synthetic rates in seriously ill patients (10 g/kg•day) using a pulse administration of ^{15}N-glycine and urinary ammonia enrichments. Prior to concluding that these observations represent real changes, similar studies will need to be conducted with additional amino acids as isotopic tracers to demonstrate that these findings are not unique to the amino acid used but represent real changes in whole body protein turnover.

STRATIFYING PATIENT POPULATIONS FOR DEGREE OF METABOLIC STRESS

The host response to injury or infection has been characterized by disturbances in amino acid metabolism which result in enhanced appearance of nitrogen, sulfur,

Table 16-8
Components of Amino Acid Flux Determined by L-(1-^{14}C)-Leucine and L-(U-^{14}C)-Tyrosine Infusions*

	L-(1-^{14}C)-Leucine	L-(U-^{14}C)-Tyrosine
Percentage of flux oxidized	87.5 ± 3.4	88.2 ± 5.1
Percentage of flux for protein synthesis	12.5 ± 3.4	11.8 ± 5.0
Percentage of flux derived from breakdown	72.6 ± 20.1	81.4 ± 9.2

*Data obtained from Desai et al. (1981).

and phosphorus in the urine. However, controversy exists whether elective operative trauma, accidental injury, sepsis, inflammation or thermal injury produce similar metabolic responses and whether amino acid requirements are similar in these different forms of injury. We have argued (Blackburn, 1981) that the metabolic response to injury or infection is a cascade of endogenous events that is remarkably constant in pattern despite the myriad of initiating processes.

Current investigation has identified an endogenous mediator, frequently called leukocyte endogenous mediator, leukocytic pyrogen, endogenous pyrogen, lymphocyte activating factor or Interleukin I, which appears to orchestrate many of the metabolic disturbances in injury and infection (Powanda and Beisel, 1982). Surgical trauma, accidental injury, and sepsis initiate a nonspecific immune response when tissue debris, whether from surgical injury or invading microorganisms, activate the complement system. The split products of the complement system modulate phagocytosis; polymorphonuclear neutrophils and tissue macrophages in their process of clearing foreign particles or tissue damage release various substances collectively called leukocyte endogenous mediator (LEM).

Administration of this peptide into healthy animals induces fever, raises serum insulin and glucose concentrations (Keenan et al., 1982a), redistributes trace minerals (Keenan et al., 1982b), increases amino acid mobilization, oxidation, skeletal and collagen protein degradation and hepatic protein synthesis (Yang et al., 1981), all similar to that seen in injury or infection. Such a biological cascade implies that the protein response at its most basic level is similar in most forms of stress. The primary difference between elective surgical injury and accidental trauma or infections would be that surgery represents a stimulus at a single point in time, whereas trauma or infection generally have a continued presence of the stimulus.

Of course, the overall response is modulated to some degree by the nutritional status of the patient and the presence of pain and hypovolemia. Although pain and accompanied sympathetic nervous system activity have profound effects on substrate mobilization and energy expenditure (Wilmore et al., 1974), their capacity to induce net protein catabolism is unclear. Experimental isoproterenol infusions actually reduce protein degradation rates in the rat hemicorpus preparation (Li and Jefferson, 1977). Although corticosteroids increase protein degradation (Nishizawa et al., 1978), their administration also stimulates endogenous LEM production (Dinarello, 1979). At the present time, we would conclude that the protein response to injury is primarily a result of endogenous protein mediators, produced by the nonspecific immune system and independent to some extent of external hormonal control.

In an attempt to stratify patients with a wide range of disease processes according to the magnitude of protein catabolism, we have promulgated the use of the "Catabolic Index" (Bistrian, 1979). The particular value of the Catabolic Index is that it integrates the level of dietary intake and degree of metabolic stress into a single number:

$$\text{Catabolic Index} = \text{UUN} - (0.5\ N_{in} + 3)$$

where a score of -5 to 0 indicates no stress or mild stress, 0 to $+5$ moderate stress, and $+5$ to $+10$ severe stress.

A major benefit of the Catabolic Index is that it relies on urine urea nitrogen (UUN) measurements which are both easy to obtain and inexpensive. The Catabolic

Index also modulates the importance of high nitrogen intake (N_{in}) on urea nitrogen production by fractional reduction. The impact of low protein intakes is minimized as well by addition of a constant 3 g of nitrogen.

The value of the Catabolic Index in determining whether patients will benefit from amino acid solutions enriched with branched-chain amino acids was recently demonstrated (Moldawer et al., 1982). In a review of previous clinical studies (Cerra et al., 1982; Echenique et al., 1982), it was suggested that in patients who were moderately to severely catabolic and as a result of fluid intolerance or organ failure had reduced protein intakes, branched-chain amino acid-enriched formulas could reduce net protein catabolism. In the unstressed patient with a Catabolic Index less than 0 or one receiving adequate intakes of dietary protein (greater than 1 g/kg•day), branched-chain amino acid supplementation would be of little added benefit.

CONCLUSIONS

The opportunity to evaluate amino acid needs with parenteral and enteral products is great, particularly given the current methodology available to investigate the metabolic consequences of such therapy. As later chapters will demonstrate, amino acid requirements in hospitalized patients will depend upon the nature of the patient's disease, presence of malnutrition, degree of stress (acute, chronic) and availability of nonprotein calories (particularly glucose), vitamins, minerals, and trace elements.

Predicting requirements and ultimate utilization of amino acids can be determined from nitrogen balance studies, and changes in amino acid metabolism will be reflected by plasma concentrations. However, determining the ultimate tissue fate of amino acids and mechanisms of nitrogen sparing will require greater use of isotopic kinetic studies and arteriovenous differences in plasma concentrations.

Although dietary-induced abnormalities in amino acid metabolism are reflected in plasma amino acid profiles, this approach is of limited value in the determination of optimal amino acid formulas. Rather, use of appropriate study designs incorporating the use of isotopically labeled amino acids, which are now widely available, will result in more precise data toward the goal of better feeding the hospitalized patient.

ACKNOWLEDGMENTS

The authors wish to acknowledge the considerable effort of Drs. S.P. Desai, M.M. Echenique, R. Martin and R.A. Keenan, as well as Brehon Laurent and Russell Yang, whose experimental work provided much of the basis for this manuscript. The authors are also grateful to Anne-Marie Leonard for her expert assistance in the preparation of this manuscript.

REFERENCES

Abumrad, N.N., Rabin, D., Wise, L.L., et al. (1982): The disposal of an intravenous administered amino acid load across the human forearm. *Metabolism* 31:463–470.

Alexander, J.W., McArthur, B.G., Stinnett, J.D., et al. (1980): Beneficial effects of aggressive protein feeding in severely burned children. *Ann. Surg.* 192:505–516.

Aoki, T.T., Brennan, M.F., Muller, W.A., et al. (1976): Amino acid levels across the normal forearm muscle and splanchnic bed after a protein meal. *Am. J. Clin. Nutr.* 29:340–350.

Augustine, S.L., Swick, R.W. (1980): Turnover of total protein and ornithine amino transferase during liver regeneration in the rat. *Am. J. Physiol.* 238:E46–52.

Aulick, L.H., Wilmore, D.H. (1979): Increased peripheral amino acid release following burn injury. *Surgery* 85:560–565.

Benotti, P. N., Blackburn, G.L. (1979): Protein and calorie or macronutrient metabolic management of the critically ill patient. *Crit. Care Medic.* 7:520–525.

Birkhahn, R.H., Long, C.L., Fitkin, D., et al. (1980): Effects of major skeletal trauma on whole body protein turnover in man, measured by L-(1-^{14}C)-leucine. *Surgery* 88: 294–300.

Bistrian, B.R., Blackburn, G.L., Hallowell, E., et al. (1974): Protein status of general surgical patients. *J. Am. Med. Assoc.* 230:858–860.

Bistrian, B.R., Blackburn, G.L., Vitale, J., et al. (1976): Prevalence of malnutrition in general medical patients. *J. Am. Med. Assoc.* 235:1567–1570.

Bistrian, B.R. (1979): A simple technique to estimate the severity of stress. *Surg. Gynecol. Obstet.* 148:675–678.

Blackburn, G.L., Flatt, J.P., Clowes, G.H.A., et al. (1979): Protein sparing therapy during periods of starvation with sepsis and trauma. *Ann. Surg.* 179:684–696.

Blackburn, G.L., Moldawer, L.L., Bothe, A., Jr, et al. (1979): Branched chain amino acid administration and metabolism during starvation, injury, and infection. *Surgery* 86:307–315.

Blackburn, G.L., Wolfe, R.R. (1981): Clinical biochemistry and intravenous hyperalimentation. In: *Recent Advances in Biochemistry* (eds: Alberti, K.G.H. and Price, B.) pp. 197–228, Churchill Livingstone, New York.

Blackburn, G.L. (1981): Protein metabolism and nutritional support. *J. Trauma* 21:707–711.

Cerra, F.B., Upson, D., Angelico, R., et al. (1982): Branched chains support post-operative protein synthesis. *Surgery* 92:192–199.

Chiasson, J.L., Liljenquist, J.E., Lacy, W.W., et al. (1977): Gluconeogenesis: Methodological approaches, in vivo. *Fed. Proc.* 36:229–235.

Clague, M.B., Carmichael, M.J., Kier, M.J., et al. (1982): Increased incorporation of an infused labeled amino acid into plasma proteins as a means of assessing the severity of injury on activity of disease in surgical patients. *Ann. Surg.* 196:53–58.

Clark, J., Bier, D.M. (1982): Interrelationship between phenylalanine and tyrosine in postabsorptive man. *Metabolism* 31:999–1005.

Clowes, G.H.A., Heidemen, M., Lindberg, B., et al. (1980a): Effects of parenteral alimentation on amino acid metabolism in septic patients. *Surgery* 88:531–543.

Clowes, G.H.A., Randall, H.T., Cha, C.J. (1980b): Amino acid and energy metabolism in septic and traumatized patients. *J. Parent. Enter. Nutr.* 4:195–205.

Clugston, G.A., Garlick, P.J. (1982): The response of protein and energy metabolism to food intake in lean and obese man. *Human Nutr. Clin. Nutr.* 36C:57–70.

Conway, J.C., Bier, D.M., Motil, K., et al. (1980): Whole body lysine flux in young adult men: Effects of reduced total protein and of lysine intake. *Am. J. Physiol.* 239:E192–230.

Crane, C.W., Picou, D., Smith, W., et al. (1977): Protein turnover in patients before and after elective orthopedic operations. *Br. J. Surg.* 64:129–133.

Desai, S.P., Moldawer, L.L., Bistrian, B.R. (1981): Amino acid and protein metabolism in humans using L-(U-^{14}C)-tyrosine and L-(l-^{14})-leucine. *Develop. in Biochem.* 18:307–313.

Desai, S.P., Bistrian, B.R., Moldawer, L.L., et al. (1982): Plasma amino acid concentrations during branched chain amino acid infusions in stressed patients. *J. Trauma* 22:747–752.

Dinarello, C.A. (1979): Production of endogenous pyrogen. *Fed. Proc.* 38:52–56.

Echenique, M.M., Bistrian, B.R., Moldawer, L.L., et al. (1983): Improvement in amino acid utilization in the critically ill with parenteral formulas enriched with branched chain amino acids. *Metabolism* 32: (In press).

Elia, M., Farrell, R., Williamson, D.H., et al. (1980): The removal of infused leucine after injury, starvation, and other conditions in man. *Clin. Sci.* 59:275–283.

Elwyn, D.H., Gump, F.E., Iles, M., et al. (1979): Protein and energy sparing of glucose added in hypocaloric amounts to peripheral infusions of amino acids. *Metabolism* 27:325–331.

Fischer, J.E., Furovus, J.M., Aguirre, A., et al. (1975): The role of plasma amino acids in hepatic encephalopathy. *Surgery* 78:276–290.

Forbes, G.B., Hursh, J.B. (1963): Age and sex trends in lean body mass calculations from K40 measurements: With a note on the theoretical basis for the procedure. *Ann. N.Y. Acad. Sci.* 110:255–263.

Forbes, G.B., Schultz, F., Cajarelli, C., et al. (1968): The effect of body size in potassium-40 measurement in the whole body. *Center Health Phys.* 15:435–442.

Freund, H.R., Hoover, H.C., Atamian, S., et al. (1979): Infusion of branched chain amino acids in post-operative patients. *Ann. Surg.* 190:18–23.

Freund, H.R., Yoshimura, N., Fischer, J.E. (1980): The role of alanine in the nitrogen conserving quality of branched chain amino acids in the post-injury state. *J. Surg. Res.* 29:23–30.

Garlick, P.J., Millward, D.J., James, W.P.T. (1973): The diurnal response of muscle and liver protein synthesis in vivo, in meal fed rats. *Biochem. J.* 136:935–945, 1973.

Garlick, P.J., Millward, D.J., James, W.P.T., et al. (1975): The effect of protein deprivation and starvation on the protein synthesis in tissues of the rat. *Biochim. Biophys. Acta* 414: 71–84.

Garlick, P.J., Clugston, G.A., Waterlow, J.C. (1980a): Diurnal pattern of protein and energy metabolism in man. *Am. J. Clin. Nutr.* 33:1983–1986.

Garlick, P.J., McNurlan, M.A., Fern, E.B., et al. (1980b): Stimulation of protein synthesis and breakdown by vaccination. *Br. Med. J.* 2:263–265.

Goldberg, A.L., Chang, T.W. (1978): Regulation and significance of amino acid metabolism in skeletal muscle. *Fed. Proc.* 37:2301–2307.

Halliday, D., McKeran, R.O. (1975): Measurement of muscle protein synthetic rate from serial muscle biopsies and total protein turnover in man by continuous infusion of L-(^{15}N)-lysine. *Clin. Sci.*49:581–590.

Harney, M.E., Swick, R.W., Benevenega, N.J. (1976): Estimation of tissue protein synthesis in rats fed diets labeled with L-(U-^{14}C)-tyrosine. *Am. J. Physiol.* 231:1018–1023.

Hill, G.L., McCarthy, I.D., Collins, J.P., et al. (1978): A new method for the rapid measurement of body composition in extremely ill surgical patients. *Br. J. Surg.* 65:732–735.

Hutson, S.M., Cree, T.C., Harper, A.E. (1978): Regulation of leucine and alpha-keto-isocaproate metabolism in skeletal muscle. *J. Biol. Chem.* 253:8126–8133.

Jackson, A.A., Golden, M.H.N. (1982): Interrelationship of amino acid pools and protein turnover. In: *Nitrogen Metabolism in Man* (eds: Waterlow, J.C., Stephens, J.M.L.) Applied Sciences Publishing, Inc., London.

James, W.P.T., Garlick, P.J., Sender, P.M. (1976): Studies of protein and amino acid metabolism in normal man with L-(U-^{14}C)-tyrosine. *Clin. Sci.* 50:525–532.

James, W.P.T. (1982): Protein and energy metabolism after trauma. *Acta Chir. Scand.* (suppl) 507:1–16.

Jeejeebhoy, K.N., Anderson, G.H., Nakhooda, A.F., et al. (1976): Metabolic studies in total parenteral nutrition with lipid in man: Comparison with glucose. *J. Clin. Invest.* 57:125–136.

Kawamura, I., Moldawer, L.L., Keenan, R.A., et al. (1982): Altered amino acid kinetics in rats with progressive tumor growth. *Cancer Res.* 42:824–829.

Kien, C.L., Young, V.R., Rohrbaugh, D.K., et al. (1978a): Whole body protein synthesis and breakdown in children before and after reconstructive surgery of the skin. *Metabolism* 27:27–34.

Kien, C.L., Young, V.R., Rohrbaugh, D.K., et al. (1978b): Whole body protein synthesis and breakdown in children recovering from burns. *Ann. Surg.* 187:383–391.

Krebs, H.A., Lund, P. (1977): Aspects of the regulation of the metabolism of branched chain amino acids. *Adv. Enz. Regul.* 15:375–394.

Li, J.B., Jefferson, L.J. (1977): Effect of isoproterenol on amino acid levels and protein turnover in skeletal muscle. *Am. J. Physiol.* 232:E243–249.

Lindberg, B.D., Clowes, G.H.A. (1981): Effects of hyperalimentation and infused leucine on the amino acid metabolism in sepsis. *Surgery* 90:278–290.

Long, C.L., Jeevanadam, M., Kim, B.M. (1977): Whole body protein synthesis and catabolism in septic man. *Am. J. Clin. Nutr.* 30:1340–1344.

Matthews, D.E., Bier, D.M., Rennie, M.J., et al. (1981): Regulation of leucine metabolism in man: a stable isotope study. *Science* 214:1129–1131.

Matthews, D.M., Schwartz, H.P., Yang, R.D., et al. (1982): Relationship of plasma leucine and ketoisocaproate during an L-(1-^{13}C)-leucine infusion in man: a method for measuring human intracellular leucine tracer enrichment. *Metabolism* (In press).

McNurlan, M.A., Fern, E.B., Garlick, P.J. (1982): Failure of leucine to stimulate protein synthesis, in vivo. *Biochem. J.* 204:831–838.

Millward, D.J., Garlick, P.J., Nnangelugo, D.O., et al. (1976): The relative importance of muscle protein synthesis and breakdown in the regulation of muscle mass. *Biochem. J.* 156:185–188.

Moldawer, L.L., O'Keefe, S.J.D., Bothe, A., et al. (1980): In vivo demonstration of the nitrogen sparing mechanisms of glucose and amino acids in the injured rat. *Metabolism* 30:173–180.

Moldawer, L.L., Bistrian, B.R., Blackburn, G.L. (1981a): Factors determining the preservation of protein status during dietary protein deprivation. *J. Nutr.* 111:1287–1296.

Moldawer, L.L., Sakamoto, A., Blackburn, G.L. (1981b): Alterations in protein kinetics produced by branched chain amino acid administration during infection and inflammation. *Develop. in Biochem.* 18:533–541.

Moldawer, L.L., Echenique, M.M., Bistrian, B.R. (1982): The importance of study design to the demonstration of efficacy with branched chain amino acid enriched solutions. 2nd Bermuda Symposium on Total Parenteral Nutrition. Plenum Press, New York.

Moore, F.D. (1959): *Metabolic Care of the Surgical Patient.* W.B. Saunders, Philadelphia.

Motil, K.J., Matthews, D.E., Bier, D.M., et al. (1981): Whole body leucine and lysine metabolism: response to dietary protein intake in young men. *Am. J. Physiol.* 240:E712–721.

Munro, H.N. (1974): Free amino acid pools and their role in regulation. In: *Mammalian Protein Metabolism* (ed: Munro, H.N.), Vol. IV, pp. 299–387. Academic Press, New York.

Nishizawa, N., Shimbo, M., Noguchi, T., et al. (1978): Effect of starvation, refeeding, and hydro-cortizone administration on turnover of myofibrillar proteins estimated by urinary excretion of 3-methylhistidine in the rat. *Agr. Biol. Chem.* 42:2083–2089.

O'Keefe, S.J.D., Sender, P.M., James, W.P.T. (1974): Catabolic loss of body nitrogen in response to surgery. *Lancet* 2:1035–1037.

O'Keefe, S.J.D., Moldawer, L.L., Young, V.R., et al. (1981a): The influence of intravenous nutrition on protein dynamics following surgery. *Metabolism* 30:1150–1158.

O'Keefe, S.J.D., Abraham, R.R., Davis, M., et al. (1981b): Protein turnover in acute and chronic liver disease. *Acta Chir. Scand.* (suppl.) 507:91–101.

Owen, O.E., Robinson, R.R. (1963): Amino acid extraction and ammonia metabolism by the human kidney during the prolonged administration of ammonium chloride. *J. Clin. Invest.* 42:263–276.

Pain, V.M., Manchester, K.L. (1970): The influence of electrical stimulation in vitro on protein synthesis and other metabolic parameters of rat extensor digitorum longus muscle. *Biochem. J.* 118:209–220.

Palombo, J.D., Maletskos, C.J., Reinhold, R.V., et al. (1981): Composition of weight loss in morbidly obese after gastric bypass. *J. Surg. Res.* 30:435–442.

Pozefsky, T., Felig, P., Tobin, J.D. (1969): Amino acid balance across tissues of the forearm in post-absorptive man. Effects of insulin at dose levels. *J. Clin. Invest.* 48:2273–2282.
Pozefsky, T., Tancredi, R.G., Moxley, R.T., et al. (1970): Effects of brief starvation on muscle amino acid metabolism in non-obese man. *J. Clin. Invest.* 57:444–459.
Rhoades, J.E., Alexander, C.E. (1955): Nutritional problems of surgical patients. *Ann. N.Y. Acad. Sci.* 63:218–275.
Rosenoer, V.M., Skillman, J.J., Hastings, P.R. (1980): Albumin synthesis and nitrogen balance in postoperative patients. *Surgery* 87:305–312.
Sakamoto, A., Moldawer, L.L., Usui, S., et al. (1979): Are the nitrogen sparing mechanisms of branched chain amino acids really unique? *Surg. Forum* 30:67–69.
Sakamoto, A., Moldawer, L.L., Palombo, J.D., et al. (1982): Alterations in tyrosine and protein kinetics produced by injury and branched chain amino acids. *Clin. Sci.* (In press).
Shenkin, A., Nauhauser, M., Wretlin, A., et al. (1980): Biochemical changes associated with severe trauma. *Am. J. Clin. Nutr.* 33:2119–2127.
Shipley, R.A., Clark, R.E. (1972): *Tracer Methods for In Vivo Kinetics.* Academic Press, New York.
Shizgal, H.M., Spanier, A.H., Humes, J., et al. (1977): Indirect measurement of total exchangeable potassium. *Am. J. Physiol.* 233:F253–259, 1977.
Skillman, J.J., Rosenoer, V.M., Smith, P.C., et al. (1976): Improved albumin synthesis in postoperative patients by amino acid infusions. *N. Engl. J. Med.* 294:1031–1040.
Sobrado, J., Maiz, A., Kawamura, I., et al. (1983): Effect of dietary protein depletion on non-specific immune responses and survival to pseudomonas pneumonia in the guinea pig. *Am. J. Clin. Nutr.* (In press).
Stein, T.P., Leskiw, M.J., Wallace, H.W., et al. (1977): Changes in protein synthesis after trauma. Importance of nutrition. *Am. J. Physiol.* 233:E348–355.
Stein, T.P., Mullen, J., Oram-Smith, J., et al. (1978): Relative rates of human gastrointestinal tumor, normal tissue, liver, and fibrinogen synthesis. *Am. J. Physiol.* 234:E648–652.
Stein, T.P., Buzby, G., Leskiw, M., et al. (1982a): Parenteral nutrition and human gastrointestinal tumor protein metabolism. *Cancer* 49:1476–1480.
Stein, T.P. (1982b): Nutrition and protein turnover, a review. *J. Parent. Enter. Nutr.* 41 (In press).
Stinnett, J.D., Alexander, J.W., Watanabe, C., et al. (1982): Plasma and skeletal muscle amino acids following severe burn injury in patients and experimental animals. *Ann. Surg.* 195:75–89.
Wahren, J., Felig, P., Hagerfeldt, L. (1976): Effect of protein ingestion on splanchnic and leg metabolism in normal man and in patients with diabetes mellitus. *J. Clin. Invest.* 57:987–999.
Wannemacher, R.W. (1977): Key role of various individual amino acids in host response to infection. *Am. J. Clin. Nutr.* 30:1269–1280.
Waterlow, J.C., Stephens, J.M.L. (1967): Lysine turnover in man measured by intravenous infusion of L-(U-^{14}C)-lysine. *Clin. Sci.* 33:507–515.
Waterlow, J.C. (1968): Observations on the mechanism of adaptation to low protein intakes. *Lancet* 2:1063–1068.
Waterlow, J.C., Garlick, P.J., Millward, D.J. (1978): *Protein Turnover in Mammalian Tissues and in the Whole Body.* Elsevier/North Holland, New York.
Waterlow, J.C., Stephens, J.M.L. (1982): *Nitrogen Metabolism in Man.* Applied Science Publishers, London.
Wheatley, D.N. (1979): Pools and protein synthesis: Studies with the D and L isomer of leucine. *Cytobio.* 25:193–216.
Wilmore, D.W., Long, J.M., Mason, A.D., et al. (1974): Catecholamines: mediator of the hypermetabolism response to thermal injury. *Ann. Surg.* 180:653–699.
Wolfe, R.R., Goodenough, R.D., Wolfe, M., et al. (1982a): Isotopic analysis of leucine and urea metabolism in exercising humans. *J. Appl. Physiol.* 52:458–466.
Wolfe, R.R., Goodenough, R.D., Burke, J.F., et al. (1982b): Response of protein and urea

kinetics in burned patients to different levels of protein intake. *Ann. Surg.* (In press).

Yang, R.D., Sakamoto, A., Keenan, R.D., et al. (1981): Leukocyte endogenous mediator alters protein dynamics in the rat. *Fed. Proc.* 40:3809A.

Young, V.R., Hussein, M.A., Murray, E., et al. (1971): Plasma tryptophan response cuve and its relationship to tryptophan requirement in young adult man. *J. Nutrition* 101:45–54.

Young, V.R., Kraisid, T., Scrimshaw N.S., et al. (1972): Plasma amino acid response curves and amino acid requirements in young men: Valine and lysine. *J. Nutrition* 102:1159–1167.

Young, V.R., Munro, H.N. (1976): 3-methylhistidine and protein turnover, a review. *Fed. Proc.* 37:2291–2300.

Young, V.R., Robert, J.J., Motil, K.J., et al. (1981): Protein and energy intake in relation to protein turnover in man. In: *Nitrogen Metabolism in Man* (eds: Waterlow, J.C., Stephens, J.M.L.) Applied Sciences Publishers, London.

17 Nutritional Consideration of Amino Acid Profiles in Clinical Therapy

Calvin L. Long

The metabolic response to injury and infection has been characterized by a number of biochemical changes that clearly interweave a number of metabolic pathways. The postinjury state is associated with an increased urinary nitrogen loss resulting from increased whole body and muscle protein breakdown as well as an increase in resting metabolic expenditure, as shown in Figure 17-1 (Long et al., 1979). Unlike starvation without injury, these hypercatabolic patients suffer profound and rapid weight loss due to the inability to "starvation adapt." Therefore, the erosion of muscle mass is thought to occur due to an energy-starved peripheral cell. As the muscle become insulin resistant (possibly more so than adipose tissue) and unable to effectively utilize glucose, and as ketones are not abundant, the muscle utilizes its own amino acids as a source of energy. This process associated with oxidation of branched-chain amino acids, with the release of large amounts of other amino acids into the circulation, has a profound effect on the patterns of blood and tissue amino acids observed during catabolic states.

The ability of the body to perform in an optimal manner depends on the availability of adequate protein and calorie intake on a daily basis. This was clearly reinforced (Rose, 1957) in defining the requirements for essential amino acids in normal man, utilizing nitrogen balance as the end point. Limited protein synthesis occurs with a deficit of any one or all essential amino acids, as shown by a number of

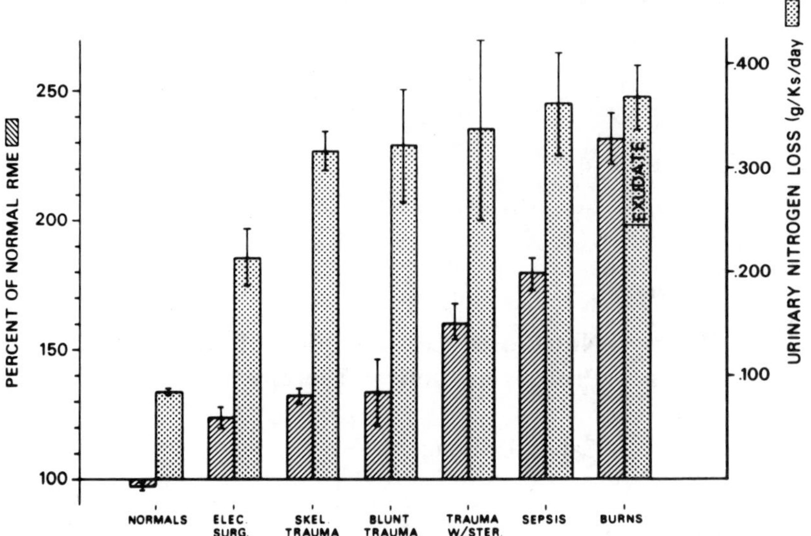

Figure 17-1 Percent increases above normal resting metabolic expenditures and increases in urinary nitrogen in g/kg/day in injured and ill patients.

investigators. On the other hand, excess amino acids, beyond those required for protein synthesis, are deaminated, and the carbon residues are used for energy. The magnitude of the free amino acid pool suggests that it would be instructive to examine the intracellular compartment of amino acids as a means of revealing changes in amino acid metabolism associated with deficits both from malnutrition as well as from demands imposed on the host during hypercatabolic responses to illness and injury. Since the pool of total free amino acids is quite small and the extracellular pool represents only about 1% of the total free amino acids, the patterns exhibited in plasma have dubious significance according to some investigators. Is this assumption really true? This presentation will discuss the observed changes in both free amino acid compartments in relation to nutritional concerns during starvation and disease states.

AMINO ACID PATTERNS IN STARVATION

The amino acid patterns seen in starvation represent an excess of certain amino acids and the absence of intake as the body rearranges its use priority of amino acids derived from endogenous protein breakdown for economy for organ function. Fasting plasma amino acid patterns as presented in Figure 17-2 (Felig et al., 1969), showing an initial increase in branched-chain amino acids, certain other amino acids as phenylalanine, tyrosine, methionine, followed by a decline after five to seven days except for phenylalanine and methionine. Similar results have been reported (Adibi, 1971). Glycine levels show an increase during this transition phase, and alanine shows a continual decrease. These changes reflect increased branched-chain amino acid utilization and increased gluconeogenesis, followed by a starvation adaptation pattern associated with decreased muscle protein breakdown. In general, plasma levels in starvation conditions show an overall decrease in plasma amino acids, an increased ratio of glycine to valine, phenylalanine to tyrosine, and low essential amino acid to nonessential ratio. These changes revert to normal patterns with the provision of adequate protein and calories.

Nutritional considerations of amino acid patterns in starvation without stress based on the plasma changes have been revealing. The plasma amino acid response of both man and animal to amino acid deficient diets has been used as a basis for assessing requirements in such states. For example, Kang-Lee and Harper (1977) showed that the plasma level of histidine in animal studies was responsive to increased levels of histidine intake. The plasma and muscle concentrations of the amino acid evolved in a change according to an S-shaped curve when the histidine intake concentration ranged from deficient levels to those exceeding the requirement. This response is not unique to histidine. McLaughlin and Illman (1967) used the changes in free plasma amino acid levels for the estimation of the requirement for various amino acids in the growing rat. Also, Zimmerman and Scott (1965) measured the response of amino acids in plasma of chicks who were given graded levels of arginine, lysine or valine to an otherwise adequate diet. When these amino acids were provided in excess of that needed to maximize weight gain, there was a rapid and linear increase of that amino acid in plasma. Similar data on the requirement for tryptophan, lysine and valine have been reported in the adult man (Young et al., 1971, 1972).

In addition to nitrogen balance and plasma amino acid concentrations as indicators of adequacy of a given essential amino acid, the concept of measuring the level of expired radioactive carbon dioxide from a labeled essential amino acid in relation to intake has been used. Since there is no storage of amino acids, any excess in intake beyond that required for protein synthesis will be oxidized. As such, the break point in the response curve $^{14}CO_2$ in the breath with increasing intakes of the test amino acid indicates the point at which the requirement has been met for maintenance of a steady state. Other techniques of amino acid nutrition have been

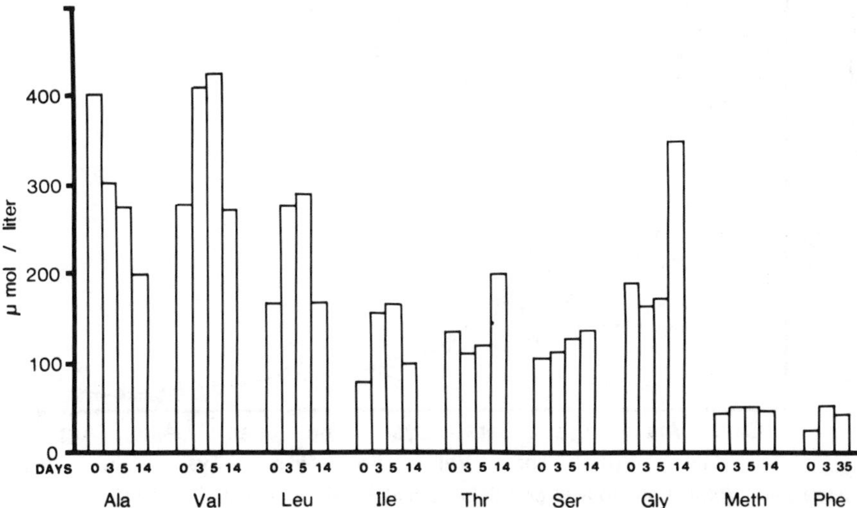

Figure 17-2 Plasma amino acid profiles during starvation. Redrawn from data of Felig et al., 1969.

useful in assessing the requirement of amino acids. The observation that the plasma lysine concentration during intake of wheat protein was below the fasting level and could be reversed by the addition of lysine, prompted Longenecker and Hause (1959) to propose a limiting order of amino acids for specific proteins of varying biological values. They postulated that those amino acids most needed by the tissues for protein synthesis would disappear most rapidly from the plasma after a test meal. The most limiting amino acid in a food protein should be the one that showed the greatest decrease or least increase in the plasma following consumption of the test protein. In these studies with dogs, the calculated plasma amino acid ratios (the difference in amino acid levels before and during intake divided by the requirement) could easily be manipulated from negative to positive ratios by varying the lysine concentration of wheat proteins.

This approach was later explored in man (Yearick and Nadeau, 1967). Using their method, we showed (Long et al., 1974, 1976) that the intravenous infusion of a protein hydrolysate, Aminosol (Abbott Laboratories, Chicago, IL), in control patients was limiting in valine, as well as phenylalanine when the hydrolysate was supplied at a rate of 10 g nitrogen per 24 hours, as shown in Figure 17-3. As indicated, the method compares the fasting plasma essential amino acids to levels taken during infusion of the hydrolysate. Any amino acid concentration during infusion that was below the fasting level suggested a limitation. The numerical ranking of the limiting order was accomplished by dividing the difference in plasma concentration by the estimated requirement for the amino acid. A negative value indicated that the requirement had not been met for that amino acid. If one compares the valine and

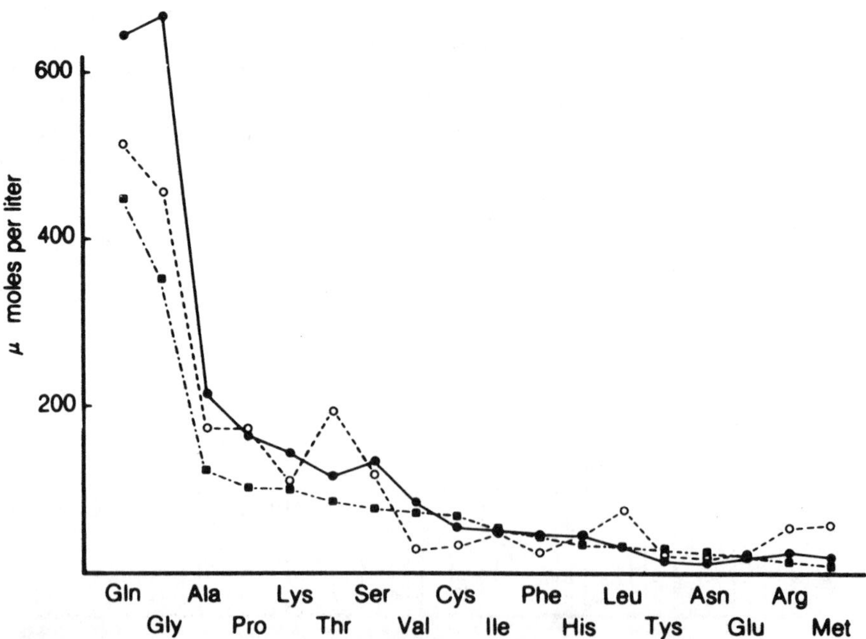

Figure 17-3 Plasma amino acid profile in normal female subject during infusion of a beef fibrin hydrolysate (○) and a crystalline L-amino acid solution (●) compared to her fasting levels (■). From Long, 1977, with permission.

phenylalanine levels in the hydrolysate as supplied by the manufacturer to the estimated requirement for the amino acids in control patients, no limitation should have been evident. However, an analysis of the free amino acids available in the hydrolysate showed that valine and phenylalanine were present to a large extent as peptides in the hydrolysate, and these were shown to be lost via the urine.

Using a variation of the limiting plasma amino acid ratio, Wells and Smits (1980) evaluated and compared the plasma amino acid changes during parenteral nutrition using Aminoplex 5 (Geistlich Sons Ltd., Chester, England) in a group of critically ill patients. They calculated a plasma amino acid elevation ratio by dividing the plasma essential amino acid level during infusion by the infusion level. This ranking order (plasma amino acid elevation ratio) of essential amino acids in these adult patients correlated quite well with the ratios of intake to requirement for the child except for threonine (Figure 17-4).

This observation is in general agreement with the suggestion by Munro (1972) that the sick adult patient may have amino acid requirements more closely related to those of a growing infant. There was a significant correlation of groups of amino acids, i.e., branched-chain group or hepatic group (aromatic), and it was suggested that amino acids that are metabolized predominantly in one tissue, for example, muscle, may also show similar plasma concentrations.

The approaches described here indicate that plasma and tissue amino acid patterns are sensitive indicators of amino acid adequacy and should be of value in establishing amino acid requirements during nutritional rehabilitation of nonstressed patients.

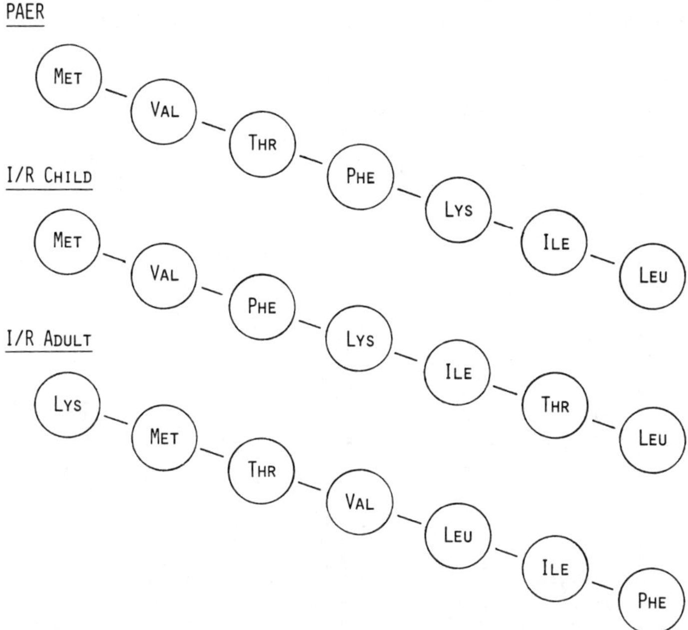

Figure 17-4 Ranking order of plasma amino acid elevation ratio (PAER) during total parenteral nutrition in sick adults as compared to the ratio of intake to requirement for the child and adult. Redrawn from data of Wells et al., 1980.

AMINO ACID PATTERNS IN STRESSED STATES

The patterns of blood amino acids in a starvation state reflect the balance between the release of amino acids and utilization in various tissues. In the early phase of starvation, prior to the increased production and utilization of ketone bodies, the glycogen reserves and carbon from the deamination of amino acids, as well as glycerol, are used for energy. The increase in the branched-chain plasma amino acids as well as the aromatic and sulfur amino acids is evident. As starvation adaptation occurs after five to ten days, the concentration of branched-chain amino acids decreases, and the aromatic and sulfur amino acids tend to stabilize. These changes accompany the conservation of the body protein as fasting is continued. The observed changes in plasma amino acid patterns during minor stress, such as elective operation, tend to follow the same patterns as observed in starvation. Thus, there is an initial rise in the branched-chain amino acids, as well as a rise in phenylalanine and methionine. A decrease is also evident for alanine.

These adaptive responses are absent in the seriously injured and septic patient. In these hypercatabolic states there is continuation of increased urinary nitrogen loss associated with an increase in whole body protein breakdown, as measured with ^{15}N alanine or ^{14}C leucine as shown in Figure 17-5 (Birkhahn et al., 1981; Long et al., 1977). The muscle contribution to this increase in whole body protein breakdown, as measured by a three- to fourfold increase in urinary 3-methylhistidine, may be as much as 40% as shown in Figure 17-6 (Long et al., 1981a,b). In addition, the septic (Clowes et al., 1976) or trauma patient (Birkhahn et al., 1981) cannot produce ketone bodies at an adequate rate during these starvation states (Figure 17-7). Even though skeletal trauma patients were maintained on lactated Ringers solution for three days posttrauma, the plasma free fatty acid and ketone body levels were not elevated, as can be seen in Figure 17-8. The respiratory quotients in these patients averaged 0.76, indicating about 68% of the energy was derived from fat oxidation.

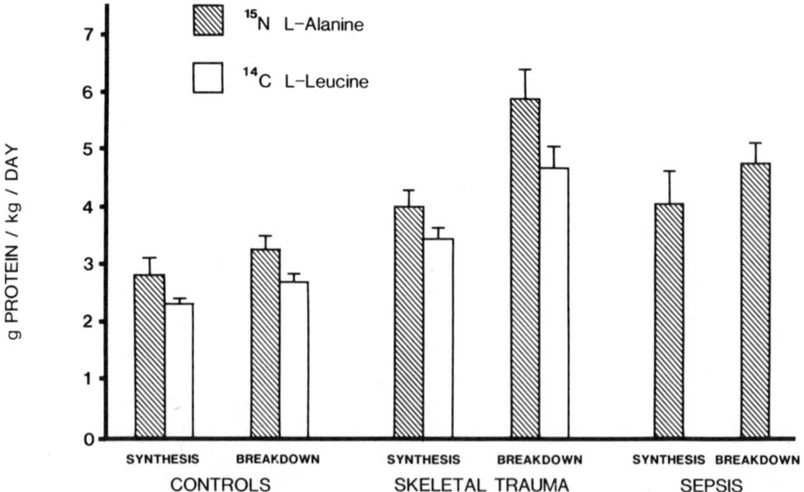

Figure 17-5 Whole body protein metabolism in controls during sepsis or following skeletal trauma using ^{15}N-L-alanine or ^{14}C-L-leucine. Redrawn from data from Long et al., 1977; Birkhahn, 1980; Birkhahn et al., 1981.

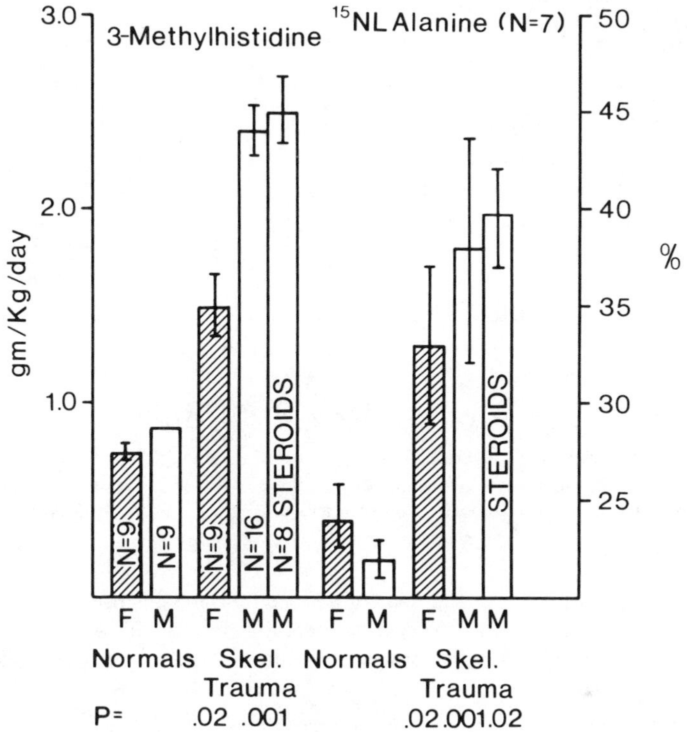

Figure 17-6 Evaluation of the contribution of muscle protein to whole body protein catabolism using 24-hour urinary 3-methylhistidine and ^{15}N-L-alanine turnover rates in the same skeletal trauma patients.

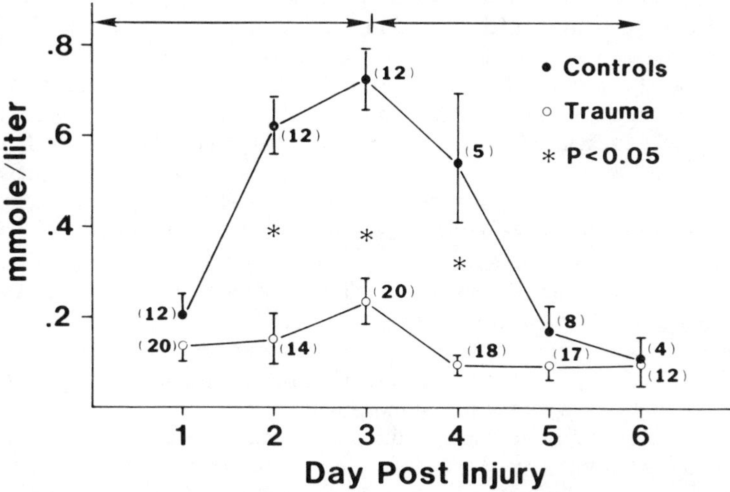

Figure 17-7 A comparison of total plasma ketones in trauma and control subjects during a three-day fast and three days of carbohydrate intake. Each point is the mean ± SEM of the number of subjects listed and * indicates significance at $p \leq .05$. From Birkhahn et al., 1981, with permission.

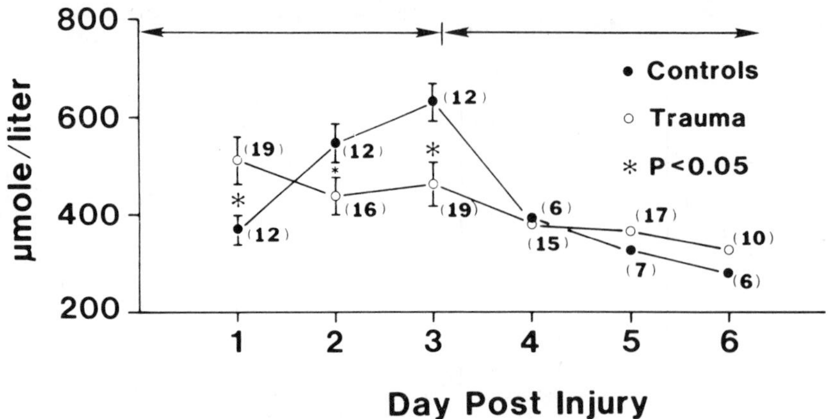

Figure 17-8 A comparison of serum free fatty acids in trauma and control subjects during a three-day fast and three days of carbohydrate intake. Each point is mean ± SEM of the number of patients and * indicates significance at p ≤ .05. From Birkhahn, 1981, with permission.

Associated with these changes is an increased plasma glucose and insulin in the trauma patient (Figure 17-9). It is evident there that fat is mobilized, but possibly its rate is diminished in the stressed state. It should be pointed out that these conclusions of nonketotic response are based on plasma concentrations. Final confirmation rests with the direct estimate of turnover rates in such catabolic states, a problem we are currently evaluating with ^{14}C-β-hydroxybutyrate infusions.

It is interesting to note that during the first five to seven days following severe injury, the provision of amino acids and calories will provide for a less negative nitrogen balance. However, regardless of the intake, using conventional amino acid solutions, it is extremely difficult, and in some cases impossible, to obtain a positive nitrogen balance. As more nitrogen is infused, there is a greater loss via the urine. The increased excretion of 3-methylhistidine in the severely traumatized patient is not reduced during total parenteral nutrition as reported (Shenkin et al., 1980) or during 3% amino acid infusions over a period of three days (Table 17-1); however, a more positive nitrogen balance with continual excretion of the same quantities of 3-methylhistidine suggest an increased synthesis of muscle and organ protein with no change in rate of muscle breakdown. Even with this reduced efficiency of amino acid utilization, it is important to ameliorate the negative nitrogen balance by the provision of amino acids and calories. Fueling the fire of catabolism and at the same time increasing protein synthesis with amino acid infusions points to a definition of increase in certain indispensable and dispensable amino acids in such stressed states. It may be more appropriate to suggest that this is a pathological requirement, as the requirement will change as the patient convalesces.

Does the extent of the insult produce a different requirement for a given amino acid or acids? Insight on this question may be drawn from the earlier studies reported by us, relative to the use of beef fibrin protein hydrolysate (Aminosol) in septic patients (Long et al., 1976). The plasma amino acid profile of a septic patient on various levels of nitrogen intake is shown in Figure 17-10. It is clear that the levels of valine, phenylalanine and methionine are below the fasting levels at 8 and 12 g

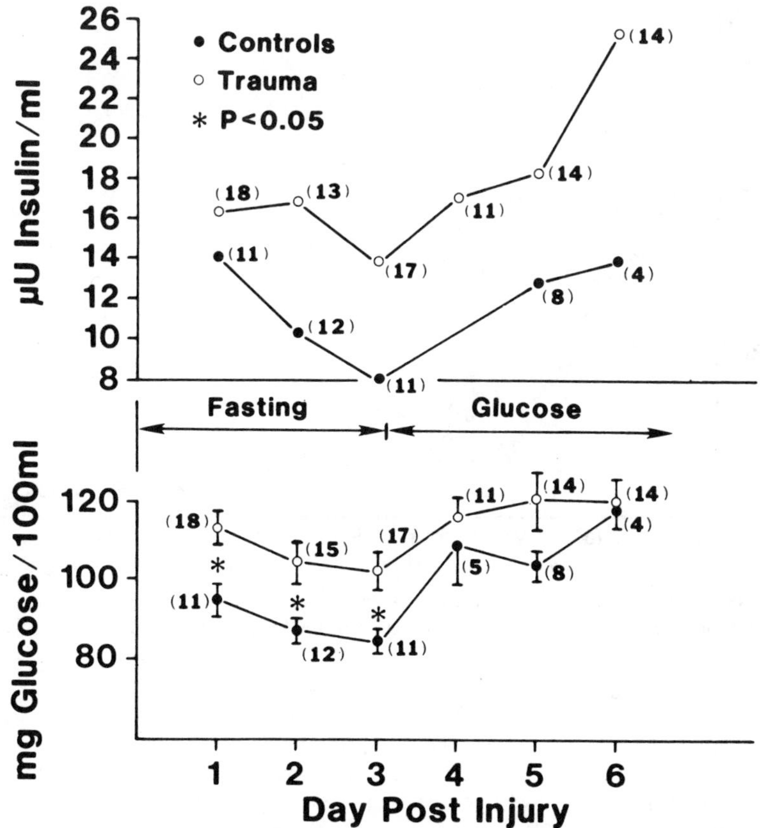

Figure 17-9 A comparison of plasma insulin and glucose in trauma and control subjects during a three-day fast and three days of carbohydrate intake. Each point is the mean of the number of patients and * indicates significance at p ≤ .05. From Birkhahn et al., 1981.

Table 17-1
Urinary Excretion of 3-Methylhistidine in Skeletal Trauma Patients on 5% Glucose or 3% Amino Acids Compared to Controls

Group	Number Patients	3-Methylhistidine 5% Glucose	μM/kg/day 3% Amino Acids
Skeletal trauma	N = 22; 5	10.1 ± 0.6	10.2 ± 0.8
Sepsis	N = 4	8.2 ± 0.6	–
Controls	N = 9; 6	3.6 ± 0.2	3.29 ± 0.1

nitrogen intake per day, but were higher at 22 g nitrogen intake. The results presented in Table 17-2 show the reliability of the method using other septic patients and also reveal that the above amino acids as well as others appear to be limiting. If all the essential amino acids were increased proportionally in sepsis, leucine should not be limiting, as it was given at 7.3 times the MDR, lysine at 2.6 times, and isoleucine at 2.1 times. Thus, it appears that the requirement for each amino acid is

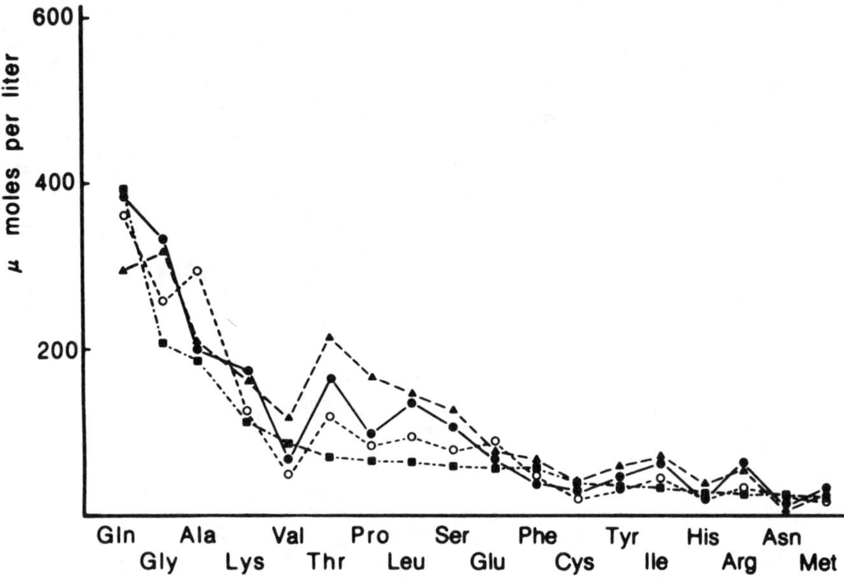

Figure 17-10 Plasma amino acid profile in a septic male patient during infusions of 8 g (○), 12 g (●), or 21 g (△) nitrogen per day compared to his fasting levels (■). From Long et al., 1977, with permission.

not altered to the same extent after injury and that the pattern of amino acid requirements is not constant under these conditions.

Abnormal plasma amino acid patterns in burns, skeletal trauma and sepsis have been reported by many investigators, and there is general agreement in regard to certain specific amino acid pattern alterations. Sepsis, trauma, and burn patients all show an increase in the concentration of plasma phenylalanine and methionine and a decrease in glutamine, glycine, and threonine. The branched-chain amino acid concentrations in plasma are variable, but most reports show that they are stable or increased during sepsis (Mylewski et al., 1982; Clowes et al., 1980; Cerra et al., 1979; Blackburn and Flatt, 1974; Freund et al., 1978). Decreased levels have also been reported (Wannemacher et al., 1977; Woolf et al., 1976) in man as well as in the dog (Woolf et al., 1979). Minimal changes have been reported in adult burned patients (Aulick and Wilmore, 1979) and a decrease in burned children (Stinnett et al., 1982). Decreased levels have also been reported in hepatic cirrhosis (Cerra et al., 1979; Fischer et al., 1975). The changes reported for the branched-chain acids in plasma following skeletal trauma are also variable; however, most indicate no change or increases (Woolf et al., 1976; Askanazi et al., 1978; Furst et al., 1979; Vinnars et al., 1976; Geiger et al., 1980; Long, 1977). Some of these variations are due to the degree of insult as well as the variations in time of blood sampling and type of infusion being received by the patient. The majority of the reports relate to studies where the patient was receiving 5% glucose solutions, although others indicate blood sampling following discontinuation of infusions for varying periods of time.

We have evaluated for plasma profiles three days following injury 21 skeletal trauma patients receiving 5% glucose and observed a trend toward an increase in the branched-chain amino acid group, but this was not statistically significant

Table 17-2
Order of Limiting Amino Acids Using Plasma Amino Acid Ratios in Patients Given Fibrin Hydrolysate

Patient	Condition	Nitrogen Intake (g)	Amino Acid Order	Ratio
LS	Normal	10	Val, phe	−
			Lys, met, leu, ile, thr	+
JC	Normal	10	Val, phe	−
			Met, ile, leu, lys, thr	+
HD-1	Septic	10	Val, lys, phe, leu	−
			Met, thr, ile	+
HD-2	Septic	10	Val, lys, phe, leu	−
			Met, ile, thr	+
HD-3	Septic	15	Val, phe	−
			Leu, met, lys, ile, thr	+
SG-1	Septic	10	Val, lys, ile	−
			Met, phe, leu, thr	+
SG-2	Septic	10	Val, ile, phe	−
			Met, lys, leu, thr	+
SG-3	Septic	15	Val, ile, thr, lys, phe	−
			Met, leu	+
GM-1	Septic	6	Val, phe, met	−
			Lys, ile, leu, thr	+
GM-2	Septic	12	Val, phe,	−
			Met, ile, leu, lys, thr	+
GM-3	Septic	22	None	
			Met, phe, val, ile, lys, leu, thr	+

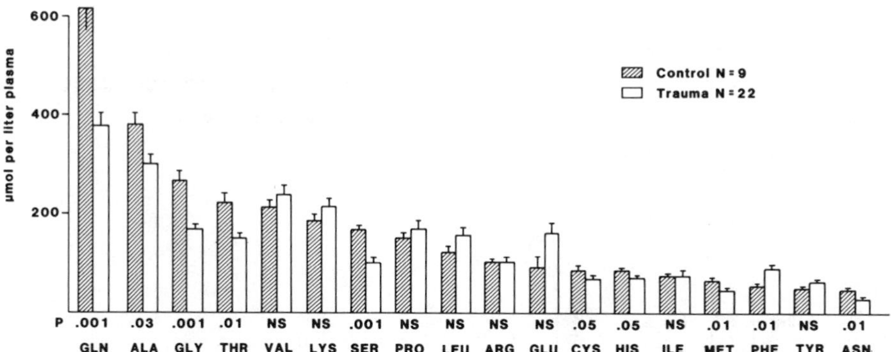

Figure 17-11 Plasma amino acid profiles on the third day following skeletal trauma in patients receiving 5% glucose solutions.

(Figure 17-11). When comparison was made to similar patients after an 18-hour postabsorptive period (Figure 17-12) or three days while receiving lactated Ringers (Figure 17-13), the increases in valine and leucine but not isoleucine were significant ($p < 0.05$).

In addition to the above possible reasons for reported variations in skeletal trauma plasma amino acid profiles as well as those during sepsis, it is possible that

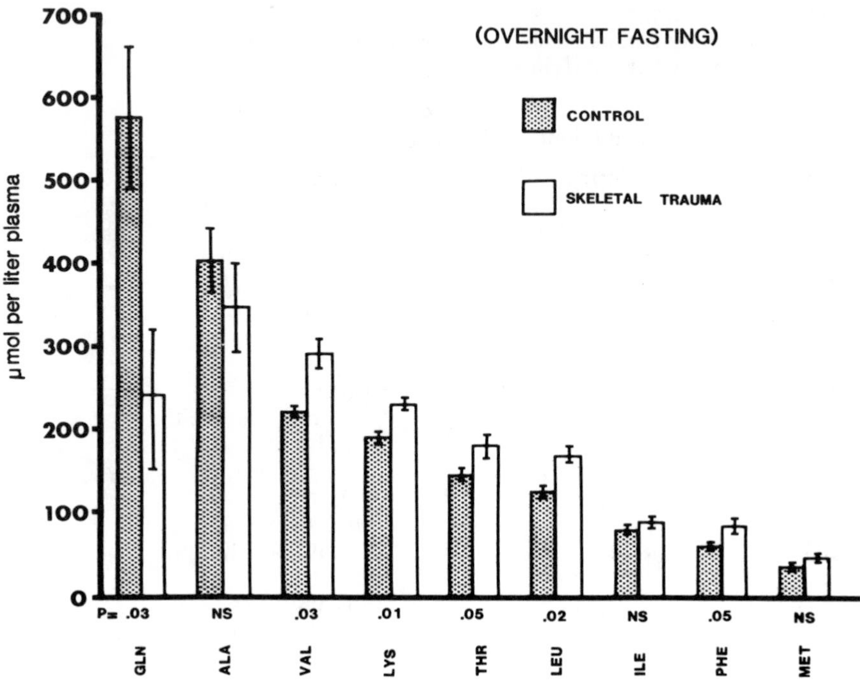

Figure 17-12 Plasma amino acid profiles on the third day following skeletal trauma in patients in an 18-hour postabsorptive state.

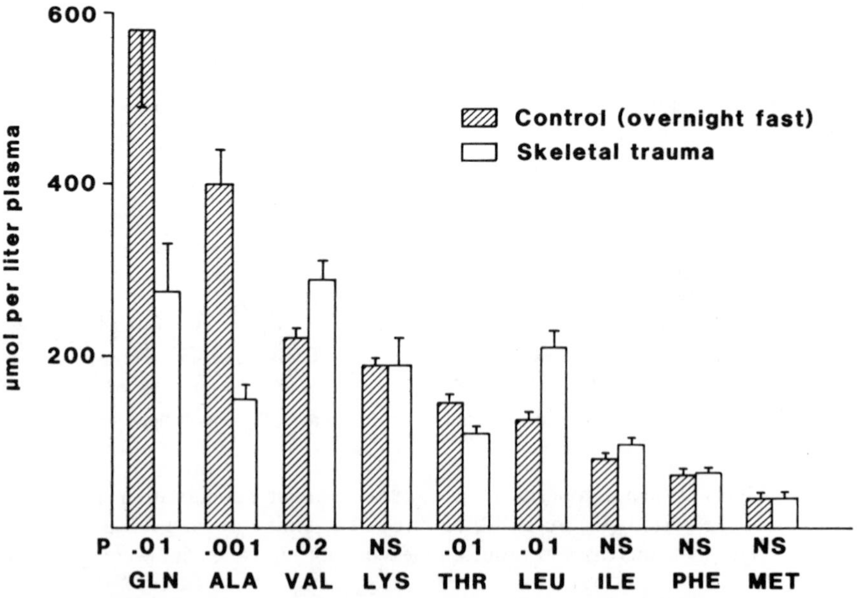

Figure 17-13 Plasma amino acid profiles on the third day following skeletal trauma in patients receiving lactated Ringers solution.

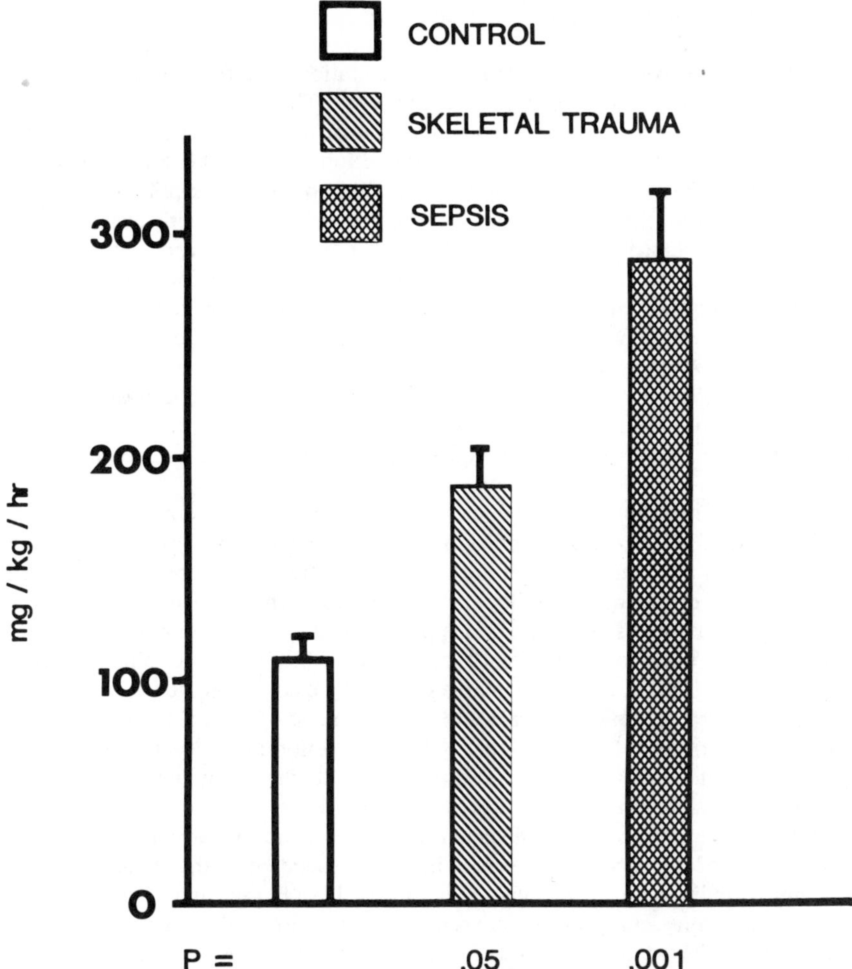

Figure 17-14 Glucose turnover rates in control, septic, and skeletal trauma patients using ^{14}C-U-L-glucose.

the substrate needs of the septic patient may be somewhat different based on the greatly increased glucose turnover rates compared to skeletal trauma as seen in Figure 17-14 (Long et al., 1971). One may conjecture that the increased need of amino acids and glucose energy for protein synthesis of acute phase proteins in liver as well as the increased energy need for glucose by the immune system and wound healing following infection determines the plasma amino acid profile format for such a picture. These considerations are compatible with the fact that septic patients invariably exhibit a higher blood glucose level and increased glucose pool size.

Measurements of muscle samples, obtained by biopsy, indicate intracellular free amino acid concentrations of all the essential amino acids are increased except lysine in sepsis and trauma (Mylewski et al., 1982; Askanazi et al., 1978; Furst et al., 1979; Vinnars et al., 1976). The variation in the plasma compartment, therefore, must be related to the extent of oxidation, gluconeogenesis and reutilization of amino acids within the intracellular compartment. On the assumption that the results obtained in the septic patients used in this comparison presentation were from those in a "high-flow" state, increased gluconeogenesis would prevail. This logically should provide a picture of an increased branched chain and a decrease in alanine concentration in the plasma compartment as in the case of early starvation. On the other hand, decreased branched-chain amino acids in the plasma compartment of septic patients, as reported by several other investigators, may be the result of increasing liver dysfunction as well as reduced release of branched-chain amino acids from the periphery (Woolf et al., 1979). In support of this changing organ function, the increased gluconeogenic reponse early in sepsis has been shown to be curtailed in endstage septicemia in rats (Wannemacher et al., 1971) and in *E. coli* shocked dogs (Woolf et al., 1979) with concomitant increases in glucogenic amino acids. Similar responses have been reported (Wilmore et al., 1976) in burned patients who develop positive blood cultures for gram-negative organisms. The decreased conversion of amino acids to glucose in these "low-flow" states was accompanied by an increased trend toward hypoglycemia.

If it is assumed that increases in certain plasma amino acids and reduced levels of others reflect abnormal or inappropriate responses, correcting such changes by manipulation of the composition of the amino acid infusion mixture is a logical step in the treatment of the injured or ill patient. This approach has been used in the formulation of a mixture of amino acids rich in branched-chain amino acids and low in aromatic amino acids to complement the plasma profile in hepatic failure (Fischer et al., 1975). This approach is acceptable only if the changes are due to the lack of ability to metabolize those amino acids that are in excess of normal levels and an increased ability to metabolize those that reduce below normal concentrations. Thus, assessment of the nutritional requirements of critically ill patients may be based, in part, on plasma amino acid profiles. However, plasma amino acid patterns in chronic uremia appear to be too divergent from their intracellular counterpart, and normalization of such profiles appears to be more dependent on the manipulation of intracellular amino acid levels (Furst et al., 1978). Low intracellular concentrations of valine, threonine and tyrosine were reported to be corrected by addition of these amino acids to the standard mixture of essential amino acids (Rose, 1957). Concerning the possible requirement of a given amino acid based on conservation of free amino acid concentrations in blood and tissue, the decrease in intracellular lysine in sepsis and trauma (Mylewski et al., 1982; Askanazi et al., 1978; Furst et al., 1979; Vinnars et al., 1976) would suggest that this amino acid may be rate limiting for protein synthesis. Provision of lysine to a complete amino acid solution and a calorie source in the stressed patient may be beneficial.

The above-noted decreases in the branched-chain amino acids in plasma in the critically ill hepatic failure patient, as well as the decrease noted for valine in the intracellular compartment of the chronic renal failure patient, speaks for the provision of branched-chain amino acids on a therapeutic basis. As noted in this presentation, the branched-chain amino acids are not decreased but more often are elevated in plasma and muscle in trauma and sepsis. From a concentration point of view, the metabolism of these amino acids for energy in the peripheral cell should result in a decrease in these compartments. The question then is why the concentrations are increased. Does this suggest that the nonadapted stressed patient is responding as in the case of early starvation? Based on these observations, one would not assume that treatment of choice is an addition of these acids to an infusion solution. In spite of these observations, it appears that the provision of a generous intake of one or more branched chain does, in fact, significantly improve nitrogen balance in patients (Freund et al., 1978a,b; Blackburn et al., 1979; Lindberg and Clowes, 1981; Eriksson et al., 1981; Elia et al., 1980; Hagenfeldt et al., 1980). These changes are associated with a normalization in plasma phenylalanine suggesting increased protein synthesis. This indicates an increased requirement for branched-chain amino acids in such stressed states, in spite of the amino acid patterns that one observes clinically.

In summary, it is clear that measurement of extracellular and intracellular patterns of amino acids observed in various stressed states suggests need to reconsider the adequacy of current mixtures of amino acids used for nutritional therapy; however, a more quantitative approach utilizing both plasma and tissue amino acid patterns, combined with additional metabolic data, is required in order to optimize formulating amino acid solutions for the nutritional care of the critically ill patient.

REFERENCES

Adibi, S.A. (1971): Interrelationships between level of amino acids in plasma and tissues during starvation. *Am. J. Physiol.* 221:829–838.

Askanazi, J., Elwyn, D.H., Kinney, J.M., Gump, F.E., Michelson, C.B., and Stinchfield, F.E. (1978): Muscle and plasma amino acids after injury: The role of inactivity. *Ann. Surg.* 188:797–803.

Aulick, L.H. and Wilmore, D.W. (1979): Increased peripheral amino acid release following burn injury. *Surgery* 85:560–565.

Birkhahn, R.H., Long, C.L., Fitkin, D., Jeevanandam, M., and Blakemore, W.S. (1981): Whole body protein metabolism due to trauma in man as estimated by ^{15}N-L-alanine. *Am. J. Physiol.* 241:E64–E71.

Birkhahn, R.H., Long, C.L., Fitkin, D.L., Busnardo, A.C., Geiger, J.W., and Blakemore, W.S. (1981): A comparison of the effects of skeletal trauma and surgery on the ketosis of starvation in man. *J. Trauma* 21:513–519.

Blackburn, G.L. and Flatt, J.P. (1974): Substrate profile in protein wasting states. In: *Protein Nutrition* (ed: Brown, H.), pp. 201–228, Charles C. Thomas, Springfield, IL.

Blackburn, G.L., Moldawer, L.L., Usui, S., Bothe, A., O'Keefe, S.J.D., and Bistrian, B.R. (1979): Branched chain amino acid administration and metabolism during starvation, injury and infection. *Surgery* 86:307–315.

Cerra, F.B., Siegel, J.H., Border, J.R., Wiles, J., and McMenamy, R.R. (1979): The hepatic failure of sepsis: Cellular vs. substrate. *Surgery* 86:409–422.

Clowes, G.H.A., Jr., O'Donnell, T.F., Blackburn, G.L., and Maki, T. (1976): Energy metabolism and proteolysis in traumatized and septic man. *Surg. Clin. N. Am.* 56:1169–1184.

Clowes, G.H.A., Randall, H.T., and Cha, C.J. (1980): Amino acid and energy metabolism in septic and traumatized patients. *J.P.E.N.,* 4:195–205.

Elia, M., Farrell, R., Ilic, V., Smith, R., and Williamson, D.H. (1980): The removal of infused leucine after injury, starvation and other conditions in man. *Clin. Sci.* 59:275–283.

Eriksson, S., Hagenfeldt, L., and Wahren, J. (1981): A comparison of the effects of intravenous infusion of individual branched-chain amino acids on blood amino acid levels in man. *Clin. Sci.* 60:95–100.

Felig, P., Owen, O.E., Wahren, J., and Cahill, G.F. (1969): Amino acid metabolism during prolonged starvation. *J. Clin. Invest.* 48:584–594.

Fischer, J.F., Funovics, J.M., Aguirre, A., James, J.H., Keane, J.M., Wesdorp, R.I.C., Yoshimura, N., and Westman, T. (1975): The role of plasma amino acids in hepatic encephalopathy. *Surgery* 78:276–290.

Freund, H.R., Ryan, J.A., and Fischer, J.E. (1978a): Amino acid derangements in patients with sepsis: Treatment with branched chain amino acid rich infusions. *Ann. Surg.* 188:423–430.

Freund, H., Yoshimura, N., Lunetta, L., and Fischer, J.E. (1978b): The role of branched chain amino acids in decreasing muscle catabolism in vivo. *Surgery* 83:611–618.

Furst, P., Ahlberg, M., Alvestrand, A., and Bergstrom, J. (1978): Principles of essential amino acid therapy in uremia. *Am. J. Clin. Nutr.* 31:1744–1755.

Furst, P., Bergstrom, J., Chao, L, Larsson, J., Liljedahl, S-O., Neuhauser, M., Schildt, B., and Vinnars, E. (1979): Influence of amino acid supply on nitrogen and amino acid metabolism in severe trauma. *Acta. Chir. Scand.* (Supp.) 494:136–138.

Geiger, J.W., Long, C.L., Birkhahn, R.H., Betts, J.E., and Blakemore, W.S. (1980): Plasma amino acid profiles in patients following major skeletal trauma. *Fed. Proc.* 39:1042.

Hagenfeldt, L, Erikkson, S., and Wahren, J. (1980): Influence of leucine on arterial concentrations and regional exchange of amino acids in healthy subjects.

Kang-Lee, Y.A. and Harper, A.E. (1977): Effect of histidine intake and hepatic histadase activity on the metabolism of histidine in vivo. *J. Nutr.* 107:1427–1443.

Lindberg, B.O. and Clowes, G.H.A., Jr. (1981): The effects of hyperalimentation and infused leucine on the amino acid metabolism in sepsis: An experimental study in vivo. *Surgery* 90:278–291.

Long, C.L., Schaffel, N., Geiger, J.W., Schiller, W.R., and Blakemore, W.S. (1979): Metabolic response to injury and illness: Estimation of energy and protein needs from indirect calorimetry and nitrogen balance. *J.P.E.N.,* 3:452–456.

Long, C.L., Zikria, B.A., Kinney, J.M., and Geiger, J.W. (1974): Comparison of fibrin hydrolysates and crystalline amino acid solutions in parenteral nutrition. *Am. J. Clin. Nutr.* 27:163–174.

Long, C.L., Crosby, F., Geiger, J.W., and Kinney, J.M. (1976): Parenteral nutrition in the septic patient: Nitrogen balance, limiting plasma amino acids, and calorie to nitrogen ratios. *Am. J. Clin. Nutr.* 29:380–391.

Long, C.L., Jeevanandam, M., Kim, B.M., and Kinney, J.M. (1977): Whole body protein synthesis and catabolism in septic man. *Am. J. Clin. Nutr.* 30:1340–1344.

Long, C.L., Birkhahn, R.H., Geiger, J.W., Betts, J.E., Schiller, W.R., and Blakemore, W.S. (1981a): Urinary excretion of 3-methylhistidine: An assessment of muscle protein catabolism in adult normal subjects and during malnutrition, sepsis and skeletal trauma. *Metabolism* 30:765–776.

Long, C.L., Birkhahn, R.H., Geiger, J.W., and Blakemore, W.S. (1981b): Contribution of skeletal muscle protein in elevated rates of whole body protein catabolism in trauma patients. *Am. J. Clin. Nutr.* 34:1087–1093.

Long, C.L. (1977): Clinical applications of amino acid patterns in injured patients with different mixtures of ideal solutions. *Clinical Nutrition Update: Amino Acids,* pp. 116–123, American Medical Association.

Long, C.L., Spencer, J.L., Kinney, J.M., and Geiger, J.W. (1971): Carbohydrate metabolism in man: Effect of elective operations and major injury. *J. Appl. Physiol.* 31:110–116.

Longenecker, J.B. and Hause, N.L. (1959): Relationship between plasma amino acids and composition of the ingested protein. *Arch. Biochem. Biophys.* 84:46–59.

McLaughlin, J.M. and Illman, W.I. (1967): Use of free plasma amino acid levels for estimation of amino acid requirements of the growing rat. *J. Nutrition* 93:21–24.

Munro, H.N. (1972): Basic concepts in the use of amino acids and protein hydrolysates for parenteral nutrition. In: *Council on Foods and Nutrition, Symposium on Total Parenteral Nutrition,* p. 7, American Medical Association.

Mylewski, P.J., Threlfall, C.J., Heath, D.F., Holbrook, I.B., Wilford, K., and Irving, M.H.

(1982): Intracellular free amino acids in undernourished patients with or without sepsis. *Clin. Sci.* 62:83–91.

Rose, W.C. (1957): The amino acid requirements of adult men. *Nutrition Abstr. Rev.* 27:631.

Shenkin, A., Neuhauser, M., Bergstrom, J., Chao, L., Vinnars, E., Larsson, E., Liljedahl, S-O., Schildt, B., and Furst, P. (1980): Biochemical changes associated with severe trauma. *Am. J. Clin. Nutr.* 33:2119–2127.

Stinnett, J.D., Alexander, J.W., Watanabe, C., Macmillan, B.G., Fischer, J.E., Morris, M.J., Trocki, O., Miskell, P., Edwards, L., and James, H. (1982): Plasma and skeletal muscle amino acids following severe burn injury in patients and experimental animals. *Ann. Surg.* 195:75–89.

Vinnars, E., Bergstrom, J., and Furst, P. (1976): The intracellular free amino acids in moderate and severe trauma. *Acta Chir. Scand.* (Suppl.) 466–76–76A.

Wannemacher, R.W., Jr., Dinterman, R.E., Rayfield, E.J., and Beisel, W.R. (1977): Effect of glucose infusion on the concentration of individual serum free amino acids during sandfly fever in man. *Am. J. Clin. Nutr.* 30:573–578.

Wannemacher, R., Jr., Powanda, M.C., Pekarek, R.S., and Beisel, W.R. (1971): Tissue amino acid flux after exposure of rats to diplococcus pneumoniae. *Infect. Immun.* 4:556–562.

Wells, F.E. and Smits, B.J. (1980): Plasma amino acid relationships during parenteral nutrition. *J.P.E.N.* 4:268–271.

Wilmore, D.W., Mason, A.D., and Pruitt, B.A. (1976): Impaired glucose flow in burn patients with gram negative sepsis. *Surg. Gynecol. Obstet.* 143:720–724.

Woolf, L.I., Groves, A.C., Moore, J.P., Duff, J.H., Finley, R.J., and Loomer, R.L. (1976): Arterial plasma amino acids in patients with serious postoperative infection and in patients with major fractures. *Surgery* 79:283–292.

Woolf, L.I., Groves, A.C., and Duff, J.H. (1979): Amino acid metabolism in dogs with E. coli bacteremic shock. *Surgery* 85:212–218.

Yearick, E.S. and Nadeau, R.G. (1967): Serum amino acid response to isocaloric test meals. *Am. J. Clin. Nutr.* 20:338–344.

Young, V.R., Hussein, M.A., Murray, E., and Scrimshaw, N.S. (1971): Plasma tryptophan response curve and its relation to tryptophan requirement in young adult men. *J. Nutrition* 101:45–59.

Young, V.R., Tontisirin, K., Ozalp, I., Lakshmanan, F., and Scrimshaw, N.S. (1972): Plasma amino acid response curves and amino acid requirements in young men: Valine and lysine. *J. Nutrition* 102:1159–1169.

Zimmerman, R.A. and Scott, H.M. (1965): Interrelationships of plasma amino acid levels and weight gain in chicks as influenced by suboptimal and superoptimal dietary concentrations of single amino acids. *J. Nutrition* 87:13–18.

18 Enteral Administration of Amino Acids in Clinical Nutrition

Yasumi Yugari
Ikuo Ohara
Hiroyuki Ohashi
Toru Takami

Since Dr. Rose's pioneering studies on the human requirements of amino acids in 1949 (Rose, 1949), extensive work with chemically defined diets has been conducted using parenteral and enteral feedings. As early as 1939, various types of protein hydrolysates were made available as a source of amino acids (Elman and Weiner, 1939) and such solutions were widely used for parenteral nutrition. In the 1950s, the synthetic manufacture of amino acids reached an industrial scale in Japan. Production of several amino acids by fermentation provided an ample supply for use in feedings of the hospitalized patient.

Amino acid solutions were first made in Japan in 1956, using an amino acid formula based on earlier studies by Dr. Rose. Crystalline L-amino acids offered distinct advantages over earlier protein hydrolysates since they were both safer and more pure. Also, crystalline amino acids could be freely mixed into any pattern desired. Over the years, various types of infusion solutions were introduced and these were influenced by the progress of research on human amino acid requirements.

The Ajinomoto Company remains the world's largest supplier of crystalline L-amino acids. In 1981, 1000 tons of amino acids were used world-wide for parenteral nutrition and approximately 60% came from Ajinomoto. To this figure, amino acids for enteral nutrition must be added.

ENTERAL FEEDINGS

Enteral amino acid nutrition was extensively studied by Greenstein and his colleagues (1957). In 1957, they proposed the term *chemically defined diet* for any diet containing water-soluble, small molecular weight components, such as amino acids, glucose, vitamins, and minerals, and essential fatty acids. Containing balanced nutrients, the chemically defined diet could support human nutrition. Because the components of these diets are readily absorbed through the intestinal wall, they are very low in residue and minimize colon flora. The chemically defined diet was chosen by NASA as a "space diet" in 1965 (Winitz et al., 1965) and then commercially marketed as a medical diet under the name Vivonex in 1968.

Unfortunately, because of its elemental nature, the taste disturbed patients on prolonged oral use, even with various attempts to flavor the product. Nausea, vomiting, and diarrhea induced by the high osmolarity were additional problems.

We have developed a chemically defined diet, Elental, which can be administered enterally (Figure 18-1). The free amino acids in the diet have been patterned after egg protein. The carbohydrate moiety is an easily digestible dextrin with an average 9-glucose polymer, which will also maintain a low osmolarity. As a total diet replacement, a 20% solution of the formula is recommended, and 2400 ml of the formula will provide 84 g of amino acids and 1800 kcal per day.

		G/100 G
AMINO ACIDS	17 AMINO ACIDS	17.61
CARBOHYDRATE	DEXTRIN	79.37
FAT	SOYBEAN OIL	0.66
VITAMINS	14 VITAMINS	0.17
MINERALS	8 MINERALS	2.02

CALORIE CONTENT	80 G/ PACKAGE
	300 CAL/ PACKAGE
	1 CAL/ ML
OSMOTIC PRESSURE	814 MOSM/L

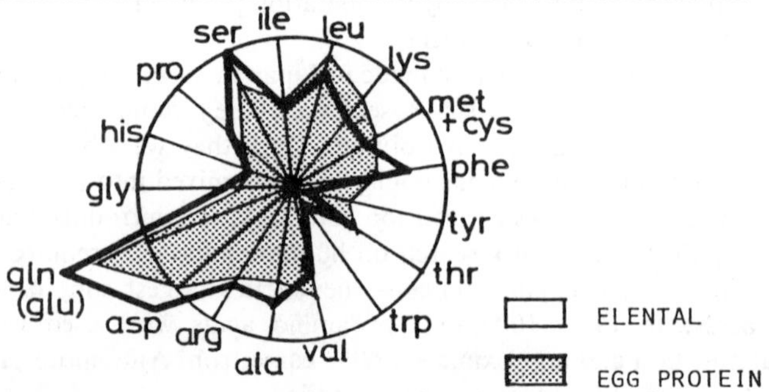

ser ile leu lys met + cys phe tyr thr trp val ala arg asp gln (glu) gly his pro

ELENTAL

EGG PROTEIN

Figure 18-1 Enteral hyperalimentation (Elental).

The efficacy of the diet was examined in rats (Nakatsuji et al., 1979), and the formula was administered by a stomach tube through an artificially created gastric fistula. The principal purpose of this diet in clinical nutrition will be its usefulness for patients undergoing the severe stress of gastrointestinal surgery. As an animal model representing the postoperative stressed state, we used rats with the first third of the small intestine resected and anastomosed end-to-end.

A feeding cannula composed of silastic tubing, 1.5 mm external diameter, tipped with a polyethylene doughnut-shaped disc, was inserted into an artificial gastric fistula and fixed to the gastric wall. The other end of the tubing was tunneled under the skin to the head of the rat. On the top of the skull, a plastic shield (Figure 18-2) was glued with Aron-X. A stainless steel tubing, 1.2 mm external diameter, ran through the shield and was connected to the cannula under the skin.

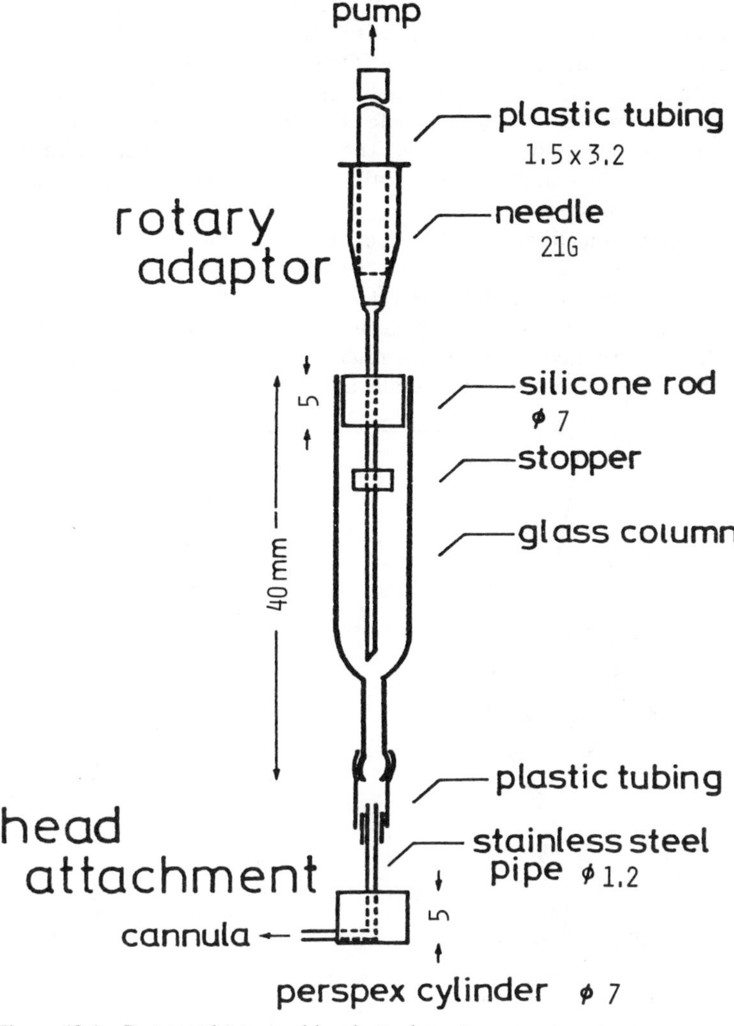

Figure 18-2 Rotary adaptor and head attachment.

The opposite end of the tubing was connected to a bottle containing the elemental diet. To prevent twisting, the tubing was passed through the top of the rat's cage and into a simple device (Ohashi et al., 1980), which kept the tubing straight during any movement of the rat (Figure 18-2). The tubing was subsequently balanced by traversing a wheel (Figure 18-3). Our experience has suggested that rats gain weight faster using this technique than with a harness (Steiger et al., 1972), because of less stress to the animal.

After partial resection of the small intestine, body weight in the rat decreases rapidly and nitrogen balance becomes negative due to accelerated protein catabolism. It is difficult to eliminate this initial catabolism by nutritional manipulation, and the purpose of nutritional support is to attenuate and shorten the duration of the catabolic phase.

In Figure 18-4, rats were force-fed various types of isocaloric liquid diets after surgery, delivering 307 kcal per kg of body weight. A diet with high molecular weight components, such as Sustagen (Japan-Bristol Laboratories), in which defatted milk was the nitrogen source, and MacEight (Ono Pharmaceuticals) with casein as the source of nitrogen, did not prevent weight loss after surgery. However, feeding the elemental diet lessened the body weight loss and shortened the recovery period similar to the parenterally fed animals. These results suggest that this formulation, when administered enterally, could be utilized to the same extent that nutrients are when administered intravenously.

To compare, quantitatively, the effect of various types of liquid diets on wound healing, 4 holes, each 8 mm in diameter, were punched in the dorsal skin of the rats that had also received a partially resected intestine. It was our belief that when nutrients administered enterally were absorbed and utilized effectively, wound healing would be accelerated and the healing rate of punched skin areas could be used as a measure of the efficacy of the enterally administered diet.

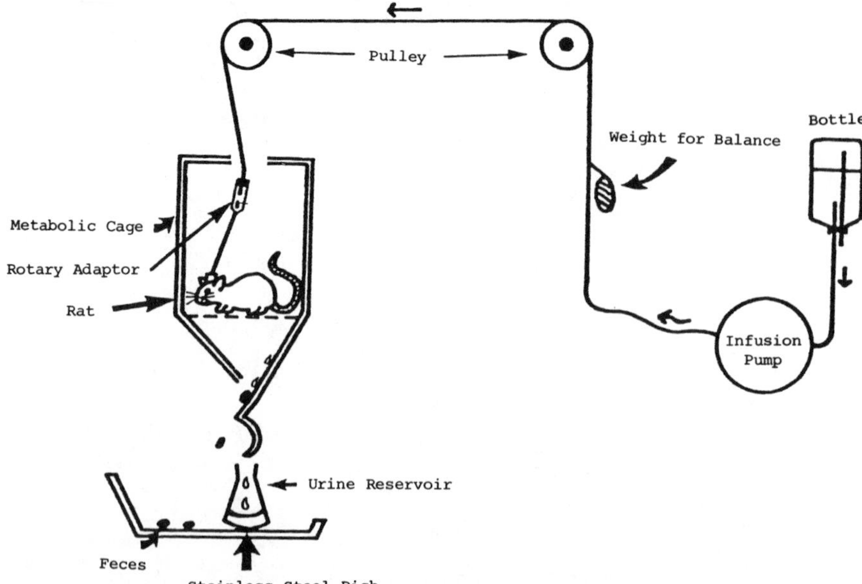

Figure 18-3 Schematic outline of continuous gastric infusion system for rat.

In Figure 18-5, skin was punched on the same day as the partial resection of intestine and enteral nutrition was started. Here again, our elemental diet produced a beneficial effect equal to parenteral feeding, whereas the high polymer liquid diets had little impact on wound healing. These results showed that our elemental diet was as effective as parenteral nutrition, provided that a certain portion of small intestine remained intact.

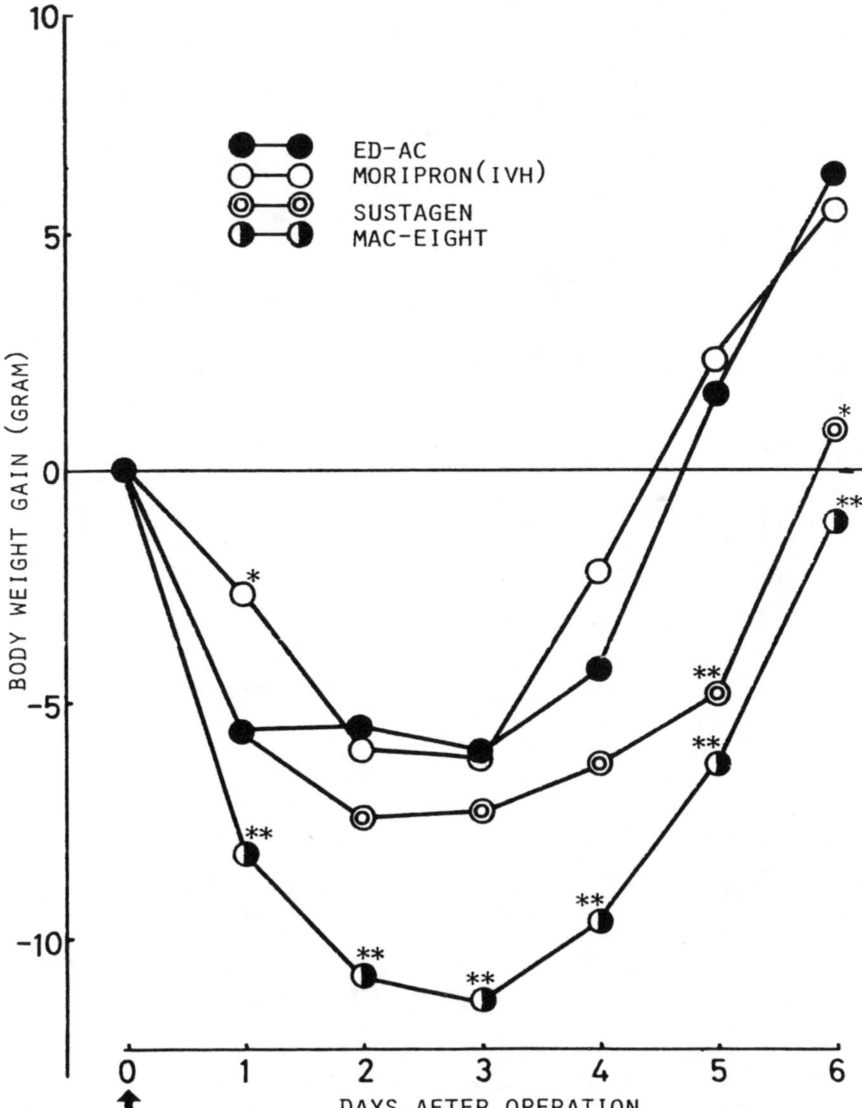

Figure 18-4 The effect of intragastric (ED-AC, Sustagen and MacEight) and intravenous (Moripron) feeding on the body weight gains in small bowel-resected rats. Fischer male rats weighing approximately 160 g received lower two thirds of small intestine resection. After the operation, continuous tube feeding was done intragastrically or intravenously for six days.

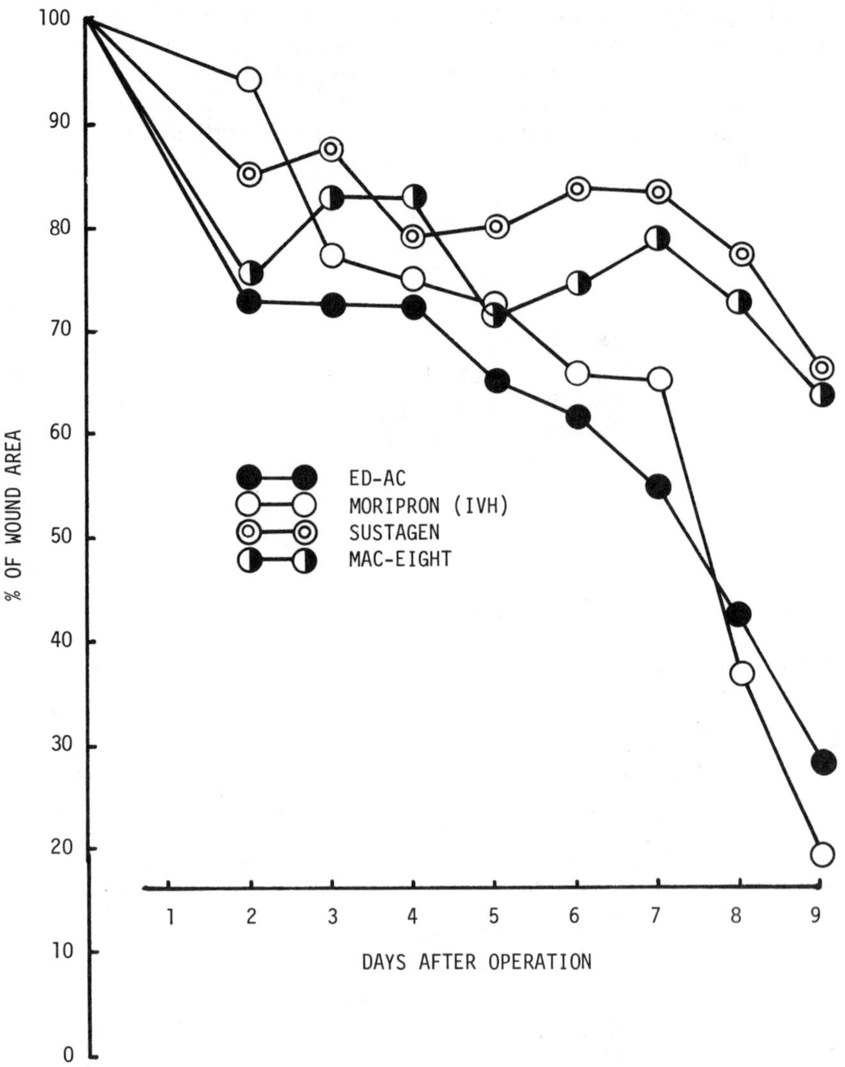

Figure 18-5 The effect of intragastric (ED-AC, Sustagen and MacEight) and intravenous (Moripron) feeding on the wound healings in small bowel resected rats. Fischer male rats weighing approximately 160 g received lower two thirds of small intestine resection. Moreover, four holes, 8 mm in diameter, were punched on the back skin. After the operation, continuous tube feeding was done intragastrically or intravenously for nine days.

Clinical trials with this formula have been performed in Japan in 539 patients from 1978 through 1979 under the management of Drs. Sato and Ogoshi, Chiba University Medical School. Twenty institutions have also collaborated. The diet has been administered under the schedule shown in Table 18-1.

The results are summarized in Figure 18-6. Two thirds of the patients who were entered into the protocol had cancer of the digestive tract. The number of pediatric patients undergoing surgery were also included. Clinical benefits of the diet were

Table 18-1
Schedule of Enteral Hyperalimentation with Elental

	Dry Weight (g)	Solution (ml)	Conc. (W/V%)	Calories (kcal/ml)	Infusion Rate (ml/hr)	Total Amount/24 hr
Schedule A	60	600	10	0.38	25	225 kcal., suppl. with I.V. injection
Schedule B	160	1200	13	0.50	50	600 kcal., suppl. with I.V. injection N: 4 g Na: 463 mg (20 mEq) K: 421 mg (11 mEq)
Schedule C	320	1800	18	0.67	75	1200 kcal N: 8 g Na: 925 mg (40 mEq) K: 842 mg (22 mEq)
Schedule D	480	2400	20	0.75	100	1800 kcal N: 12 g Na: 1388 mg (60 mEq) K: 1263 mg (33 mEq)
Schedule E	640	2760	23	0.87	115	2400 kcal N: 16 g Na: 1850 mg (80 mEq) K: 1684 mg (43 mEq)
Schedule F	800	3000	27	1.00	125	3000 kcal N: 20 g Na: 2313 mg (100 mEq) K: 2105 mg (54 mEq)

Note: 1) Start the enteral hyperalimentation on the day of the operation according to Schedule A and change the Schedule to B, C, D, E or F every one or two days based on the physician's judgment.
2) For maintenance dose (adult), employ Schedule D; Schedule E or F may be employed in some cases.

evaluated by nitrogen balance, body weight change, plasma aminogram, blood chemistries including serum proteins, general performance and presence of side effects. These data were summarized into five grades. If the cases of "slightly improved" were included in the total number of responses, this new elemental diet proved to be beneficial in at least 85% of the patients. Complications were found in only 1.8% of the cases and the principal difficulty was either vomiting or diarrhea.

Table 18-2
Contraindications of Elental

1. Less than three months-old infant	4. Metabolic disorder of carbohydrates
2. Short bowel syndrome, in acute stage	5. Hepatic insufficiency
3. Ileus, in acute stage	6. Renal failure

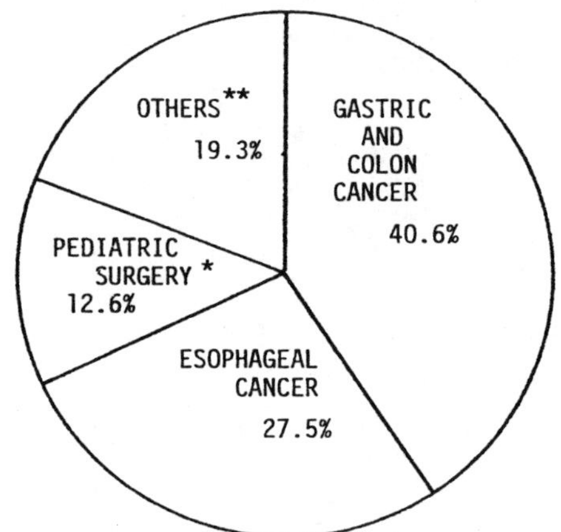

*: INTESTINAL OBSTRUCTION, HIRSCHSPRUNG'S DISEASE, ANAL ATRESIA, EXTENSIVE AGANGLINOSIS, etc.

**: ULCER, COLITIS, CROHN'S DISEASE, etc.

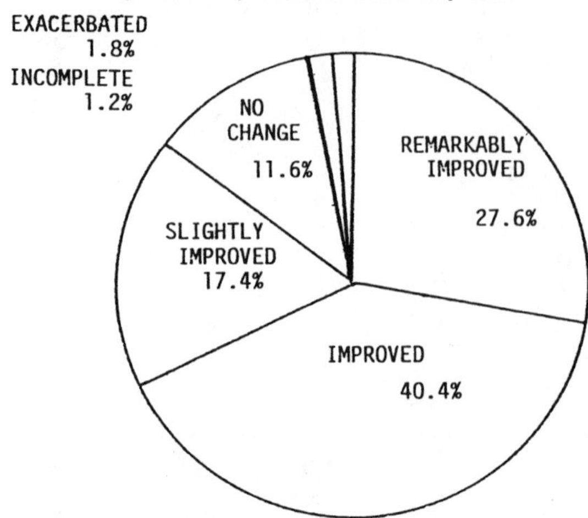

Figure 18-6 Summary of the clinical trials of Elental in 539 patients in Japan (1978–1979).

In Table 18-2, the contraindications for use of the elemental diet are listed. In summary, the clinical applications for this product are listed in Table 18-3.

Table 18-3
Clinical Applications of Elental

1. Nutritional management before and after surgery
2. Management of gastric and intestinal fistulas
3. Improvement of malabsorption and maldigestion; postgastrectomy, etc
4. Inflammatory intestinal disease and other diarrhea; Crohn's disease, ulcerative colitis, etc
5. Congenital metabolic disorders
6. Nutritional management of cancer patients
7. Acceleration of metabolism; severe injury
8. Miscellaneous

NUTRITIONAL THERAPY WITH ELEMENTAL DIET

Recently, the characteristic metabolic changes that occur in individual disease states have drawn attention. Such metabolic deviations are expressed in the plasma amino acid profile (Figure 18-7). Pathological aminograms have been observed in patients with malnutrition, metabolic disturbances, protein catabolism, and a variety of miscellaneous disease processes (Yugari, 1979, 1982).

The aminogram of the undernourished patient is characterized by low levels of essential amino acids. The changes in amino acid levels in patients with metabolic disturbances are reflected by an increase of certain amino acids, in which their metabolism is impaired. Liver failure is a prime example (Fischer et al., 1974) in which most amino acid levels are elevated, such as tyrosine, phenylalanine, methionine, aspartate, and glutamate. Low birth-weight babies are often too immature to be able to metabolize tyrosine, phenylalanine, cysteine, and methionine (Abitbol et al., 1975) and their levels are frequently affected. The aminogram of catabolic patients is characterized by high levels of branched-chain amino acids.

Each deviation of the amino acid profile is a result of a specific metabolic disturbance produced by the disease. Nutritional treatment must not only provide nutrients, but also should normalize aminogram and relieve symptoms.

Elemental Diet for Hepatic Failure

The plasma aminogram in hepatic failure (Fischer et al., 1974) is diagrammed in Figure 18-7. It is characterized by its low branched-chain amino acid concentrations and high concentration of amino acids which are metabolized in liver, such as tyrosine, phenylalanine, methionine, aspartate, and glutamate. In these clinical conditions, Dr. Josef Fischer has proposed a unique infusion solution (FO-80) to treat and prevent hepatic coma. FO-80 is characterized by its high content of branched-chain amino acids and low content of aromatic amino acids. The amino acid profile of FO-80 is complementary to the plasma aminogram and the FO-80 showed remarkable effects in reversing the clinical symptoms of hepatic coma.

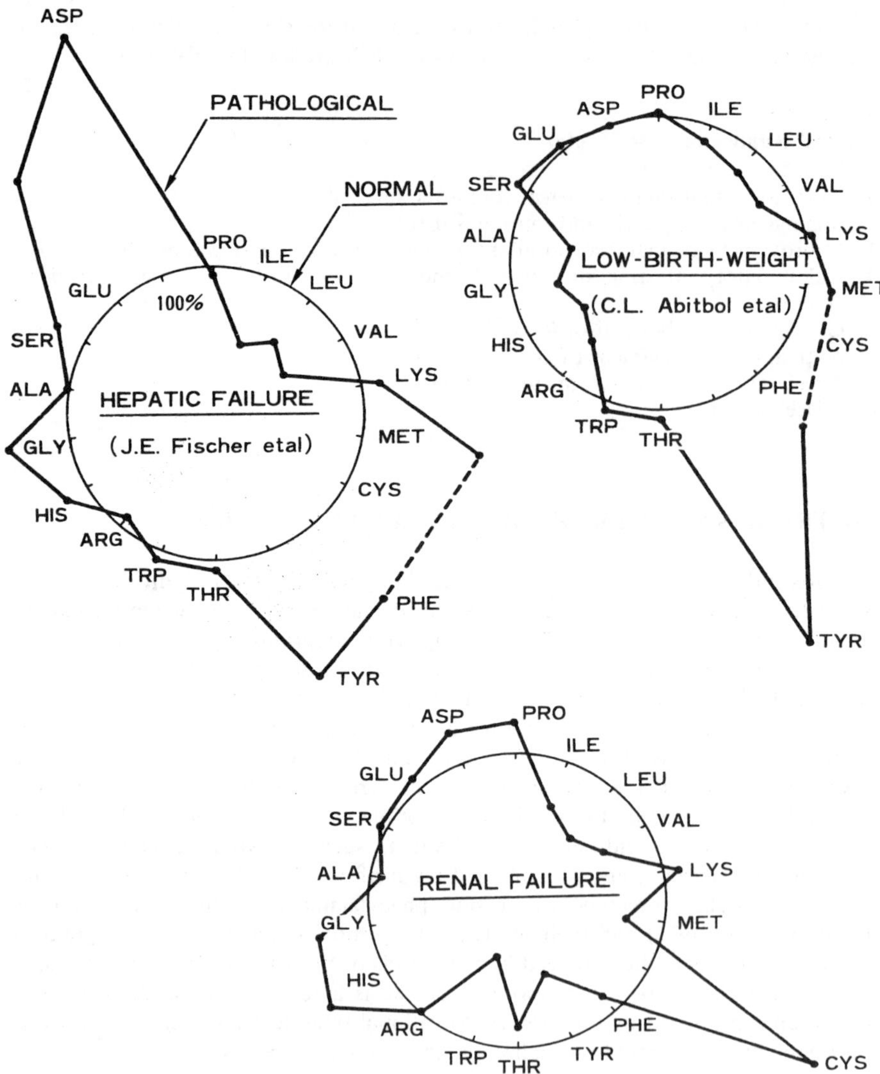

Figure 18-7 Deviations of plasma aminogram in pathological conditions.

Based on similar findings to Fischer, we have proposed a new formula for an elemental diet to support the patient with hepatic failure. This formula is characterized by its high content of branched-chain amino acids (50%), increased proportion of arginine (15.5%), and low percentage of aromatic amino acids, such as phenylalanine, tyrosine, and tryptophan (Figure 18-8). This diet is very different from the earlier egg pattern formula and also varies from Fischer's pattern, especially in the quantities of branched-chain amino acids and arginine. To examine its effect on hepatic failure, we chose to study rats with liver cirrhosis.

Cirrhotic liver failure was induced by subcutaneous injection of 1 ml per kg of 43% carbon tetrachloride in olive oil twice a week for ten successive weeks in

Sprague-Dawley rats. Histologically, diffuse fibrosis of hepatic tissue was observed.

To induce coma in these rats, 70% of the liver was resected and 48 hours after the operation, a 10% solution of ammonium chloride was injected. Coma was diagnosed by the loss of ortho-positional reflex. The elemental diet was administered immediately after hepatectomy. Figure 18-9 shows the duration of coma and mortality in rats administered various amounts of this elemental diet. With our new formula, the duration of coma was the shortest and mortality was lowest, compared to Hepatic Aid (American McGaw Laboratories) (BCAA: 34.6%; arginine: 7.3%), and our previous formula (BCAA: 17.1%; arginine: 7.08%). Plasma aminograms in those rats are shown in Figure 18-10. When fed the new diet, plasma branched-chain

		G/100G
AMINO ACIDS	14 AMINO ACIDS	14.40
CARBOHYDRATE	DEXTRIN	74.32
FAT	SOYBEAN OIL	3.50
VITAMINS	14 VITAMINS	0.16
MINERALS	10 MINERALS	6.23
CALORIE CONTENT		386
CAL/N		175

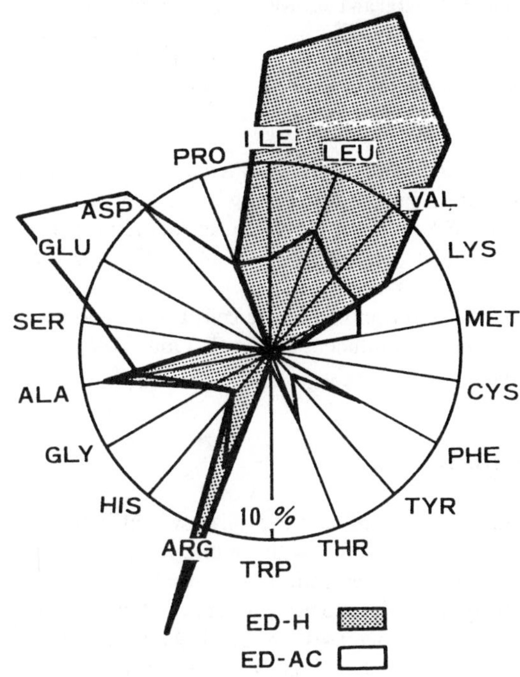

Figure 18-8 Elemental diet for hepatic insufficiency (ED-H).

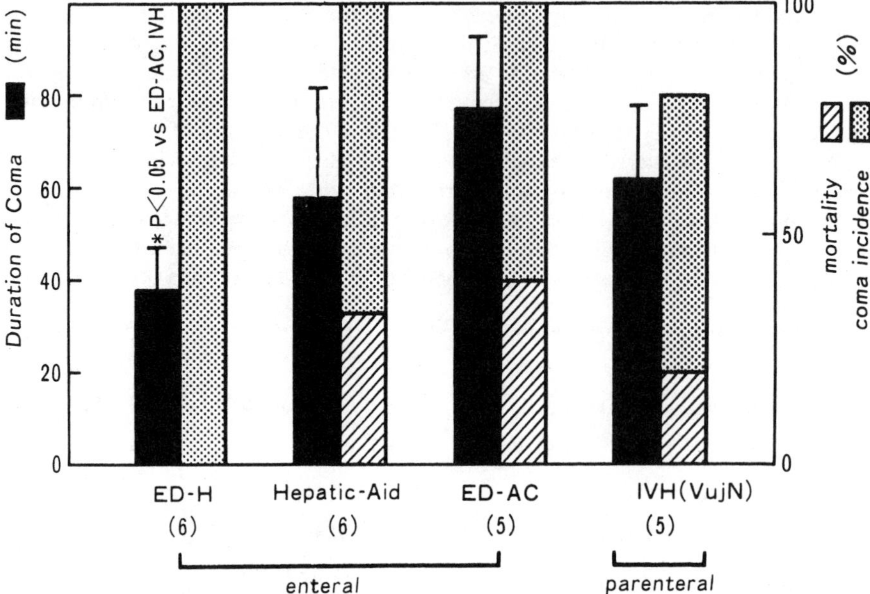

Figure 18-9 The effect of elemental diet on the duration of coma and mortality in partially hepatectomized rats with coma by 10% NH_4Cl. Sprague-Dawley male rats weighing approximately 200 g received 70% hepatoectomy and, after 48 hours, coma was induced by the intraperitoneal injection of 2.6 ml/kg of 10% NH_4Cl solution. Coma was diagnosed by the loss of ortho-positional reflex. Enteral and intravenous nutrition was started immediately after the hepatectomy. Duration of coma (■) was shown by the time (min) between the loss and recovery of ortho-positional reflex. Mortality (▨) means the ratio of the number of rats that did not recover from the coma to the total number of rats in each group.

amino acids and arginine levels were elevated and phenylalanine, tyrosine, tryptophan, and methionine concentrations were low compared to that of normally fed rats. Fischer's ratio, BCAA/Phe + Tyr + Trp, in rats fed our new formula, Hepatic Aid, or our previous diet were 1.99 ± 0.14, 1.75 ± 0.10, and 1.56 ± 0.10, respectively.

Examining the regeneration of hepatic cells is now underway. Clinical trials of this product are also being conducted by Dr. T. Oda, Tokyo University and Dr. H. Sato, Chiba University.

Elemental Diets for Infants

The plasma amino acid profile in low birth-weight babies is characterized by a general hypoaminoacidemia but with high levels of methionine. Plasma phenylalanine and tyrosine concentrations in low birth-weight babies are also altered (Abitbol et al., 1975), because hepatic p-hydroxy-phenylpyruvate oxidase activity which is initially very low increases progressively with gestational development. Tyrosine concentrations may be reduced in low birth-weight babies because of limited activity of phenylalanine hydroxylase (Freedland et al., 1962).

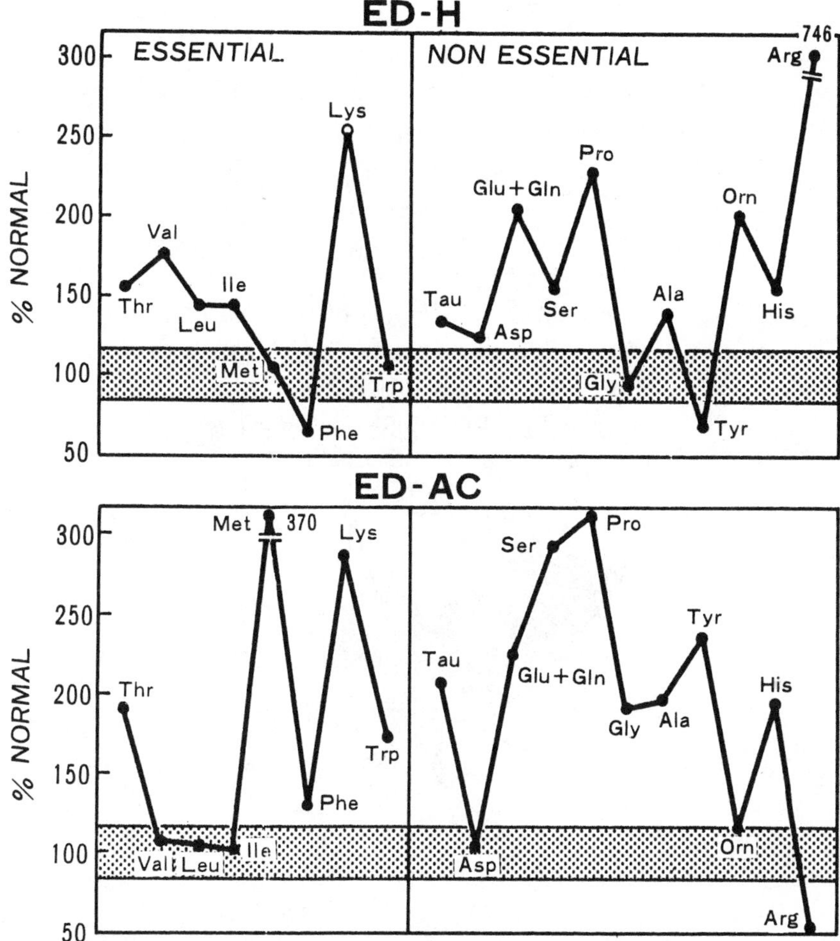

Figure 18-10 The effect of elemental diet on the plasma-free amino acids in partially hepatectomized rats with coma by 10% NH_4Cl. See the experimental conditions in Figure 18-9. The blood was drawn immediately after the arousal from coma.

Figure 18-11 shows the amino acid patterns of a new formulation for preterm infants. Amino acid composition of the product was modified from the pattern found in human breast milk. The branched-chain amino acid intake was increased to stimulate muscle protein synthesis. Ratios of dietary methionine/cysteine and of phenylalanine/tyrosine were less than 1.0 because cysteine and tyrosine formation from methionine and phenylalanine are impaired in newborn babies (Sturman et al., 1970). To supply enough essential fatty acids, the fat content was also increased.

To evaluate the feeding, gastric fistula were made and fine silastic tubing catheters, 0.97 mm in external diameter, were inserted in 2- to 10-day-old rats. The tubing was fixed at the lateral abdominal skin and on the back of the neck. Rats were housed individually in a small wire cage and placed in an incubator, where temperature, humidity, and oxygen consumption were controlled. By feeding this

		G/100 G
AMINO ACIDS	17 AMINO ACIDS	13.10
CARBOHYDRATE	DEXTRIN	77.50
FAT	SOYBEAN OIL	3.50
VITAMINS	14 VITAMINS	0.16
MINERALS	9 MINERALS	5.08

CALORIE CONTENT	80 G/ PACKAGE
	300 CAL/ PACKAGE
	0.8 CAL/ ML
OSMOTIC PRESSURE	596 MOSM/ L

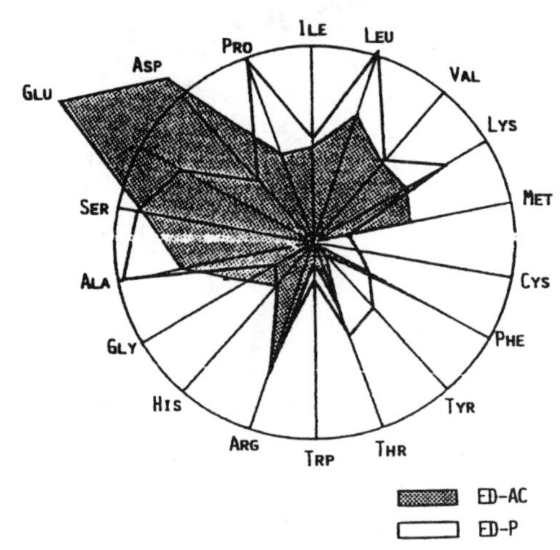

Figure 18-11 Elemental diet for infant use (ED-P).

product, survival rate of weanling animals was 100% for 10-day-old animals. However for 2-day-old rats, only 20% survived.

Body weight gain in 18-day-old rats fed the diet for eight days from the tenth day following birth is shown in Figure 18-12. A 15% solution of this new formula and our original one have been administered so as to be isocaloric and isonitrogenous. The amount of nutrients that could be administered safely was considerably less than observed in mother-fed rats. Body weight gains in these rats were also less than in mother-fed rats. However, among rats receiving the elemental diets, the new product produced better weight gain and growth than previous ones. A comparison between this product and a human milk pattern is now being studied.

The protein efficiency ratio (PER) of the two elemental diets in 18-day-old rats was calculated from the data over the previous eight-day feeding period. The PER for the new product and our previous one was 3.72 and 2.15, respectively (Figure 18-13). Total serum protein levels in mother-fed, new product-fed, and previous

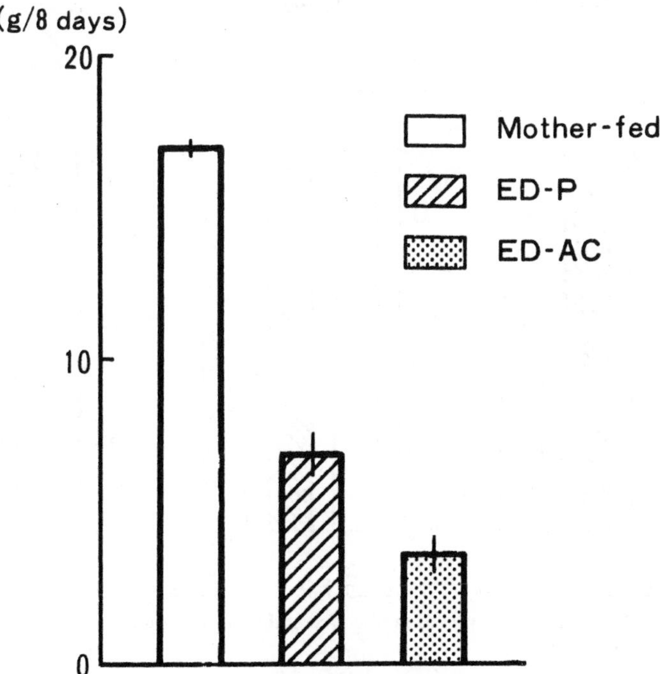

Figure 18-12 Body weight gains of mother-fed and tube-fed infant rats. Ten-day-old unsexed Sprague-Dawley rats weighing approximately 20 g were gastrostomized. After the operation, continuous gastric infusion of 15% elemental diet solutions was performed for eight days. Mother-fed rat pups were used as the control.

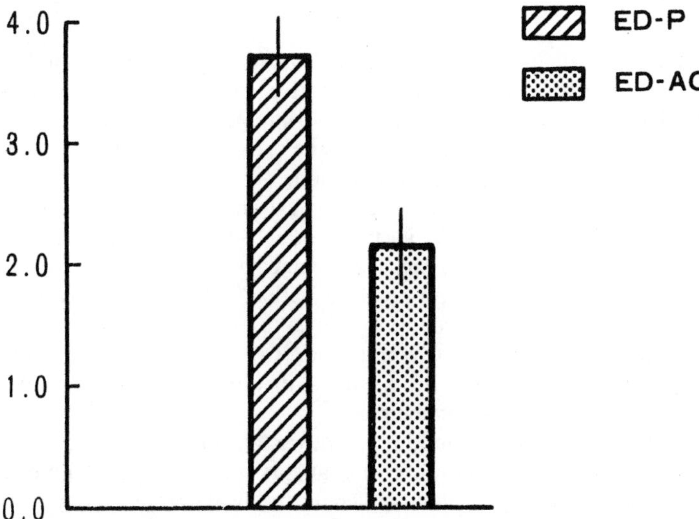

Figure 18-13 Protein efficiency ratios (PER) of tube-fed infant rats. See the experimental conditions in Figure 18-12. PER (weight gain in grams/nitrogen × 6.25 consumed in grams) were compared between ED-AC and ED-P.

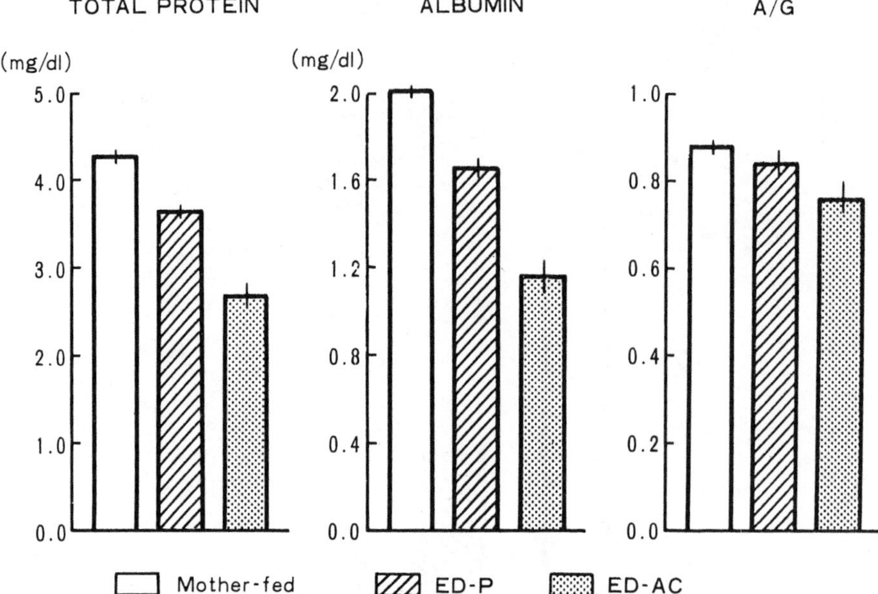

Figure 18-14 Serum protein levels of mother-fed and tube-fed infant rats. See the experimental conditions in Figure 18-12.

product-fed rats were 4.27, 3.65, and 2.68 g/dl, respectively (Figure 18-14). A clinical trial of this new product in Japan is now scheduled.

SUMMARY

Adequate dietary intake is the goal of nutritional support and is essential for treating the hospitalized patient. In practice, many patients become anorectic and clinical nutritionists must remember the importance of palatability, the personal likes and dislikes of each patient, and the effects of cooking on the acceptance of food served, as well as its nutritional value.

To those patients whose appetite is extremely suppressed, or to those whose digestive ability is impaired by gastrointestinal surgery, nutrients must be prescribed and administered under a physician's management. An easily digestible liquid diet of polymeric nutrients is effective for those patients whose digestive ability is essentially intact and such diets can provide ample calories and nitrogen.

In patients whose digestive and absorptive ability is markedly impaired, use of total parenteral nutrition or the elemental diet in which small portions of remaining intestine are utilized is recommended.

Total parenteral nutrition has the advantage in that administration of nutrients can be closely regulated. However, in patients with suppressed immune competence, such as cancer or in aged patients, there is the always present danger of infection and sepsis. To avoid infection, sanitary facilities and well-trained medical teams are required.

In contrast, elemental diets can supply sufficient energy and nitrogen for long periods of time through the residual part of the small intestine. If the elemental diet is administered under a schedule of gradually increasing concentration and total volume, many of the adverse side effects can be reduced or eliminated. The elemental diet also can have its composition freely designed to deal with various diseases and altered metabolism. Examples are special formulas designed for renal, liver failure, cancer, coronary insufficiency, and others. Thus, in the near future, we will be able to create specific nutritional therapies not only to supply sufficient nutrient to support the host, but also to restore altered metabolism to normal.

REFERENCES

Abitbol, C.L., Feldman, D.B., Ahman, P. and Pudman, D. (1975): Plasma amino acid patterns during supplemental intravenous nutrition of low-birth-weight infants. *J. Pediatr* 86:766–822.

Daabees, T.T. and Stegink, L.D. (1978): L-Alanyl-L-tyrosine as a tyrosine source during intravenous nutrition of the rat. *J. Nutr.* 108:1104–1113.

Dudrick, S.J., Wilmore, D.W., Vars, H.M. and Rhoads, J.E. (1968): Quantitative nutritional studies with water-soluble, chemically defined diets. 1. Growth, reproduction and lactation in rats. *Surgery* 64:134–142.

Elman, R. and Weiner, D.O. (1939): Intravenous alimentation with specific reference to protein (amino acid) metabolism. *JAMA* 112:796–802.

Fischer, J.E., Yoshimura, N., Aquirre, A., James, J.H., Cummings, M.G., Abel, R.M. and Deindoerfer, F. (1974): Plasma amino acids in patients with hepatic encephalopathy. Effects of amino acid infusions. *Am. J. Surgery* 127:40–47.

Freedland, R.A., Krakowski, M.C. and Waisman, H.A. (1962): Effect of age, sex, and nutrition on liver phenylalnine hydroxylase activity in rats. *Am. J. Physiol.* 202:145–148.

Greenstein, J.P., Birnbaum, S.M., Winitz, M. and Otey, M.C. (1957): Quantitative nutritional studies with water-soluble, chemically defined diets. 1. Growth, reproduction and lactation in rats. *Arch. Biochem. Biophys.* 72:396–416.

Nakatuji, H., Sato, O., Saito, F., Kurata, S., Otsuka, S., Yugari, Y. and Yanagimoto, Y. (1979): Nutritional evaluation of elemental diet (ED-AC) in small bowel resected rats. *Basic Pharmacol. Ther.* (Japanese) 7:3471–3498.

Nakatuji, H., Sato, O., Saito, F., Otsuka, S. and Yugari, Y. (1979): The effect of elemental diet (ED-AC) on the wound healing in small bowel resected rats. *Basic Pharmacol. Ther.* (Japanese) 7:3547–3550.

Nakatuji, H., Sato, O., Saito, F., Kurata, K., Otsuka, S., Yugari, Y. and Yanagimoto, Y. (1979): Nutritional evaluation of elemental diet (ED-AC) by the continuous gastric infusion technique in small bowel resected rats. *Basic Pharmacol. Ther.* (Japanese) 7:3499–3545.

Ohashi, H., Sugiyama, Y. and Takami, T. (1980): Continuous intravenous infusion to unrestrained rats; improved method. *Igaku No Ayumi* (Japanese) 112:30–32.

Rose, W.C. (1949): Amino acid requirements of man. *Fed. Proc.* 8:546–552.

Steiger, E., Vars, H.M. and Dudrick, S.J. (1972): A technique for long-term intravenous feeding in unrestrained rats. *Arch. Surg.* 104:330–332.

Sturman, J.A., Gaull, G. and Raiha, N.C.R. (1970): Absence of cystathionase in human fetal liver. Is cystine essential? *Science* 169:74–75.

Yugari, Y. (1979): The effect of branched-chain amino acids. *Trends Parent. Nutr.* (Japanese) 3:1–6.

Yugari, Y. (1982): Amino acids infusion for various diseased states. *J. Jpn. Soc. Nutr. Food Sci.* (Japanese) 35:1–13.

Winitz, J., Graff, J., Gallagher, N., Narkin, A. and Seedman, D.A. (1965): Evaluation of chemical diets as nutrition for man—in space. *Nature* 205:741–743.

19 Parenteral Amino Acid Nutrition in Infants

Robert W. Winters
William C. Heird
Ralph B. Dell

This brief presentation will concentrate upon the historical development of amino acid mixtures for use in parenteral nutrition of infants. However, this particular subject has implications beyond the immediate pediatric one. For example, since the human infant is the most sensitive model for assessing safety as well as efficacy of any parenteral amino acid mixture, it follows that an amino acid solution designed specifically to promote growth of the human infant should be close if not identical to the optimal amino acid mixture for promoting anabolism or "regrowth" of depleted adults. Thus, even those not charged with the immediate care of infants are well advised to pay close attention to developments concerning amino acid metabolism of infants during parenteral nutrition. It is likely that such developments will be qualitatively and perhaps quantitatively applicable to the problem of promoting "regrowth" of the depleted adult.

PROTEIN HYDROLYSATES

A brief review of the historical development of present-day amino acid solutions used for parenteral nutrition in infants reveals some interesting and important changes in our thinking about the basis for the development of amino acid solutions generally.

What may be called the first generation of amino acid sources for parenteral nutrition were two protein hydrolysates—casein hydrolysate and fibrin hydrolysate. These two products, introduced over three decades ago, had two basic rationales: they could be produced in large quantity at reasonable cost and, in reasonable amounts, they met most of the essential amino acid requirements of adults.

The hydrolysates suffered from several deficiencies, most notably the uncertain metabolic fate of peptides (which constituted about 50% of the total amino acid content), the uncontrollable batch-to-batch variation in composition, the production of a generally mild, asymptomatic hyperammonemia, especially in infants, and occasional production of a rather severe, allergic-type reaction.

The problem of hyperammonemia attracted a good deal of attention among pediatric investigators (Ghadimi, 1975). In the opinion of many, the hyperammonemia seen in infants receiving hydrolysates was attributable to the preformed ammonia content which resulted from the deamination of glutamine in the manufacturing process. Values for preformed ammonia content of up to 2000 μg/dl were reported. The problem with this relatively simple explanation was that it failed on quantitative grounds. Thus, a reasonable intake of hydrolysate delivered only about 1 mmol/Kg-d of free ammonia, an amount which can easily be metabolized by an infant. For example, infants with metabolic alkalosis due to pyloric stenosis have received up to 6 mmol/Kg-d of ammonium chloride without showing any clinical signs of hyperammonemia (Kildeberg, 1964).

A clue to the etiology of hydrolysate-induced hyperammonemia was provided by the observation of Sunshine and colleagues (unpublished) that infants with hydrolysate-induced hyperammonemia showed profuse orotic aciduria. Based on studies of inborn errors of the urea cycle, this finding suggested an arginine deficiency which results in a large load of ammonia being shunted toward the pyrmidine biosynthetic pathway of which orotic acid is a prominent intermediate. This explanation became even more obvious, largely in hindsight, after our studies of hyperammonemia in infants receiving a crystalline amino acid mixture (see below).

CRYSTALLINE AMINO ACID SOLUTIONS

Once it became possible to produce large amounts of pure crystalline L-amino acids at reasonable cost, a new second generation of amino acid mixtures appeared. These are the solutions that are most widely used today—FreAmine III (American McGaw), Aminosyn (Abbott Laboratories), and Travasol (Travenol Laboratories).

Available technology for the production of reproducible amino acid mixtures did not solve the problem of defining an optimal amino acid formulation. Several approaches were tried. One mixture that did not make it beyond the investigational stage was based on the free amino acid pattern of one of the hydrolysates, apparently on the incorrect notion that the peptides of the hydrolysates were not metabolically available. Another serious flaw in the formulation of this mixture was that it included the cationic amino acids, arginine, histidine and lysine, as the hydrochloride salts. This resulted in a large load of preformed acid being delivered by the solution. In infants, a rather profound hyperchloremic metabolic acidosis ensued (Heird et al., 1972a). In older children and adults, a less severe variety of the same acid-base disturbance was seen. This experience proved valuable in that all subsequent formulations of amino acid mixtures have incorporated the cationic amino acids as acetate salts. This maneuver results in a final solution which is "neutral" from an acid-base point of view, i.e., the H^+ resulting from the metabolism of the cationic amino acids is exactly offset by production of HCO_3^- from the acetate anion.

Actually, as subsequent work has shown, the acid-base problems associated with parenteral nutrition have not been completely solved. Many of the presently available "neutral" solutions (as defined above) seem to produce metabolic alkalosis, particularly in older infants and children (Heird, 1977). It is uncertain whether a similar phenomenon occurs in adults since the search has not been thoroughly carried out as yet. The mechanism of this effect is obscure, but fundamentally it must represent an excretion of urinary H^+ (as TA + NH_4^+) that is inappropriately large in relation to the ongoing metabolic production of acid.

Most of the second generation amino acid solutions (FreAmine, Aminosyn and Travasol) seem to have been based upon the amino acid composition of high quality dietary proteins but modified to replace the glutamate and aspartate with glycine. These mixtures meet the known essential amino acid requirements as defined from oral nutrition for infants (Holt and Snyderman, 1967; Fomon and Filer, 1967).

The metabolic effects of these second generation amino acid mixtures have been intensively studied by our group and others. These effects are summarized below:

1. Each amino acid mixture, when provided with an adequate caloric intake, produces a predictable gain in body weight and positive nitrogen balance in metabolically stable infants; however, no significant differences have been documented with respect to either of these variables among the three currently available solutions, provided they are administered isonitrogenously and isocalorically. In infants, no crystalline mixture has ever been shown to be clearly superior with respect to nitrogen retention or weight gain.

2. Each second generation amino acid solution produces a characteristic amino acid pattern in the plasma (Winters et al., 1977). These patterns, however, are not a simple reflection of the composition of the infusate; rather they show many differences indicating that, even though the liver and intestine are largely by-passed, metabolic changes and renal excretion conspire to alter the infusate pattern so as to produce a characteristic amino acid plasma pattern.

3. Each amino acid solution is associated with several significant and characteristic plasma aminogram abnormalities, i.e., a deviation outside the 95% postprandial plasma limits of normal, enterally fed infants (Winters et al., 1977). All infants, regardless of the mixture received, have low plasma values for cystine and tyrosine. Another consistent abnormality is hyperglycinemia; the plasma glycine level varies in a linear fashion in relation to glycine intake.

4. Attempts to counter the low plasma cystine levels with cysteine•HCl supplementation have led to conflicting results with respect to plasma levels. This problem, however, is complicated by some complex methodological problems, which are only now being solved (Winters et al., 1977). Nitrogen balance seems unaffected by cysteine•HCl supplementation (Zlotkin et al., 1981), but since all such studies have been carried out in infants who are also deficient in tyrosine, as indicated by very low plasma tyrosine levels, these results may not be conclusive.

5. One second generation solution, FreAmine, has undergone several successive modifications, each based upon direct study of the parenterally fed infant. The first

of these modifications consisted of replacing some of the hydrochloride salts of cationic amino acids with corresponding acetate salts. Subsequently, the D,L-methionine, which produced hypermethioninemia as we had shown earlier (Winters et al., 1977), was replaced with an isomolar amount of L-methionine which resulted in normal plasma methionine levels. Another change, based on our observation of an unexpected severe hyperammonemia in four infants receiving the "original" FreAmine, was the substitution of part of excess glycine with arginine (Heird, et al., 1972b). The hyperammonemia, which was associated with orotic aciduria as well as excretion of other unidentified nitrogenous compounds (Figure 19-1) and a corresponding decrease in urinary urea, was readily responsive to arginine supplementation.

The above observations on hyperammonemia provided the basis for the postulation that hydrolysate-induced hyperammonemia was probably due to arginine deficiency rather than to any preformed ammonia load. A comparison of the arginine content of the hydrolysates with that of FreAmine confirms this suspicion (see Figure 19-2). This hypothesis could be tested critically by ascertaining the effects of arginine supplementation of hydrolysates, but to the authors' knowledge, such a study has not been carried out.

One of the primary concerns of parenteral amino acid therapy in the infant is the possible adverse effects upon development of the nervous system. This concern stems largely from the association of inborn errors of amino acid metabolism with mental retardation. In addition, there is the general question of whether parenteral nutrition alone will support completely normal brain growth.

We have studied some of these questions in newborn beagle puppies who received only parenteral nutrition for various periods during the first six weeks of life. The chemical growth of the brain and other organs of these puppies was compared to that of suckled puppies of the same age. Brain DNA, RNA and most groups of brain

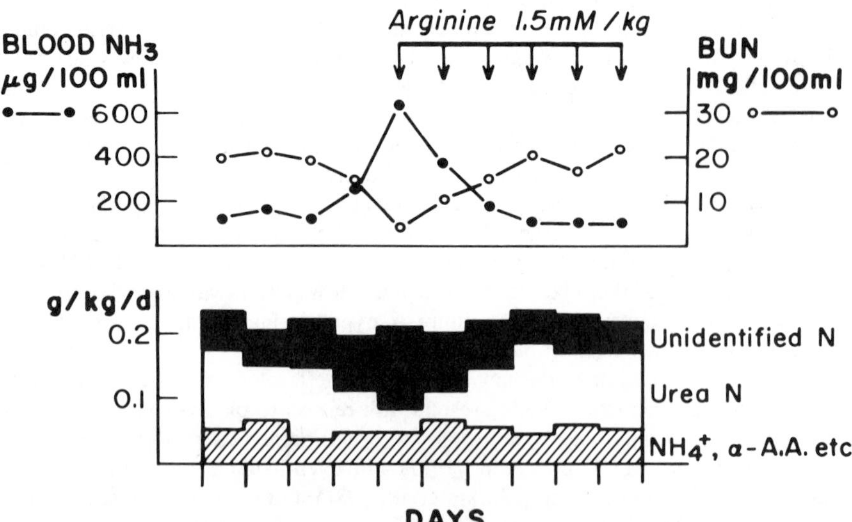

Figure 19-1 Changes in blood NH_3 and Urea-N (top) and urinary nitrogen fractions (bottom) in an infant who developed hyperammonemia while receiving FreAmine as part of the TPN regimen and who was treated with arginine supplementation (Bohles, unpublished).

lipids were similar in the two groups. However, the free amino acid pattern of the brain tissue of the animals receiving TPN was grossly abnormal. The brain weight and protein content of these animals were lower than controls (Heird, 1979). In addition, animals deprived of an exogenous source of essential fatty acids (EFA) developed not only an abnormal plasma lipid fatty acid pattern but also an abnormal brain ethanolamine phosphoglyceride fatty acid pattern.

The free amino acid abnormalities of the brain reflect the abnormal pattern of the plasma amino acids. This is one of the reasons why we feel that a completely normal plasma amino acid pattern during parenteral nutrition is the optimal end-point for defining both the safety and efficacy of amino acid solutions used for parenteral nutrition in infants.

NEWER CRYSTALLINE AMINO ACID SOLUTIONS

The third generation of amino acid solutions is already clearly in sight. These mixtures are based upon the principle of first defining a set of biochemical abnormalities that are characteristic of a given metabolic state and then devising a solution to correct these abnormalities. Mixtures for renal failure and hepatic failure have already been developed following this principle. We have been involved in developing an amino acid mixture to support anabolism by attempting to reproduce the characteristic postprandial plasma amino acid patterns of healthy, rapidly growing enterally fed infants. Finally, to round out this picture, work is underway in several laboratories to devise a solution to counter the metabolic abnormalities of the hypermetabolic, hypercatabolic patient. Such a solution might be most useful in patients suffering from trauma, burns and sepsis.

To mimic a given plasma pattern of amino acids requires a great deal of background data concerning the effects of variable intakes of each amino acid on the

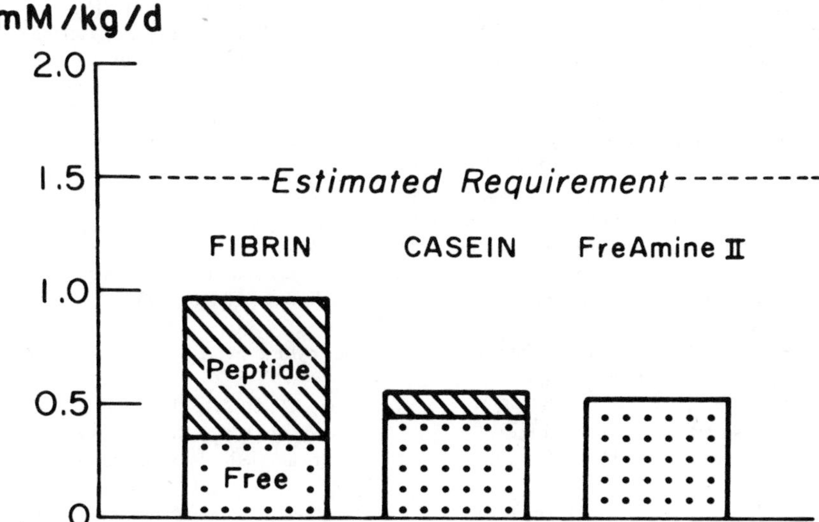

Figure 19-2 Arginine, free and peptide-bond, in fibrin and casein hydrolysate and FreAmine II, compared to estimated arginine requirement.

plasma level of that amino acid. In addition, the possible interrelationships between the intake of several amino acids on the plasma level of any single amino acid must be determined. Once a large data base is in hand, predetermined end-points for the plasma level of each amino acid can be selected and the probable intake required to meet each end-point determined.

SUMMARY

Looking to the future, it seems increasingly likely that more and more "special purpose" amino acid solutions will be developed as specific metabolic abnormalities, amenable to correction by parenteral amino acid solutions, are uncovered. In other words, the days of the single "general purpose" amino acid solution are limited; as metabolic sophistication increases so also will metabolic therapy. These advances, which we have every reason to believe will result in better patient care, are possible only because of the technology of such organizations as the Ajinomoto Company.

REFERENCES

Fromon, S.J. and Filer, L.J., Jr. (1967): Amino acid requirements for normal growth. In: *Amino Acid Metabolism and Genetic Variation* (ed: W.L. Nyhan), McGraw-Hill, New York.

Ghadimi, H. (1975): Conventional amino acid solutions for parenteral use. In: *Total Parenteral Nutrition: Premises and Promises* (ed: H. Ghadimi), Vol. 19, pp. 373–392, John Wiley & Sons, New York.

Heird, W.C. (1977): Studies of pediatric patients receiving Aminosyn® as the nitrogen source of total parenteral nutrition. In: *Current Approaches to Nutrition of the Hospitalized Patient,* pp. 45–49, Abbott and Ross Laboratories, Chicago and Columbus, IL.

Heird, W.C., and Malloy, M.H. (1979): Brain composition of beagle puppies receiving total parenteral nutrition. In: *Nutrition and Growth of the Fetus and Infant* (ed: H.K.A. Visser), pp. 365–375, Martinus Nijhoff Publishers BV, The Hague/Boston/London.

Heird, W.C., Dell, R.B., Driscoll, J.M., Jr., Grebin, B., and Winters, R.W. (1972a): Metabolic acidosis resulting from intravenous alimentation mixtures containing synthetic amino acids. *N. Engl. J. Med.* 287:943–948.

Heird, W.C., Nicholson, J.F., Driscoll, J.N., Jr., Schullinger, J.N., and Winters, R.W. (1972b): Hyperammonemia resulting from intravenous alimentation using a mixture of synthetic L-amino acids: A preliminary report. *J. Pediatr.* 81:162–165.

Holt, L.E., Jr. and Snyderman, S.E. (1967): The amino acid requirements for children. In: *Amino Acid Metabolism and Genetic Variation* (ed: W.L. Nyhan), McGraw-Hill, New York.

Kildeberg, P. (1964): Metabolic alkalosis in hypertrophic pyloric stenosis. Clinical significance and treatment. *Acta Paediatr. Scand.* 53:132–142.

Winters, R.W., Heird, W.C., Dell, R.B., and Nicholson, J.F. (1977): Plasma amino acids in infants receiving parenteral nutrition. In: *Clinical Nutrition Update* (eds: H.L. Greene, M.A. Holliday and H.N. Munro), pp. 147–157, American Medical Association Publishers; Chicago, IL.

Zlotkin, S.H., Bryan, H. and Anderson, G.H. (1981): Cysteine supplementation to cysteine-free intravenous feeding regimens in newborn infants. *Am. J. Clin. Nutr.* 34:914–923.

20 Nutritional Considerations and the Elderly Patient

William P. Steffee

If one wishes to discuss the role of nutritional support for the elderly hospitalized patient, one immediately begins to have problems with definition of what constitutes an elderly patient. For the purpose of this discussion, an elderly patient will be defined as an individual greater than 60 years of age who requires admission to a hospital for treatment of a disease state. There are several questions immediately encountered, a series of important ones being:

1. Do the elderly constitute a significant proportion of hospitalized patients?
2. Are the elderly treated by nutrition support teams?
3. Can we define the nutritional status of the elderly patient?
4. Can we estimate nutrient requirements in the elderly, stressed patient?
5. Does nutrition intervention make a difference in clinical outcome?
6. Are there cost/effectiveness considerations?

In the sections that follow, we will discuss briefly each of the questions in an attempt to highlight the need for research and new knowledge and in order to achieve a more effective and rational approach to the nutritional support of elderly patients.

ELDERLY POPULATION

Of all "minority" groups, the elderly represent one of the most rapidly increasing groups within the U.S. population. As can be seen from data derived from the National Center of Health Statistics, the U.S. population is growing older (Figure 20-1). In 1900, approximately 4% of individuals were greater than 65 years of age. This has increased to approximately 11% at the current time, and projections place this value at 12% at the end of this century. Within this group, the very old, defined as those individuals greater than 85 years of age, are also increasing at a rate proportional to the total elderly (Figure 20-2).

How does this translate into the cost for the delivery of health care? In 1974, the estimated cost of health care for the elderly was $26.8 billion. Of that, nearly 50% related to hospital care, most of which was supported by public funds (Figure 20-3). There is reason to believe that not only the amount but the portion paid by public funds is increasing. An indication of this can be gained from a recent survey of the patient population in an urban hospital, St. Vincent Charity Hospital and Health Center, in Cleveland, Ohio.

In Figure 20-4, the age distribution of all patients admitted to this hospital for the past three years is presented. The preponderance of elderly patients within the population is evident. More importantly is the increased trend toward an older population during the last three years. This change is of concern to hospital administrators.

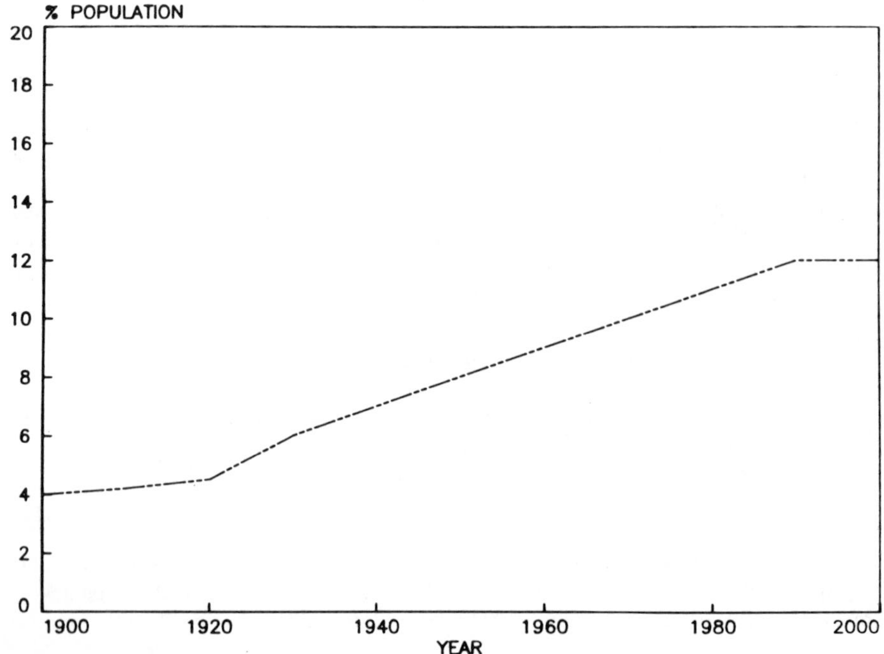

Figure 20-1

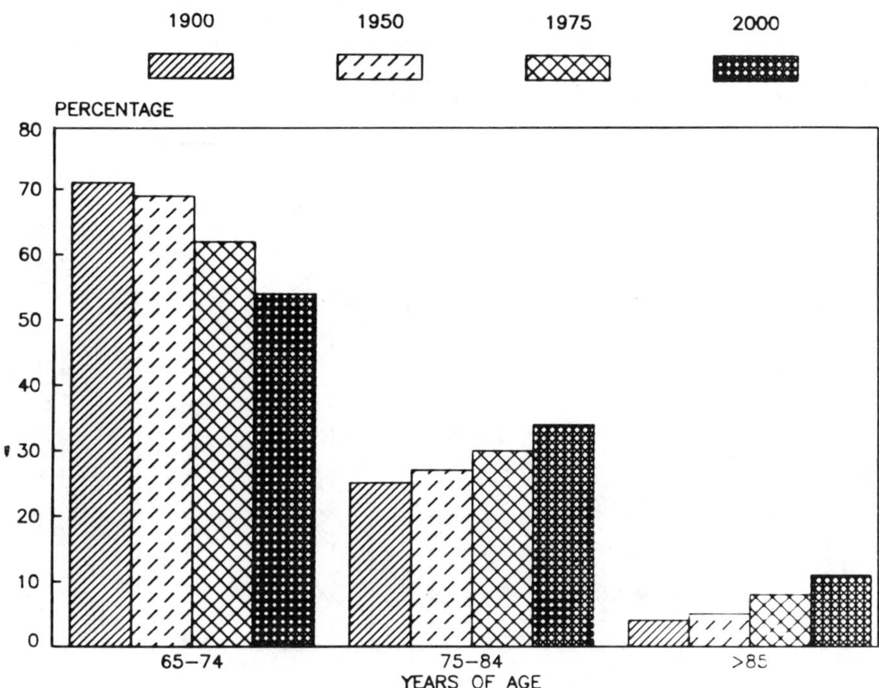

Figure 20-2

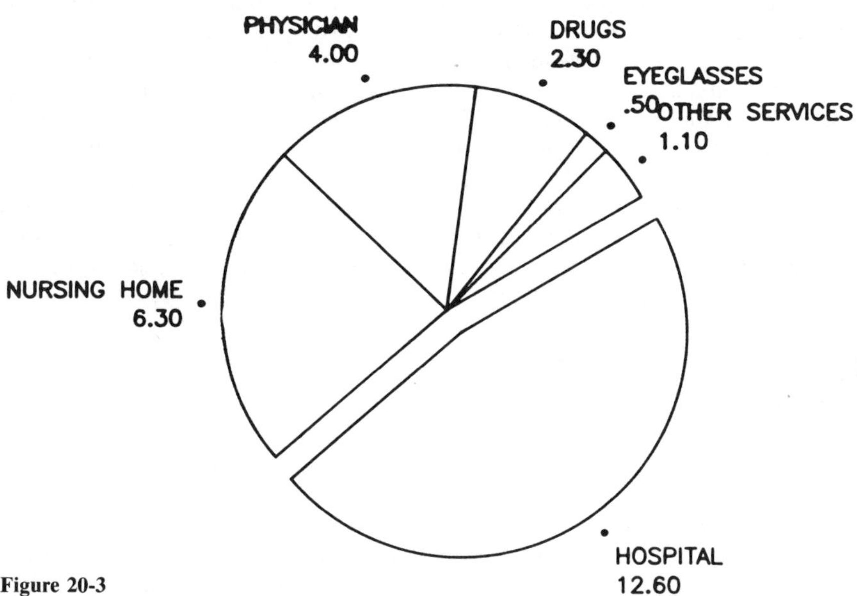

Figure 20-3

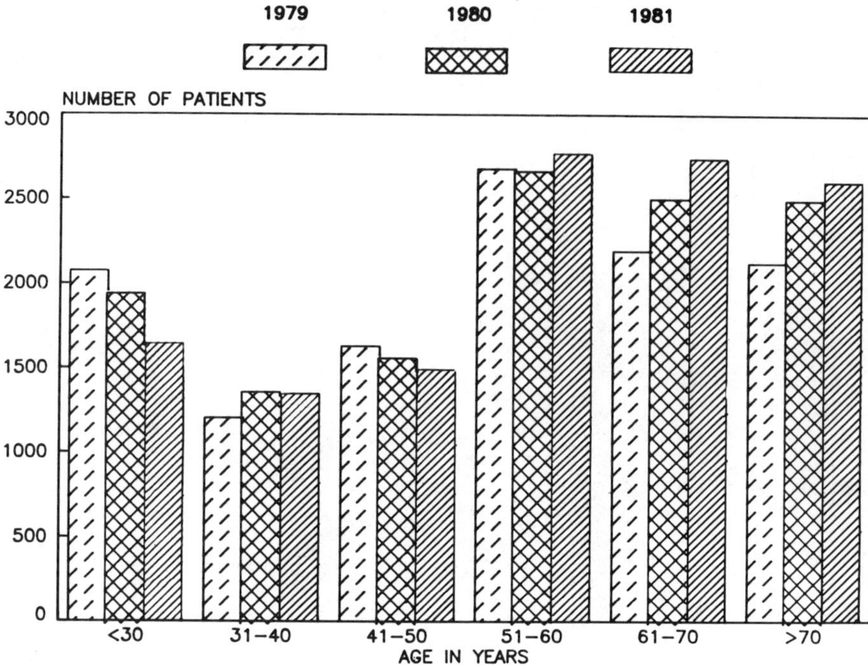

Figure 20-4

In 1971, 57,978 patient days were covered by Blue Cross and only 41,122 by Medicare. By 1981, a dramatic reversal occurred with only 35,439 patient days covered by Blue Cross and 65,513 by Medicare. Medicare, by definition, deals with elderly patients. These changes in the sources of funds used to cover cost of hospitalization and treatment offer considerable insight into the significance of the elderly patient for this particular hospital. Undoubtedly, such changes are experienced by the majority of urban hospitals in the United States. Of course, these trends are not due only to the increased proportion of the elderly in our population. Other factors may include changes in the population structure of the inner city, movement to the suburbs by younger families, and the changing economy. For whatever reason, those involved in the clinical practice of nutrition in large urban hospitals must be prepared to deal with the elderly patient.

IMPACT OF THE ELDERLY ON NUTRITION SUPPORT SERVICES

While at University Hospital in Boston, I had the opportunity to review an entire year's experience of the Clinical Nutrition Unit. We found that of a total of 260 patients, 48.7 were greater than 60 years of age (Figure 20-5). This pattern is also emerging in the experience of the new Nutrition Intervention Team at St. Vincent Charity Hospital and Health Center. During the first four weeks of its operation, a total of 29 patients were treated, with average age 53.9 years and with 55% being greater than 60 years of age (Figure 20-6). With this trend expected to continue, it will be crucial to be able to assess adequately both nutritional status and requirements in this patient population group.

ASSESSMENT OF NUTRITIONAL STATUS

An assessment of the nutritional status of any hospitalized patient, particularly in relation to the effects of stress on lean body mass, is exceptionally difficult. Our inability to assess nutritional status with any degree of reproducibility, sensitivity or precision is perhaps one of the greatest stumbling blocks to the acceptance of the discipline of Clinical Nutrition as a credible medical speciality. Such considerations are compounded in the elderly subject, to a great extent, because we have no standards for "normal" for these individuals, particularly the very old. To say that an individual patient is malnourished implies that we can define an adequate state of nutrition. All of us who treat patients have been confronted by the apparently frail but spry 75-pound old woman who, by anthropometric standards, should be near death. Yet, from a functional and biochemical point of view, the patient appears to be "normal." To be malnourished is to be abnormal; but what is the definition of normal?

For those of us who ponder such questions, it would be instructive to refer to

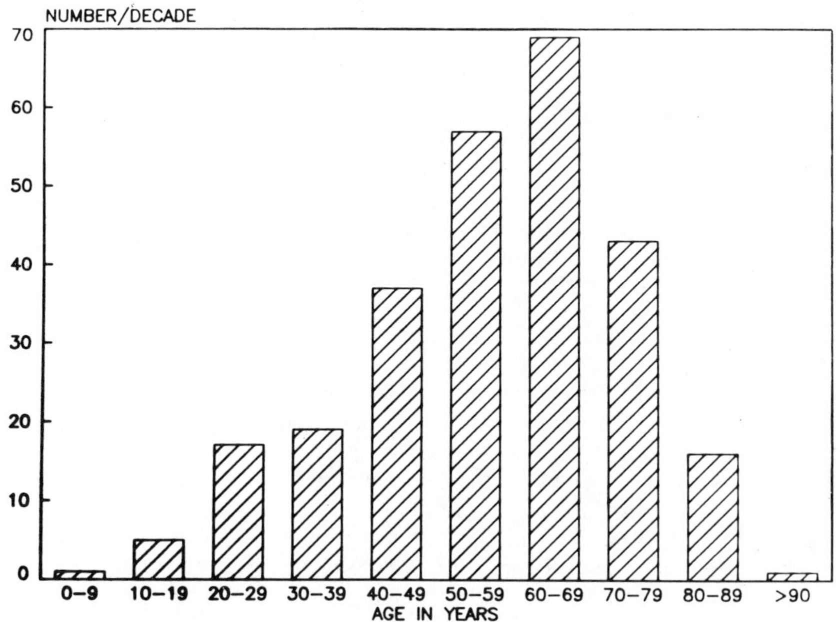

Figure 20-5

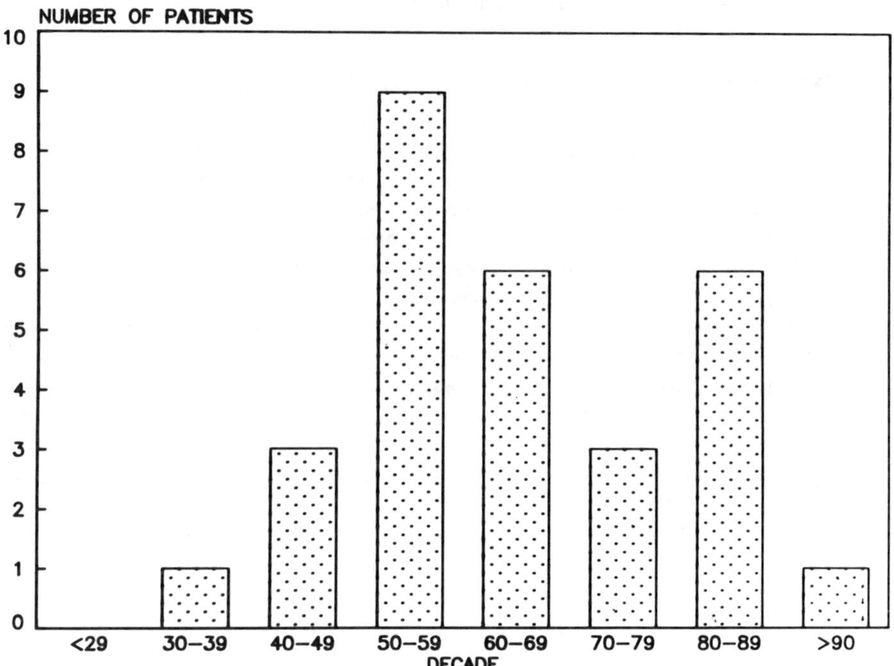

Figure 20-6

the article "Plato and Clementine," written by a champion of "normal" renal physiology, Homer W. Smith (1943). He states that normal is

> a formless, limitless, insubstantial ghost not to be captured by any trap set by the anatomist, physiologist or statistician. There is no such thing as an ostensibly normal person—only persons who show no ostensible danger of pain, disability or death. The word normal is useful in only one sense—as a tag for ignorance.

Nearly all parameters used for assessing nutritional status have some drawbacks when the patient is elderly, particularly the very old.

Decreased weight for a given height is not a reliable means for assessing nutritional status. Loss of lean body mass with aging is an accepted fact, yet there are no norms for older people that help to define an appropriate body weight, or the proportion of weight represented by fat or lean body tissue.

Body height is used to select an ideal body weight, as it is used to establish a creatinine/height index. What height is appropriate for a kyphotic individual who has lost inches due to both the spinal deformity and perhaps compressed vertebral bodies and/or intervertebral discs? His measured height? His "physiologic" height prior to the onset of physical deformities?

Determination of the midarm muscle circumference has gained favor with those individuals who are trying to quantify the extent of cachexia. Again, the reference values available are for a young adult population from which the elderly may deviate, due to age, rather than malnutrition or disease. Of course, regardless of the degree of deviation from "normal," a decrease may represent muscular inactivity *per se* rather than either malnutrition or a physiological factor relating to the aging process.

Changes in plasma protein may be a valid index of protein nutritional status regardless of age (Lipschitz, 1982). This is true, of course, if no other cause for abnormality is present. For example, after the nephrotic syndrome, liver failure or protein-losing enteropathy are ruled out, the greatest influence on plasma albumin levels is the patient's state of hydration. Unfortunately, many patients who are afflicted with a disease that has the tendency to create malnutrition, also tend to be dehydrated on admission to the hospital, sometimes severely so. In such instances, plasma volume can be reduced to a level that falsely elevates the plasma albumin concentration, making its measurement an unreliable indicator of nutritional status.

The application of skin tests to assess the patient's immune response is routinely used for the evaluation of nutritional status. Whereas this technique is questioned by some, questions arise about the elderly patient who is described as developing "immune senescence" (Twomey et al., 1982). It may be that the elderly are all protein malnourished; however, such correlations are unwarranted.

From my perspective as a clinician, it is imperative that nutritional science provide a means for assessing a patient's nutritional status, particularly from the perspective of protein nutritional status. More often than not, we stand by the bedside of an elderly stressed, ill patient and wonder how malnourished he/she might be. This becomes a critical issue because one's first impulse is to assign the cachexia to simple "old age," implying that it cannot be corrected by parenteral or enteral nutrition therapies. However, if the patient simply appears terminal due to correctable state of malnutrition, then every effort should be instituted to correct the condition of protein malnutrition.

Of course, what the clinician is really asking—from a protein nutritional point of view—is whether the individual has the capacity to accelerate rates of tissue and organ protein synthesis to levels equal to or above those in healthy subjects that would allow wounds to heal, appropriate immune responses to develop, and health to be restored. Protein malnutrition involves profound changes in whole body and organ protein dynamics. Even though protein turnover might slow with age (Winterer et al., 1976), it must be accelerated to allow a successful response to a specific disease process. Thus, nutritional assessment for the stressed, hospitalized patient should involve a determination of such capacities, and hopefully improved diagnostic tools will become available for use by clinicians, with advances in the research described elsewhere in this volume.

NUTRIENT REQUIREMENTS

With the ability to deliver nutrients in variable amounts to any individual, it should be obvious that we need to obtain better estimates of what an individual's nutritional requirements might be. This is particularly true of the very old, since even under the most severe stress, caloric requirements need not be great. Likewise, amino acid requirements to support optimal rates of protein synthesis may be less than in healthy young adults. The fact remains that we really do not know what these requirements are in a stressed individual. Much work is still required to define both the total amount of protein required and, in particular, the mixture of specific amino acids that is of greatest benefit to the stressed, elderly patient.

EFFECT OF NUTRITION SUPPORT ON CLINICAL OUTCOME

There have been few studies to define the effectiveness of nutrition interventions on the eventual outcome of the hospitalized geriatric patient. Should the patient who has suffered a major cerebrovascular accident, resulting in an inability to eat, be supported nutritionally? If unsupported, is return of cerebral function impaired by nutrient lack? If nutrition intervention is undertaken, what end-point is chosen for nutritional rehabilitation? Obviously, we should nourish the old patient to the point of normalcy, but again what is normal?

A common scene in the hospital setting is the elderly patient who has exhibited marginal recovery from a particular disaster, lying quietly or sleeping in bed or sitting in a chair, marginally responsive to external stimuli, refusing to eat, and awaiting nursing home placement. Most all of us who have dealt with such individuals have a strong clinical impression that when these patients are force fed, either by total parenteral nutrition or, most commonly, by enteral hyperalimentation, these patients become more alert, more responsive to stimuli, more receptive to even routine tasks such as eating an acceptable diet. One can anticipate a dramatic effect of nutritional therapy only if the patient is malnourished to begin with. But how does one diagnose malnutrition? How much and for how long should the feedings, enteral or parenteral, be administered?

It is with considerable frustration that we deal with such issues. I recently submitted the results of an extensive prospective, randomized and controlled study to the National Institutes of Health in an attempt to gain some insights into whether nutrition intervention made any difference to clinical outcome in the elderly patient. The response was brief and brusque. I was informed that first of all everyone knew that the elderly were malnourished; second, everyone knew that total parenteral nutrition corrected malnutrition; and third, for these reasons, there was little reason to perform such a study. It is my fervent desire that the Nutrition Study Section of the NIH recognizes the major gaps in knowledge, as outlined above, and that it recommends clinically oriented research to narrow these gaps in correct knowledge.

COST/EFFECTIVENESS CONSIDERATIONS

In view of today's economy, and in the many regulations imposed on hospital practice, how can we possibly afford to impose upon hospital administrations the cost required to intervene nutritionally (in the more vigorous sense) for a patient whose lifestyle may or may not benefit appreciably? An obligation has been made by St. Vincent Charity Hospital and Health Center for the development of a Nutrition Intervention Team, amounting to $1.2 million for the first year. Of this cost, the greatest proportion is for amino acids. They will be administered by knowledgeable and caring individuals whose main objective is to return these individuals, principally elderly, to a reasonable state of nutritional health. We proceed with the full realization that whereas prevention of malnutrition would have been a relatively inexpensive and short-term task, the repair of deficits that have been allowed to develop will result in enhanced costs, prolonged lengths of hospital stay, critical questions from Utilization Reviewers, discouragement of family, concerns raised by the Administration, and constant worry about meeting hospital budget requirements. Until criteria are firmly in hand relative to the assessment of both nutritional status and nutritional requirements, we will be forced to proceed, more with the concept that "food is good" and life is important no matter what the age in years, rather than relying upon a sound scientific basis.

CONCLUSION

The patient mix for which the practicing clinical nutritionist is responsible reflects the increasing age of the U.S. population. A good physician must be prepared to deal with the elderly patient. In so doing, however, the physician must be aware that nutritional science and its application in medicine has not reached that point where it is possible to evaluate adequately and treat the malnourished elderly patient, with the full knowledge that clinical outcome will be favorably modified in a cost-effective manner.

REFERENCES

Lipschitz, D.A. (1982): Protein calorie malnutrition in the hospitalized elderly. In: *Primary Care* (ed: W.P. Steffee), W.B. Saunders Co., New York (In Press).

Smith, H.W. (1943): Plato and Clementine. *N.Y. Acad. Med.* 23:352–377.

Twomey, P. et al. (1982): Utility of skin testing in nutritional assessment: A critical review. *J.P.E.N.* 6:50–58.

Winterer, J.C. et al. (1976): Whole body protein turnover in aging man. *Exp. Gerontol.* 11: 79–87.

Urinary Excretion of Carnitine, a Lysine Catabolite, in Patients on Partial Parenteral Nutrition

Vichai Tanphaichitr, Alice Thienprasert, Siroj Kanjanapanjapol, and Auchai Kanjanapitak

Carnitine in the body is derived from the dietary intake of preformed carnitine and biosynthesized carnitine via transformation of lysine and methionine metabolism (Tanphaichitr and Broquist, 1973a; 1973b). It is the purpose of this study to assess carnitine status in patients receiving carnitine-free and amino acid-free partial parenteral nutrition (PPN).

MATERIALS AND METHODS

The study was conducted on two groups: 41 normal adults with a mean age of 35.6 ± 1.7 (± SEM) years and 15 patients with gallstones. The clinical data on the six male and nine female patients are shown in Table 1. Prior to surgery (D-1), the patients consumed an oral diet. On the day of surgery (D0), they received intravenous dextrose which provided 200 to 600 kcal. During the five-day postoperative period (D1-D5), each patient received PPN which provided a daily supply of 1200 kcal, derived entirely from dextrose.

Venous blood was obtained from the 41 normal adults after a 12- to 14-hour fast and from each patient between 7 and 8 AM on D-1, D1, D2, and D6. Twenty-four-hour urine samples were collected from normal adults one day prior to the venipuncture. For hospitalized patients, the samples were collected daily during the study. The carnitine contents in serum and urine were determined by the enzymatic-radioisotopic method (McGarry and Foster, 1976). Each serum and urine sample was analyzed for both free and total carnitine contents. The acylcarnitine concentration was obtained from the difference between the total and free carnitine values. The Student's test (one-tailed) was used to establish statistical significance (Colton, 1974).

RESULTS

Table 2 shows the mean ± SEM of urinary carnitine excretion in normal adults and hospitalized patients. Urinary free carnitine excretion on D0 and D1 and urinary total carnitine excretion on D1 were significantly higher than those on D-1, respectively. Urinary free carnitine excretion on D0-D3 and urinary acylcarnitine and total carnitine excretion on D1-D5 were significantly higher than those in normal adults, respectively.

Table 1
Clinical Data in 15 Patients on PPN

Patient	Age (yr)	Diagnosis	Operation
Male			
1	49	Gallstone	Cholecystectomy
2	59	Gallstone	Cholecystectomy and appendectomy
3	47	Gallstone and chronic pancreatitis	Cholecystectomy
4	50	Gallstone and peptic ulcer	Cholecystectomy
5	49	Gallstone	Cholecystectomy, exploration of common bile duct with T-tube drainage, and appendectomy
6	48	Gallstone	Cholecystectomy and exploration of common bile duct
Female			
7	60	Gallstone	Cholecystectomy
8	60	Gallstone	Cholecystectomy
9	42	Gallstone	Cholecystectomy
10	58	Gallstone	Cholecystectomy
11	54	Gallstone, common bile duct stone, and diabetes mellitus	Cholecystectomy and exploration of common bile duct
12	30	Gallstone and thalassemia	Cholecystectomy
13	46	Gallstone and left lower calyceal stone	Cholecystectomy
14	51	Gallstone	Cholecystectomy
15	46	Gallstone	Cholecystectomy

Table 3 presents the mean ± SEM of serum carnitine levels in normal adults and hospitalized patients. Serum free, acyl and total carnitine levels in patients did not significantly differ from those in normal adults. Serum free carnitine levels on D1 and D2 were significantly lower than those on D-1.

DISCUSSION

Serum and urinary carnitine levels are regulated by nutritional and endocrine factors. Decreased serum carnitine concentration and urinary carnitine excretion have been reported in subjects with protein-calorie malnutrition (Mikhail and Mansour, 1976; Khan and Bamji, 1977; Rudman et al., 1977; Tanphaichitr et al., 1980; Khan-Siddiqui and Bamji, 1980) and hypothyroidism (Maebashi et al., 1977). Tanphaichitr and Pakpeankitvatana (1981) have shown the effects of protein intake on

Table 2
Mean ± SEM of Urinary Carnitine Excretion in Normal Adults and Patients

Subject		Urinary Carnitine, μmol/day		
Group	*No.*	*Free*	*Acyl*	*Total*
Normal	41	162 ± 19	165 ± 13	328 ± 28
patient				
D-1	15	167 ± 39	343 ± 132	510 ± 157
D0	15	347 ± 44[*,∥]	315 ± 62[¶]	662 ± 83[∥]
D1	15	429 ± 86[†,∥]	543 ± 109[∥]	997 ± 132[‡,§]
D2	15	321 ± 90[∥]	335 ± 52[∥]	656 ± 98[∥]
D3	15	330 ± 75[¶]	407 ± 80[∥]	737 ± 106[∥]
D4	14	185 ± 44	277 ± 60[#]	462 ± 59[¶]
D5	15	198 ± 37	356 ± 80[¶]	554 ± 63[§]

*Significant difference from D-1: $p < 0.01$.
†Significant difference from D-1: $p < 0.005$.
‡Significant difference from D-1: $p < 0.025$.
§Significant difference from normal adults: $p < 0.0005$.
∥Significant difference from normal adults: $p < 0.005$.
¶Significant difference from normal adults: $p < 0.025$.
#Significant difference from normal adults: $p < 0.05$.

Table 3
Mean ± SEM of Serum Carnitine Levels in Normal Adults and Patients

Subject		Serum Carnitine, μmol/l		
Group	*No.*	*Free*	*Acyl*	*Total*
Normal patient	41	65 ± 2	53 ± 4	118 ± 4
D-1	15	72 ± 5	64 ± 11	136 ± 12
D1	15	65 ± 4*	88 ± 37	154 ± 37
D2	14	61 ± 2[†]	66 ± 10	127 ± 11
D6	15	70 ± 2	62 ± 9	131 ± 10

*Significant difference from D-1: $p < 0.025$.
†Significant difference from D-1: $p < 0.01$.

urinary carnitine excretion in adult males. In that study individuals were fed diets adequate in total energy but limited in carnitine and containing different levels of egg protein. The means ± SEM of urinary free and total carnitine excretion in subjects on a protein-free diet were 276 ± 13 and 517 ± 19 μmol/day, respectively, which were significantly higher than normal values. The stress stimuli, i.e., lack of dietary protein and carnitine with adequate fat consumption, were alleviated when egg protein was added to the protein-free diet. The means ± SEM of urinary free and total carnitine excretion in subjects on 0.65 g egg protein per kg body weight per day were 8 ± 1 and 70 ± 7 μmol/day, respectively. The data suggested that lysine and methionine present in the egg protein were effectively utilized for carnitine biosynthesis. This, in turn, decreased carnitine mobilization from skeletal muscle which is the major storage site of carnitine (Tanphaichitr and Broquist, 1973b; Tanphaichitr and Broquist, 1974; Tanphaichitr et al., 1976).

Infection or tissue injury increases the pituitary production of adrenocorticotrophic hormone which, in turn, stimulates the adrenocortical release of cortisol (Moore, 1976). These endocrine responses result in the increase in serum carnitine levels and urinary carnitine excretion (Maebashi et al., 1976; Maebashi et al., 1977). In this study, all of the patients underwent surgery listed in Table 1 and received a carnitine-free and amino acid-free PPN postoperatively. Their significant increase in urinary carnitine excretion during the postoperative period (Table 2) can be explained by the endocrine responses to the stress phenomenon and indicates a catabolic response by skeletal muscle. These findings agree with our previous studies in patients on total parenteral nutrition (Tanphaichitr and Lerdvuthisopon, 1981) and adult males on protein-free diet (Tanphaichitr and Pakpeankitvatana, 1981). The significant decrease in serum free carnitine level on D1 and D2 (Table 3) was due to an increase in the urinary free carnitine excretion on Day 0 and D1 (Table 2). Since carnitine is involved in long-chain fatty acid oxidation (Bressler, 1970) and oxidative utilization of ketone bodies, glucose and amino acids (Siliprandi and Ramacci, 1980) the significant loss of urinary carnitine, a lysine catabolite, could impair energy metabolism.

ACKNOWLEDGMENTS

This work was supported by a grant from the Faculty of Medicine, Ramathibodi Hospital, Ajinomoto Co (Thailand) Ltd., and Revlon Health Care Group Asia/Pacific.

REFERENCES

Bressler, R. (1970): Fatty acid oxidation. In: *Comprehensive Biochemistry* (eds: M. Florkin and E.H. Stotz), Vol. 18, pp. 331–359, Elsevier Publishing Co., New York.

Colton, T. (1974): *Statistics in Medicine.* (1st edition), Little Brown and Co., Boston, Mass.

Khan, L.A., and Bamji, M.S. (1977): Plasma carnitine levels in children with protein-calorie malnutrition before and after rehabilitation. *Clin. Chim. Acta* 75:163–166.

Khan-Siddiqui L., and Bamji, M.S. (1980): Plasma carnitine levels in adult males in India: effects of high cereal low fat diet, fat supplementation, and nutritional status. *Am. J. Clin. Nutr.* 33:1259–1263.

Maebashi, M., Kawamura, N., Sato, M., Yoshinaga, K., and Suzuki, M. (1976): Urinary excretion of carnitine in man. *J. Lab. Clin. Med.* 87:760–766.

Maebashi, M., Kawamura, N., Sato, M., Imamura, A., Yoshinaga, K., and Suzuki, M. (1977): Urinary excretion of carnitine in patients with hyperthyroidism and hypothyroidism: augmentation by thyroid hormone. *Metabolism* 26:351–356.

Maebashi, M., Kawamura, N., Sato, M., Imamura, A., Yoshinaga, K., and Suzuki, M. (1977): Urinary excretion of carnitine and serum concentrations of carnitine and lipids in patients with hypofunctional endocrine diseases: involvement of adrenocorticoid and thyroid hormones in ACTH-induced augmentation of carnitine and lipid metabolism. *Metabolism* 26:357–361.

McGarry, J.D., and Foster, D.W. (1976): An improved and simplified radioisotopic assay for the determination of free and esterified carnitine. *J. Lipid Res.* 17:277–281.

Mikhail, M.M., and Mansour, M.M. (1976): The relationship between serum carnitine levels and the nutritional status of patients with schistosomiasis. *Clin. Chim. Acta* 71:207–214.

Moore, F.D. (1976): La maladie post-operatoire: is there order in variety? The six stimulus-response sequences. *Surg. Clin. North Am.* 56:803–815.

Rudman, D., Sewell, C.W., and Ansley, J.D. (1977): Deficiency of carnitine in cachectic cirrhotic patients. *J. Clin. Invest.* 60:716–723.

Siliprandi, N., and Ramacci, M.T. (1980): Carnitine as a "drug" affecting lipid metabolism. In: *Drugs Affecting Lipid Metabolism* (eds: R. Fumagalli, D. Kritchevsky, and R. Paoletti), pp. 381–392, Elsevier Publishing Co., New York.

Tanphaichitr, V., and Broquist, H.P. (1973a): Lysine deficiency in the rat: concomitant impairment in carnitine biosynthesis. *J. Nutr.* 103:80–87.

Tanphaichitr, V., and Broquist, H.P. (1973b): Role of lysine and ε-N-trimethyllysine in carnitine biosynthesis. II. Studies in the rat. *J. Biol. Chem.* 248:2176–2181.

Tanphaichitr, V., and Broquist, H.P. (1974): Site of carnitine biosynthesis in the rat. *J. Nutr.* 104:1669–1673.

Tanphaichitr, V., Zaklama, M.S., and Broquist, H.P. (1976): Dietary lysine and carnitine: relation to growth and fatty livers in rat. *J. Nutr.* 106:111–117.

Tanphaichitr, V., Lerdvuthisopon, N., Dhanamitta, S., and Broquist, H.P. (1980): Carnitine status in Thai adults. *Am. J. Clin. Nutr.* 33:876–880.

Tanphaichitr, V., and Pakpeankitvatana, R. (1981): Effects of egg protein intake on urinary carnitine excretion in adult males. *XII International Congress of Nutrition,* p. 114, San Diego, California.

Tanphaichitr, V., and Lerdvuthisopon, N. (1981): Urinary carnitine excretion in surgical patients on total parenteral nutrition. *J. Parent. Enter. Nutr.* 5:505–509.

MALNUTRITION

21 Clinical Impact of Protein Malnutrition on Organ Mass and Function

John P. Grant

Since recorded time man has faced episodes of starvation threatening his survival. The availability of food has been a factor in natural selection. In spite of long experience, much remains to be learned of the impact of acute and chronic starvation on organ function. What we do know has come from five main sources. The first is records of more than 400 natural famines which have occurred throughout the world and ongoing studies in impoverished or poorly developed areas. The second is medical records of military detention camps, in particular those in Europe in the early 1940s. The third source is from human volunteer studies of semi-starvation. The first such study was the Carnegie Nutrition Laboratory Experiment of 1917 in which 24 men were placed on a 120-day semi-starvation diet. Results were published by Benedict et al. (1919). The second study was the Minnesota Experiment done in 1944. In this study 32 men and women, who were conscientious objectors, underwent 24 weeks of semi-starvation followed by a 12-week program of rehabilitation. This study was reported by Keys et al. (1950). The fourth source of information on the impact of malnutrition on organ function has been fasting of experimental animals. The final experience has been from studies of hospitalized patients over the past 20 years. All these sources will be drawn upon in this monograph, but it must be recognized that more detailed investigation of this devastating disease is needed.

The current incidence of protein-calorie malnutrition in the world is difficult to determine. In the United States it has been estimated that between 20% and 60% of hospitalized patients have significant malnutrition (Bistrian et al., 1974; Willcutts, 1977; Weinsier et al., 1979; Shaver et al., 1980). This number appears to be increasing as the average age increases and as noncurative therapies become more commonly employed such as renal dialysis, chemotherapy for malignant diseases, and new techniques of cardiopulmonary support. Recent studies have correlated loss of body weight, decreased serum albumin, and other nutritional assessment parameters with increased morbidity and mortality (Studley, 1936; Cruse and Foord, 1973; Reinhardt et al., 1980; Mullen, 1981). It is, therefore, important to review current knowledge of interactions between protein-calorie malnutrition, organ mass, and function. This discussion will deal with the consequences of simple starvation alone. Others will address the significant nutritional challenges to body homeostasis of stress and sepsis.

BODY COMPOSITION CHANGES WITH STARVATION

Krieger (1921) reviewed changes in body and organ weight at autopsy of severely emaciated patients who died of various diseases (Table 21-1). Death occurred after loss of 38% to 42% of total body weight regardless of whether due to starvation, malignant tumor, or chronic infection. Various organs lost differing amounts of

Table 21-1
Weight Loss at Autopsy of Emaciated Bodies

	Cause of Death		
	Cachexia	*Tumor*	*Chronic Infection*
Body Weight	38.8*	38.0	43.9
Heart	34.7	33.2	30.7
Liver	42.1	32.8	28.0
Kidney	36.0	27.5	15.5
Brain	4.6	3.4	2.8

*percent loss
Modified from Krieger, 1921

Table 21-2
Loss of Organ Mass in Seven-day Starved Rats

	Percent Loss	
Organ	*Jackson, 1915*	*Ross and Grant, 1982**
Body weight	33	23
Musculature	31	—
Gastrointestinal tract	57	19
Heart	28	17
Kidneys	26	25
Liver	58	27
Lungs	31	17
Brain	5	—

*Rats fed protein-free oral diet for seven days. Unpublished data.

Table 21-3
Relative Losses of Protein from Various Organs and Tissues in Rats (Seven-day Fast)

Organ or Tissue	% Loss
Liver	40
Gastrointestinal tract	28
Kidneys	20
Heart	18
Muscle and skin	8
Brain	5

Modified from Addis et al., 1936

weight. In cachexia of chronic starvation, the liver lost the greatest percentage, with the kidney next, then the heart, and finally the brain. In the experimental rat model, seven days of starvation likewise results in significant loss of organ masses (Table 21-2). That this loss of mass is due to loss of organ protein content and not just water or fat has been shown in the rat (Table 21-3).

Studies by Kinney et al. (1968), Moore and Ball (1952), and Cahill et al. (1966) have demonstrated nitrogen losses of 5 to 40 g per day during stress and sepsis in the human reflecting endogenous utilization of 30 to 240 g protein per day. Depending on the clinical setting and hormonal influences, this protein is derived from muscle, internal organs, or from both sources.

IMPACT OF PROTEIN DEPLETION ON ORGAN MASS AND FUNCTION

Skeletal Muscle Mass and Function

Skeletal muscle mass depletion during chronic semi-starvation was estimated in the Minnesota Experiment from measurements of upper arm muscle area and thigh muscle area subtracting bone area (Table 21-4). A progressive decrease in muscle mass was seen with a 46% loss of upper arm muscle area and 37% loss of thigh muscle area after 24 weeks of semi-starvation. Over the same period, there was a 23% decrease in body weight. Studies in the rat (Table 21-2) have demonstrated a 31% decrease in muscle mass with 33% body weight loss after seven days of starvation (Jackson, 1915). Histological sections of muscle during starvation demonstrate a decrease in fiber diameter proportional to the decrease in body weight with crowding of nuclei. With extreme starvation there is an actual loss of muscle cells.

Table 21-4
Change in Muscle Mass After 12 and 24 Weeks of Semi-Starvation

	C	S12	S24	% Loss
Upper arm muscle area – bone	61 cm^2	40	33	46
Thigh muscle area – bone	171 cm^2	123	108	37
Body weight	69 kg	57	53	23

Modified from Keys et al., 1950

Alteration in the capacity to perform work during chronic semi-starvation was evaluated in the Minnesota Experiment by the Harvard Fitness Test comparing mean scores during starvation and rehabilitation (Table 21-5). Through starvation, a progressive decline in the quality of fitness was observed, with all volunteers being of poor fitness after 24 weeks. Recovery of normal function was delayed, remaining incomplete even after 12 weeks of refeeding. This demonstrates, as is true of other organs, that recovery from starvation requires at least as much if not more time. The clinical expression of chronic muscle wasting is weakness, easy fatigability, and decreased ambulation.

Table 21-5
Mean Harvard Fitness Scores During Semi-Starvation and Refeeding (Minnesota Experiment)

General Fitness	C	S12*	S24	R3†	R12
Average-to-Good	29‡	7	0	2	9
Poor	3	25	32	30	23
Average Harvard Fitness Score	64	33	18	22	35

*Weeks of semi-starvation
†Weeks of refeeding
‡Number of patients with good, average, or poor function in testing
Modified from Keys et al., 1950

The impact of acute starvation as seen in the hospitalized patient has been less well studied. Tui et al. (1944) evaluated endurance of the upper extremities in patients following gastrointestinal surgery using a bedside ergograph. They reported postoperative "asthenia" in patients which persisted through the 12th postoperative day if 50 to 150 g negative nitrogen balance occurred.

We have measured grip strength in 187 hospitalized patients using a hand dynamometer comparing strength to mid-triceps arm muscle circumference and area, creatinine excretion and creatinine–height index, and body weight (Moran et al., 1980). We found no correlation with a wide range of function associated with various indicators of muscle mass. The best correlation with muscle function was serum transferrin and prealbumin, suggesting function during the early stages of poor nutrition to be more sensitive to energy and structural substrates than actual muscle mass. Interpretation of standard anthropometric measurements must, therefore, be made with caution in "early" starvation, realizing complications due to poor muscle function may well occur irrespective of muscle mass.

Gastrointestinal Tract Mass and Function

Postmortem studies of children and adults with protein-calorie malnutrition have demonstrated significant atrophy of the gastrointestinal tract (Tejada and Restrepo, 1962). The Warsaw Ghetto Hospital autospy reports in cachectic patients related "paper-thin" bowels through which newsprint could be read (Apfelbaum, 1946). Gastroscopy has shown atrophy of gastric mucosa in starvation (Bebray et al., 1946). In seven-day starvation of rats, Jackson (1915) demonstrated a 57% decrease in the gastrointestinal tract mass associated with a 33% body weight loss, and we have found a 19% decrease in mass with a protein-free diet yet adequate calories (Table 21-2). Histological changes during starvation include a loss of fat, thinning of the gastrointestinal wall with atrophy of the mucosa, and moderate to marked muscular atrophy with decreased cell size, some cellular degeneration, and some vacuolization (Schneider and Viteri, 1972; Mayoral et al., 1972). Gastric mucosa demonstrates cytoplasmic and nuclear degeneration of the parietal and chief cell populations.

Clinically, diarrhea, pseudodysentery, colic, and flatulence are universal observations of all famine periods, as well as in detention centers in Europe. In addition there has been an increased incidence of intestinal ulcers reported, in particular of the stomach (Lipscomb, 1945). Evidence from the Minnesota Experiment and from other reports paradoxically demonstrate decreased acid production as starvation progresses (Adesola, 1968; Mata et al., 1972; Gracey et al., 1973). Malabsorption is a typical finding in severe malnutrition. D-xylose absorption and glucose absorption are decreased as is fat absorption (Mayoral et al., 1972; Viterie et al., 1973; Viteri and Schneider, 1974). In addition, contrary to animal experiments, protein absorption in man is impaired by *in vivo* and *in vitro* testing (Adibi and Allen, 1970; Steiner and Gray, 1969). Impaired B_{12} absorption, unresponsive to intrinsic factor supplementation, and increased fecal loss of bile acids suggests impaired terminal ileal absorption as well (Alvarado et al., 1973). The malabsorption can be attributed to several factors. Hypoproteinemia may result in significant bowel wall edema with decreased passage of nutrients across the mucosal membrane. Decreased absorptive surface and decreased brush border enzyme concentrations are also important factors (Adibi and Allen, 1970; Levine et al., 1974). Bacterial proliferation in the upper intestine and stomach during chronic malnutrition, thought due to impaired defense mechanisms in general and breakdown of normal intrinsic defense mechanisms of the gastrointestinal tract in particular, including loss of gastric acid secretion, is felt to contribute to the malabsorption and diarrhea (Mata et al., 1972; Gracey et al., 1973; Gracey et al., 1975). Finally, significantly decreased gastric emptying and prolonged intestinal transit time is common in malnutrition (Keys et al., 1950; Viteri and Schneider, 1974). Recovery of normal motility with refeeding is slow.

The impact of acute starvation on the gastrointestinal tract is less well studied. Recent investigation has indicated the small intestine to be an important site of drug metabolism, containing both cytochrome P-450 and glutathione 5-transferases. Exclusion of oral nutrients in the rat reduces metabolism of pentobarbitol (Knodel et al., 1980). Whether similar alterations occur in fasted man and whether it is of clinical significance remain to be determined.

Pancreatic exocrine function is reduced during protein-calorie malnutrition with lower lipase, trypsin, chymotrypsin, and amylase production in that order (Veghelyi, 1948; Thompson and Trowell, 1952; Viteri and Schneider, 1974). Zymogen granules are decreased and the response to secretin and cholecystokinin are reduced. Recovery of pancreatic function with adequate nutrition may require several months (Barbezat and Hansen, 1968).

Cardiac Mass and Function

In 1866 Voit evaluated cardiac mass in starved cats (Voit, 1866). He found relative preservation of cardiac mass and proposed that the heart was spared during starvation. His concept remained unchallenged through 1924 when Vaquez stated: ". . . inanition has no harmful action on the heart" (Vaquez, 1924). Subsequent studies, however, have demonstrated starvation to have significant impact upon cardiac mass and function. Keys reported that the human heart atrophied proportional to body weight loss (Keys et al., 1950). Abel found a 20% to 30% decrease in myofiber diameter with starvation, and Heymsfield found all chamber volumes decreased with starvation proportional to loss of body weight (Abel et al., 1977; Heymsfield et al., 1978). It has been recognized that in the hypercatabolic patient, starvation does not result in as significant cardiac atrophy likely due to work stimulation of the muscle mass. Reference to Table 21-1 demonstrates 30% to 35% decrease in cardiac weight upon death associated with severe cachexia. In the rat, the heart was found to lose 17% to 28% of its mass and 18% of its total protein content with seven days of starvation (Tables 21-2 and 21-3).

Recent studies have attempted to better define cardiac function during starvation. In general, decreased cardiac output and stroke volume have been demonstrated proportional to the decrease in body weight. This response may only reflect adaptation to decreased demands on the heart with decreased body size. However, Kyger et al. (1978) demonstrated the decreased cardiac contractility and stroke volume of isolated perfused hearts of starved rats worsened with increasing left atrial pressure, suggesting an underlying functional defect. Abel demonstrated decreased cardiac compliance and contractility in dogs with decreased force velocities following starvation (Abel et al., 1977). Nutter et al. (1978), however, found little change in cardiac function in starved rat hearts. Clinically, patients present with bradycardia, hypotension, and occasional arrhythmias which may contribute to the sudden death associated with progressive protein-calorie malnutrition. Congestive heart failure is unusual during starvation and rare during slow refeeding, but common with rapid refeeding, consistent with Kyger's findings. The decreased metabolic state with starvation places little load on the heart, but with rapid refeeding the stress can become significant leading to cardiac failure.

Renal Mass and Function

Decrease in kidney size is consistently found in chronic starvation. In the report of Krieger (Table 21-1), kidney mass decreased 36% during chronic starvation, with body weight loss of 39%. In rat studies, seven days of starvation or protein-free diets has been associated with 25% to 26% loss of mass and 20% loss of kidney protein content (Tables 21-2 and 21-3). Histologically, there is thinning of the renal cortex, with cloudy swelling of the cells of the tubules and Bowman's capsule. In severe starvation there is degeneration and desquamation of tubular epithelium.

Renal function in starvation has been characterized by gradual deterioration of the ability to excrete titratable acid, which renders the starving patient susceptible to metabolic acidosis (Klahr et al., 1970). This abnormality is corrected in part with administration of phosphorus. Commonly, polyurea and nocturia occur with starvation, which is felt to be due to decreased urea concentration in the medulla and subsequent impairment of renal concentrating ability (Klahr et al., 1967). Renal dilution ability appears unaltered. In children, glomerular filtration rate and renal plasma flow are decreased with chronic malnutrition, which can lead to impaired drug excretion (Pullman et al., 1954; Klahr and Alleyne, 1973; Buchanan et al., 1979). In adults the data is less clear.

Liver Mass and Function

The liver is the most sensitive organ to starvation with respect to loss of mass. In the study of Krieger (Table 21-1) the liver lost 42% of its weight compared to a body weight loss of 39% with death from chronic starvation. In rats, the liver lost 58% of its mass and 40% of its protein content during a seven-day fast (Tables 21-2 and 21-3). Filkins (1970) demonstrated in a seven-day fast of rats that there was a 39% decrease in body weight and a 66% decrease in liver weight with 74% loss of liver protein mass. We have recently found a seven-day protein-free diet in rats to result in 23% body weight loss, 27% loss of liver mass, and 59% decrease in liver protein content. The organ weight loss inaccurately reflected the protein loss due to significant fatty infiltration. Histologically, there is cloudy swelling and atrophy of the hepatocytes along with hemosiderosis and vacuolization. Degenerative changes in mitochondria and microsomes have been demonstrated (Bernhard and Rouiller, 1956). Typically, a fatty infiltration of the liver occurs, especially with diets that are low in protein and moderate to high in carbohydrate content. Filkins demonstrated nuclear crowding, with a twofold increase in nuclei present on histological sectioning per gram wet weight of tissues in rats.

The function of the liver during starvation has been only partly evaluated. Biochemical studies have demonstrated increases in selective enzymes: glucose 6-phosphatase, tyrosine transaminase, tryptophan pyrollase, and the gluconeogenic series of enzymes. Other enzymes are significantly decreased, including fructose diphosphatase, phosphohexose isomerase, LDH phosphoglucomutase, 6-phosphoglucodehydrogenase, xanthine oxidase, and cytochrome oxidase (Onicescu and Radu, 1969; Filkins, 1970). Several studies of drug metabolism have demonstrated clearance, suggesting impaired enzyme function (Dixon et al., 1960; Kato et al., 1968). Antipyrine is a drug cleared by the microsomal mixed oxidation enzyme system. Buchanan demonstrated in children approximately one year of age with kwashiorkor that the half-life of antipyrine was 7.9 hours, and after 21 days of feeding reduced to 4.3 hours (Buchanan et al., 1979). Similar data was demonstrated by Krishnaswami and Naidu (1977). Hepatic microsomal glucuronidation was shown to be decreased by Buchanan as measured by d-glucaric acid excretion in children (Buchanan et al., 1979). The prefeeding clearance was 60.6 μmol per 24 hours, whereas after 21 days of feeding, 121.8 μmol per 24 hour of d-glucaric acid was excreted. Metabolism of other drugs by microsomal enzymes may be similarly altered (Brodie et al., 1958).

Finally, studies with indocyanine green have demonstrated decreased clearance in protein-depleted patients (Paumgartner et al., 1970; Grant and Curtas, 1980). This dye is transported into the hepatocyte by a surface receptor and then excreted into the bile requiring little metabolic activity. The hepatocyte surface receptor appears to be sensitive to protein nutrition. Albumin synthesis has been studied by several authors (Eckart et al., 1972; Rothschild et al., 1972). Normal albumin synthesis is between 130 to 200 mg/kg/day, with a maximal synthetic rate reported as 860 mg/kg/day. In patients treated with protein deficient diets, albumin synthesis decreases by as much as 50%. The decreased synthetic rate persists until protein intake is increased.

Repiratory Mass and Function

Most human studies have demonstrated little change in pulmonary mass during chronic starvation. In studies of rats, however, lung weight decreased 17% to 31% after seven days of a protein-free diet or starvation (Table 21-2). Histological changes during starvation include decreased mucous production, dry chronic bronchitis, and an unusually high incidence of emphysematous changes which may approach 13%, a third of these changes appearing in patients less than 30 years of age (Stein and Fenigstein, 1946). There appears to be an increased tendency to nontubercular lung cavitation such as following minor pulmonary infarcts.

Pulmonary function testing during chronic semi-starvation demonstrated a significant decrease in vital capacity, rate of respiration, tidal volume, and respiratory efficiency after 24 weeks (Table 21-6). Only incomplete recovery was recognized after 12 weeks. The minute ventilation and the ventilatory efficiency during aerobic and anerobic work also decreased significantly as starvation progressed. Recovery with feeding was slow (Keys et al., 1950).

Table 21-6
Changes in Resting Pulmonary Function During Semi-Starvation (Minnesota Experiment)

	C	S12*	S24	R12†
Vital capacity (liters)	5.17	4.97	4.78	5.00
Respirations (per minute)	11.4	9.9	9.9	10.5
Tidal volume (liters)	421	353	340	381
Liters per minute	4.8	3.5	3.3	4.0

*Weeks of semi-starvation
†Weeks of re-feeding
Modified from Keys et al., 1950

We have studied the effects of short-term starvation on pulmonary muscle function by measuring maximal expiratory pressure and inspiratory vaccum in over 200 hospitalized patients. No correlation was found between pulmonary muscle function and any parameter of body muscle mass. Significant correlation was found, however, with serum albumin, transferrin and prealbumin concentrations, suggesting respiratory muscle function is dependent on energy and protein substrate availability in early starvation rather than actual muscle mass. Sahebjami and Vassallo (1979) found ten-day semi-starvation of rats significantly increased lung surface elastic forces, decreased tissue elasticity of the lung, and increased airspace. One week after refeeding, surface forces were restored but tissue elasticity and airspace enlargement were only partially corrected.

The function of pulmonary chemoreceptors appears to be significantly altered early in starvation. Benedict et al. (1917) first showed decreased sensitivity to carbon dioxide in 1917. Recently, Weissman et al. (1982) confirmed these findings, demonstrating a blunted ventilatory response to breathing 2% and 4% carbon dioxide in the inspired air after a seven-day protein-free diet in healthy volunteers. The sensitivity to carbon dioxide was easily restored after one day of intravenous amino acid administration but was unaffected by carbohydrate infusion. Doekel et al. (1976) demonstrated a significant decrease in the respiratory response to hypoxia after four to ten days of starvation in normal volunteers.

The potential clinical implications of altered respiratory mass and function in hospitalized, malnourished patients remains speculative but of major importance.

Brain Mass and Function

The brain appears to be the least sensitive to starvation of all organs in the body. Krieger (Table 21-1) demonstrated only a 4.6% decrease in brain mass associated with a 39% decrease in body weight. Rats subjected to seven-day starvation demonstrated only a 5% decrease in mass and protein content of the brain (Tables 21-2 and 21-3). Histologically, increased pericellular space with frequent vacuoles are identified on cut sections. With severe starvation, cloudy swelling occurs as well as chromatolysis. Although there is little change in mass, function does appear to be sensitive to starvation. The Minnesota Experiment evaluated mental changes during chronic semi-starvation and reported a variety of symptomatologies as indicated in Table 21-7. A prominent adaptive response to short-term starvation in the hospitalized patient is lethargy, loss of mental alertness, and occasional confusion. This adaptive response as well as the acute psychosis observed in intensive care units might in part be related to the poor nutritional state typically present.

Table 21-7
Mental Changes During Semi-Starvation (Minnesota Experiment)

Symptom	Score	Direction
Tiredness	3.5	+
Appetite	3.1	+
Irritability	1.8	+
Apathy	1.8	+
Concentration	1.7	−
Mental alertness	1.5	−
Depression	1.4	+
Apprehension	0.4	+

0 = normal, 5 = extreme, n = 32
Modified from Keys et al., 1950

CONCLUSIONS

We are only beginning to understand the impact of short-term and chronic starvation on organ mass and function. Much work remains to be done. Attention must be placed not only upon disruption of normal organ function during starvation but the impact of abnormal organ function on subsequent nutrition with further deterioration. As the consequences of starvation become clearer, the importance of nutritional rehabilitation and, in particular, prevention of malnutrition in clinical practice is obvious.

REFERENCES

Abel, R.M., Alonso, D.R., Grimes, J., and Gay, W.A., Jr. (1977): Biochemical, ultrastructural, and hemodynamic changes in chronic protein-calorie malnutrition in dogs. *Circulation* 56:55A.

Addis, T., Poo, L.J., and Lew, W. (1936): The quantities of proteins lost by the various organs and tissues of the body during a fast. *J. Biol. Chem.* 115:111–116.

Adesola, A.O. (1968): The influence of severe protein deficiency on gastric acid secretion in Nigerian children. *Br. J. Surg.* 55:866.

Adibi, S.A., and Allen, E.R. (1970): Impaired jejunal absorption rates of essential amino acids induced by either dietary, calorie or protein deprivation in man. *Gastroenterology* 59:404–413.

Alvarado, J., Vargas, W., Diaz, N., and Viteri, F.E. (1973): Vitamin B-12 absorption in protein-calorie malnourished children and during recovery: influence of protein depletion and of diarrhea. *Am. J. Clin. Nutr.* 26:595–599.

Apfelbaum, E. (ed.) (1946): *Maladie de Famine. Recherches Cliniques sur la Famine Executees dans la Ghetto de Varsovie en 1942.* Am. Joint Distribution Committee, Warsaw.

Barbezet, G.O. and Hansen, J.D.L. (1968): The exocrine pancreas and protein calorie malnutrition. *Pediatrics* 42:77–92.

Benedict, F.G., Miles, W.R., Roth, P., and Smith, H.M. (1919): *Human Vitality and Efficiency Under Prolonged Restricted Diet.* Carnegie Inst. Washington Publ. No. 280.

Bernhard, W., and Rouiller, C. (1956): Close topographical relationship between mitochondria and ergastoplasm of liver cells in a definite phase of cellular activity. *J. Biophys. Biochem. Cytol.* 2(Suppl.):73–78.

Bistrian, B.R., Blackburn, G.L., Hallowell, E., and Hadelle, R. (1974): Protein status of general surgical patients. *JAMA* 230:858–860.

Brodie, B.B., Gillette, J.R., and LaDu, B.N. (1958): Enzymatic metabolism of drugs and other foreign compounds. *Ann. Rev. Biochem.* 27:427–454.

Buchanan, N., Davis, M.D., and Eyberg, C. (1979): Gentamycin pharmacokinetics in kwashiorkor. *Br. J. Clin. Pharmacol.* 8:451–453.

Buchanan, N., Eyberg, C., and Davis, M.D. (1979): Antipyrine pharmacokinetics and D-glucaric excretion in kwashiorkor. *Am. J. Clin. Nutr.* 32:2439–2442.

Cahill, G.F., Jr., Felig, P., and Marliss, E.P. (1966): Some physiological principles of parenteral nutrition. In: *Body Fluid Replacement in the Surgical Patient* (eds: G. Nahas and C. Fox), Part IV, pp. 286–295, Grune and Stratton, Inc., New York.

Cruse, P.J.E., and Foord, R. (1973): A five-year prospective study of 23,649 surgical wounds. *Arch. Surg.* 107:206–210.

Debray, C., Zarakovitch, M., Ranson, B., Jacquemin, J., Robert, J., and Siraga, M. (1946): Contribution a l'etude de la pathologie des deportes. *Sem. Hop. Paris* 22:863–870.

Dixon, R.L., Shultice, R.W., and Fouts, J.E. (1960): Factors affecting drug metabolism by liver microsomes. IV. Starvation. *Proc. Soc. Exp. Biol. N.Y.* 103:333–335.

Doekel, R.C., Zwillich, C.W., Scoggin, C.H., Kryger, M., and Weil, J.V. (1976): Clinical semi-starvation: Depression of the hypoxic ventilatory response. *N. Engl. J. Med.* 295:358–361.

Eckart, J., Tempel, G., Schreiber, V., Schaaf, H., Oeff, K., and Schurubrand, P. (1972): The turnover of I-125-labelled serum albumin after surgery and injury. In: *Parenteral Nutrition.* (ed: A.W. Wilkinson), pp. 288–298, Churchill Livingstone, Edinburgh.

Filkins, J.P. (1970): Lysosomes and hepatic regression during fasting. *Am. J. Physiol.* 219:923–927.

Gracey, M., Suharjono, Sunoto, and Stone, D.E. (1973): Microbial contamination of the gut; another feature of malnutrition. *Am. J. Clin. Nutr.* 26:1170–1174.

Gracey, M., Burke, V., Thomas, J.A., and Stone, D.E. (1975): Effect of micro-organisms isolated from the upper gut of malnourished children on intestinal sugar absorption in vivo. *Am. J. Clin. Nutr.* 28:841–845.

Grant, J.P., and Curtas, S. (1980): Visceral proteins as a measure of liver function. *JPEN* 4:583 (abstract).

Heymsfield, S.B., Bethel, R.A., Ansley, J.D., Gibbs, D.M., Felner, J.M., and Nutter, D.O. (1978): Cardiac abnormalities in cachectic patients before and during nutritional repletion. *Am. Heart J.* 95:584–594.

Jackson, C.M. (1915): Effect of acute and chronic inanition upon the relative weights of the various organs and systems of adult albino rats. *Am. J. Anat.* 18:75–116.

Kato, R., Oshima, T., and Tomizawa, S. (1968): Toxicity and metabolism of drugs in relation to dietary protein. *Jap. J. Pharmac.* 18:356–366.

Keys, A., Brozek, J., Henschel, A., Mickelsen, O., and Taylor, H.L. (1950): *The Biology of Human Starvation.* University of Minnesota Press, Minneapolis, Minn.

Kinney, J.M., Long, C.L., Gump, F.E., and Duke, J.H. (1968): Tissue composition of weight loss in surgical patients. I. Elective operation. *Ann. Surg.* 168:459–474.

Klahr, S., Tripathy, K., Garcia, F.T., Mayoral, L.G., Ghitis, J., and Bolanos, O. (1967): On the nature of the renal concentrating defect in malnutrition. *Am. J. Med.* 43:84–96.

Klahr, S., Tripathy, K., and Lotero, H. (1970): Renal regulation of acid-base in malnourished man. *Am. J. Med.* 48:325–331.

Klahr, S., and Alleyne, G.A.O. (1973): Effects of chronic protein-calorie malnutrition on the kidney. *Kidney Int.* 3:129–141.

Knodell, R.G., Spector, M.H., Brooks, D.A., Keller, F.X., and Kyner, W.T. (1980): Alterations in pentobarbitol pharmacokinetics in response to parenteral and enteral alimentation in the rat. *Gastroenterology* 79:1211–1216.

Krieger, M. (1921): Ueber die Atrophie der menschlichen Organe bei Inanition. *Z. angew. Anat. Konstitutional.* 7:87–134.

Krishnaswamy, K., and Naidu, A.N. (1977): Microsomal enzymes in malnutrition as determined by plasma half life of antipyrine. *Br. Med. J.* 1:538–540.

Kyger, E.R., Block, W.J., Roach, G., and Dudrick, S.J. (1978): Adverse effects of protein malnutrition on myocardial function. *Surgery* 84:147–156.

Levine, G.M., Deren, J.J., Steiger, E., and Zinno, R. (1974): Role of oral intake in maintenance of gut mass and disaccharidase activity. *Gastroenterology* 67:975–982.

Lipscomb, F.M. (1945): Medical aspects of Belsen concentration camp. *Lancet* 2:313–315.

Mata, L.J., Jimenez, F., Cordon, M., Rosales, R., Prera, E., Schneider, R.E., and Viteri, F. (1972): Gastrointestinal flora of children with protein-calorie malnutrition. *Am. J. Clin. Nutr.* 25:1118–1120.

Mayoral, L.G., Tripathy, K., Bolanos, O., Lotero, H., Duque, E., Garcia, F.T., and Ghitis, J. (1972): Intestinal, functional, and morphologic abnormalities in severely protein-malnourished adults. *Am. J. Clin. Nutr.* 25:1084–1091.

Moore, F.D., and Ball, M.R. (1952): *The Metabolic Response to Surgery.* Charles C. Thomas, Springfield, IL.

Moran, L., Custer, P., Murphy, G., and Grant, J. (1980): Nutritional assessment of lean body mass. *JPEN* 4:595 (abstract).

Mullen, J.L. (1981): Consequences of malnutrition in the surgical patient. *Surg. Clin. North Am.* 61:465–487.

Nutter, D.O., Heymsfield, S.R., Murray, T.G., and Fuller, E.O. (1980): Cardiac dynamics and myocardial contractility in chronic protein-calorie undernutrition. *Clin. Res.* 26:256A.

Onicescu, D., and Radu, A. (1969): Histochemical researches of the hepatocyte in experimental starvation conditions. I. On the activity of some oxido-reducing enzymes. *Acta Histochemica* 32:418–424.

Paumgartner, G., Probst, P., Kraines, R., and Leevy, C.M. (1970): Kinetics of indocyanine green removal from the blood. *Ann. N.Y. Acad. Sci.* 170:134–147.

Pullman, T.N., Alving, A.S., Dern, R.J., and Landowne, M. (1954): The influence of dietary protein intake on specific renal functions in normal man. *J. Lab. Clin. Med.* 44:320–332.

Reinhardt, G.F., Myscofski, J.W., Wilkens, D.B., Dobrin, P.B., Mangan, J.E., Jr., and Stannard, R.T. (1980): Incidence and mortality of hypoalbuminemic patients in hospitalized veterans. *JPEN* 4:357–359.

Rothschild, M.A., Oratz, M., and Schreiber, S.S. (1972): Albumin synthesis. *N. Engl. J. Med.* 286:748–757, 816–821.

Sahebjami, H., and Vassalo, C.L. (1979): Effects of starvation and refeeding on lung mechanics and morphometry. *Am. Rev. Respir. Dis.* 119:443–451.

Schneider, R.E., and Viteri, F.E. (1972): Morphological aspects of the duodenojejunal mucosa in protein-calorie malnourished children and during recovery. *Am. J. Clin. Nutr.* 25:1091–1102.

Shaver, H.J., Loper, J.A., and Lutes, R.A. (1980): Nutritional status of nursing home patients. *JPEN* 4:367–370.

Stein, J., and Fenigstein, H. (1946): Anatomie pathologique de la maladie de famine. In: *Maladie de Famine. Rescherches Cliniques sur la Famine Executees dans la Ghetto de Varsovie en 1942.* pp. 21–77, Am. Joint Distribution Committee, Warsaw.

Steiner, M., and Gray, Ś.J. (1969): Effect of starvation on intestinal amino acid absorption. *Am. J. Physiol.* 217:747–752.

Studley, H.O. (1936): Percentage of weight loss: A basic indicator of surgical risk in patients with chronic peptic ulcer. *JAMA* 106:458–460.

Tejada, C., and Restrepo, C. (1962): Effect of malnutrition on the gastrointestinal tract and on the pancreas. Proceedings of the Eighth Pan American Congress of Gastoenterology, New York.

Thompson, M.D., and Trowell, H.C. (1952): Pancreatic enzyme activity in duodenal contents of children with a type of kwashiorkor. *Lancet* 1:1031–1035.

Tui, C., Wright, A.M., Mulholland, J.H., Carabba, V., Barcham, I., and Vinci, V.J. (1944): Studies on surgical convalescence. *Ann. Surg.* 120:99–122.

Vaquez, H. (1924): *Diseases of the Heart* (ed: G.F. Laidlaw), p. 291, W.B. Saunders, Philadelphia.

Veghelyi, P.V. (1948): Pancreatic function in nutritional oedema. *Lancet* 1:497–498.

Viteri, F.E., Flores, J.M., Alvarado, J., and Behar, M. (1973): Intestinal malabsorption in malnourished children before and during recovery. Relation between severity of protein deficiency and the malabsorption process. *Am. J. Dig. Dis.* 18:201–211.

Viteri, F.E. and Schneider, R.E. (1974): Gastrointestinal alterations in protein-calorie malnutrition. *Med. Clin. North Am.* 58:1487–1505.

Voit, C. (1866): Ueber die Verschiedenheiten der Eiweisszersetzung beim Hungern. *Ztscher. F. Biol.* 2:308–365.

Weinsier, R.L., Hunker, E.M., Krumdieck, C.L., and Butterworth, C.E., Jr. (1979): Hospital malnutrition. A prospective evaluation of general medical patients during the course of hospitalization. *Am. J. Clin. Nutr.* 32:418–426.

Weissman, C., Askanazi, J., and Rosenbaum, S.H. (1982): Amino acids and respiration. In press.

Willcutts, H.D. (1977): Nutritional assessment of 1000 surgical patients in an affluent suburban community hospital. *JPEN* 1:25A.

22 Repletion of the Malnourished Patient

David H. Elwyn

Protein-calorie malnutrition remains an important problem among hospitalized adult patients. Since a major cause of this malnutrition is partial or complete malfunction of the gastrointestinal tract, repletion and subsequent maintenance frequently involve total parenteral nutrition (TPN) for periods ranging from a week or two up to the lifetime of the patient. Many of the problems of providing adequate intravenous nutrition have been solved during the past four decades. The result is that TPN is becoming ever more widely available, and the incidence and extent of malnutrition in hospitals is undoubtedly decreasing. Nevertheless, there remain substantial numbers of such patients, who lose 10% or more of their body weight prior to or during their hospital stay, for whom repletion is a necessary and in some cases an imperative requirement.

While adequate TPN can now be provided for a wide range of patients, there are considerable gaps in our knowledge, and some controversy, when it comes to defining optimal amounts of nutrients. The present chapter will deal with some of these questions as they apply to the macronutrients, protein, carbohydrate, and fat. It should be understood, nevertheless, that any repletion diet must contain adequate amounts of all nutrients, including vitamins, electrolytes and trace elements. The importance of this is illustrated in Figure 22-1. Elimination of either nitrogen, potassium or phosphate from an otherwise adequate diet causes parallel and immediate changes (within one day) in both K^+ and N balances, from markedly positive to markedly negative. Sodium, which is an extracellular constituent, has a smaller effect. As of the present, all essential nutrients can be obtained commercially for intravenous use, except for a few of the trace elements. General guidelines for their use may be obtained from a number of manuals (Mullen et al., 1981; Shils, 1980; AMA, 1979; Shenkin and Wretlind, 1978; Wilmore, 1977; Fischer, 1976; Ballinger, 1975).

The major concern in nutritional treatment of depleted patients is restoration and subsequent maintenance of lean body mass (LBM). Associated and interrelated goals are restoration or preservation of host defense functions and restoration of full physical capabilities without undue fatigue. A major interest of the Surgical Metabolism Program at Columbia University in the last few years has been to quantify the relation between energy and nitrogen intake and restoration of LBM.

TECHNICAL PROBLEMS OF NITROGEN BALANCE METHODS

A variety of ways have been employed for estimating changes in lean body mass or body cell mass (BCM). These include measurements of daily balances of N or K^+, and sequential determination of total body content of K^+, N, or other elements by isotope dilution techniques, whole body counting, or neutron activation analysis. Each has its own virtues, faults and particular assumptions. The method we have used is to measure daily N balance, together with O_2 production and CO_2 consumption, in order, also, to elucidate energy expenditure and balance.

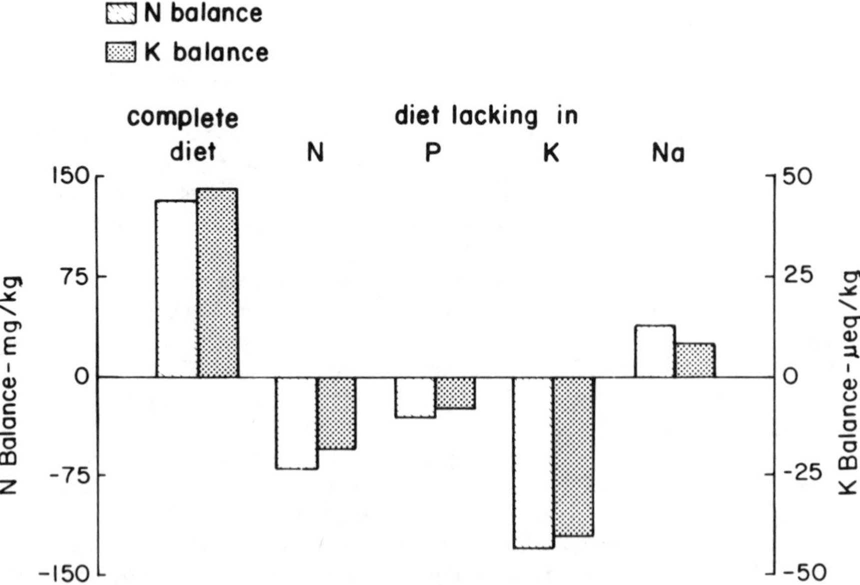

Figure 22-1 Effect of eliminating various dietary components on N and K^+ balance in depleted patients. Data from Rudman et al. (1975). Reproduced with permission of *Crit. Care Med.* (Elwyn, 1980).

One problem which hinders N balance studies, is the length of time required to reach steady state after a dietary change. When large changes in N intake are made, with no change in energy intake, it will take several weeks before a new steady state is reached in normal adults (Oddoye and Margen, 1979). In depleted patients an approximate steady state is reached sooner. The effect of changing intake from 5% dextrose to TPN is to abruptly change N balance which then remains fairly constant for two weeks or more (Figure 22-2). There are no statistically significant changes with time, although the large day-to-day variability may mask small trends. With changes in energy intake, a steady state of N balance is achieved rapidly, even in normal subjects (Munro, 1964). This is illustrated for depleted patients (Figure 22-3) given isonitrogenous diets which supplied 75% or 150% of resting energy expenditure (REE). There is no discernible trend with time on either diet.

Another problem is the large variability in N balance, both between patients and from day to day. Standard deviations for studies of depleted patients in our laboratory range between 1 and 2 g N per day and are similar to values found by other investigators. These are much higher than are found in studies of normal subjects (Oddoye and Margen, 1979) and presumably reflect that depleted patients are an inhomogeneous group of severely ill patients and that their degree of illness is continuously changing.

Another problem which applies to both normal subjects and ill patients is the difficulty in accurately measuring absolute values of N balance. Intake tends to be overestimated and output underestimated. Intake errors can be minimized by careful, exclusive use of parenteral nutrition. In our laboratory, total N is measured in urine, stool, drainages and vomitus, and recoveries are monitored by measuring urinary creatinine and urea (Elwyn et al., 1979). However, integumental losses are not measured but are estimated from data on normal subjects (Calloway et al., 1971). Blood losses for sampling, or blood gains by transfusions, are difficult to handle in short-term balance studies since the bulk of nitrogen is present in the form of

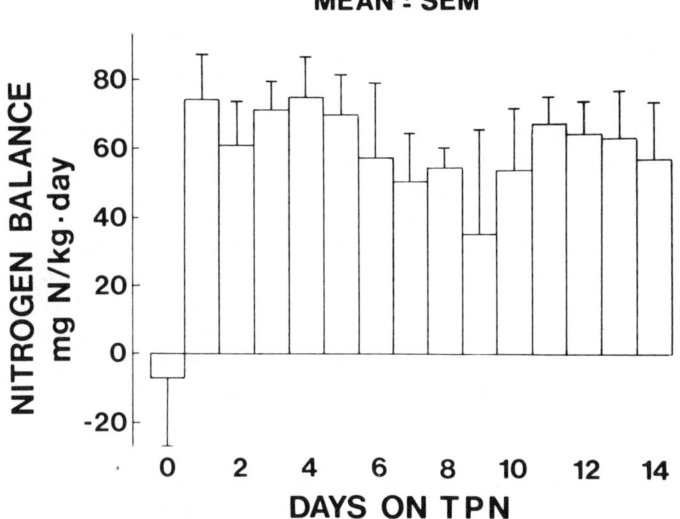

Figure 22-2 Nitrogen balance in depleted patients given 5% dextrose (day 0) or TPN supplying 266 mg N and 35.2 kcal per kg•day. Data adapted from Elwyn et al. (1980).

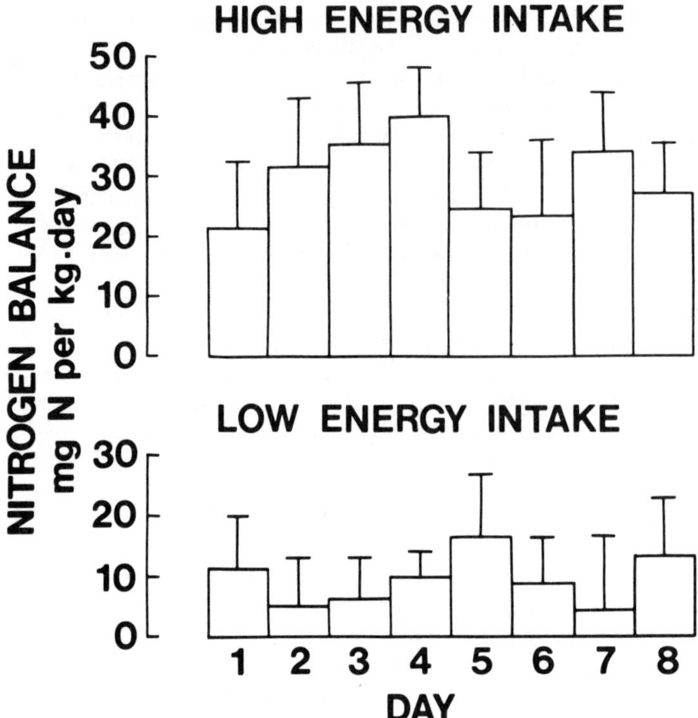

Figure 22-3 Effect of changing energy intake on N balance using a moderate N intake averaging 170 mg/kg•day. Patients were randomly assigned to start either the low (75% of REE) or high (150% of REE) energy diet, and were then given the other diet for periods of eight days each.

red blood cell and plasma proteins with long turnover times, an unpredictable portion of which are denatured and are therefore degraded much more rapidly. Thus, it becomes important to carefully control for blood losses and infusions.

A final problem to be considered is that of estimating energy expenditure. We make use of a noninvasive canopy system for measuring CO_2 production and O_2 consumption which was developed in this program (Kinney et al., 1964; Spencer et al., 1972). This gives accurate values for resting gas exchange and energy expenditure and is highly suitable for bedridden patients. However, many depleted patients are ambulatory, and estimation of energy expenditure due to physical activity is a more difficult problem. One approach is to use a simplified daily log of activities in and out of bed, based on tables of activity energy expenditures (Durnin and Passmore, 1967). Another approach, which requires further documentation, is the estimation of activity energy expenditure from the apparent carbohydrate balance at rest, under conditions in which glycogen stores can be assumed constant (Elwyn et al., 1979; Elwyn and Kinney, 1980).

Despite these problems, useful quantitative information can be obtained relating nitrogen and energy intakes to nitrogen and energy balances in depleted patients. But, it is well to keep in mind the limits on the accuracy and precision of this type of information.

THEORETICAL RELATIONS BETWEEN NITROGEN AND ENERGY INTAKE AND NITROGEN BALANCE IN DEPLETED PATIENTS

Nitrogen requirements for the normal adult average 80 mg/kg•day when given as an ideal protein (Nat. Res. Council, 1980) and at zero energy balance. Increasing N intake above this level causes a temporary deposition of what has been termed "labile protein," but subsequently N balance returns to or toward zero. It has generally been considered that at any intake above minimum requirements adult subjects will in time "drift to equilibrium" (Allison, 1951). However, this does not appear to hold true with very high N intakes. Recent studies indicate that N balance does not differ significantly from zero at an N intake of 12 g/day or 158 mg/kg•day. However, with a threefold increase in N intake, N balance at steady state increased by 23 mg/kg•day, which accounted for 7% of the increment in intake. This persisted for 57 days (the length of the experiment), suggesting sustained accretion of nitrogen over long periods in the normal adult (Oddoye and Margen, 1979).

The effect of increasing energy intake, at energy intakes close to or above normal and with adequate N intake, is to increase N balance. The effect on the normal adult persists and lasts as long as the increased energy intake is maintained (Munro, 1964). Thus, at energy intakes above requirements a positive N balance is maintained indefinitely. At moderate N intake the increment in N balance lies between 1 and 2 mg/kcal. The composition of tissue deposited as a result of overfeeding energy is about one-half part of lean body mass to one part of fat (Elwyn et al., 1979; Keys et al., 1955).

The depleted patient would be expected to differ from the normal in response to changes in N intake in that a positive N balance should be achievable even at zero energy balance, as illustrated in Figure 22-4. Furthermore, N balance should continue to increase as N intake increases. The response to increasing energy intake should be qualitatively similar in the depleted as in the normal subject; however, the quantitative responses need to be determined independently.

In Figure 22-4, N balance is related to energy balance rather than energy intake. This seems preferable on theoretical grounds, since both N and energy intake independently affect N balance, and without taking account of energy expenditure it is impossible to assign definite amounts of change in N balance to each of the two factors. The difference in plotting N balance against energy intake or energy balance is shown in Figures 22-5 and 22-6. Nitrogen balance, for ten patients at three different energy intakes but constant N intake, is plotted against energy intake in Figure 22-5, to give a slope of 1.4 mg N/kcal. When the same data is plotted against energy balance, Figure 22-6, the slope increases to 1.7 and a number of aberrant points, those with markedly negative values for N balance, are brought into line. These changes result from two factors: one, that the energy requirements of these patients vary markedly, from 80% to 150% of predicted values; the other, that increasing energy intake also increases energy expenditure (Elwyn et al., 1979).

In Figure 22-7 lines for fat balance have been superimposed on the grid in Figure 22-4. Since energy balance is the sum of nitrogen and fat balance, expressed in energy equivalents, and assuming steady state with respect to glycogen stores, an increase in N balance at any given energy balance will cause a corresponding decrease in fat balance.

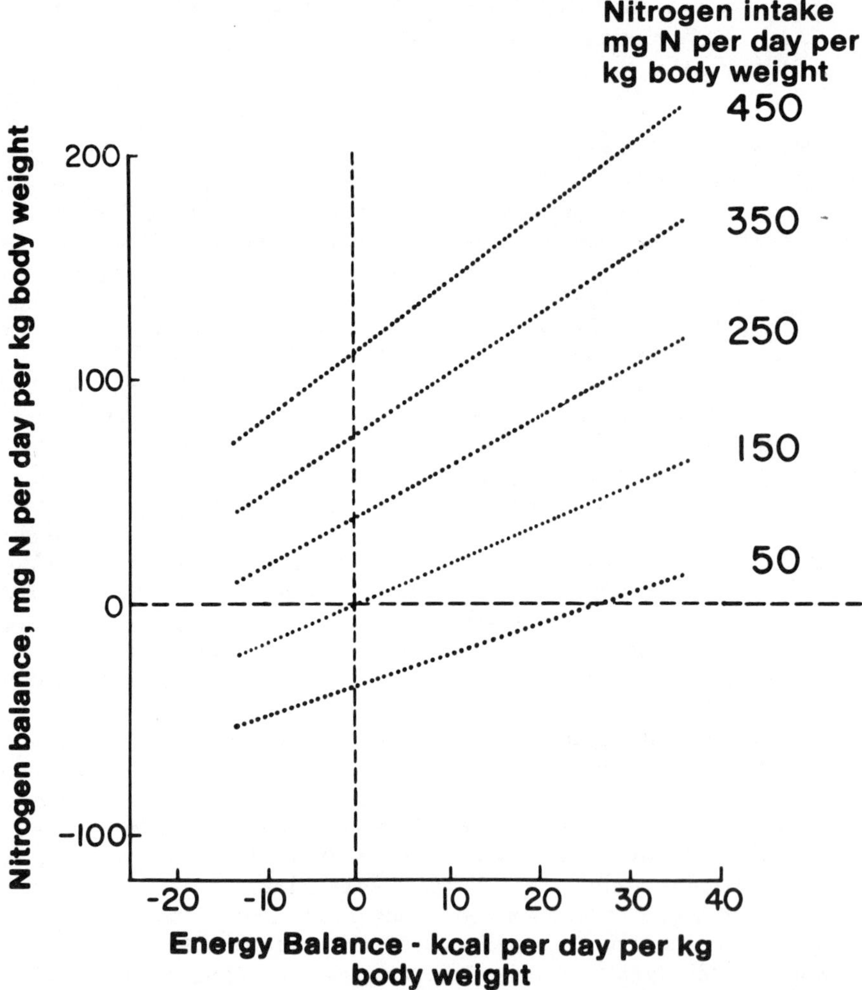

Figure 22-4 Theoretical relations between nitrogen intake, nitrogen balance and energy balance in depleted patients. Constructed from data of Elwyn et al. (1979), Bozetti (1977), Rudman et al. (1975), and Plough et al. (1956).

MEASUREMENTS OF THE EFFECTS OF N AND ENERGY INTAKE ON N BALANCE IN DEPLETED PATIENTS

Data on the effects of both N and energy intake on N balance are shown in Figure 22-8, superimposed on the grid shown in Figure 22-7. Very few studies have been performed with depleted patients in which the effects of N or energy intake can be separated from each other. The solid line is taken from the data in Figure 22-6 (Elwyn et al., 1979) after correcting for integumental losses. The solid circles are taken from a study of Rudman et al. (1975) in which depleted patients were given six different diets, sequentially for six days each, containing varying N intakes, from 0

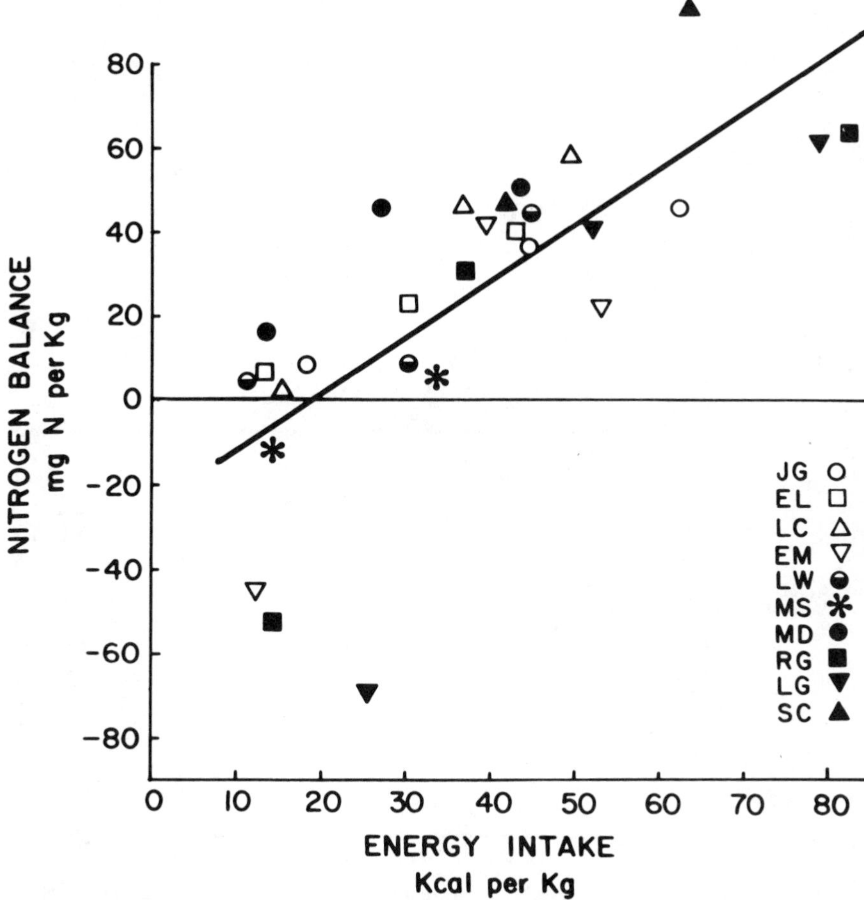

Figure 22-5 Nitrogen balance as a function of energy intake for ten depleted patients on constant N and variable glucose intake. Each point represents the daily mean for the third and fourth day of one or more four-day periods at constant energy intake for one subject. Slope of the regression line is 1.4 ± .17 (SE) mg N/kcal. Reprinted with permission of *Am. J. Clin. Nutrition* (Elwyn et al., 1979).

to 400 mg N/kg•day, but a constant energy intake of 60 kcal/kg•day. Energy expenditure was not measured; for inclusion in Figure 22-8 it was assumed to be 32 kcal/kg•day. The solid triangles are taken from a study by Shaw et al. (1982) in which depleted patients were maintained on isocaloric diets containing either 180 or 364 Mg N/kg•day. The solid square is from a study comparing fat and glucose as energy sources (Elwyn et al., 1980). Data from a number of other studies in which the effects of N and energy intake and energy balance were not separated (Dudrick et al., 1968; Patel et al., 1973; Anderson et al., 1974; Jeejeebhoy et al., 1976; Bozetti, 1976; Paradis et al., 1978) are in reasonable quantitative agreement with Figure 22-8.

The experimental data are consistent with the hypothetical grid except that the lines for N intake for 350 and 450 mg N are probably too high and not steep enough. The data indicate that depleted patients require 150 mg N/kg•day to attain zero N

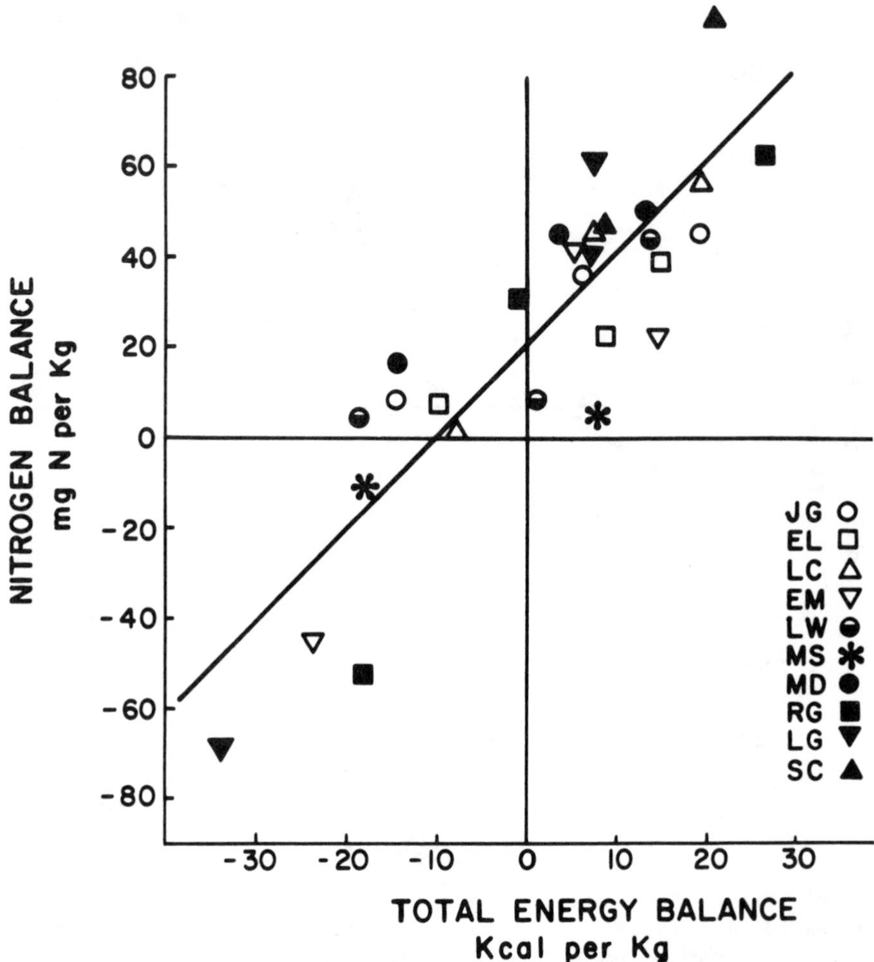

Figure 22-6 Nitrogen balance as a function of energy balance. Identical data to that in Figure 22-5 except for changes in units of abscissa. Slope of the regression line is 1.7 ± .19 mg N/kcal. Reprinted with permission of *Am. J. Clin. Nutrition* (Elwyn et al., 1979).

balance at zero energy balance. This is twice the minimum requirement of 80 mg N/kg•day for normal adults (Nat. Res. Council, 1980). This increased requirement, together with the large variability noted above and shown in Figure 22-6, reflects most likely that depleted, adult patients who require TPN tend to be severely ill with varying degrees of hypercatabolism. In addition, intravenous requirements may be greater than with enteral intake (Rowlands et al., 1977), and the amino acid compostition of the crystalline amino acid solutions used for intravenous feeding may not be optimal.

Nevertheless, increasing N intake at zero energy balance causes markedly positive N balance. In the experiment represented by the solid triangles in Figure 22-8, increasing N intake from 180 to 364 mg/kg•day resulted in increased N retention which amounted to 22% of the increment in intake. This is substantially higher

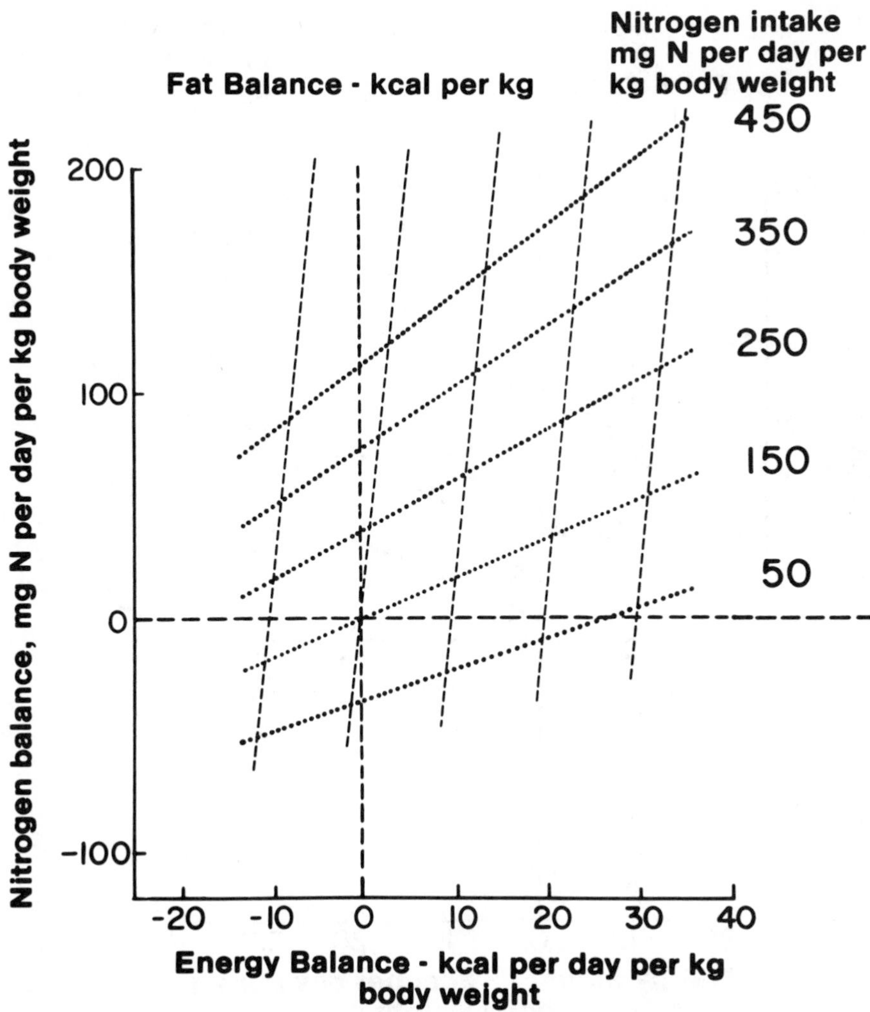

Figure 22-7 Theoretical relation between nitrogen intake, nitrogen balance, energy balance and fat balance. Same as Figure 22-4 with addition of isocaloric lines for fat balance.

than that for normal adults noted above. At high energy intake, a larger proportion of added N is retained. In the studies of Rudman et al. (solid circles in Figure 22-8), 40% of the added N was retained in going from an intake of 160 to 400 mg N/kg• day. Thus, as has been previously shown (Plough et al., 1956), there is a synergism between N and energy intake. The effect on N balance of a simultaneous increase in both is greater than the sum of the effects of each given separately. Further information is needed to complete this grid, and a study is now in process to determine the effect of increasing energy intake at a high constant value of N intake.

The grid in Figure 22-8 can be used as a general guide for the effects of energy and N intake on N and fat balance, taking into account that it represents mean values derived from studies of depleted, adult hospitalized patients, all of whom

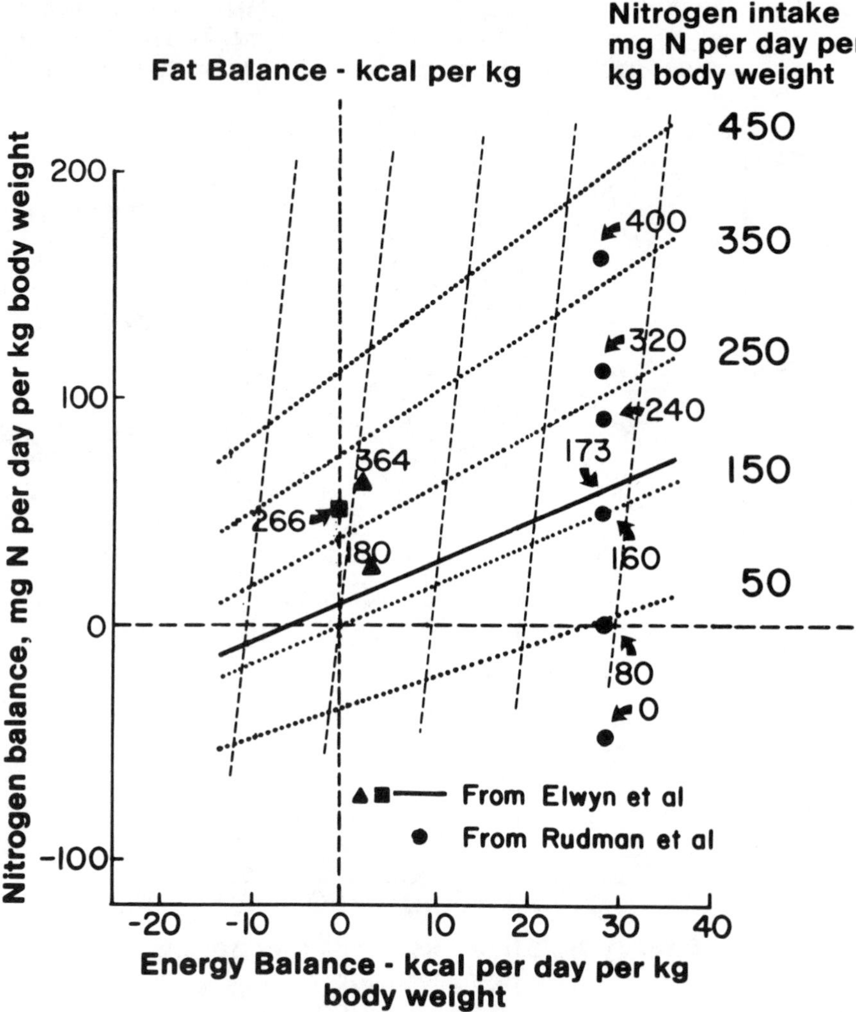

Figure 22-8 Experimental data relating N balance, N intake, energy balance and fat balance superimposed on grid of Figure 22-7 Numbers associated with solid line and figures refer to N intake. For origins of data see text.

required TPN and among whom there was considerable individual variability. Starting at zero energy and N balances (Figure 22-8), increasing energy intake alone will increase deposition of fat and lean body mass in the proportion of one-half part LBM to one part fat. This would be suitable for the patient who has had excessive fat losses but has maintained LBM reasonably well. Increasing N intake alone would deposit LBM with a net loss of fat and might be suitable for a previously obese individual who had lost considerable amounts of protein. For most depleted patients, the compostition of tissue losses ranges from two parts LBM to one part fat in fasting (Benedict, 1914) or after elective injury (Kinney et al., 1968) to four parts to one after major injury (Kinney, 1977). This range, in terms of the units in Figure

22-8, is 7 to 14 mg N/kcal fat. Thus, for most depleted patients, it would seem desirable to increase both energy and N intake above that required to maintain zero N balance at zero energy balance in order to replenish both fat and LBM in appropriate proportions.

In order to use the grid in Figure 22-8 some estimate must be obtained for N expenditure and energy balance. With parenteral, or chemically defined enteral diets, accurate estimates of intake are readily made. Accurate measurements of N excretion and energy expenditure, although essential for research purposes, are neither necessary nor suitable for clinical evaluation of patients. Energy expenditure may be estimated from standard tables of basal metabolic rate, modified for the degree of hypercatabolism, as shown in Figure 22-9. An adequate value for N excretion may be

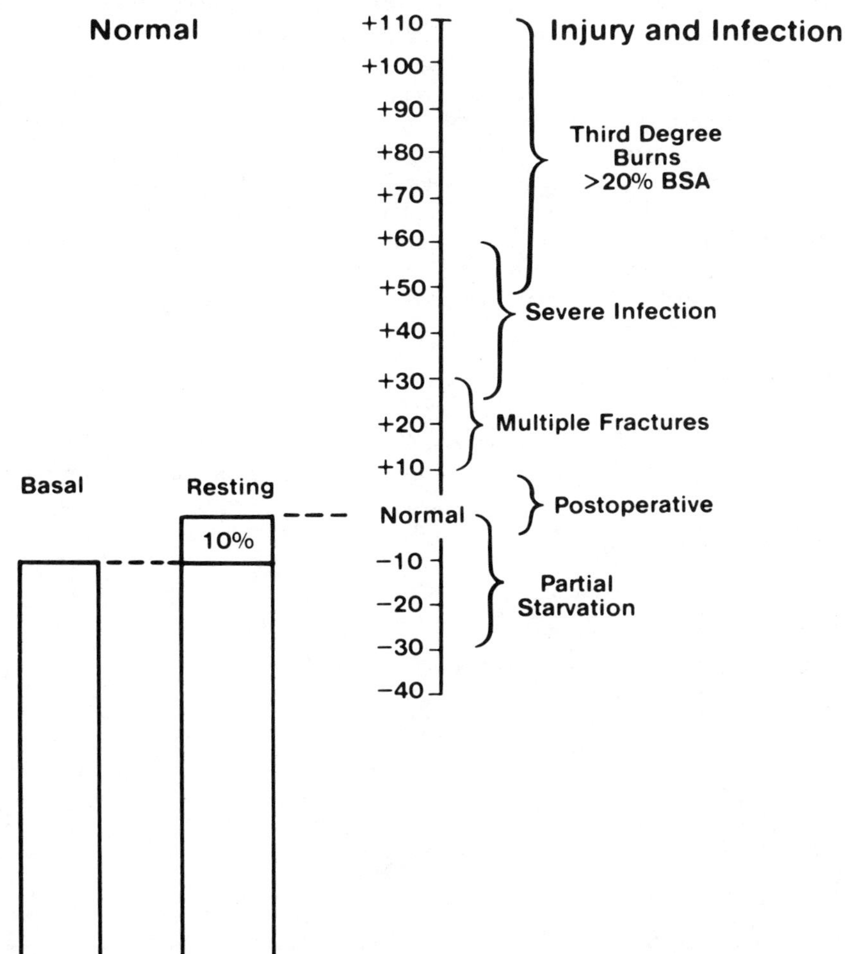

Figure 22-9 Effects of injury, sepsis, and starvation on energy expenditure. Resting energy expenditure is taken to be 10% higher than basal metabolic rate for fed subjects to account for the specific dynamic action of foods. Adapted from Kinney et al. (1970). Reprinted with permission of *Crit. Care Med.* (Elwyn, 1980).

obtained by measuring 24-hour urinary urea output and adding appropriate estimates for other N losses (Wilmore, 1977; Mullen et al., 1981). Alternatively, 24-hour urinary K^+ excretion may be measured, in order to calculate K^+ balance as an estimate of repletion of LBM.

INTERCHANGEABILITY OF FAT AND CARBOHYDRATE AS NONPROTEIN ENERGY SOURCES

It has been known for a long time that carbohydrate has a much greater protein-sparing effect than fat, but this difference holds only for low intakes. If 100 to 150 g glucose is given to a normal adult, further increases in energy intake are equally effective in sparing N, whether given as carbohydrate or fat (Munro, 1964). Furthermore, this difference is transitory and dependent on the protein content of the diet. When a normal mixed diet is replaced by an isonitrogenous, isocaloric diet containing only or mostly fat as the nonprotein energy source, there is an abrupt increase in urinary N which peaks at two to four days and then returns toward normal (Figure 22-10; Silwer, 1937). On the high protein diet, 2.35 g/kg•day, urinary N excretion returned to control values by 12 days. On the moderate intake, 1.20 g/kg•day, N excretion remained above control values, until the end of the study. On the low intake, 0.31 g/kg•day, N excretion returned to control values by 16 days; but on this diet there was a significant carbohydrate intake, 0.62 g/kg•day, compared with 0.10 to

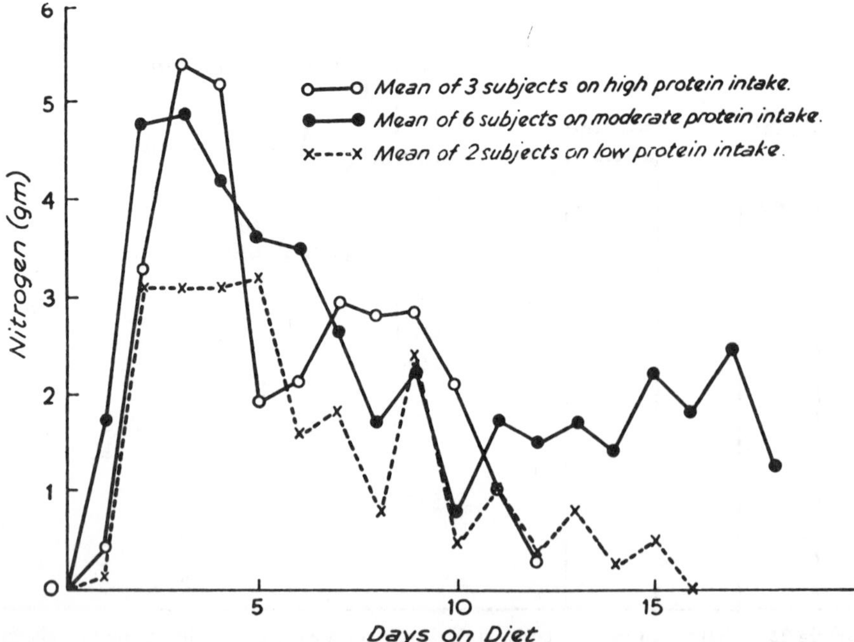

Figure 22-10 Change in urinary nitrogen output in human subjects on constant protein intake, with dietary carbohydrate largely replaced by an isocaloric amount of fat. Adapted from data of Silwer (1937). Reprinted with permission of *Academic Press* (Munro, 1964).

0.12 on the other diets. There was increased ketone body excretion with all diets, which reached a maximum in five to seven days (Silwer, 1937). These data are quantitatively consistent with the obligatory requirement of the brain for glucose (Cahill and Owen, 1968). On a normal mixed diet this is approximately 2 g/kg•day. On low carbohydrate diets this requirement is reduced but not eliminated, due to the availability of ketone bodies, and must be met largely from protein. If dietary protein is insufficient, the required glucose will be synthesized mainly from muscle protein, causing a negative N balance. From Silwer's experiment it appears that an intake of 2.35 g protein/kg•day is sufficient to supply brain glucose requirements, but that an intake of 1.20 g/kg•day is not.

The amount of carbohydrate intake above which fat and carbohydrate have equal effects on N balance has not been exactly determined in depleted patients. In one study (Jeejeebhoy et al., 1976) depleted patients were given TPN with all nonprotein energy as glucose, 10.7 g/kg•day, or with one-sixth the amount, only 1.78 g as glucose, with the remaining nonprotein energy supplied as a lipid emulsion. There was a transient decrease in N balance on the high fat diet and a transient increase on the high glucose diet, but after four days both diets were equivalent. In a number of other studies in which glucose contributed at least 50% of nonprotein energy, there were no significant differences in the effects of additional glucose or fat on N balance (Bark et al., 1976; Elwyn et al., 1980; MacFie et al., 1981a). These data suggest that at least 2 g glucose/kg•day should be given to depleted patients, and that above this the effects of fat and glucose on N balance are not markedly different. A minimum of fat is also needed, 0.2 to 0.3 g/kg•day, to prevent essential fatty acid deficiency. In severely hypercatabolic patients, the minimum amount of glucose required before fat and glucose are equal may be much higher (Long et al., 1977; Woolfson et al., 1979).

This greater N sparing effect of glucose is mediated mainly by insulin and its effect is primarily to conserve muscle protein. In the absence of adequate protein intake, muscle protein is conserved, by glucose, at the expense of visceral and blood proteins (Munro, 1964), an effect which is detrimental to the organism and similar to that seen in kwashiorkor.

CHANGES IN POTASSIUM AS AN INDICATOR OF REPLETION

Whole body exchangeable K^+, calculated from measurements of total body water with ^3H_2O, exchangeable Na^+ using $^{22}Na^+$, and K^+ and Na^+ concentration in whole blood, has been used as an index of LBM repletion in extensive studies of malnourished patients (Shizgal and Forse, 1980). In agreement with the N balance data discussed above, they found that carbohydrate had a greater effect on repletion of BCM than did fat, but, above 50% of nonprotein energy given as glucose, additional fat and glucose were equally effective. However, in apparent disagreement with our N balance data, the authors concluded that increasing N intake, from 209 to 366 mg N/kg•day, had no effect on the rate of repletion of BCM. Their data do indicate a small increase in the rate of K^+ repletion at the higher N intake, which would correspond to approximately 13 mg N/kg•day or 8% of the additional intake. This is not significantly different from zero but also may not be significantly different from twice this value. Nevertheless, it appears to be substantially smaller than would be expected from measurements of N balance, which at the energy intake of 50 kcal/kg used in their study, should be about 30% of the additional nitrogen intake (Figure 22-8). This is not necessarily surprising, for, although both K^+ and N are used as indices of BCM and although the normal composition of BCM may be relatively constant, changes in K^+ and N in ill patients are frequently dissociated (MacFie et al., 1981b; Mernagh et al., 1981). Unpublished observations from this laboratory indicate that malnourished patients often show more depletion of K^+ than of N and that repletion of K^+ is much more sensitive to the glucose content of the diet than is repletion of N. This dissociation of changes in N and K^+ balance in ill patients may result from several factors. Decreases in cell membrane potential due to disease and malnutrition would cause relatively faster loss of K^+ than of N, with relatively faster repletion of K^+ as membrane potentials return to normal. Deposition or loss of glycogen is accompanied by large changes in K^+ content of cells with no change in N (Fenn and Haege, 1940). We may conclude that in severe illness there is no simple index of changes in BCM. The components of BCM change, in part, independently. To measure changes in body protein, one must measure nitrogen. To measure changes in body potassium one must measure potassium. Both of these constituents are important, and nutritional therapy should be aimed at restoring both, but measurements of one component are not necessarily good predictors of the other.

UPPER LIMITS OF NUTRIENTS FOR REPLETION OF DEPLETED PATIENTS

Since restoration of LBM is a major goal of repletion therapy, it would be desirable to know the optimal rates for nutrient administration. For a number of reasons, such information is hard to come by. In terms of restoration of organ function, particularly muscle function and host defense, we have little idea as to whether faster or slower rates of protein repletion are better or worse. In the patient with an intact gastrointestinal tract, appetite plays an important role in regulating intake. Observations of patients undergoing oral repletion suggest that intakes tend to be moderate. With TPN, there are few checks, other than self-restraint, on the therapist's ability to provide an excessive amount of nutrients. Until we have more solid information as to the benefits to be obtained, it is probably wise to avoid very high intakes of either energy or nitrogen. A major factor in the return of skeletal muscle function is the amount of physical activity of the patient. This is as important as diet. There is no doubt that physical activity should be encouraged in depleted patients. However, there is too little information on the interrelations between diet and physical activity, particularly at the low levels suitable for ill patients, to provide any precise quantitative guidelines in this area.

There are certain situations in which an excess of one or another nutrient can be demonstrated and should be avoided. From Figure 22-8, it is clear that too high a proportion of energy to nitrogen will cause excessive deposition of fat. In patients with prior hypertriglyceridemia, fat emulsions should be administered with caution. Other adverse effects of fat emulsions have been observed, but are very rare at intakes below 1500 kcal/day (Pelham, 1981). Nitrogen intake should be carefully monitored in patients with renal failure. High amounts of glucose have been implicated in development of fatty liver and other signs of liver malfunction (Sheldon,

1980). Both glucose and amino acids have marked effects on respiration which in some situations may cause pulmonary problems.

Increasing glucose intake from that given as 5% dextrose to the amount given in high glucose TPN can double CO_2 production (Elwyn, 1980; Elwyn, 1981; Askanazi et al., 1980). Increasing amino acid intake increases the respiratory sensitivity to CO_2 (Askanazi, 1982). Thus, when both are increased together, as in glucose-based TPN, they act synergistically to markedly increase ventilatory rate. This is well tolerated in many patients. In some patients with inadequate pulmonary reserve severe respiratory distress may result, sometimes immobilizing an otherwise ambulatory patient and interfering with weaning from the respirator. Reduction of glucose intake and replacement with fat emulsion will often solve this problem.

TENTATIVE CONCLUSIONS

Intravenous repletion of the depleted patient should be carried out with a complete diet containing between 200 and 350 mg N/kg•day and energy to supply 10 to 15 kcal/kg•day in excess of resting requirements. Fat and glucose should each supply at least one-fourth of nonprotein energy. Urinary urea output should be monitored to determine whether or not N balance is in the appropriate range.

REFERENCES

Allison, J.B. (1951): Interpretation of nitrogen balance data. *Fed. Proc.* 10:676–683.

AMA Department of Foods and Nutrition. (1979): Guideline for essential trace element preparation for parenteral use. *JAMA* 241:2051–2054.

Andersen, G.H., Patel, D.G., and Jeejeebhoy, K.N. (1974): Design and evaluation by nitrogen balance and blood aminograms of an amino acid mixture for total parenteral nutrition of adults with gastrointestinal disease. *J. Clin. Invest.* 53:904–912.

Askanazi, J., Carpentier, Y.A., Elwyn, D.H., Nordenström, J., Jeevanandam, M., Rosenbaum, S.H., Gump, F.E., and Kinney, J.M. (1980): Influence of total parenteral nutrition on fuel utilization in injury and sepsis. *Ann. Surg.* 191:40–46.

Askanazi, J., Weissman, C., Rosenbaum, S.H., Hyman, A.I., Milic-Emili, J., and Kinney, J.M. (1982): Nutrition and the respiratory system. *Crit. Care Med.* 10:163–172.

Ballinger, W.F., Collins, J.A., Drucker, W.R., Dudrick, S.J., and Zeppa, R. (1975): *Manual of Surgical Nutrition.* W.B. Saunders Co., Philadelphia, PA.

Bark, S., Holm, I., Håkansson, I., and Wretlind, A. (1976): *Acta Chir. Scand.* 142:423–427.

Benedict, F.G. (1914): *A Study of Prolonged Fasting.* Publication 203, Carnegie Institute, Washington, D.C.

Bozetti, F. (1976): Parental nutrition in surgical patients. *Surg. Gynecol. Obstet.* 142:16–20.

Cahill, G.F., Jr., and Owen, O.E. (1968): Some observations on carbohydrate metabolism in man. In: *Carbohydrate Metabolism and Its Disorders* (eds: F. Dickens, P.J. Randle, and W.J. Whelan), Vol. 1, pp. 497–522, Academic Press, New York.

Calloway, D.H., Odell, A.C.F., and Margen, S. (1971): Sweat and miscellaneous losses in human balance studies. *J. Nutr.* 101:775–786.

Dudrick, S.J., Wilmore, D.W., Vars, H.M., and Rhoads, J.E. (1968): Long-term total parenteral nutrition with growth, development, and positive nitrogen balance. *Surgery* 64: 134–142.

Durnin, J.V.G.A., and Passmore, R. (1967): *Energy, Work and Leisure.* Heinemann, London.

Elwyn, D. (1980): Nutritional requirements of adult surgical patients. *Crit. Care Med.* 8:9–20.

Elwyn, D.H., Askanazi, J., Kinney, J.M., and Gump, F.E. (1981): Kinetics of energy substrates. *Acta Chir. Scand. (Suppl.)* 507:209–219.

Elwyn, D.H., Gump, F.E., Munro, H.N., Iles, M., and Kinney, J.M. (1979): Changes in nitrogen balance of depleted patients with increasing infusions of glucose. *Am. J. Clin. Nutr.* 32:1597–1611.

Elwyn, D.H., and Kinney, J.M. (1980): A unique approach to measuring total energy expenditure by indirect calorimetry. In: *First Ross Conference on the Assessment of Energy Metabolism in Health and Disease* (ed: J.M. Kinney), pp. 54–61.

Elwyn, D.H., Kinney, J.M., Gump, F.E., Askanazi, J., Rosenbaum, S.H., and Carpentier, Y.A. (1980): Some metabolic effects of fat infusions in depleted patients. *Metabolism* 29:125–132.

Fenn, W.O. and Haege, L.F. (1940): The deposition of glycogen with water in the livers of cats. *J. Biol. Chem.* 136:87–101.

Fischer, J.E. (1976): *Total Parenteral Nutrition.* Little, Brown and Co., Boston, MA.

Jeejeebhoy, K.N., Andersen, G.H., Nakhooda, A.F., Greenberg, G.R., Sanderson, I., and Marliss, E.B. (1976): Metabolic studies in total parenteral nutrition with lipid in man. Comparison with glucose. *J. Clin. Invest.* 57:125–136.

Keys, A., Andersen, J.T., and Brozek, J. (1955): Weight gain from simple overeating. I. Character of tissue gained. *Metabolism* 4:427–432.

Kinney, J.M. (1977): The tissue composition of surgical weight loss. In: *Advances in Parenteral Nutrition* (ed: I.D.A. Johnston), pp. 511–518, MTP Press, London.

Kinney, J.M., Duke, J.H., Jr., Long, C.L., and Gump, F.E. (1970): Tissue fuel and weight loss after injury. *J. Clin. Path.* 23(Suppl. 4):65–72.

Kinney, J.M., Long, C.L., Gump, F.E., and Duke, J.H., Jr. (1968): Tissue composition of weight loss in surgical patients. I. Elective Operation. *Ann. Surg.* 168:459–474.

Kinney, J.M., Morgan, A.P., Dominguez, F.J., and Gildner, K.J. (1969): A method for continuous measurement of gas exchange in acutely ill patients. *Metabolism* 13:205–211.

Long, J.M., III, Wilmore, D.W., Mason, A.D., Jr., and Pruitt, B.A., Jr. (1977): Effect of carbohydrate and fat intake on nitrogen excretion during total intravenous feeding. *Ann. Surg.* 185:417–422.

MacFie, J., Smith, R.C., and Hill, G.L. (1981a): Glucose or fat as nonprotein energy source? A controlled clinical trial in gastroenterological patients requiring intravenous nutrition. *Gastroenterology* 80:103–107.

MacFie, J., Yule, A.G., and Hill, G.H. (1981b): Effect of added insulin on body composition of gastroenterologic patients receiving intravenous nutrition—a controlled clinical trial. *Gastroenterology* 81:285–289.

Mernagh, J.R., McNeill, K.G., Harrison, J.E., and Jeejeebhoy, K.N. (1981): Effect of total parenteral nutrition in the restitution of body nitrogen, potassium and weight. *Nutr. Res.* 1:149–157.

Mullen, J.L., Crosby, L.O., and Rombeau, J.L. (1981): Symposium on surgical nutrition. *Surg. Clin. North Am.* 61:1–761.

Munro, H.N. (1964): General aspects of the regulation of protein metabolism by diet and hormones. In: *Mammalian Protein Metabolism* (eds: H.N. Munro and J.B. Allison), Vol. 1, pp. 382–482, Academic Press, New York.

National Research Council (1980): *Recommended Dietary Allowances.* (9th edition), Nat. Acad. Sci., Washington, D.C.

Oddoye, E.A. and Margen, S. (1979): Nitrogen balance studies in humans: long term effect of high nitrogen intake on nitrogen accretion. *J. Nutr.* 109:363–377.

Paradis, C., Spanier, A.H., Calder, M., and Shizgal, H.M. (1978): Total parenteral nutrition with lipid. *Am. J. Surg.* 135:164–171.

Patel, D., Andersen, G.H., and Jeejeebhoy, K.N. (1973): Amino acid adequacy of parenteral casein hydrolysate and oral cottage cheese in patients with gastrointestinal disease as measured by nitrogen balance and blood aminograms. *Gastroenterology* 65:427–437.

Pelham, L.D. (1981): Rational use of intravenous fat emulsions. *Am. J. Hosp. Pharm.* 38: 198–208.

Plough, I.C., Iber, F.L., Shipman, M.E., and Chalmers, T. (1956): The effects of supplementary calories on nitrogen storage at high intakes of protein in patients with chronic liver disease. *Am. J. Clin. Nutr.* 4:224–230.

Rowlands, B.J., Giddings, A.E., Johnston, A.O.B., Hindmarsh, J.T., and Clark, R.G. (1977): Nitrogen sparing effects of different feeding regimes in patients after operation. *Br. J. Anaesth.* 49:781–787.

Rudman, D., Millikan, W.J., Richardson, T.J., Bixler, T.J., II, Stackhouse, W.J., and McGarrity, W.C. (1975): Elemental balances during intravenous hyperalimentation of underweight adult subjects. *J. Clin. Invest.* 55:94–104.

Shaw, S.N., Schwarz, Y., Iles, M., Elwyn, D.H., Askanazi, J., and Kinney, J.M. (1981): Effect of varying nitrogen intake on nitrogen and energy balance. *JPEN* 5:559.

Sheldon, G.F., and Baker, C. (1980): Complications of nutritional support. *Crit. Care Med.* 8:35–37.

Shenkin, A., and Wretlind, A. (1978): Parenteral nutrition. *World Rev. Nutr. Dietet.* 28: 1–111.

Shils, M.E. (1980): Parenteral nutrition. In: *Modern Nutrition in Health and Disease* (6th edition) (eds: R.S. Goodhart and M.E. Shils), pp. 1125–1152, Lea and Febiger, Philadelphia, PA.

Shizgal, H.M., and Forse, R.A. (1980): Protein and calorie requirements with total parenteral nutrition. *Ann. Surg.* 192:562–569.

Silwer, H. (1937): Studien über die N-Ausscheidung im Harn bei einshrankung des Kohlehydrates der Nahrung ohne wesentliche Veränderung des Energiengehaltes derselben. *Acta Med. Scand. Suppl.* 79:1–273.

Spencer, J.L., Zikria, A.B., Kinney, J.M., Broell, J.R., Michailoff, T.M., and Lee, A.B. (1972): A system for the continuous measurement of gas exchange and respiratory functions. *J. Appl. Physiol.* 33:523–528.

Wilmore, D.W. (1977): *The Metabolic Management of the Critically Ill.* Plenum Press, New York.

Woolfson, A.M., Heatley, R.V., and Allison, S.P. (1979): Insulin to inhibit protein catabolism after injury. *N. Engl. J. Med.* 300:14–17.

TRAUMA AND INFECTION

23 Amino Acid Support in the Hypercatabolic Patient

John M. Kinney

The hypercatabolic patient is characterized by a variety of changes in resting metabolism, but the best known is the increase in nitrogen excretion which roughly parallels the severity of an injury or an infection. The role of amino acids in the support of such patients received great impetus from the work of Elman (1937) and Lindstrom and Wretlind (1952) who pioneered in the development of protein hydrolysates for clinical use. Schuberth and Wretlind (1961) then introduced total parenteral nutrition in Sweden which included a satisfactory lipid emulsion. The concept of amino acids, given as a fat-free mixture with hypertonic glucose, was then introduced by Dudrick et al. (1966). Despite these advances in parenteral nutrition, most hospitalized patients were still receiving only isotonic dextrose solution by peripheral vein when Blackburn et al. (1973a) emphasized the importance of administering amino acids even in the absence of a nonprotein calorie source.

While the basic importance of providing amino acids is now well accepted, major questions remain about the amount and composition of amino acid solutions which should be provided to the hypercatabolic patient and how the benefit resulting from their administration should be measured. A major difference of opinion at the present time relates to the optimum balance between amino acids and nonprotein calories for such patients. Some investigators emphasize the increase in energy expenditure, which is usually present and, hence, believe such patients might benefit from an intake with a high calorie-to-nitrogen ratio. Other investigators emphasize the increase in nitrogen loss of such patients and urge that the amino acid content of the intake be increased, with a resultant lowering of the customary calorie-to-nitrogen ratio.

The technique of daily nitrogen balance has been the standard methodology for evaluating calorie and nitrogen intake in most clinical conditions. The technique of nitrogen balance was first demonstrated by Boussingault (1842), when he conducted a series of painstaking experiments on the role of carbohydrate versus fat on the metabolic balance of cows and other farm animals. The technique was an obvious outgrowth of early European advances in chemistry and has remained essentially unmodified to the present time, although it is subject to several kinds of errors which have been reviewed by Allison and Bird (1964).

The major part of the increase in the nitrogen loss of the acutely catabolic patient is thought to be due to the deamination of amino acids, resulting from muscle protein breakdown. Thus, an important aspect of providing amino acid therapy to such patients is to improve muscle protein synthesis and thereby improve daily nitrogen balance. When the influence of amino acid intake is being studied by nitrogen balance techniques in the hypercatabolic patient, it is important to remember that increased urea nitrogen can result from the breakdown of necrotic tissue or from protein sequestered in a hematoma, as well as from the deamination of normally occurring protein. In the presence of a major hematoma, catabolic weight loss is delayed because of secondary water retention, while urinary nitrogen excretion is increased well beyond the extent of muscle protein breakdown. Therefore, the importance of administering amino acids may be obscured by the apparent failure to improve nitrogen balance when enhanced protein synthesis may actually be taking place.

NITROGEN LOSS IN THE HYPERCATABOLIC PATIENT

The role of amino acid therapy in the support of the hypercatabolic patient must be considered in the perspective of the altered nitrogen metabolism which occurs in such patients. The term *hypercatabolic* indicates a level of tissue breakdown which exceeds that which is associated with uncomplicated partial starvation. In the latter condition, urinary nitrogen excretion commonly begins to decrease after the first two to three days. This is in contrast to the hypercatabolic patient where the urinary nitrogen excretion is increased during the first week or more following injury or during infection. The elevated nitrogen loss usually diminishes toward normal in parallel with the decreasing stimulus to catabolism. The daily urinary loss commonly decreases to levels below normal if extensive tissue loss occurs during the hypercatabolic phase.

The nitrogen composition of the 24-hour urine of a normal subject is presented in Table 23-1, taken from Peaston (1974). The dominant role of urea nitrogen is emphasized in pathological conditions. The urinary urea decreases in starvation, while it is increased in hypercatabolic states. Urinary urea is a measurement which is sometimes available when total urinary nitrogen is not measured, thus leading to the suggestion that nitrogen balance can be estimated by measuring urinary urea and multiplying by a factor based on the urea representing a fixed proportion of the total nitrogen excretion. The range of error that may be introduced by this approach has been studied in our laboratory. Daily measurements in a variety of hypercatabolic patients have shown that the urea nitrogen content varies from less than 60% to over 90% of the daily urinary nitrogen excretion. Efforts have been made to determine whether this proportion of urine nitrogen as urea could be correlated with the stage of convalescence, or the level of nitrogen intake, but no correlation could be identified.

Table 23-1
Typical Nitrogen Composition of Normal Urine on 90 g Protein Diet (g/24h)

Total	14.40
Urea	12.50
Creatinine	0.67
Ammonia	0.44
Uric acid	0.23
Other	0.56

From Peaston (1974) with permission.

It has been suggested that the deterioration of patients, following major injury or infection, may be directly related to the progressive loss of body protein and that death may occur when some threshold amount, or function, of protein has been exceeded. Patients undergoing elective surgical operation will lose from 40 to 80g of N during the postoperative period before resuming oral intake if no amino acids have been administered. These cumulative nitrogen losses can be minimized by the intravenous administration of amino acids alone, although the total nitrogen loss is usually not obliterated. Major accidental injury, or extensive sepsis, is commonly associated with cumulative nitrogen losses of 100 to 200 g without the aggressive administration of total parenteral nutrition. These losses of body nitrogen should be thought of in terms of a normal 70 kg adult man (Moore et al., 1963). This individual could be expected to have approximately 15% of his body weight as crude protein, representing 10,500 g of protein, or 1700 g of body nitrogen. This total body nitrogen can be considered to be divided into approximately 15% as blood proteins and visceral proteins, 40% as muscle protein, and approximately 45% associated with extracellular supporting structures. Therefore, a nitrogen loss of 100 g in this theoretical individual would represent approximately one-eighth of his intracellular protein stores. Reports from Hill et al. (1978) and McNeill et al. (1979) describe techniques with neutron activation to obtain a measure of body nitrogen. Such studies should begin to provide insight into cumulative nitrogen losses in relation to normal body stores and, therefore, a better understanding of how much protein can be lost before survival is threatened. Such information should be of special importance in determining how aggressive to be in the administration of total parenteral nutrition to patients during the early catabolic phase of injury, or infection.

INFLUENCE OF NITROGEN INTAKE ON NITROGEN BALANCE

The classic relationship between nitrogen balance and nitrogen intake can be presented as a diagonal line crossing the horizontal axis in the neighborhood of 8 to

12 g/N per day. The normal individual will begin to reduce his nitrogen excretion after two to three days of starvation and can be expected to decrease to approximately 5 g/day during a period of one to two weeks of no nitrogen intake (Wretlind, 1981). The opposite changes occur in the hypercatabolic patient in which there is a "shift to the right" so that the nitrogen excretion on zero intake is increased and the nitrogen intake to achieve equilibrium is increased to an amount which can be roughly correlated with the magnitude of the injury or infection. The study of Soroff et al. (1961) demonstrated the severe right shift in seriously burned patients which progressively moved back toward the normal range as the neuroendocrine stimulus to catabolism became less severe and the burn wound was progressively excised and grafted.

The widespread acceptance of a negative nitrogen balance as characterizing the hypercatabolic state has led to suggestions that a large proportion of the weight loss at that time is associated with protein breakdown and that a correspondingly large proportion of the energy expenditure at this time has arisen from the oxidation of protein. Metabolic balance studies, which included daily resting calorie balance as well as daily nitrogen balance following major injury, were analyzed to determine the correlation between weight loss and body nitrogen loss. During the first three to five days following injury, protein was found to contribute only 7% to 9% of the weight loss and thereafter slowly increased to a contribution of 12% to 15% by the third week (Kinney, 1976). It was of special interest that the relationship in total starvation was of very similar magnitude when the same measurements were performed on an obese patient undergoing total starvation for weight reduction.

It has been suggested that the large energy requirements associated with injury or infection exceeded the ability of fat stores to provide this energy. Therefore, the increased nitrogen excretion seen in these conditions probably reflected the deamination of amino acids from muscle protein that were being degraded to provide extra two-carbon fuel. This concept was examined by Duke et al. (1970) who analyzed the energy contribution of protein to the resting energy expenditure of various categories of acute surgical patients. Protein normally contributed 10% to 15% of the resting energy expenditure (REE) in patients before and during the early days after elective operation. If the postoperative patients were continued on a nutritional intake of only 400 kcal per day of dextrose, the contribution of protein calories would decrease to 7% or 8% of the total REE. In more severe forms of major injury, protein contributed from 15% to 22% of the daily REE. However, even in the most severe conditions body fat was the major tissue constitutent, together with exogenous nutrients, for meeting daily energy demands. This relatively small contribution of protein to resting energy expenditure suggested that the increased urea excretion in the hypercatabolic state was to provide amino acid carbon for synthethic purposes, such as gluconeogenesis, and the carbohydrate intermediates of connective tissue for wound healing, rather than simply serving to provide two-carbon fragments for tissue fuel.

USE OF PERIPHERAL AMINO ACIDS WITHOUT A CALORIE SOURCE

When one considers the nutritional requirements for amino acids in the hypercatabolic patient, there is the possibility of increased amino acid requirements for increased synthetic needs, in addition to the neuroendocrine stimulus causing increased amino acid breakdown. It is common to observe that the elevated urea nitrogen in the hypercatabolic state is increased even further by the administration of amino acids at this time. Therefore, some investigators have proposed that amino acid administration be postponed or given at only minimal levels until the major catabolic stimulus has passed. The early work of Blackburn et al. (1973a) was important to call attention to the fact that amino acid intake was needed even during periods when their administration might increase urinary nitrogen loss, since the overall nitrogen balance was regularly improved. Further work is needed to demonstrate the efficiency with which amino acid intake may support the synthesis of high priority body proteins, despite the fact that an overall negative nitrogen balance may exist at the same time.

The quantitative effects of glucose and amino acids on nitrogen balance remain somewhat controversial when given as isotonic solutions by peripheral vein. It is possible that the nitrogen-sparing effect of amino acid infusions may be related to the degree of the hypercatabolic state. In normal subjects and in those undergoing elective operation, peripheral amino acid infusions improve nitrogen balance when compared with peripheral glucose infusions. Blackburn et al. (1973a) demonstrated a beneficial effect of amino acids infused by peripheral vein on nitrogen balance, whereas added glucose appeared to be detrimental. Hoover et al. (1975) confirmed the nitrogen-sparing effect of peripheral amino acids, as have other investigators (Blackburn et al., 1973b, Greenberg et al., 1976, Freeman et al., 1975). However, several reports have appeared in which adding hypocaloric glucose infusions to the amino acid intake did not have a detrimental effect but tended to improve the negative nitrogen balance (Howard et al., 1976; Elwyn et al., 1978). In a study of patients undergoing total hip replacement, there was no difference between the nitrogen balance of the patients who received peripheral amino acids for the first six postoperative days and the patients who received peripheral glucose for the same period (Elwyn, 1970). These patients were at total bedrest during the period of study and, therefore, the inactivity of skeletal muscle may have contributed to lack of improvement in cumulative nitrogen balance when amino acids were given alone, when compared with glucose.

FREE AMINO ACIDS OF PLASMA AND MUSCLE

A study was conducted by Elwyn of the influence of a large meat meal on the plasma amino acids of the dog (Elwyn, 1970). In these studies, Elwyn emphasized the importance of the liver in regulating peripheral plasma amino acid concentrations. In a recent study by Bark (1980), the enteral and parenteral administration of amino acids were examined in regard to plasma concentrations in both dog and man. In the fasting dog, several essential and nonessential amino acids were released from peripheral tissue, while the gut took up glutamine and released some nonessential amino acids which were then taken up by the liver. This was accompanied by the release of leucine and isoleucine from the liver. Gastrointestinal administration of the same amino acid solution resulted in an uptake of most amino acids, both in peripheral tissue and in the liver. The glutamine release from peripheral tissues in the fasting state was continued during the gastrointestinal administration. When the same amino acids were given by intravenous infusion, a lesser number of amino acids were taken up by the liver in spite of higher arterial plasma concentrations when compared with enteral intake. Glutamine was released from peripheral tissues simultaneously with the uptake of branched-chain amino acids and methionine. Bark (1980) recommended an oral amino acid loading test for investigation of protein malnutrition in selected patients.

The pattern of circulating amino acids in plasma and in muscle has been studied utilizing the percutaneous needle biopsy technique of Bergstrom (1962). Patients undergoing total hip replacement were treated with either 90 g/day of glucose, 70 g/day of amino acids, or both intakes together (Askanazi et al., 1980a). The pattern on the fourth postoperative day of amino acids in both muscle and plasma could be summarized as elevated levels of the branched-chain amino acids, phenylalanine, tyrosine, and methionine. There was a marked decrease in muscle glutamine and smaller decreases in the basic amino acids of both muscle and plasma. The muscle-to-plasma concentration ratios increased for the neutral amino acids, decreased for glutamine and the basic amino acids, and were unchanged for the acidic amino acids. There was little effect of either postoperative glucose or amino acids on the free amino acid concentrations in muscle. In plasma, the concentrations of the branched-chain amino acids and proline were higher in the group given peripheral amino acids than in the other groups. Thus, a particular abnormal amino acid pattern is associated with elective operation which is relatively unaffected by the type of hypocaloric intravenous nutrition. This pattern of amino acids is almost identical to that seen after colectomy or major accidental injury.

Because the metabolic response to injury is commonly studied while the patient is on bedrest and receiving only hypocaloric nutrition by periphral vein, 21 normal volunteers were studied on a metabolic ward for a five- to six-day period of strict bedrest (Askanazi et al., 1978). Dietary intake was divided between regular meals, 5% dextrose, 3½% amino acids, or total fasting. Muscle and plasma amino acids were essentially unchanged in the patients receiving a regular diet, while those receiving peripheral dextrose and amino acids showed changes in plasma and muscle which were in the same direction as the changes following injury, but the extent of the change was less marked. These findings are consistent with the view that the abnormalities in the amino acid concentrations of plasma and muscle seen after injury are a summation of the metabolic response to the injury, superimposed upon a lack of nutritional intake.

Patients were studied by Askanazi et al. (1980b) who were resuscitated after emergency admission for major injury. Free amino acids were measured in plasma and muscle from the second to the fourth postinjury day. Similar measurements were made in five of the patients at the height of major secondary infection and in five of the patients in late convalescence, just before discharge. The pattern described above in the postoperative patients was again seen following major injury. At the time of serious infection, the abnormal pattern became more accentuated, but no unique changes were observed which would serve as a metabolic marker for infection when compared with injury.

AMINO ACIDS, THERMOGENESIS AND VENTILATION

The thermic effect, or specific dynamic action associated with the intake of protein or amino acids, has been recognized since the days of Rubner a century ago

(Kleiber, 1975), but remains poorly understood. It is now generally believed that this thermic effect is not the result of digestion or absorption in the gastrointestinal tract, but seems to be most evident when amino acids are degraded with urea formation in the liver. It has not been clear as to whether there was a thermic effect related to giving isotonic amino acids by peripheral vein. In a recent study of patients undergoing total hip replacement (Askanazi, 1981), we observed that patients who were given only peripheral dextrose had no change in their resting energy expenditure over the first six postoperative days, while patients receiving peripheral amino acids showed an increase of 10% to 15% in their REE over the same period. When similar studies are conducted in normal volunteers on bedrest to mimic the postoperative condition, the REE slowly decreased from 10% to 15% during six days of peripheral dextrose by vein, while the volunteers who received amino acids by peripheral vein showed no decrease during the same period. Therefore, peripheral amino acids appeared to have a distinct thermic effect when compared with peripheral dextrose in both normal subjects and postoperative patients.

Total parenteral nutrition consisting of glucose and amino acids has been observed by Askanazi et al. (1980c) to have a thermogenic effect of 15% to 30%, when administered to hypercatabolic patients, while administration of the same TPN to depleted patients produced no thermogenic effect. Current studies are underway to determine the proportion of this thermic effect which is the result of amino acid administration versus any thermic effect due to the high glucose load.

Various investigators working with TPN solutions have observed that occasional patients appeared to be "doing less well" when receiving a conventional amount of TPN than prior to beginning the increased intake. This clinical impression was often difficult to define, but sometimes the patients appeared to have increases in their respiratory rate or an increase in the effort to breathe. We observed several patients who were acutely ill and responded to TPN with increases in minute ventilation of 3 to 6 liters/minute. Such observations have prompted a prospective clinical study to examine the relationship between the increased CO_2 excretion which resulted from the high carbohydrate load and the increase in minute ventilation (Askanazi et al., 1980d). The evidence seems clear that the increase in minute ventilation is correlated with the increase in CO_2 production; however, the increase in ventilation is much greater in the acutely ill patient than in the depleted patient. This finding led us to conclude that the acutely ill patient shows an increase in CO_2 production from carbohydrate, plus the thermogenic effect of the TPN; both of which are stimulating ventilation. The depleted patient has less stimulus to ventilation from TPN, because his CO_2 production is not increased as much as in the acutely ill patient, and also has no thermogenic response to the TPN.

We have recently been involved in a series of studies to examine the influence of amino acids alone on ventilation. Depleted patients have a blunted ventilatory response to breathing 2% and 4% CO_2 in the inspired air. This response can be restored to normal by infusion of amino acids by peripheral vein for only one day (Weissman et al., in press). Therefore, intravenous amino acids appear to stimulate ventilation by increasing the responsiveness of the ventilatory center to any given level of CO_2. Consequently, the amino acid component of TPN exerts a stimulatory effect on ventilation which is independent of that seen by the increased CO_2 resulting from carbohydrate loads.

CONCLUSION

The effect of the metabolic response to injury includes providing the body with a rapidly available source of amino acids at the expense of muscle protein. This process appears to guarantee amino acids for the increased synthesis of new proteins for host defense, coagulation, and wound healing as well as for gluconeogenesis. The result is a rapid drain upon the protein stores of the body which in normal situations can be repaired during the anabolic phase of late convalescence. Peaston (1974) has observed that the body exchanges the value of immediate amino acid availability for the disadvantage of a subsequent "nitrogen debt," very similar teleologically to the oxygen debt incurred in muscle tissue during severe exercise. This hypercatabolic state can be viewed as an asset to survival when its duration is limited, but when it persists beyond a certain ill-defined point because of calorie deprivation or the extra demands of infection, the total debt incurred may exceed the body's capacity to reverse the trend which must inevitably be fatal if continued long enough. This hypercatabolic response can be modified by parenteral nutrition and by an increased ambient temperature. In the most severely catabolic states, the body's protein reserves may only be sufficient to provide the requirements for three to four weeks. In such clinical situations, it may be life saving to diminish the protein losses by every means possible lest the patient succumb to the effect of acute post-traumatic depletion.

Future studies are awaited with interest to learn whether special amino acid mixtures can assist the body in healing injured or infected tissue. It is conceivable that repair of a mucosal injury of the intestinal tract or of a damaged liver may each have special amino acid needs which differ from that of the person recovering from an injury to the musculoskeletal system.

REFERENCES

Allison, J.B. and Bird, J.W.C. (1964): Elimination of nitrogen from the body. In *Mammalian Protein Metabolism* (eds: H.N. Munro and J.B. Allison) Vol. 1, p. 483. New York-London, Academic Press.

Askanazi, J., Carpentier, Y.A., Elwyn, D.H., Nordenstrom, J., Jeevanandam, M., Rosenbaum, S.H., Gump, F.E., and Kinney, J.M. (1980c): Influence of total parenteral nutrition on fuel utilization in injury and sepsis. *Ann. Surg.* 191:40–46.

Askanazi, J., Carpentier, Y.A., Jeevanandam, M., Michelsen, C.B., Elwyn, D.H., and Kinney, J.M. (1981): Energy expenditure, nitrogen balance, and norepinephrine excretion after injury. *Surgery* 89:478–484.

Askanazi, J., Carpentier, Y.A., Michelsen, C.B., Elwyn, D.H., Furst, P., Kantrowitz, L.R., Gump, F.E., and Kinney, J.M. (1980b): Muscle and plasma amino acids following injury: Influence of intercurrent infection. *Ann. Surg.* 192:78–85.

Askanazi, J., Elwyn, D.H., Kinney, J.M., Gump, F.E., Michelsen, C.B., and Stinchfield, F.E. (1978): Muscle and plasma amino acids after injury: The role of inactivity. *Ann. Surg.* 188:797–803.

Askanazi, J., Furst, P., Michelsen, C.B., Elwyn, D.H., Vinnars, E., Gump, F.E., Stinchfield, F.E., and Kinney, J.M. (1980a): Muscle and plasma amino acids after injury: Hypocaloric glucose vs amino acid infusion. *Ann. Surg.* 191:465–472.

Askanazi, J., Rosenbaum, S.H., Hyman, A.I., Silverberg, P.A., Milic-Emili, J., and Kinney,

J.M. (1980d): Respiratory changes induced by the large glucose loads of total parenteral nutrition. *JAMA* 243:1444–1447.

Bark, S. (1980): Enteral and parenteral administration of crystalline amino acids. Thesis in *Acta Chir. Scand.* Suppl 497.

Bergstrom, J. (1962): Muscle electrolytes in man. *Scand. J. Clin. Lab. Invest.* 14:1(Suppl 68).

Blackburn, G.L., Flatt, J.P., Clowes, G.H.A., and O'Donnell, T.F. (1973a): Peripheral intravenous feeding with isotonic amino acid solutions. *Am. J. Surg.* 125:447–454.

Blackburn, G.L., Flatt, J.P., Clowes, G.H.A., Jr., O'Donnell, T.F., and Hensle, T.E. (1973b): Protein sparing during periods of starvation with sepsis or trauma. *Ann. Surg.* 177:588–594.

Dudrick, S.J., Vars, H.M., Rawnsley, H.H., and Rhoads, J.E. (1966): Total intravenous feeding and growth in puppies. *Fed. Proc.* 25:481A.

Duke, J.H., Jr., Jørgensen, S.B., Broell, J.R., Long, C.L., and Kinney, J.M. (1970): Contribution of protein to caloric expenditure following injury. *Surgery* 68:168–174.

Elman, R. (1937): Urinary output of nitrogen as influenced by intravenous injection of a mixture of amino-acids. *Proc. Soc. Exp. Biol. Med.* 37:610–613.

Elwyn, D.H. (1970): The role of the liver in regulation of amino acid and protein metabolism. In *Mammalian Protein Metabolism* (ed: H.N. Munro), vol. 4, p. 523. New York-London, Academic Press.

Elwyn, D.H., Gump, F.E., Iles, M., Long, C.L., and Kinney, J.M. (1978): Protein and energy sparing of glucose added in hypocaloric amounts to peripheral infusions of amino acids. *Metabolism* 27:325–331.

Freeman, J.B., Stegink, L.D., Fry, K.L., Sherman, B.M., and Denbesten, L. (1975): Evaluation of amino acid infusions as protein-sparing agents in normal adult subjects. *Am. J. Clin. Nutr.,* 28:477–481.

Greenberg, G.R., Marliss, E.B., Anderson, G.H., Langer, B., Spence, W., Tovee, E.B., and Jeejeebhoy, K.N. (1976): Protein-sparing therapy in postoperative patients. *N. Engl. J. Med.* 294:1411–1416.

Hill, G.L., McCarthy, D., Collins, J.P., and Smith, A.H. (1978): A new method for the rapid measurement of body composition in critically ill surgical patients. *Br. J. Surg.* 65:732–735.

Hoover, H.C., Grant, J.P., Gorschboth, C., and Ketcham, A.S. (1975): Nitrogen sparing intravenous fluids in postoperative patients. *N. Engl. J. Med.* 293:172–175.

Howard, L., Dobbs, A., and Chodus, R. (1976): A comparison of administering protein alone and protein plus glucose on nitrogen balance. *Clin.* 24:501A.

Kinney, J.M. (1976): Surgical diagnosis, patterns of energy, weight and tissue change. In *Metabolism and the Response to Injury* (eds: A.W. Wilkinson and D. Cuthbertson), p. 121. Kent, England, Pitman Medical.

Kleiber, M. (1975): *The Fire of Life,* pp. 272–284. Huntington, New York, Robert E. Krieger.

Lidstrom, F., and Wretlind, A. (1952): Effect of dialyzed casein hydrolysate. The effect of intravenous administration of a dialyzed, enzymatic casein hydrolysate (Aminosol) on the serum concentration and on the urinary excretion of amino acids, peptides and nitrogen. *Scand. J. Clin. Lab. Invest.* 4:167–178.

McNeill, K.G., Mernagh, J.R., Jeejeebhoy, K.N., Wolman, S.L., and Harrison, J.E. (1979): In vivo measurements of body protein based on the determination of nitrogen by prompt gamma analysis. *Am. J. Clin. Nutr.* 32:1955–1961.

Moore, F.D. (1963): *The Body Cell Mass and Its Supporting Environment.* Philadelphia-London, WB Saunders.

Munro, H.N. (1964): Historical introduction: The origin and growth of our present concepts of protein metabolism. In *Mammalian Protein Metabolism* (eds: H.N. Munro and J.B. Allison), Vol. 1, p. 13. New York-London, Academic Press.

Peaston, M.J.T. (1974): Protein and amino acid metabolism—Response to injury. In *Parenteral Nutrition in Acute Metabolic Illness* (ed: H.A. Lee), p. 139. New York-London, Academic Press.

Schuberth, O., and Wretlind, A. (1961): Intravenous infusion of fat emulsions, phosphatide and emulsifying agents. *Acta. Chir. Scand. (Suppl)*. 278:1–21.
Soroff, H.S., Pearson, E., and Artz, C.P. (1961): An estimation of the nitrogen requirements for equilibrium in burned patients. *Surg. Gynecol. Obstet.* 132:159–172.
Weissman, C., Askanazi, J., and Rosenbaum, S.H. (in press): Amino acids and respiration.
Wretlind, A. (1981): Parenteral nutrition. *Nutr. Rev.* 39:257–265.

24 Altered Amino Acid Concentrations and Flux Following Traumatic Injury

Douglas W. Wilmore
David C. Brooks
Ferdinand Muhlbacher
C. Raja Kapadia
Thomas T. Aoki
Robert Smith

The metabolic response to injury was first characterized by Cuthbertson who noted marked alterations in nitrogen metabolism, manifested by increased urinary nitrogen excretion in patients with long bone fractures (Cuthbertson and Tilstone, 1969). Since that time, studies of 3-methylhistidine excretion (Long et al., 1975) and total body nitrogen flux (Herrmann et al., 1980; Birkhahn et al., 1981) support the concept that a moderate to severe accidental injury increases the rate of protein breakdown—skeletal muscle accounts for the major portion of protein mass undergoing accelerated degradation. Amino acid residues liberated from skeletal muscle are transported via the bloodstream to visceral tissues and utilized for protein synthetic purposes (for example, the synthesis of acute phase protein by the liver) or undergo deamination, with the carbon skeleton used to synthesize new glucose (Wilmore et al., 1980). The nitrogen residues from this latter process are converted to urea and excreted. The increased urea appearance and loss in the urine accounts for most of the increased nitrogen loss following injury. Wound losses occur, but this is primarily exudation loss of plasma protein. The process is distinctly different from the hypercatabolic response of injury.

The dynamic loss of body protein following accidental injury is thus characterized by a translocation of nitrogen from the carcass (i.e., skeletal muscle) to visceral tissue (liver and kidney). With wound healing and convalescence, a time usually accompanied by adequate enteral nutrition and increasing patient mobility and exercise, restoration of normal protein metabolism occurs associated with a rebuilding of skeletal muscle mass.

Because of the profound changes observed in body nitrogen following injury, interest has focused on amino acid metabolism. These investigations have aided understanding of the pathophysiologic mechanisms involved in this hypercatabolic process. Some of the information derived from these investigations has provided the bases for treatment modalities which attempt to offset the protein catabolic changes that occur following injury. This chapter will review the amino acid alterations that occur in humans following traumatic injury.

DEFINITION AND SCOPE

Injury to humans, whether accidental or following elective surgical procedures, initiates a variety of changes that are altered with time following the traumatic event. For example, when Cuthbertson described the metabolic alterations that occurred following long bone fracture, he noted an early "ebb" phase associated with hypovolemia. With restoration of blood volume and adequate tissue perfusion, this initial phase was followed by a later "flow phase," a period associated with hypermetabolism and increased nitrogen loss (Cuthbertson and Tilstone, 1969). This discussion will primarily focus on the flow phase of accidental injury when metabolic alterations are not confounded by inadequate perfusion.

A variety of studies of amino acid metabolism have been performed in surgical patients, and many investigations have been performed in patients following elective operative procedures. With modern day care, patients undergoing elective operative procedures undergo minimal stress, and their protein metabolic response differs quite markedly from that observed following moderate to severe accidental injury (Wilmore et al., 1982). Therefore, data from studies in patients following elective operations should not be interpreted as reflecting changes that occur following major accidental injury. In patients being studied following elective operative procedures, such variables as the underlying disease process, medications, type of anesthesia, and postoperative analgesia should all be standardized so that these treatment variables do not confound the response being studied.

Investigators studying patients following accidental injury have frequently failed to standardize their study conditions. Blood samples are obtained for analysis at various times throughout the day (or night), and under a variety of conditions (the most common confounding variable is the infusion of dextrose-containing intravenous solutions). In general, few reports standardize other treatment variables such as the use of ventilators, cardiotropic agents or analgesic medication. Entry criteria for patients into an investigation are frequently unclear, and in many reports patients are studied only because they are in a similar geographic area—that is, they are all together in a common intensive care unit.

Another common problem is the inclusion of data from patients following accidental injury who develop infection. The responses in these individuals do not represent post-traumatic changes nor do they demonstrate the effect of infection. Rather, the physiological and biochemical alterations are the result of an interaction between injury and infection and should be viewed as such. In this review, only patients documented to be free of infection will be discussed.

Finally, animal studies are useful, yet injured animal models are difficult to maintain, and variables, such as mobility, pain, and food intake, are almost impossible to standardize. Therefore, this review will highlight human investigations and will cite animal studies when these investigations support patients' studies, add detail to pertinent research questions, or point directions for further investigations.

CHANGES IN PLASMA AMINO ACID CONCENTRATIONS

Postoperative Patients

In the 1940s, Man and associates (1946) monitored plasma α-amino acid nitrogen in patients undergoing operative procedures. In patients who were previously in good health and well nourished, amino acid nitrogen was normal before operation (> 4 mg/100 dl), but fell following the operative procedure and returned slowly to normal during convalescence. Sicker or more malnourished patients had lower preoperative α-amino nitrogen concentrations, and these volumes remained depressed for a longer period of time following operation. Others have confirmed the postoperative decline of most plasma amino acids following operation (Hoover-Plow et al., 1980; Dale et al., 1977). Dale, Johnson, Tweedle, and associates (1977), in a very carefully designed study, noted that postoperative patients receiving only saline infusions maintained total amino acid concentrations following vagotomy and pyloroplasty for duodenal ulcer disease; although, with time, nonessential amino acid levels fell and essential amino acid concentrations rose. In contrast, patients receiving glucose during the postoperative period were found to decrease plasma amino acid concentrations. Individuals receiving intravenous amino acids or fat emulsions during the postoperative period maintained normal or supernormal amino acid concentrations, especially the essential amino acids as a group. The changes in amino acid concentrations could not be attributed to starvation, anesthesia or tissue damage alone. For example, Owen et al. (1969) observed only a 12% decrease in α-amino nitrogen in obese patients fasted for 28 days, and Dale and associates (1977) noted no alterations in amino acid concentration following anesthesia associated with cystoscopy.

Accidental Injury

In patients following accidental injury, amino acid concentrations have been reported to rise, fall, and/or remain within normal limits. In reports of measurements obtained during the flow phase of injury under defined conditions greater than three to four days following the traumatic event, a more consistent response emerges. Aulick and Wilmore (1979) determined amino acid concentrations in 18 noninfected burn patients studied during the second to third week following injury. These patients had received vigorous nutritional support during their hospitalization, but were postabsorptive at least six hours, and resting comfortably during the morning of study. Concentrations of most amino acids were below normal levels, although phenylalanine was elevated. Branched-chain amino acid concentrations were not distinguishable from control values. Similar findings during comparable study conditions had been reported by others (Clowes et al., 1980). However, even when plasma samples are obtained during the fed state, total plasma amino acid concentrations may be low. Thus, Alexander et al. (1980) monitored plasma amino acid concentrations in patients receiving a variety of nutrient intakes, calculated to maintain body weight in thermally injured children. In spite of near continuous protein and amino acid feeding (via enteral or parenteral routes), total amino acid concentrations in the injured children were low when compared with control studies. In additional studies these investigators noted that most individual amino acid concentrations fell, but there was an elevation in phenylalanine, aspartate, glutamate, hydroxyproline, and methionine (Stinnett et al., 1982). The concentration of phenylalanine (or the phenylalanine:tyrosine ratio) was related to the severity of the catabolic state and postinjury mortality.

In summary, it appears that plasma amino acid concentrations fall after operation if the patient receives glucose-containing solutions. Following accidental injury, amino acid concentrations are low during the flow phase of injury, even during protein or amino acid feedings. Phenylalanine is the exception and is elevated in all studies reported.

AMINO ACID FLUX

Concentration in the plasma compartment is dependent upon the rate of inflow into this distribution space and the rate of outflow from this compartment. A low concentration of plasma amino acids could result from diminished amino acid inflow, increased amino acid outflow or both. Investigators have frequently concluded that skeletal muscle breakdown is accelerated, although precise studies have rarely been performed. The most common problem is the measurement of limb AV concentration difference across an extremity without simultaneous bloodflow measurements. When both extremity flow and concentration measurements were performed simultaneously in postabsorptive, noninfected burn patients studied two to three weeks following injury, the release of amino acid nitrogen was approximately two to three times greater than that found in normal controls (Aulick and Wilmore, 1979). Using alanine flux as a marker of nitrogen catabolism, the release of alanine was generally related to the extent of injury and the oxygen consumption of the patient. Another study of traumatized individuals using estimates of limb bloodflow in a more heterogeneous study population supports these observations (Clowes et al., 1980).

If influx of amino acids into the plasma compartment from skeletal muscle is increased during steady state conditions, there should be a comparable outflow of amino acids from the plasma into visceral tissue. Such is the case (Wilmore et al., 1980). A comparable group of noninfected burn patients was studied following hepatic vein catheterization. Plasma amino acid uptake calculated from measurements of splanchnic bloodflow and arterial-hepatic vein concentration differences demonstrated an accelerated uptake of amino acids when compared to postabsorptive normals (Table 24-1). Because arterial concentrations were approximately the same and extraction ratio for the amino acids was similar to that observed in normal individuals, the increased uptake was primarily the result of increased splanchnic bloodflow which augmented delivery of amino acids to the liver. Measurements of amino acid released from peripheral tissue (skeletal muscle) compared favorably

Table 24-1
Splanchnic Bloodflow and Alanine Exchange (Range or Mean ± S.E.)

	Control Subjects	Burn Patients
Splanchnic bloodflow (L/minute•m^2)	0.63–0.85	1.54 ± 0.12
Arterial alanine concentration (μM/L)	250–400	345 ± 51
Arterial-hepatic vein difference (μM/L)	80–100	119 ± 28
Extraction ratio (%)	34–38	34 ± 5
Alanine splanchnic uptake (μM/minute•m^2)	30–45	124 ± 31

Table 24-2
Estimate of Peripheral Amino Acid Release and Splanchnic Uptake*
(Mean or Range)

Net Release	Control Subjects	Burn Patients
100 ml leg volume (μmol/100 ml leg volume•minute)	0.08	0.35
Whole leg (μmol/minute)	8–10	35–40
Total skeletal muscle (μmol/minute)	48–58	210–240
Splanchnic alanine uptake (μmol/minute)	53–79	164–270

*From measurements of patients with comparable burn size. (≅ 45% total body surface).

with the measurements of splanchnic uptake (Table 24-2), and confirm the marked translocation of amino acid nitrogen from carcass to viscera.

LIVER AMINO ACID HOMEOSTASIS – ROLE OF GLUCAGON

The uptake of amino acids by the liver is carefully matched by amino acid release from skeletal muscle. Hepatic perfusion of isolated organs demonstrates the hepatic amino acid uptake increases in direct proportion to plasma concentration, yet in injured patients concentration of most amino acids is low, not elevated. The mechanism which may explain this increased hepatic amino acid uptake may be related to the known effects of glucagon, a hormone elaborated from the α-cell of the pancreas in increasing quantities following injury (Wilmore et al., 1974). Studies from glucagon infusion demonstrate that this hormone causes hypoaminoacidemia (Liljenquist et al., 1981), augments splanchnic bloodflow, and increases hepatic α-amino nitrogen uptake (Kibler et al., 1964).

REGULATION OF MUSCLE PROTEOLYSIS

Release of amino acids from the periphery does not appear to be a direct glucagon effect (Wolf et al., 1979; Marliss et al., 1970), but may be related to other factors such as alterations in concentration gradients, the effects of cortisone, and decreased nutritional intake. The role of endogenous pyrogens arising from the inflammatory response associated with injured tissue and increased body temperature may also exert an effect on skeletal muscle protein degradation (F. Goldberg, personal communication, 1982). (See also Ekman and Lundholm, p. 212.)

PHENYLALANINE AS A MARKER OF SKELETAL MUSCLE CATABOLISM

Serum concentrations of phenylalanine are consistently elevated in injured patients. This essential amino acid is an index of skeletal muscle catabolism and is solely catabolized by the liver. However, increased concentrations of phenylalanine may not indicate altered hepatic handling of this amino acid following uncomplicated injury. Studies of the rate of appearance of tyrosine, the phenylalanine metabolite, assessed following an oral phenylalanine load was normal in uncomplicated trauma patients (Herndon et al., 1978), and the rate of hepatic uptake was increased following injury (Wilmore et al., 1980). Thus, the elevation of serum phenylalanine concentrations and the increased flux of phenylalanine through the plasma compartment reflect the rapid skeletal muscle catabolism that occurs following injury and does not necessarily reflect decreased hepatic uptake of this amino acid. Similar kinetic studies have been performed following the infusion of leucine, and the half-life of the infused dose was shortened in the patients who sustained accidental injury, despite increased blood concentrations (Elia et al., 1980).

MUSCLE INTRACELLULAR FREE AMINO ACID CONCENTRATIONS

Amino acids move through the plasma compartment as they are transported from skeletal muscle to viscera. The plasma amino acids are supported by efflux from the free amino acid pool located within skeletal muscle. Concentrations in this pool are determined by skeletal muscle protein degradation, intracellular metabolic pathways, and efflux into the plasma compartment. Bergstrom and associates developed techniques to analyze intracellular amino acids in the small quantity of skeletal muscle tissue obtained by needle biopsy. Vinnars reported changes in the free amino acids of muscle tissue following an uncomplicated elective operation and more severe injury (Vinnars et al., 1975). In these patients, typical changes following operation include increases in the branched-chain amino acids, phenylalanine, tyrosine, methionine, glycine, and alanine, and decreases in concentrations of glutamine. The changes occurred at a time when no major alterations were observed in plasma amino acid concentrations.

In more severely injured patients, the essential amino acid pool was reduced in both plasma and intracellular water, and the intracellular fluid compartment was expanded (Vinnars et al., 1980). In muscle, phenylalanine was increased, and lysine and glutamine were decreased. In additional studies in patients undergoing elective operative procedures, the effect of various hypocaloric parenteral nutrient infusions on the intracellular amino acid composition was assessed (Askanazi et al., 1980). There was little effect of diet on free amino acid concentrations in muscle, although dietary alterations often exerted changes in some plasma amino acid levels as previously reported.

Because glutamine represents approximately two thirds of the free amino acid pool and falls dramatically following a variety of catabolic diseases, we have examined a variety of factors which could explain the decreased intracellular glutamine concentration following injury. After developing appropriate analytical procedures for the analysis of glutamine synthetase and glutaminase, glutamine changes were monitored following a single perturbation, the administration of steroids to a dog. With steroid, all animals developed marked negative nitrogen balance (– 7.1 g N/day). Whole blood glutamine concentrations remained relatively constant, but intracellular concentrations of glutamine were dramatically reduced from 22.1 mmol/L intracellular water to 10.0 within two weeks. Muscle tissue analysis, however, demonstrated no alteration in the enzyme activity, and, hence, alterations in enzyme activity could not explain the changes that were observed in intracellular glutamine concentrations. Preliminary flux studies demonstrated increased glutamine outflow from the muscle compartment during steroid administration. Other studies are currently in progress to determine molecular mechanisms which explain alteration in intracellular amino acid concentrations.

THE ROLE OF EXOGENOUS AMINO ACIDS ON PROTEIN ANABOLISM IN TRAUMA PATIENTS

Injured patients have been studied during the flow phase of their post-traumatic course and require increased quantities of exogenous nitrogen and energy in order to maintain nitrogen equilibrium during the catabolic phase of injury (Moore, 1959; Wilmore, 1977). Studies using N^{15} kinetic methodology to determine rates of protein synthesis and catabolism demonstrate that the administration of adequate calories and nitrogen primarily supports protein synthesis in the injured patient and exerts minimal impact on rate of degradation (Herrmann et al., 1980). Thus, in the severely injured patient feeding supports the increased flux of nitrogen through the body—this accelerated turnover rate only returns to normal with resolution of the disease process.

Because branched-chain amino acids studied *in vitro* exert regulatory effects on synthesis and degradation of skeletal muscle protein, investigators have been attracted toward the use of these substances to minimize protein loss following injury. Animal studies suggest that the administration of single or all three branched-chain amino acids provides net anabolic effects as determined by total nitrogen balance (Freund and Fischer, 1978; Blackburn et al., 1979). Studies in normals and postoperative patients demonstrate that branched-chain amino acid infusions achieve nitrogen balance comparable to that observed with infusion of a "balanced" amino acid solution (Wolf, 1980; Freund et al., 1975). A variety of clinical trials are now in progress, and the available reports do not allow firm conclusions as to the safety and efficacy of infusion of these substances into patients who have sustained severe injury.

Aoki and associates (1981) have recently reported that a leucine meal administered by the oral route to normals results in net negative nitrogen balance across the skeletal muscle bed of the forearm. Certainly, more work is necessary to establish if there is clear benefit from using specialized solutions when compared to the usual balanced amino acid formulas.

REFERENCES

Alexander, J.W., MacMillan, B.G., Stinnett, J.D., Ogle, C., Bozian, R.C., Fischer, J.E., Oakes, J.B., Morris, M.J., and Krummel, R. (1980): Beneficial effects of aggressive protein feeding in severely burned children. *Ann. Surg.* 192:505–507.

Aoki, T.T., Brennan, M.F., Fitzpatrick, G.F., and Knight, D.C. (1981): Leucine meal increases glutamine and total nitrogen release from forearm muscle. *J. Clin. Invest.* 68: 1522–1528.

Askanazi, J., Furst, P., Michelsen, C.B., Elwyn, D.H., Vinnars, E., Gump, F.E., Stinchfield, F.E., and Kinney, J.M. (1980): Muscle and plasma amino acids after injury. Hypocaloric glucose versus amino acid infusion. *Ann. Surg.* 191:465–472.

Aulick, L.H., and Wilmore, D.W. (1979): Increased peripheral amino acid release following burn injury. *Surgery* 85:560–565.

Birkhahn, R.H., Long, C.L., Fitkin, D., Jeevanandam, M., and Blakemore, W.S. (1981): Whole-body protein metabolism due to trauma in man as estimated by L-[N^{15}] alanine. *Amer. J. Phys.* 241:E64–E71.

Blackburn, G.L., Moldawer, L.L., Usui, S., Bothe, A., O'Keefe, J.D., and Bistrian, B.R. (1979): Branched chain amino acid administration and metabolism during starvation, injury, and infection. *Surgery* 86:307–315.

Clowes, G.H.A. Jr., Randall, H.T. and Cha, C.J. (1980): Amino acid and energy metabolism in septic and traumatized patients. *JPEN* 4:195–205.

Cuthbertson, D. and Tilstone, W.J. (1969): Metabolism during the postinjury period. *Adv. Clin. Chem.* 12:1.

Dale, G., Young, G., Latner, A.L., Goode, A., Tweedle, D., and Johnston, I.D.A. (1977): The effect of surgical operation on venous plasma free amino acids. *Surgery* 81:295–301.

Elia, M., Farrell, R., Ilic, V., Smith, R., and Williamson, D.H. (1980): The removal of infused leucine after injury, starvation and other conditions in man. *Clin. Sci.* 59:275–283.

Freund, H., and Fischer, J.E. (1978): Nitrogen-conserving quality of branched-chain amino acids: possible regulator effect of valine in post-injury muscle catabolism. *Surg. Forum* 24:69–71.

Freund, H., Hoover, H.C., Atamian, S., and Fischer, J.E. (1975): Infusion of the branched chain amino acids in postoperative patients. *Ann. Surg.* 190:18–23.

Herrmann, V.M., Clark, D., Wilmore, D.W., and Moore, F.D. (1980): Protein metabolism: effect of disease and altered intake on the stable 15N curve. *Surg. Forum* 31:92–94.

Herndon, D.N., Wilmore, D.W., Mason, A.D. Jr., and Pruitt, B.A., Jr. (1978): Abnormalities of phenylalanine and tyrosine kinetics: Significance in septic and nonseptic burned patients. *Arch. Surg.* 113:133–135.

Hoover-Plow, J.L., Clifford, A.J., and Hodges, R.E. (1980): The effects of surgical trauma on plasma amino acid levels in humans. *Surg. Gynecol. Obstet.* 150:161–164.

Kibler, R.F., Taylor, W.J., and Meyers, J.D. (1964): The effect of glucagon on net splanchnic balances of glucose, amino acid nitrogen, urea ketones, and oxygen in man. *J. Clin. Invest.* 43:904–915.

Liljenquist, J.E., Lewis, S.B., Cherrington, A.D., Sinclair-Smith, B.C., and Lacy, W.W. (1981): Effects of pharmacologic hyperglucagonemia on plasma amino acid concentrations in normal and diabetic man. *Metabolism* 30:1195–1199.

Long, C., Haverberg, L.N., Young, V.R., Kinney, J.M., Munro, H.N., and Geiger, J.W. (1975): Metabolism of 3-methylhistidine in man. *Metabolism* 24:929–935.

Man, E.B., Bettcher, P.G., Cameron, C.M., and Peters, J.P. (1946): Plasma α-amino acid nitrogen and serum lipids of surgical patients. *J. Clin. Invest.* 25:701–708.

Marliss, E.B., Aoki, T.T., Unger, R.H., Soeldner, J.S., and Cahill, G.F., Jr. (1970): Glucagon levels and metabolic effects in fasting man. *J. Clin. Invest.* 49:2256–2270.

Moore, F.D. (1959): *Metabolic Care of the Surgical Patient.* Philadelphia, W.B. Saunders Company.

Owen, O.E., Felig, P., Morgan, A.P., Wahren, J., and Cahill, G.F., Jr. (1969): Liver and kidney metabolism during prolonged starvation. *J. Clin. Invest.* 48:574–583.

Stinnett, J.D., Alexander, J.W., Watanabe, C., MacMillan, B.G., Fischer, J.E., Morris, M.J., Trocki, O., Miskell, P., Edwards, L., and James, H. (1982): Plasma and skeletal muscle amino acids following severe burn injury in patients and experimental animals. *Ann. Surg.* 195:75–89.

Vinnars, E., Bergstom, J., and Furst, P. (1975): Influence of the postoperative state on the intracellular free amino acids in human muscle tissue. *Ann. Surg.* 182:665–671.

Vinnars, E., Furst, P., and Liljedahl, S.O. (1980): Effect of parenteral nutrition on intracellular free amino acid concentration. *JPEN* 4:184–187.

Wilmore, D.W. (1977): Energy requirements for maximum nitrogen retention. *Proceedings of a Symposium on Amino Acids* (eds: H.L. Green, M.A. Holliday and H.N. Munro) pp. 47–57. American Medical Association.

Wilmore, D.W., Black, P.R., and Muhlbacher, F. (1982): Injured man: trauma and sepsis. In *Nutritional Management of the Seriously Ill Patient* (ed: R.W. Winters). Bristol-Meyers, Syracuse, New York.

Wilmore, D.W., Goodwin, C.W., Aulick, L.H., Powanda, M.C., Mason, A.D., and Pruitt, B.A., Jr. (1980): Effect of injury and infection on visceral metabolism and circulation. *Ann. Surg.* 192:491–504.

Wilmore, D.W., Lindsay, C.A., Moylan, J.A., Faloona, G.R., Pruitt, B.A., and Unger, R.H. (1974): Hyperoglucagonemia after burns. *Lancet* 1:73–75.

Wolf, B.M. (1980): Substrate-endocrine interaction and protein metabolism. *JPEN* 4:188–193.

Wolf, B.M., Culebras, J.M., and Aoki, T.T. (1979): The effects of glucagon on protein metabolism in normal man. *Surgery* 86:248–257.

Protein Dynamics in Stress

Robert R. Wolfe, Richard D. Goodenough, John F. Burke, and Marta H. Wolfe

Most methods that have been used to assess protein metabolism in burned patients require many hours or days to complete. Since it is not ethical to deny nutritional support to a severely burned patient for a prolonged time, studies of protein or amino acid metabolism in postabsorptive burn patients are limited. Therefore, we undertook the following study to assess leucine kinetics and oxidation in postabsorptive burn patients by means of the prime-constant infusion of 1-^{13}C-leucine. From the determination of the rate of $^{13}CO_2$ excretion and the plasma enrichments of leucine and α-ketoisocaproic acid, we were able to distinguish the oxidation of leucine derived from protein catabolism within the cell in which deamination occurred ("intracellular leucine") from the oxidation of leucine taken up by cells from the plasma. We then applied the data to a model of whole-body protein synthesis and catabolism that we have described in detail elsewhere (Wolfe et al., 1982).

It can be argued that resting volunteers are not appropriate controls for burn patients, because the level of energy expenditure is greater in burn patients. We, therefore, have compared the response of burn patients not only to the corresponding values from resting volunteers, but also to the responses elicited in normal volunteers subjected to other stimuli for increased energy expenditure, namely, exercise and cold exposure.

Finally, we have used this methodology to assess two aspects of the response to different levels of protein intake in burn patients: (1) Can the balance between protein synthesis and catabolism be improved by increasing the protein intake from 1.4 to 2.2 g protein/kg•day when calories are held constant? and (2) Is the alteration in basal protein metabolism induced by burn injury affected by the protein content of the diet?

METHODS

Burn Patients

Six severely burned patients were studied. No patient was diagnosed as systemically septic at the time of the study, and the studies were performed when the patients were in a relatively stable condition. Each patient was studied at the end of two three-day dietary control periods. The same amount of calories were provided during the two periods ($\overline{X}$ = 40.8 Kcal/kg•d). In one regimen (high protein) the protein intake averaged 2.20 ± 0.13 g protein/kg•d, and in the other regimen (low protein) the protein intake was an average of 1.43 ± .06 g protein/kg•day. Patients were studied in both the fed state and after 10 to 12 hours of fasting.

(1-^{13}C)-Leucine was infused as the tracer (0.15 μmol/kg•min) with priming doses of 9.1 μmol/leucine/kg and 2.1 μmol/kg of $NaH^{13}CO_3$. Oxygen consumption

($\dot{V}O_2$) and carbon dioxide production ($\dot{V}CO_2$) were determined in each subject during the isotope infusion, and expired air and blood samples were collected for mass spec analysis of the enrichment of CO_2, plasma leucine, and plasma α-KICA (Wolfe et al., 1982).

Volunteer Studies

The volunteers were studied twice, each time after an overnight fast. Dietary intake in each subject over the three-day period before the study was approximately equivalent to that of the patients on the 1.5 g protein diet. Each study consisted of two periods. The protocol for the first two hours (Period 1) was identical to that for the studies in the patients. Following Period 1, and without interruption of the isotope infusion, the subjects either exercised moderately for 100 minutes or were exposed to cold for the same length of time. The cold exposure was achieved by the rapid cooling of the temperature-controlled room in which the experiments were performed. The exercise intensity averaged 360 kpm•min (approximately 30% $\dot{V}O_2$ max), and the cold exposure was 10° C.

CALCULATIONS

Details of the calculations of leucine and α-KICA kinetics have been published recently (Wolfe et al., 1982). Leucine oxidation was divided into the oxidation of leucine that has appeared in the plasma and that which never left the cell of origin prior to deamination ("intracellular leucine"). From the leucine and α-KICA flux and oxidation data, rates of whole-body protein synthesis and catabolism were calculated as described previously.

RESULTS

The leucine kinetics and oxidation data are presented in Table 1. Ra leucine was significantly elevated in burned patients as compared to resting volunteers, and the % of α-KICA flux derived from plasma leucine was significantly reduced. Both total leucine oxidation and "intracellular leucine" oxidation were also significantly elevated.

The patterns of response of normal volunteers to cold exposure and exercise were different in some aspects, and also differed in some respects from the response to burn injury (Table 1). When the results were extrapolated to rates of whole-body protein synthesis and catabolism, injured patients were unique in having significant increases in both synthesis and catabolism (Table 2). Protein catabolism also increased in both cold exposure and exercise, but in cold there was no significant change in synthesis, and in exercise synthesis was decreased.

When the burn patients were studied on different levels of protein intake, no differences in endogenous leucine flux or "intracellular leucine" oxidation were evident. Protein synthesis was elevated in the fed state as opposed to the corresponding fasting study, and synthesis was higher on the high protein intake (Table 3). A net balance between synthesis and catabolism was achieved during the 1.5 g protein diet, and no significant improvement in net balance was noted on the high protein diet, although the absolute rates of both synthesis and catabolism were elevated.

Table 1
Leucine Kinetics in Different States of Increased Energy Expenditure

	Control	Burned	Cold	Exercise
VO_2 (μmol/kg•min)	152 ± 10.4	200 ± 42.4	345 ± 42.4	680 ± 38.4
Ra Leucine flux (μmol/kg•min)	1.63 ± 0.13	2.40 ± 0.53	2.08 ± 0.16	1.45 ± 0.05
α-KICA flux derived from plasma leucine (%)	78.7 ± 1.94	57.3 ± 4.70	90.4 ± 4.70	64.0 ± 6.66
Total Leucine Oxidation (μmol/kg•min)	0.37 ± 0.07	0.60 ± 0.17	0.61 ± 0.15	1.41 ± 0.14
"Intracellular leucine" Oxidation (μmol/kg•min)	0.08 ± 0.01	0.24 ± 0.03	0.07 ± 0.03	0.63 ± 0.06

Table 2
Protein Turnover in Exercise, Cold Exposure, and Burn Injury

	Control	Burned	Cold	Exercise
Synthesis	136 ± 8.2	192 ± 32.8	157 ± 14.9	66 ± 7.4
Catabolism	174 ± 14.4	260 ± 10.3	219 ± 18.0	204 ± 7.1
Net breakdown	38 ± 7.3	61 ± 7.9	61 ± 8.3	138 ± 13.4

Units are mg protein/kg•h.

Table 3
Effect of Protein Intake on Protein Synthesis and Catabolism in Burn Patients

	HP Fed	HP Fast	LP Fed	LP Fast
Synthesis	.346 ± .019	.245 ± .017	.280 ± .019	.193 ± .036
Catabolism	.336 ± .072	.321 ± .050	.280 ± .061	.254 ± .103
Net	+ .010 ± .031	− .076 ± .012	.000 ± .015	− .061 ± .008

Units are g protein/kg•h.

DISCUSSION

The results of this study using an isotopic tracer of protein metabolism demonstrate that net protein breakdown is increased in postabsorptive burn patients due to a marked increase in protein catabolism that is not accompanied by as large an increase in the rate of synthesis. From the leucine and α-KICA kinetic and oxidation data it can be inferred that muscle protein catabolism contributes significantly to the overall increase in the rate of protein catabolism after burn injury. Since the branch-chain transaminase activity is high in muscle relative to that in other tissues (Shinnick and Harper, 1976), and because of the large muscle mass in the body, it is reasonable to assume that most of the deamination of leucine to α-KICA occurs in muscle. Thus, the decrease in the percent of α-KICA flux derived from plasma leucine after injury, considered in light of the increase in the rate of plasma leucine flux, suggests an increased rate of catabolism of muscle protein.

Although the hypermetabolic response to injury is different in nature than the hypermetabolic response to cold exposure or exercise, certain interesting points arise from the comparison of these situations. Thus, it seems that the increased rate of protein synthesis in burn patients was a response to injury rather than a nonspecific response induced by the increased breakdown of protein. In both cold exposure and exercise, protein catabolism also were accelerated, yet there was no concomitant increase in synthesis in cold exposure, and in exercise synthesis was actually decreased.

Although net protein catabolism was accelerated in burn patients, we found that a balance between protein synthesis and catabolism could be achieved with 1.4 g protein/kg•day and approximately 40 kcal/kg•day. The failure of the higher protein intake to further stimulate net protein synthesis is consistent with the findings of Shizgal and Forse (1980) in normally nourished or malnourished surgical patients in whom body composition was measured during different diets. The question as to whether achieving balance between whole-body protein synthetic and catabolic rates should be the ultimate goal of nutritional therapy is not addressed by these data. Perhaps the stimulation of the overall rate of protein flux observed with the higher protein intake resulted in the preferable metabolic state for the patient.

Finally, it is of interest that the level of protein intake had no effect on endogenous leucine flux or "intracellular leucine" oxidation. Thus, even though a balance between protein synthesis and catabolism was observed in burned patients given a normal level of protein intake, nutritional therapy did not affect the underlying alteration of protein metabolism that occurred as a response to the injury. It, therefore, seems likely that there is a limitation of the extent to which nutrition alone can optimize the burned patient's metabolic status and, thus, ability to respond appropriately to other modes of therapy.

REFERENCES

Shinnick, F.L., and Harper, A.E. (1976): Branched-chain amino acid oxidation by isolated rat tissue preparations. *Biochem. Biophys. Acta* 437:477–486.

Shizgal, H.M., and Forse, R.H. (1980): Protein and caloric requirements with total parenteral nutrition. *Ann. Surg.* 192:562–568.

Wolfe, R.R., Goodenough, R.D., Wolfe, M.H., Royle, G.T., and Nadel, E.R. (1982): Isotopic analysis of leucine and urea metabolism in exercising humans. *J. Appl. Physiol.* 52(2):458–466.

Protein Turnover in Severely Ill Patients as Measured with ^{15}N Glycine

Samuel D. Ang and T. Peter Stein

In recent years there has been considerable interest in the determination of the whole-body protein synthesis rate (PSR), particularly in man. One reason for this is the availability of new analytical methods, most of which were developed by Waterlow, Garlick and their collaborators (1980) from the pioneering studies of Rittenberg and his students at Columbia. While much is known about the metabolic behavior of individual tissues down to the level of specific enzymes and substrates, only *in vivo* whole body experiments can indicate how the system functions as a whole. Biochemistry defines the available mechanisms and pathways, but whole body experiments are needed to assess their relative physiological importance.

The newer methods use amino acid tracers, labeled with stable isotopes, and rely on analyses of the plasma amino acids, expired air or urine. With such limited sampling, verification of the methodology is difficult. The problem is to decide whether the results from a particular method in a given experimental situation are best interpreted in terms of the metabolism of the amino acid used as the tracer rather than the whole body PSR. The validity of a method can be investigated by 1) comparison against a more rigorous method such as carcass analysis, and 2) comparison against other methods, using the argument that if two or more methods based on different assumptions give the same result, then it follows that both are correct. However, the problem here, as for example comparison of flux and end-point methods, is that some of the assumptions are still common to both approaches and the error may occur in one of the common assumptions or approximations. This article reports our attempts to measure whole-body protein synthesis rate in a series of stressed, but not post-trauma patients. ^{15}N glycine was used as the tracer and the flux was determined from the mean enrichment of the urinary ammonia in the 10 hours following the administration of a single pulse of 400 mg of ^{15}N glycine. In other studies on essentially healthy individuals this approach was found to give results in good agreement with values obtained by using ^{14}C leucine and ^{15}N lysine as tracers (Garlick et al., 1980; Waterlow, et al., 1978).

Figure 1 shows a scatter plot of the results. It is apparent that the results from the patients are much higher than is found in normals and there is a very wide range. Furthermore, it appears that a very high "apparent" PSR is associated with increased mortality. Elevated protein turnover rates have been reported post-trauma and postsepsis as being part of the normal response of protein metabolism to an acute stress (James et al., 1976). However, in this study we took care to ensure that none of the patients were studied in the immediate post-trauma phase. In fact, most of the patients were studied prior to surgery, although a few were studied some weeks after surgery.

The most obvious feature of the plot is the large number of patients with apparently elevated synthesis rates, and the apparent correlation with mortality. It is unlikely that very sick patients at bed rest are hypermetabolic. Parallel determination of the resting energy and basal energy expenditures revealed no evidence of hypermetabolism. We have previously reported that such very high PSRs are due to the concomitant presence of liver dysfunction which invalidates the one amino acid pool

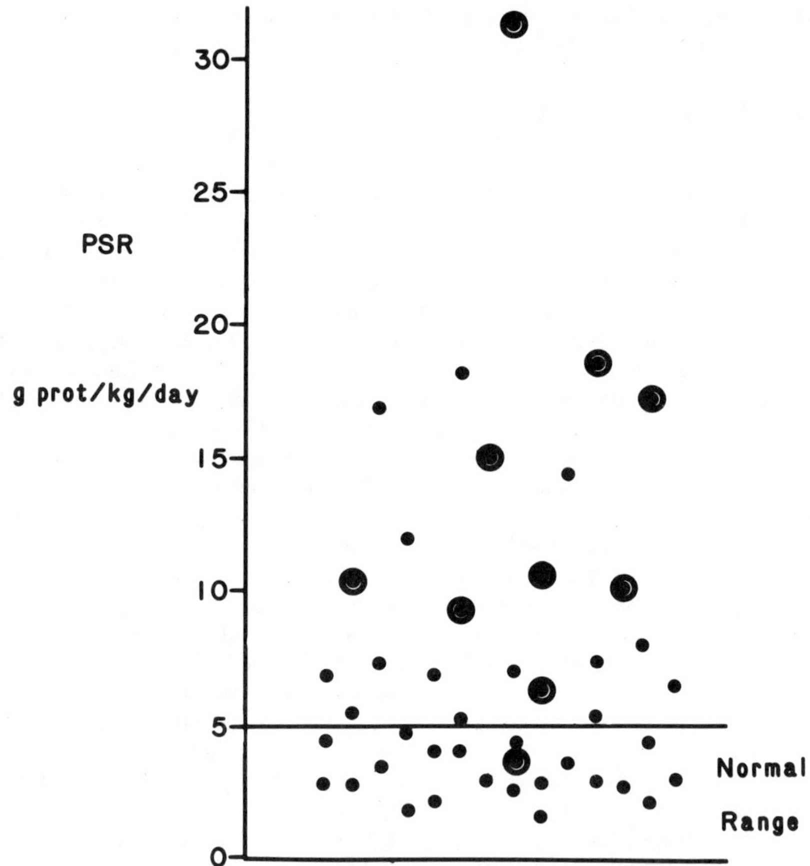

Figure 1 Distribution pattern for the PSRs (in g protein/kg body wt./day) for a series of chronically ill patients. None of the patients were in the immediate post-trauma state. Their clinical status ranged from undergoing bowel rest to critically ill, with some organ systems failure. In general, the more seriously ill the patient, the higher the PSR. The double circles indicate that the patient died within three weeks of the study. The PSR was determined by the single pulse ^{15}N glycine method and analysis of the mean ^{15}N enrichment of the urinary ammonia excreted over the next 10 hours.

assumption of the Rittenberg-San Pietro scheme (Ang et al., 1982). It would appear that there is no longer equilibration of nitrogen in the body, and the urinary ammonia becomes disproportionately derived from a colder pool, i.e., there is some segregation of amino acid pools within the body. Muscle is the most likely source for the cold amino acid nitrogen. Segregation is incompatible with the Rittenberg-San Pietro scheme because the model only allows for one amino acid pool in the body.

There is some evidence that supports a compartmentation hypothesis (James et al., 1976; Tarunga et al., 1979). James pointed out that ^{15}N glycine may overestimate the contribution of the liver, and animal experiments have shown that glycine nitrogen does become compartmentized under certain circumstances; for example, when there is a severe deficit in exogenous nitrogen with an excess of energy (Stein et al., 1976).

A plausible hypothesis for the correlation between morbidity, an "apparently high" PSR and the compartmentation of amino acid metabolism is as follows. The normal response to a metabolic stress is an increase in protein turnover (Stein et al., 1977). The metabolic stress in patients, such as those depicted in Figure 1, is from their disease. The stress is an additional metabolic load on the liver. Potential contributing factors are a diseased liver, increased peripheral demands from the wound, sepsis, or an excess or imbalance of nutrients, etc.

If the liver is damaged or liver function otherwise impaired, there will be metabolic burden above which the liver cannot cope. The liver no longer has the capacity to supply substrate, process all the waste products and interconvert metabolites which have been partially metabolized by one tissue and are necessary for normal periphery metabolism. The result is an imbalance between the demands of the periphery and the liver's metabolic capacity (Ansley et al., 1978).

This analysis and the observation of a good correlation between an apparently very high PSR and mortality suggests that the single pulse ^{15}N glycine method could be used to monitor a patient's clinical progress (Ang et al., 1982). Three examples are described briefly in the following paragraphs. The first patient had no evidence of liver failure, was adequately nourished, and underwent an uneventful elective procedure (coronary artery bypass graft). He had a normal response to elective surgery, with the protein turnover rate being low preoperatively, high postoperatively, and then, a week later just before discharge, the protein turnover rate dropped back to the preoperative value (Figure 2).

The second patient was unable to eat due to midesophageal carcinoma. He was studied four times (Figure 3). The first study was prior to the institution of parenteral nutrition, the second after three days of TPN at 1440 kcal/day, 15.84

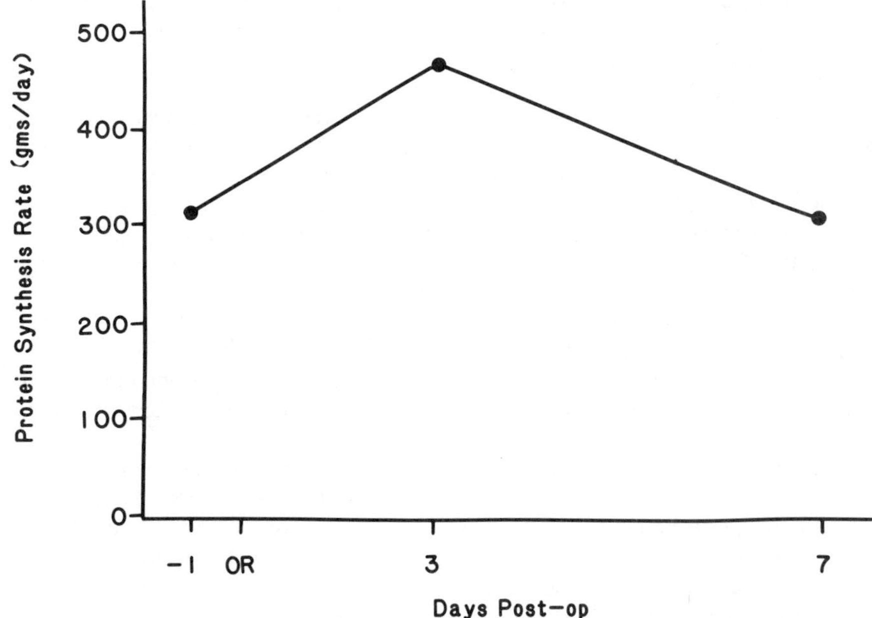

Figure 2 Changes in protein synthesis with trauma. Three studies were done, one prior to surgery, a second three days later, and a third on recovery, the day before discharge.

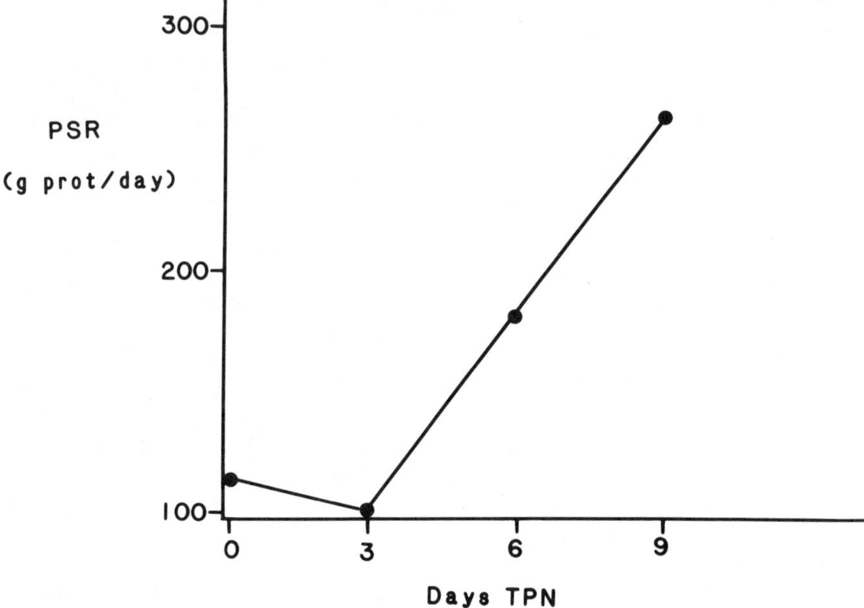

Figure 3 The effect of increasing TPN on the PSR. A data point was obtained preTPN, and then TPN given at 15.8 gN and 1440 kcal/day for three days, increased to 23.7 gN/day 2160 kcal/day for three days, and finally increased to 31.6 gN and 2880 kcal/day.

gN/day (60 ml/hr), the third study three days later at 90 ml/hr and the fourth study three days later at 120 ml/hr. For this patient who had a healthy liver the PSR increased as intake increased.

The third patient, a 58-year-old female with a huge ovarian tumor (> 15 kg), had a low PSR and no evidence of liver disease. The association between a low PSR and a large tumor suggests that for this patient, at least, the tumor burden did not lead to an elevated PSR. Following surgery, the PSR was elevated, she became septic and developed respiratory insufficiency requiring prolonged ventilatory support, but eventually recovered and the PSR returned to the preoperative value. Her liver function tests, SGOT and SGPT, paralleled the changes in the PSR. Removal of the tumor had little, if any, effect on the whole-body PSR (Figure 4).

The question of whether there is a relationship between tumor size or burden and the whole-body PSR is unclear at present. Recently, Carmichael et al. (1980) suggested that there was such a correlation. Sixteen of the 43 patients depicted in Figure 1 had malignancies, six had PSRs > 7 (mean 11.7 ± 2.1 SEM), five of whom had elevated function tests (SGOT > 45 IU).

We recently published a set of PSR values for malnourished patients with gastrointestinal malignancies and reported markedly elevated PSRs (Stein et al., 1981). Retrospective examination of the patients' charts showed that five out of seven patients whose charts could be located had elevated liver function tests (mean PSR = 14.4 ± 1.6, SGOT > 45 IU). The PSR was determined by a constant-infusion-cumulative excretion method, using ^{15}N glycine as a tracer. A very similar method was recently described by Fern et al. (1981) and shown to give results in agreement with other methods for healthy controls. In the method used, good plateaus in the

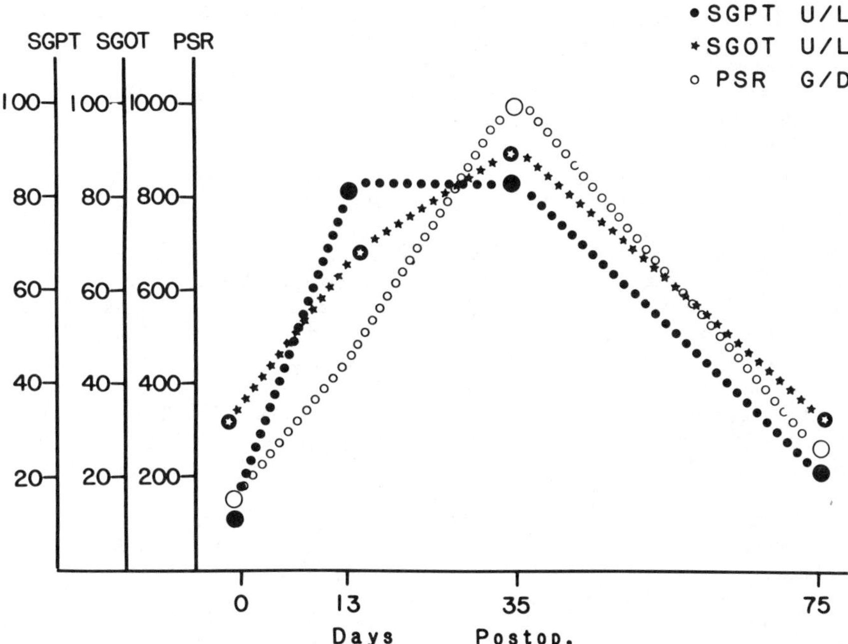

Figure 4 Changes in the PSR, serum glutamate-oxaloacetate transferase (SGOT) and serum pyruvate transaminase (SGPT) in a patient undergoing surgical removal of an ovarian tumor, who had a difficult postoperative period, but eventually made a full recovery.

urinary ammonia were obtained, and the synthesis rate was determined from the total amount of ^{15}N excreted into urea and ammonia rather than from the urinary ammonia enrichment done. Finding anomalously high results with both a urea-plus-ammonia and an ammonia-based method indicates that the findings with ^{15}N glycine are independent of the end product used for analysis.

It would seem that with ^{15}N glycine as a tracer, elevated PSRs in cancer-bearing patients are often associated with the simultaneous presence of liver insufficiency. Thus, what is measured in patients with very high PSRs is glycine metabolism rather than the true PSR. Whether this relationship also applies to other tracers, such as carbon-labeled leucine, is an unanswered question. The liver insufficiency could be aggravated by the metabolic demands of the tumor, but in this case the degree of PSR elevation will depend on both the demands of the tumor and the liver's functional capacity. Thus, an otherwise healthy liver will be able to accommodate a large tumor, whereas a small tumor may prove excessive for a diseased liver.

In summary, it would appear that although it is a relatively simple matter to measure the whole-body synthesis rate with ^{15}N glycine, interpretation of the results may be complex. Nevertheless, interesting information about a patient's metabolic status can be obtained.

REFERENCES

Ang, S.D., Stein, T.P., Leskiw, M.J., and Nusbaum, M. (1982): Protein synthesis as determined with [^{15}N] glycine and clinical outcome. *Fed. Proc.* 41:536.

Ansley, J.D., Isaacs, J.W., Rikkers, L.D., Kutter, M.H., Nordliger, B.M., and Rudman, D. (1978): Quantitative tests of nitrogen metabolism in cirrhosis relation to other manifestations of liver disease. *Gastroenterology* 75:570–579.

Carmichael, M.J., Clague, M.B., Keir, M.J., and Johnston, I.D.A. (1980): Whole body protein turnover, synthesis and breakdown in patients with colorectal carcinoma. *Br. J. Surg.* 67:736–739.

Fern, E.B., Garlick, P.J., McNurlan, M.A., and Waterlow, J.C. (1981): The excretion of isotope in urea and ammonia for estimating protein turnover in man with ^{15}N glycine. *Clin. Sci.* 6:217–228.

Garlick, P.J., Clugston, G.A., and Waterlow, J.C. (1980): Influence of low energy diets on whole body protein turnover in obese subjects. *Am. J. Physiol.* 238:E235–E244.

James, W.P.T., Sender, P.M., Garlick, P.J., and Waterlow, J.C. (1976): The choice of label and measurement technique in tracer studies of body protein metabolism in man. In *Dynamic Studies with Radioisotopes in Medicine,* pp. 461–472. Vienna International Atomic Energy Agency.

Stein, T.P., Oram-Smith, J.C., Leskiw, M.J., and Wallace, H.W. (1976): The effect of nitrogen and calorie restruction on protein synthesis in the rat. *Am. J. Physiol.* 20:1321–1325.

Stein, T.P., Leskiw, M.J., Oram-Smith, J.C. (1977): Changes in protein synthesis after trauma. Importance of nutrition. *Am. J. Physiol.* 233:1321–1325.

Stein, T.P., Buzby, G.P., Rosato, E.F., and Mullen, J.L. (1981): Effect of nutrition on protein synthesis in adult cancer patients. *Am. J. Clin. Nutr.* 34:1484–1488.

Tarunga, M., Jackson, A.A., and Golden, M.H.N. (1979): Comparison of ^{15}N labeled glycine, aspartate, valine and leucine for measurement of whole body protein turnover. *Clin. Sci.* 57:281–283.

Waterlow, J.C., Golden, M.H.N., and Garlick, P.J. (1978): Protein turnover in man measured with ^{15}N: comparison of end products and dose regimens. *Am. J. Physiol.* 255: E165–E174.

Nutritional and Metabolic Response to Intravenous Hyperalimentation in Severely Stressed Surgical Patients

Joel Faintuch, Jacob J. Faintuch, Marcel C.C. Machado, and Arrigo A. Raia

The nutritional effects of intravenous hyperalimentation (IVH) have been measured by a variety of techniques, including nitrogen balance (Lowry and Brennan, 1979; Peters and Fischer, 1980), indirect calorimetry (Long et al., 1979), exchangeable body potassium (Spanier and Shizgal, 1977), and simple body weight curve (Bozzetti, 1979).

In both nonstressed and severely stressed surgical patients, a correlation usually can be established between input of calories and a measurable response reflecting body anabolism (Lowry and Brennan, 1979; Peters and Fischer, 1980; Spanier and Shizgal, 1977). The intersection of the regression line thus obtained furnishes the minimal caloric requirements for those patients, a value of practical application in the planning of IVH needs for a given population.

We have prospectively evaluated the response to IVH in critically ill surgical patients by means of two simple parameters, namely body weight and serum albumin concentration. These results were compared with the clinical condition, the caloric load, and certain indices of metabolic abnormalities (SGOT, SGPT, alkaline phosphatase, total bilirubin, and amylase), in order to verify whether: 1) these nutritional measurements would correlate with the caloric intake; 2) they would anticipate the correct needs for this population, adjusted for their particular diagnoses and functional derangements; and 3) they would imply an association between excessive calorie administration and biochemical abnormalities.

METHODS

Only cases without edema or liver failure were admitted to this study. Careful daily water balance and weight measurements indicated no abnormal gains or losses.

Patients in shock or requiring transfusions of blood or plasma were excluded, and interpretation of serum albumin was not done if human albumin concentrate was prescribed during IVH.

Body weight was determined daily in early morning, and albumin was calculated by automated methods, together with SGOT, SGPT, amylase, alkaline phosphatase and total bilirubin. Estimations of the basal energy expenditure (BEE) were performed according to the formulas of Harris and Benedict, without correction for fever or other factors (Blackburn et al., 1977).

The presence of liver enzyme abnormalities, cancer and infection was not considered a contraindication for investigation in this study. Indeed, among the 40 patients studied, 70% were septic, 37.5% had cancer of the digestive tract, and 30% suffered from significant liver abnormalities (one test increased above twice the upper normal limit, or three tests increased to any degree) (Lowry and Brennan, 1979). Initial aberration of serum amylase was detected just once (2.5%).

All patients received a standard mixture of amino acids and hypertonic glucose providing 118 kcal per gram of nitrogen. Mean caloric intake in this series was 41 ± 14 kcal/kg/day, and duration of treatment was 44 ± 42 day (mean ± SEM).

RESULTS

Weight and albumin responses showed a modest correlation with caloric input, expressed either as a function of BEE or body weight (Figures 1 and 2), but they did not correlate between themselves ($r = 0.177$; $p > 0.05$). Regression analysis indicated that minimum requirement for weight equilibrium was 1.57 BEE (40 kcal/kg/day), and for albumin maintenance was 1.35 BEE (33 kcal/kg/day). The lower estimate for albumin stabilization is possibly due to the very high content of nitrogen in our mixture (6.4 g), in contrast with a comparatively modest energy load (748 kcal).

When these patients were divided according to the presence or absence of cancer, infection and liver dysfunction, all individuals with such limitations exhibited a weaker nutritional response with much higher minimum requirements (Figures 3, 4, and 5). This difference was obtained even within the group of cancer cases, when patients resected for cure were faced with tumor-bearing controls (Figure 3).

Alkaline phosphatase and amylase significantly increased by the end of the rehabilitation procedure (Figure 6). This modification was more marked in cases receiving caloric loads either higher or lower than 35 to 51 kcal/kg/day (Figure 7).

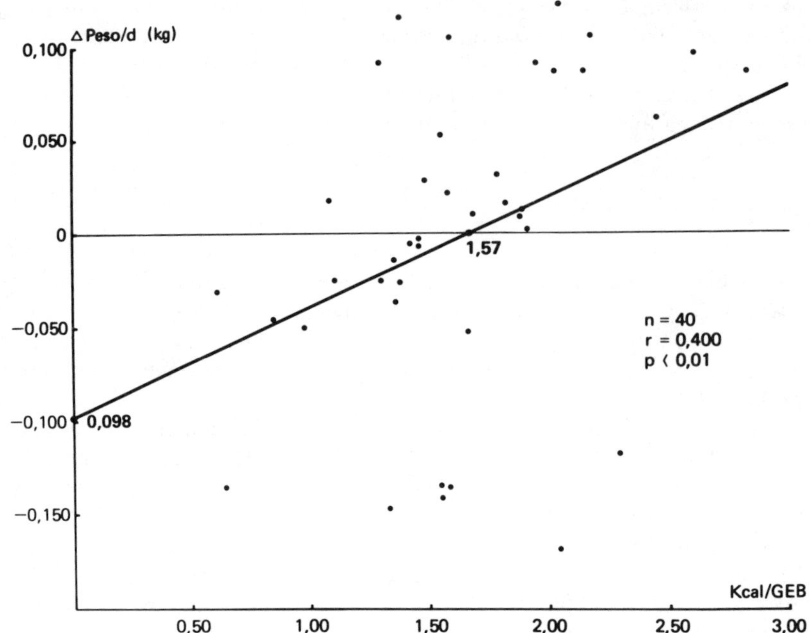

Figure 1 Correlation between weight gain and caloric intake (weight in kg/day, intake in kcal/BEE).

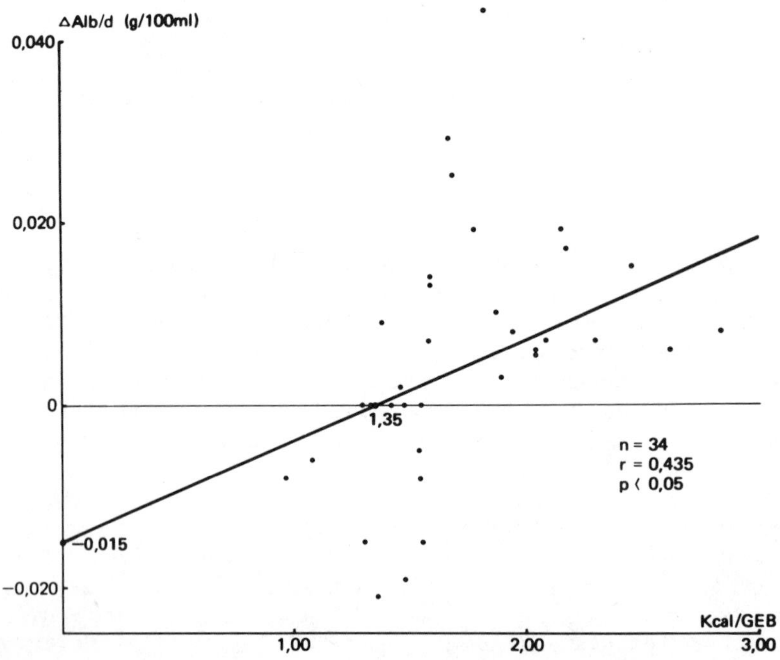

Figure 2 Correlation between albumin concentration increase and caloric intake (albumin in g/100 ml/day, intake in kcal/BEE).

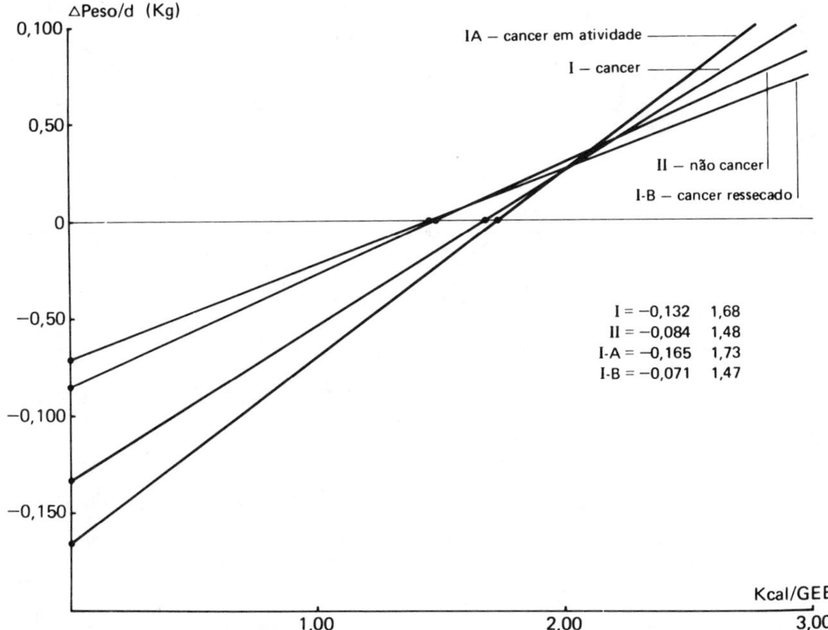

Figure 3 Correlation between weight increase and caloric input in patients with and without cancer. Group I: All cancer patients; Group II: Noncancer; Group I-A: Tumor-bearing cases; Group I-B: Tumor resected for cure.

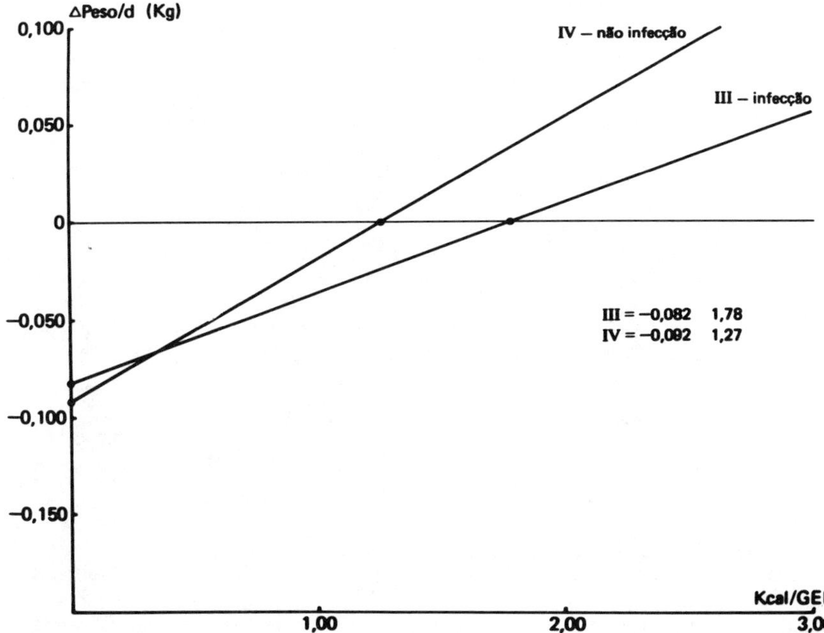

Figure 4 Correlation between weight gain and caloric input in patients with and without infection. Group III: Septic cases; Group IV: Nonseptic.

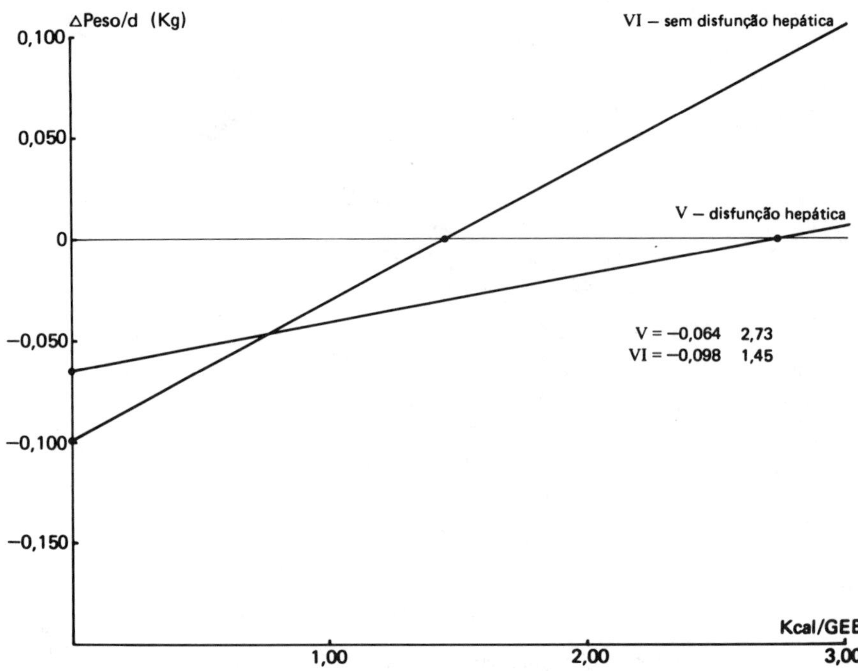

Figure 5 Correlation between weight gain and caloric intake in patients with and without liver dysfunction. Group V: Dysfunction present; Group VI: No significant dysfunction.

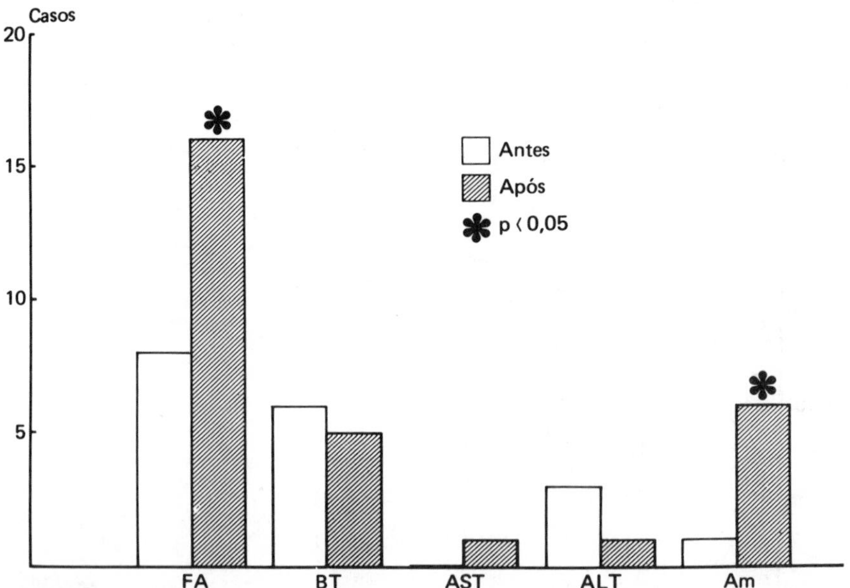

Figure 6 General profile of biochemical tests before and after IVH. Alkaline phosphatase (FA) and amylase (Am) suffered an increase during this therapy, but not SGOT (AST), SGPT (ALT) or total bilirubin (BT).

An analysis of weight and albumin regression lines in those circumstances revealed that prescriptions between 35 and 51 kcal/kg/day were accompanied by the best anabolic results (Figures 8 and 9).

DISCUSSION

The energy requirements of surgical and gastroenterological patients undergoing IVH seem to vary widely. Zohrab et al. (1973) discovered that 32.5 kcal/kg/day could be enough, and Peters and Fischer (1980) achieved nitrogen equilibrium with even less (24 kcal/kg/day). On the other hand, Spanier and Shizgal (1977) recommended minimum intakes of 45 kcal/kg/day (approximately 1.5 BEE), for patients with sepsis and injuries, and Rutten et al. (1975) as well as Bozzetti (1979) advocated even more, up to 1.76 to 2.00 BEE in those conditions.

Our results align better with those of Lowry and Brennan (1979), where 1.39 BEE was the mean input that produced nutritional stabilization of the patients. Furthermore, we also noticed that much higher prescriptions are not advised, since this exposes the patient to a greater risk of liver functional damage. In our experience those individuals given less than 35 kcal/kg/day also exhibited a higher incidence of metabolic abnormalities with poorer nutritional performance, but these were the sickest cases in the whole series, which did not tolerate ordinary amounts of fluid or glucose.

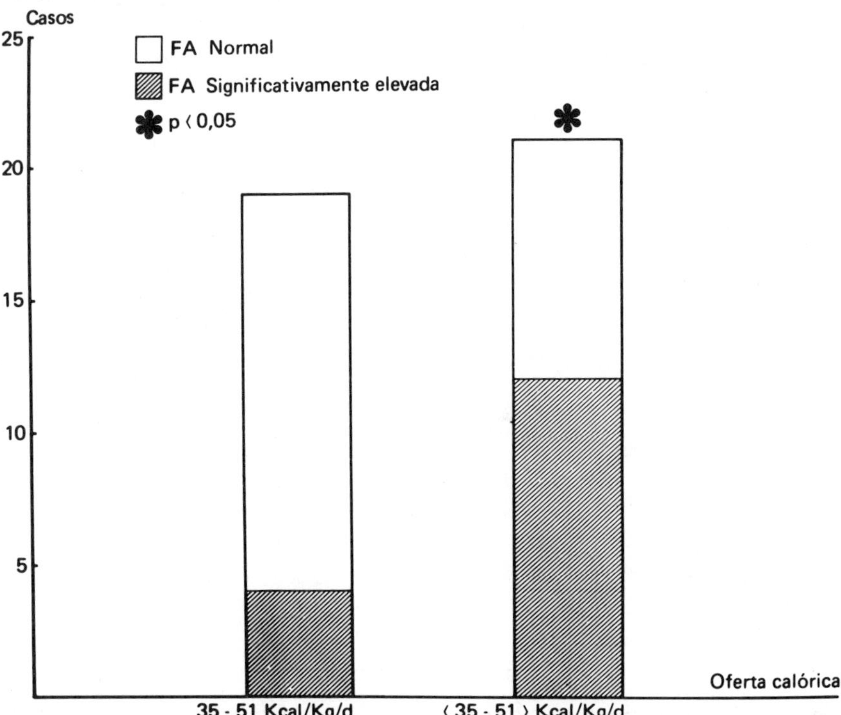

Figure 7 Final values of alkaline phosphatase in patients receiving prescriptions within 35 to 51 kcal/kg/day and out of this range. Only in the second situation was a significant increase demonstrated.

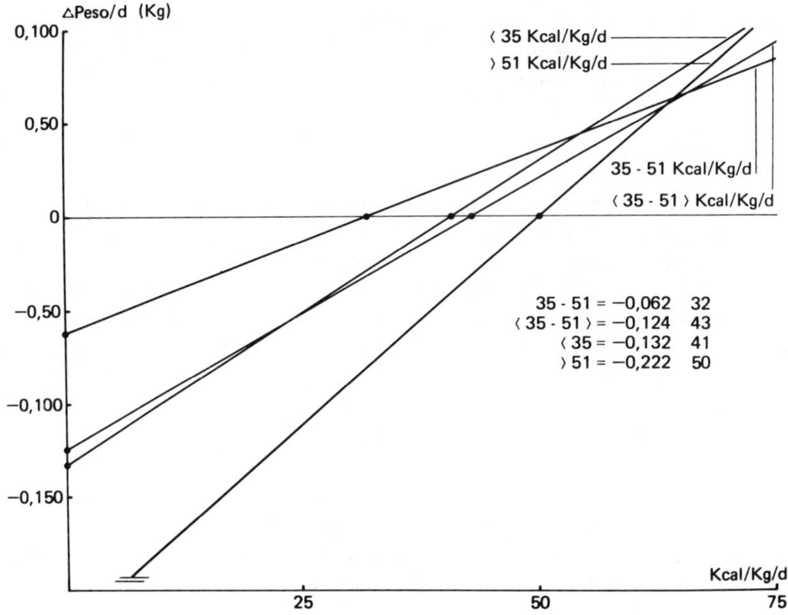

Figure 8 Weight gain in patients receiving various amounts of calories. The best results were with administration of 35 to 51 kcal/kg/day.

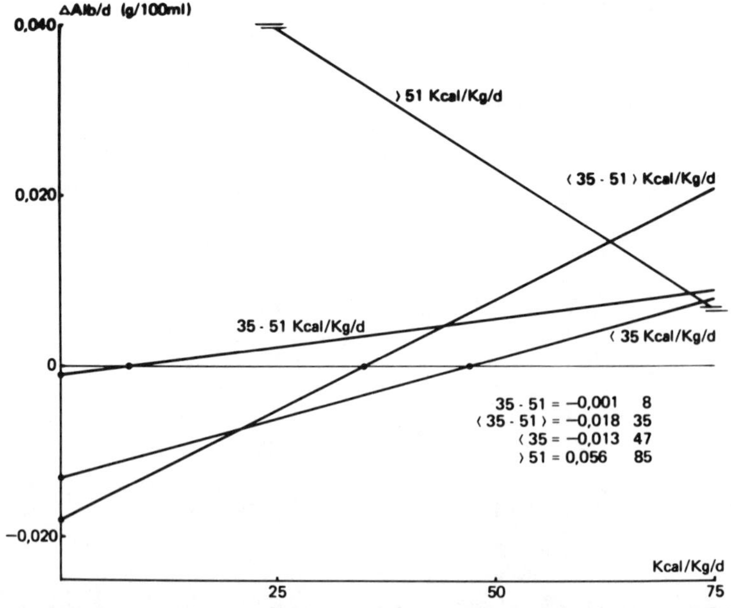

Figure 9 Albumin increase in patients receiving various caloric intakes. Again, the best results corresponded to the population given 35 to 51 kcal/kg/day. Correlation was negative for those receiving more than 51 kcal/kg/day, although statistical confirmation was not obtained ($r = -0.449$; $p > 0.05$).

As anticipated by Iapichino et al. (1981), Peters and Fischer (1980), Rutten et al. (1975) and several others, we found that energy requirements decrease and nutritional response is more encouraging in the absence of sepsis, cancer and liver dysfunction.

The finding that high caloric intakes in the form of carbohydrates are associated with potential danger has been further explored by Wolfe et al. (1980). In their experience with postoperative patients, not more than 35 kcal/kg/day of glucose were fully oxidized by the liver, the balance being converted into triglycerides. This lipogenesis can predispose, in addition to biochemical derangements, to fatty metamorphosis and to hypercapnia, but these last complications were not specifically sought in this study.

CONCLUSIONS

In the conditions of this investigation, it is concluded that: 1) weight and albumin concentration correlate with caloric intake during IVH of severely stressed patients; 2) minimum caloric needs were similar to those found in other studies, but increased markedly in the presence of cancer, infection or liver dysfunction; 3) alkaline phosphatase and amylase increased at the end of IVH. The former changed significantly less in cases receiving 35 to 51 kcal/kg/day than in all other patients; and 4) response of body weight and serum albumin was best when the selected prescription range was 35 to 51 kcal/kg/day.

REFERENCES

Blackburn, G.L., Bistrian, B.R., Maini, B.S., Schlamm, H.J., and Smith, M.F. (1977): Nutritional and metabolic assessment of the hospitalized patient. *J. Parent. Ent. Nutr.* 1:11–22.

Bozzetti, F. (1979): Determination of the caloric requirement of patients with cancer. *Surg. Gynecol. Obstet.* 149:667–670.

Iapichino, G., Solca, M., Radrizzani, D., Zucchetti, M., and Damia, G. (1981): Net protein utilization during total parenteral nutrition of injured critically ill patients: An original approach. *J. Parent. Ent. Nutr.* 5:317–321.

Long, C.L., Schaffel, N., Geiger, J.W., Schiller, W.R., and Blakemore, W.S. (1979): Metabolic response to injury and illness: Estimation of energy and protein needs from indirect calorimetry and nitrogen balance. *J. Parent. Ent. Nutr.* 3:452–456.

Lowry, S.F., and Brennan, M.F. (1979): Abnormal liver function during parenteral nutrition. Relation to infusion excess. *J. Surg. Res.* 26:300–307.

Peters, C., and Fischer, J.E. (1980): Studies on calorie to nitrogen ratio for total parenteral nutrition. *Surg. Gynecol. Obstet.* 151:1–8.

Rutten, P., Blackburn, G.L., Flatt, J.P., Hallowell, E., and Cochran, D. (1975): Determination of optimal hyperalimentation infusion rate. *J. Surg. Res.* 18:477–483.

Spanier, A.H., and Shizgal, H.M. (1977): Caloric requirements of the critically ill patient receiving intravenous hyperalimentation. *Am. J. Surg.* 133:99–104.

Wolfe, R.R., O'Donnell, T.F., Stone, M.D., Richmond, D.A., and Burke, J.F. (1980): Investigation of factors determining the optimal glucose infusion rate in total parenteral nutrition. *Metabolism* 29:892–900.

Effect of Diet and Pneumococcal Infection on Protein Dynamics of Blood Lymphocytes in Cynomolgus Monkeys

Robert W. Wannemacher, Jr., George A. McNamee, Jr., Richard E. Dinterman, and David L. Bunner

In a recent workshop, it was stressed that there is a need for nutrient support in patients with life-threatening infections and who had lost 10% of their body weight (Wilmore and Kinney, 1981). These authors also stressed importance of development of support therapy that would optimally stimulate host defense against infectious disease. It was recommended that research on nutritional support during infection be performed in both animals and man. An important factor in developing a rational approach to nutritional supportive therapy in infected individuals is knowledge of effects of various nutrients on protein dynamics in various cells and tissues of the body. It has been previously demonstrated that adequate calories and amino acids will prevent protein wasting during sepsis in the monkey (Wannemacher et al., 1978). This conclusion is based on nitrogen balance data, which represent the algebraic sum of the protein dynamics in various tissue compartments. Nutrient support therapy can improve the immune response in a protein-calorie depleted patient. There is, however, very little data on the comparative effects of amino acid and dextrose calories on stimulating immune response or protein dynamics of leucocytes in either infected or noninfected monkeys.

EXPERIMENTAL PROCEDURE

Thirty-six male cynomolgus monkeys were divided into three groups of 12 each. All monkeys had catheters implanted in the jugular and femoral veins and were maintained in metabolic cages via a jacketed-tethering system. On day three after surgery the monkeys were infused via the jugular vein with either 8% dextrose (34 kcal/kg), 4.25% amino acids (16 kcal/kg), or dextrose plus amino acid (50 kcal/kg/day). In addition, each solution contained similar amounts of vitamins, electrolytes and trace elements. One day after starting the nutrient support solutions, six monkeys in each group received an intravenous dose of 2×10^8 live *S. pneumoniae* or 2×10^8 heat-killed *S. pneumoniae*. The monkeys receiving the heat-killed organisms served as noninfected controls. Two days after receiving the microorganisms, ^{14}C leucine was infused over a six-hour time period. Six hours after ^{14}C infusion, the specific activity of the leucine in the protein-free filtrate of plasma had reached a plateau indicative of a constant precursor pool. At this six-hour time period a blood sample was removed and specific activity of leucine was measured in samples of mixed leukocyte proteins. Lymphocytes were separated by sedimentation of the red cells in dextran, followed by centrifugation in lymphocyte separating media. Specific activity was measured in the mixed proteins of this cellular pool. A second sample of blood removed after six hours was utilized to measure mitogen stimulation of lymphocyte blastogenesis by concanavalin A (Con A), phytohemagglutin (PHA), or pokeweed mitogen (PWM).

Table 1
Effect of Intravenous Amino Acids and/or Glucose on Total Body Protein Dynamics, Mitogen Stimulation of Lymphocyte Blastogenesis, and Mixed Lymphocyte Protein Dynamics

Treatment	Leucine Turnover (μmols/kg•hr^{-1})	Stimulation Index*			Fractional Synthetic Rate of Lymphocyte Protein (%/day)
		Con A	*PHA*	*PWM*	
			4.25% Amino acids[†]		
Control	438 ± 37[‡]	10.69 ± 1.19	40.52 ± 7.16	24.43 ± 2.51	33.1 ± 5.1
Infected	614 ± 96[§]	4.29 ± 1.13[‡]	5.09 ± 2.05[‡]	4.80 ± 1.17[§]	42.1 ± 8.4
			8% Dextrose		
Control	62 ± 11	5.38 ± 1.30	15.16 ± 2.23	12.66 ± 3.37	2.76 ± 1.17
Infected	90 ± 9	2.05 ± 0.52	3.49 ± 1.05[‡]	2.9 ± 0.85[§]	2.08 ± 0.74
			4.25% Amino acid + 8% dextrose		
Control	348 ± 14	5.06 ± 0.92	15.39 ± 1.81	30.74 ± 8.70	19.2 ± 4.1
Infected	406 ± 18	1.95 ± 0.30	5.62 ± 1.01	4.28 ± 0.98	16.5 ± 3.9

*Stimulation index = $\frac{\text{DPM in mitogen stimulated lymphocytes}}{\text{DPM in nonstimulated lymphocytes}}$

[†] Leucine intake 243 μmols/kg•hr^{-1}
[‡] Mean ± SE of six monkeys.
[§] $P < 0.01$ compared to control.

RESULTS

Infusion of 8% dextrose solution significantly reduced leucine turnover and release from breakdown of total body protein as compared to infusion of 4.25% amino acids (Table 1). Amino acid plus dextrose infusion tended to be intermediate between the other two groups. In all three groups, presence of infection increased the rate of leucine turnover and breakdown of total body protein. Nitrogen balance was poorest in the dextrose group and best in the amino acid plus dextrose group. Infectious disease decreased nitrogen imbalance in all three groups; however, the dextrose plus amino acid group was still in positive balance.

No differences were observed between dextrose or amino acid infusion on blood lymphocyte concentrations, but pneumococcal sepsis did result in a decrease in blood lymphocyte counts. The stimulation index for lymphocytes by all three mitogens was significantly greater in monkeys receiving intravenous amino acids compared to those infused with dextrose (Table 1). In all three groups pneumococcal sepsis markedly reduced the stimulation produced by the various mitogens.

The protein content of lymphocytes from control monkeys infused with amino acids was significantly greater than those infused with dextrose or dextrose plus amino acids. Infection tended to reduce total lymphocyte protein content in all three groups. The fractional rate of synthesis of mixed lymphocyte proteins was significantly lower in monkeys infused with dextrose as compared to amino acids (Table 1). The amino acid plus dextrose group tended to fall intermediate between the two other groups.

CONCLUSIONS

Intravenous infusion of amino acids and/or dextrose has marked effects on breakdown of total body protein and synthesis of mixed lymphocyte proteins. While dextrose infusion tended to conserve body protein by decreasing the rate of turnover of total body protein, it markedly inhibited the immune response and fractional rate of synthesis of mixed lymphocyte proteins. Infusion of amino acids resulted in a greater turnover of body protein but resulted in a marked increase in lymphocyte blastogenesis and mixed protein synthesis as compared to dextrose infusions. The amino acid plus dextrose infusions tended to fall intermediate between the other two nutrient support therapies. Infectious disease increased leucine release and protein breakdown in all three nutrient support therapies. Only the addition of amino acids plus dextrose prevented severe wasting of body protein. Pneumococcal sepsis tended to reduce mitogen stimulation in lymphocytes but had no effect on its fractional rate of protein synthesis. These observations raise the question as to whether measurements of only protein loss can be used as a criteria for assessing the value of nutrient support therapy in stimulating host defense against infectious disease.

REFERENCES

Wannemacher, R.W., Jr., Kaminski, M.V., Jr., Neufeld, H.A., Dinterman, R.E., Bostian, K.A., and Hadick, C.L. (1978): Protein sparing therapy during pneumococcal infection in rhesus monkeys. *J.E.P.N.* pp. 507–518.

Wilmore, D.W., and Kinney, J.M. (1981): Panel report on nutritional support of patients with trauma or infection. *J. Am. Clin. Nutr.* 34:1213–1222.

Intravenous Alanine Tolerance in Conscious Septic and Nonseptic Rats

John J. Spitzer, Gregory J. Bagby, Owen P. McGuinness, and Charles H. Lang

Alanine, the predominant gluconeogenic amino acid released by the skeletal muscle, is an important contributor to hepatic gluconeogenesis. Following endotoxin administration (Kuttner and Spitzer, 1978) or in sepsis (Clowes et al., 1980), alanine assumes an even greater importance in supporting the needs of the organism for gluconeogenesis. Plasma alanine concentrations alone are not necessarily indicative of the rate of alanine turnover, as changes in turnover are not always accompanied by similar alterations in arterial alanine concentration. In septic patients plasma alanine concentration has been found to be elevated (O'Donnell et al., 1976), decreased (Royle et al., 1978, and Clowes et al., 1980), or unchanged (Swaminathan et al., 1981). In spite of the decreased (Royle et al., 1978) or unchanged (Swaminathan et al., 1981) alanine concentration, the half-time of administered alanine was not significantly altered. The aim of this study was to compare the kinetics of alanine removal (half-time, clearance rate and volume of distribution) in septic and sham-operated rats in order to determine the ability of septic animals to handle an exogenous load of alanine in the course of the septic episode. Additionally, the effects of an alanine load on plasma lactate and glucose concentrations were also compared in septic versus nonseptic rats.

Male Sprague-Dawley rats (350 to 400 g) were anesthetized with ether, and under sterile operating conditions an arterial catheter (PE-50) was chronically implanted in the arch of the aorta. Following catheterization sepsis was induced by intraperitoneal administration of 0.5 ml of a pooled fecal inoculum; controls received equal volumes of sterilized inoculum. All animals were allowed food and water ad libitum and were monitored for five consecutive days following infection. The pooled fecal inoculum, which was used to insure a uniform inoculation of bacteria to all rats, was progressively lethal with 3%, 24%, 53%, 67%, and 76% of the animals dying at one, two, three, four, and five days postinfection. Quantitative bacteriology of the peritoneal fluid and blood from septic animals indicated an infection that was polymicrobial with gram-negative bacteria predominating. Control animals had negative blood and peritoneal fluid cultures. During the five-day observation period, septic animals were normotensive, tachycardic and exhibited a febrile response on days two through four. L-alanine, 2.8 mmols per kg in 2 ml of sterile distilled water, was infused at time 0 for 2 minutes into the arterial catheter. Serial blood samples (0.2 ml) were obtained 10 minutes prior to and 5, 10, 15, 20, 30, 40, 50, and 60 minutes after alanine injection. Alanine, lactate and glucose were determined enzymatically on each sample (Lowry and Passoneau, 1972).

The alanine concentration in control animals gradually increased over the five-day period, while levels in the septic animals declined slightly. By days four and five, septic rats had alanine concentrations that were more than 40% below control (Table 1). In sham-operated controls, plasma lactate concentrations were stable, averaging 0.9 mM over the five-day observation period. Throughout most of this period, plasma lactate was approximately doubled in the septic rats. Control animals

Table 1
Arterial Substrate Concentrations in Septic and Nonseptic Rats

	Time, Postinoculation (Days)				
	1	*2*	*3*	*4*	*5*
Alanine (μM)					
Control	275 ± 18* (8)	273 ± 19 (8)	334 ± 28 (8)	378 ± 29 (7)	394 ± 56 (4)
Septic	257 ± 19 (7)	251 ± 16 (8)	302 ± 31 (7)	216 ± 24† (7)	229 ± 21† (3)
Lactate (mM)					
Control	0.96 ± 0.13 (8)	0.95 ± 0.15 (8)	0.99 ± 0.12 (8)	0.93 ± 0.09 (7)	0.90 ± 0.13 (4)
Septic	1.35 ± 0.09† (7)	1.04 ± 0.11 (8)	1.82 ± 0.12† (7)	1.87 ± 0.28† (7)	1.65 ± 0.32 (3)
Glucose (mM)					
Control	6.65 ± 0.27 (8)	7.36 ± 0.12 (8)	6.91 ± 0.25 (8)	6.58 ± 0.24 (7)	7.10 ± 0.17 (4)
Septic	8.40 ± 0.66† (7)	6.23 ± 0.22† (8)	5.84 ± 0.17† (7)	5.89 ± 0.21 (7)	4.99 ± 0.41† (3)

*Results expressed as mean ± standard error (n).
†Values significantly different ($p < 0.05$) from control values.

maintained their blood glucose concentration, while septic animals showed a mild increase on day one and a subsequent decrease on days two through five.

The half-time ($T_{1/2}$, min) was calculated from the semilogarithmic regression line of the excess alanine concentration versus time, where the difference between the alanine concentration at any time and the preinjection alanine value represents the excess alanine concentration. The volume of alanine distribution (Vd, $ml \cdot kg^{-1}$) was estimated by dividing the quantity of alanine infused by the extrapolated alanine concentration at time zero. The alanine clearance rate ($ml \cdot min^{-1} \cdot kg^{-1}$) was taken to be the product of Vd and the fractional disappearance rate, k, where k equals $\ln 2/T_{1/2}$.

The half-time of the injected alanine load in sham-operated rats was approximately 18 minutes, which was similar to that observed in man (Swaminathan et al., 1981). However, the $T_{1/2}$ of injected alanine was prolonged (about 50%) on days two through five in septic rats as compared to sham-operated controls. The alanine clearance rate in the septic animals was about 20% slower on days two and three than in nonseptic rats. Alanine distribution volume tended to be greater in the septic animals.

Both groups of animals showed a transient hyperlactacidemia which peaked 15 minutes postalanine injection and then gradually returned toward normal by 60 minutes. However, the lactate peak was more pronounced in septic than in sham-operated animals (Table 2), which is consistent with the decreased ability of septic rats to handle the alanine load. Blood glucose in the septic rats fell rapidly (10 to 15 min) following the alanine injection, but thereafter continually increased resulting in mild hyperglycemia by 60 minutes. There was no hypoglycemia and only a minimal elevation of glucose concentration (less than 5%) following the alanine load in nonseptic animals. The initial drop in blood glucose concentrations in septic rats is consistent with the increased release of insulin seen after physiologic stimulation following the administration of endotoxin (Blackard et al., 1976, and Yelich and Filkins, 1980). Alternatively, the hypoglycemia may be the result of increased glucose utilization by peripheral tissues in the septic animals. This phenomenon would be similar to that found by Romanosky et al. (1980) and Raymond et al. (1981) following endotoxin administration. On the other hand, several investigators have observed insulin resistance in the septic state (O'Donnell et al., 1974, Ryan et al., 1974, and Wichterman et al., 1979).

No significant changes in alanine, lactate, or glucose were seen in septic and nonseptic animals that received saline injections in place of alanine. Therefore, changes in these blood substrates following alanine injection appear to be a direct consequence of the alanine and are not due to the stress of repeated blood sampling.

These investigations indicate that septic rats have an impaired ability to handle an injected alanine load. This depressed ability may be related to altered gluconeogenesis, or to competition with other gluconeogenic precursors which share a common pathway.

ACKNOWLEDGMENTS

These studies were supported by NIH Grants GM07029 and HL07098.

Table 2
Arterial Substrate Changes During Alanine Tolerance Test in Septic and Nonseptic Rats

	Time, Postinoculation (Days)				
	1	*2*	*3*	*4*	*5*
*Lactate Peak**					
Control	1.00 ± 0.24‡ (8)	0.92 ± 0.23 (8)	0.80 ± 0.16 (8)	0.29 ± 0.21 (7)	0.00 ± 0.11 (4)
Septic	1.35 ± 0.22 (7)	1.36 ± 0.20 (8)	1.19 ± 0.30 (7)	1.27 ± 0.27‖ (7)	1.26 ± 0.24‖ (3)
*Glucose Drop**					
Control	+ 0.03 ± 0.18§ (8)	− 0.30 ± 0.17 (8)	+ 0.28 ± 0.18 (8)	+ 0.25 ± 0.18 (7)	+ 0.50 ± 0.15 (4)
Septic	− 0.92 ± 0.38‖ (7)	− 0.06 ± 0.15 (8)	− 0.83 ± 0.18‖ (7)	− 0.90 ± 0.20‖ (7)	− 1.03 ± 0.37‖ (3)
Glucose Rise†					
Control	0.60 ± 0.19 (8)	− 0.18 ± 0.19 (8)	− 0.09 ± 0.23 (8)	− 0.02 ± 0.11 (7)	− 0.25 ± 0.14 (4)
Septic	1.52 ± 0.64 (7)	0.66 ± 0.24‖ (8)	0.63 ± 0.16 (7)	0.29 ± 0.12 (7)	0.68 ± 0.54 (3)

*mM change in concentration from baseline at 15 minutes after alanine injection.
†mM change in concentration from baseline at 60 minutes after alanine injection.
‡Results expressed as mean ± standard error (n).
§Positive numbers indicate an increase from baseline; negative numbers indicate decrease from baseline.
‖Values significantly different ($p < 0.05$) from control values.

REFERENCES

Blackard, W.G., Anderson, J.H., and Spitzer, J.J. (1976): Hyperinsulinism in endotoxin shock dogs. *Metabolism* 25:675–684.

Clowes, G.H., Randall, H.T., and Cha, C.J. (1980): Amino acid and energy metabolism in septic and traumatized patients. *J. Parent. Enter. Nut.* 4:195–205.

Kuttner, R.E. and Spitzer, J.J. (1978): Gluconeogenesis from alanine in endotoxin-treated dogs. *J. Surg. Res.* 25:166–173.

Lowry, O.H., and Passoneau, J.V. (1972): *A Flexible System of Enzymatic Analysis.* Academic Press, New York.

O'Donnell, T.F., Clowes, G.H., Blackburn, G.L., and Ryan, N.T. (1974): Relationship of hind limb energy fuel metabolism to the circulatory responses in severe sepsis. *J. Surg. Res.* 16:112–123.

O'Donnell, T.F., Clowes, G.H., Blackburn, G.L., Ryan, N.T., Benotti, P.N., and Miller, J.D. (1976): Proteolysis associated with a deficit of peripheral energy fuel substrates in septic man. *Surgery* 80:192–200.

Raymond, R.M., Harkema, J.M., and Emerson, T.E. (1981): Direct effects of gram-negative endotoxin on skeletal muscle glucose uptake. *Am. J. Physiol.* 240:H342–347.

Romanosky, A.J., Bagby, G.J., Bockman, E.L., and Spitzer, J.J. (1980): Increased muscle glucose uptake and lactate release after endotoxin administration. *Am. J. Physiol.* 239: E311–E316.

Royal, G., Kettlewell, M., Ilic, V., and Williamson, D. (1978): The metabolic effects of alanine infusion in prolonged sepsis. *Br. J. Surg.* 65:363.

Ryan, N.T., Blackburn, G.L., and Clowes, G.H. (1974): Differential tissue sensitivity to elevated endogenous insulin levels during experimental peritonitis in rats. *Metabolism* 23: 1081–1089.

Swaminathan, R., Morgan, D.B., Hill, G.L., and Bradley, J.A. (1981): Blood concentration and disappearance of injected alanine and β-hydroxybutyrate in surgical patients. *Horm. Metab. Res.* 13:383–386.

Wichterman, K.A., Chaudry, I.H., and Baue, A. (1979): Studies of peripheral glucose uptake during sepsis. *Arch. Surg.* 114:740–745.

Yelich, M.R., and Filkins, J.P. (1980): Mechanism of hyperinsulinemia in endotoxicosis. *Am. J. Physiol.* 239:E156–E161.

Branched-Chain Amino Acid Solutions Enhance Nitrogen Accretion in Postoperative Cancer Patients

Michael M. Meguid, Aurora Landel, Chun-Chih Lo, Chun-Rong Chang, Daniel Debonis, and L. Robert Hill

Exogenous leucine has been shown to a) promote protein synthesis by enhancing leucine uptake, b) be oxidized by muscle for energy, and c) stimulate insulin secretion which inhibits amino acid efflux from muscle (Manchester, 1965; Goldberg and Chang, 1978; Buse and Reid, 1975). During acute stress, the branched-chain amino acids (BCAA) in general, but leucine in particular, appear to be preferentially oxidized by skeletal muscle and used for gluconeogenesis (Ryan et al., 1974; Freund et al., 1978). Low molar insulin-glucagon ratios (Meguid et al., 1974) result in muscle breakdown which is reflected by a negative nitrogen balance. These findings may explain our observations, reported in this study, of low plasma branched-chain amino acid levels in our depleted cancer patients who are in a catabolic state after surgery.

Whether an improvement in the distorted amino acid profile with a concomitant enhancement of nitrogen accretion as shown by positive nitrogen balance could be obtained, was investigated in a prospective trial comparing standard TPN solution to one enriched with branched-chain amino acids.

METHOD AND MATERIALS

Forty undernourished cancer patients, predominantly with malignancies of the gastrointestinal tract, undergoing major surgery were studied. The type of patients, the degree of malnutrition, and their diagnosis is detailed in Table 1.

After surgery, these patients were randomized to receive isocaloric isonitrogenous amounts of either standard TPN in the form of 25% dextrose/4.25% crystalline amino acid containing a ratio of BCAA:nonBCAA of 25:75, or a crystalline amino acid solution enriched with BCAA in the form of 25% dextrose/10% fat/3.5% amino acid containing a BCAA:nonBCAA ratio of 45:55.

Serial plasma samples were analyzed for amino acids (Beckman 121MB) in fasting conditions on postoperative day one (preinfusion) and compared to plasma amino acid profile of 10 normal fasting volunteers, aged 23 to 68 years (mean 43.2).

Thereafter, the patients in both groups received a mean nutrient intake of 34 ± 14 kcal and 0.18 ± 0.03 g $N \cdot kg^{-1} \cdot d^{-1}$ (M ± S.E.). The daily and weekly TPN additives in the form of vitamins, minerals, and trace elements were given to each patient according to the Medical Center TPN protocol. Serial plasma amino acid profiles were obtained on days seven and 14 while on TPN. Twenty-four-hour urine was collected continuously during the 14-day period for total nitrogen measurement (Technicon Analyzer) and true nitrogen balance calculated.

The baseline total amino acid levels and the levels of the different amino acid groups were compared to those of the fasting volunteers. The amino acid profile changes for the two groups were sequentially compared using a multiple comparison procedure based on the two-sample t-test. The calculated true nitrogen balance data for each patient group was compared in a similar manner. The data expressed in the text represents the mean ± S.E.

RESULTS

Low total amino acid levels as well as essential, nonessential, glycogenic and branched-chain amino acid levels were observed in postoperative cancer patients in both groups on day one compared to normals ($p < 0.01$) (Figures 1 and 2). A significant increase ($p < 0.001$) in these values was observed by the first week in both groups. The relatively higher glycogenic values for the standard TPN group compared to the BCAA/TPN group may be due to the higher day one values for the former. The amino acid levels decreased significantly in the standard TPN group ($p < 0.01$), but remained elevated in the BCAA/TPN group by the second week.

A net negative nitrogen balance occurred in most patients in both groups on day one, while positive nitrogen balance was seen by the first week in both groups with a sustained improvement ($p < 0.01$) occurring during the second week in only the BCAA/TPN group (Figure 3).

Table 1
Demographic Data Pertaining to Population Studied

Solution Type	n	Sex	Age Range	Mean	Diagnosis	Nutrition Status
Standard TPN	20	10 M 10 F	24–79	59	17 Gastrointestinal CA 3 Genitourinary CA	– 13 undernourished
BCAA/TPN	20	10 M 10 F	22–78	56	17 Gastrointestinal CA 2 Genitourinary CA 1 Bronchogenic CA	– 14 undernourished

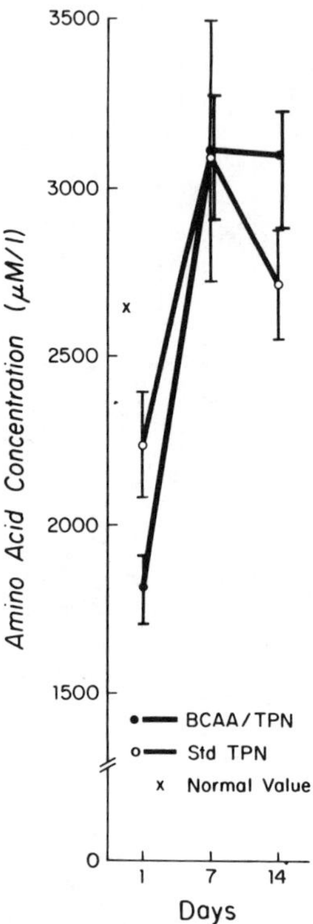

Figure 1 Total amino acid (AA) levels (± S.E.) in postoperative patients.

DISCUSSION

These data show low total amino acid concentration following elective surgery. This is secondary to low concentrations of essential, nonessential, glycogenic, branched-chain amino acid and other amino acid groups. The quantitative contribution to this low state by the depleted cancer patient, as compared to the stress of surgery, is currently being explored by us.

The sustained increase in the total, essential, nonessential, glycogenic and branched-chain amino acid levels in the 20 postoperative cancer patients who received the BCAA-enriched TPN solutions is reflected in the improved nitrogen accretion and the positive nitrogen balance. These data suggest that branched-chain amino acids spare body protein by reducing amino acid efflux from skeletal muscle (Freund et al., 1978) associated with increased protein synthesis and decreased protein breakdown (Hutson et al., 1978).

The metabolic dilemma of the postoperative cancer patient is twofold. First, the clinical course of a cancer-bearing patient is largely reflected by the cell type, stage, and extent of the tumor. Concomitant malnutrition can not only greatly enhance the risk of a serious complication and prejudice ultimate survival but also alter the bio-

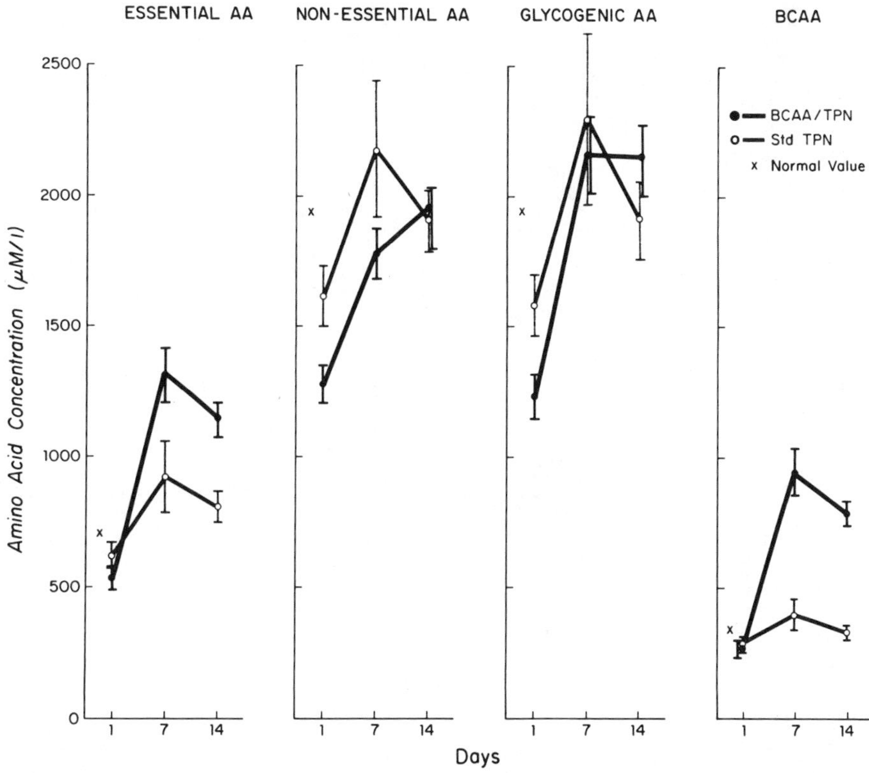

Figure 2 Essential, nonessential, glycogenic (ala, arg, asp, cys, glu, gly, his, met, ser, thr, trp, val, pro) and branched-chain (leu, ileu, val) AA levels (± S.E.) in postoperative patients on day one (preinfusion) and days seven and 14 after continuous infusion with standard TPN (○) and BCAA/TPN (●); total AA levels of normal volunteers (x).

chemical profile. Of our total hospitalized cancer patient population, approximately 25% are malnourished. Of those who underwent surgery, we found in this study that 65% were malnourished, suffering from protein energy malnutrition of the marasmic variety (Howard and Meguid, 1981; Meguid, 1981). This is the primary indication for TPN.

Although there have been relatively few studies of energy requirements of cancer patients, the data suggest that resting energy metabolism is increased in many patients with cancer (Young, 1977). Numerous studies have demonstrated a close relationship between body protein metabolism and energy metabolism in experimental animals and in man (Waterlow, 1968; Munro, 1969). Thus changes in energy expenditure in cancer patients would be expected to reflect parallel changes in body protein metabolism, accounting for the high frequency of marasmus seen in our cancer patients associated with the failure to meet increased requirements.

Secondly, following surgery or trauma, there is an increase in urinary nitrogen excretion that persists despite zero nitrogen intake. Skeletal muscle appears to be the principal source of small molecular weight nitrogen compounds that are metabolized in increased quantity to meet the increased energy need via gluconeogenesis after surgical stress. The concomitant increases in the excretion of creatine and creatinine,

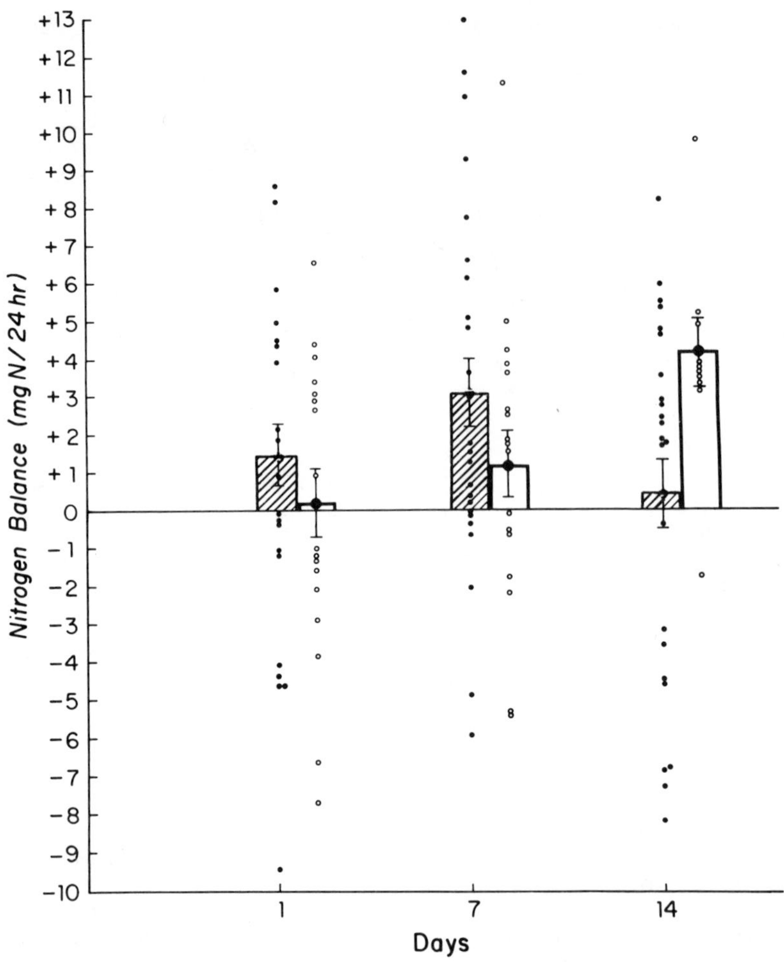

Figure 3 Nitrogen balance in postoperative patients on day one (preinfusion) and days seven and 14 after continuous infusion with Std TPN (▨) and BCAA/TPN (□).

as well as the bulk wasting of skeletal muscle, support such a view. The hormone milieu induced by the stress of surgery is one of increased catecholamine and glucagon secretion, and inhibition of insulin secretion (Meguid et al., 1974), increased urine insulin loss (Meguid et al., 1976), a shortened insulin half-life (Meguid et al., 1981) resulting in low insulin-to-glucagon molar ratio. This hormonal milieu is consistent with increased substrate mobilization and utilization leading to hyperglycemia, hypertriglyceridemia, increased amino acid efflux from muscle (Meguid and Moore, 1978), and the preferential oxidation of leucine by skeletal muscle (Ryan et al., 1974).

It is now apparent that this dual metabolic predicament can be redressed by the provision of adequate nutrients to patients during hospitalization, which has two main functions: 1) to stimulate insulin secretion and inhibit glucagon secretion altering the catabolic hormone milieu to one of anabolism, and 2) to provide calories, essential amino acids, nitrogen and micronutrients needed for increased body protein metabolism associated with anabolism.

This study suggests that the provision of adequate calories in the form of glucose and fat, together with a branched-chain amino acid-enriched crystalline amino acid solution, enhances nitrogen accretion in depleted cancer patients who undergo major stress in the form of abdominal surgery.

ACKNOWLEDGMENTS

We acknowledge the contributions of Susan Jeffers, R.N., M.S., Laura Dorr, R.D., Lee Ganteaume, Michael Akahoshi, Pharm. D., and Robert Hayashi, Pharm. D., who assisted in conducting this study, and Violet Kaufman for her editorial assistance.

REFERENCES

Buse, M.G., and Reid, S.S. (1975): Leucine: A possible regulator of protein turnover in muscle. *J. Clin. Invest.* 56:1250–1261.

Freund, H., Yoshimura, N., Lunetta, L., Fischer, J.B. (1978): The role of the branched-chain amino acids in decreasing muscle catabolism in vivo. *Surgery* 83:611–618.

Goldberg, A.L., and Chang, T.W. (1978): Regulation and significance of amino acid metabolism in skeletal muscle. *Fed. Proc.* 37:2301–2307.

Howard, L., and Meguid, M.M. (1981): Nutritional assessment in total parenteral nutrition. *Clin. Lab. Med.* 1:611–630.

Hutson, S.M., Cree, T.C., and Harper, A.E. (1978): Regulation of leucine and α-ketoisoceproate metabolism in skeletal muscle. *J. Biol. Chem.* 253:8126–8133.

Manchester, K.L. (1965): Oxidation of amino acids by isolated rat diaphragm and the influence of insulin. *Biochim. Biophys. Acta* 100:295–298.

Meguid, M.M. (1981): Protein: The essence of life. *City of Hope Quarterly* 10(3):305.

Meguid, M.M., Aun, F., and Soeldner, J.S. (1976): The effect of severe trauma on urine loss of insulin. *Surgery* 79:177–181.

Meguid, M.M., Aun, F., Soeldner, J.S., Albertson, D.A., and Boyden, C.M. (1981): Insulin half-life in man after trauma. *Surgery* 89:650–653.

Meguid, M.M., Brennan, M.F., Aoki, T.T., Muller, W.A., Ball, M.R., and Moore, F.D. (1974): Hormone-substrate interrelationships following trauma. *Arch. Surg.* 109:776–783.

Meguid, M.M., and Moore, F.D. (1978): Homeostasis and Nutrition in the Surgical Patient. In *Practice of Surgery,* Chapter 15, Harper and Row Co., Baltimore, MD.

Munro, H.N. (1969): Evolution of protein metabolism in mammals. In *Mammalian Protein Metabolism* (ed: H.N. Munro), Vol. 4, pp. 3–130. Academic Press, New York.

Ryan, N.T., George, B.C., Odessey, R., and Egdahl, R.H. (1974): The effect of hemorrhagic shock, fasting, and glucocorticoid administration on leucine oxidation and incorporation into protein by skeletal muscle. *Metabolism* 23:901–904.

Waterlow, J.C. (1968): Observations of the mechanism of adaptation to low protein intakes. *Lancet* 2:1091–1097.

Young, V.R. (1977): Energy metabolism and requirements in the cancer patient. *Cancer Res.* 37:2336–2347.

CANCER

25 Protein and Amino Acid Metabolism in Cancer-Bearing Man: The Effects of Total Parenteral Nutrition on Alanine Kinetics

Murray F. Brennan
Michael E. Burt

Weight loss is a common accompaniment of malignancy, and is a prognostic indicator of outcome in many cancer patients. Widespread use of nutritional support in an effort to prevent or reverse this weight loss in the cancer patient is, however, controversial. The center of this controversy seems to depend upon the ability of total parenteral nutrition (TPN) to reverse the deficits observed in cancer patients and to favorably impact on treatment and outcome. We have taken the approach that unless nutritional support can reverse the metabolic abnormalities identified in the cancer-bearing host, the possible impact of such nutritional support on the response to antineoplastic therapy and thereby long-term survival would be minimal (Brennan, 1981). With the availability of TPN, any nutritional defects in the cancer-bearing host can be reversed, if they are due to either lack of intake or failure of the gastrointestinal tract to digest or absorb normally. If, however, there are specific or nonspecific abnormalities of substrate metabolism independent of route of intake, but related to the tumor-bearing state, then it will be important to identify them and demonstrate that they can be reversed by TPN. Because of the limitation placed upon survival by the dissolution of lean tissue mass by starvation (Brennan, 1978), we have placed emphasis on examining protein and amino acid kinetics in cancer-bearing man and the effect of TPN on intermediary metabolism in these patients.

There are numerous approaches for determination of protein and amino acid metabolism in cancer-bearing man (Table 25-1). Our laboratory has been involved in studies that address the majority of methods listed in the table with the exception of total body nitrogen by neutron activation (Lukaski et al., 1981); ^{14}C-amino acids (Carmichael et al., 1980; O'Keefe et al., 1981), other than alanine; direct antibody production and albumin degradation.

Table 25-1
Protein and Amino Acid Metabolism in Cancer-bearing Man

- Methods
  - Whole body:
    - Nitrogen balance
    - Body composition
      - Potassium–^{40}K
      - Nitrogen–neutron activation
    - Kinetic studies
      - Protein flux
        - ^{15}N-Glycine, lysine, alanine
        - ^{14}C-Leucine, tyrosine
        - Albumin degradation
        - Gluconeogenesis
        - ^{14}C-Alanine to ^{14}C-glucose
    - Muscle metabolism
      - 3-Methyl-histidine
      - Tumor-bearing limb
    - Plasma markers
      - Serum albumin
      - Antibody production

Hradec in 1958 suggested that radiolabeled methionine-albumin had a decreased half-life in tumor-bearing compared to nontumor-bearing animals. However, Waldmann, in 1963, demonstrated in patients with lymphoma a relatively normal catabolic rate for albumin with some decrease in synthesis compared to nontumor-bearing controls. The suggestion that in patients with cancer there was a relatively normal breakdown of albumin but decreased synthesis conflicted with the study in animals. Other authors have suggested that albumin catabolism is increased and synthesis decreased in patients with cancer. There is minimal information on amino acid and protein metabolism in patients receiving total parenteral nutrition (O'Keefe et al., 1981; Sauerwein et al., 1981).

The present report summarizes some of our studies on alanine kinetics and the conversion of alanine to glucose in the cancer-bearing host prior to and following nutritional support (Burt et al., 1982). We were interested in determining if there was an obligate need for gluconeogenesis in the cancer-bearing host that might not be reversed by nutritional support as has been suggested in septic man (Long et al., 1976), thereby providing a contributing cause for the cachexia of malignancy. The present studies have been based on our prior work in small animals, examining the influence of glucose infusion on rates of gluconeogenesis from alanine (Lowry et al., 1980). In these studies we demonstrated minor differences in the peak percentage of ^{14}C alanine dose recovered as ^{14}C glucose when comparing fasting tumor-bearing and nontumor-bearing rats; specific rates of gluconeogenesis were not determined, as alanine and lactate specific activity was not measured directly.

A subsequent study (Burt et al., 1981) demonstrated an increased rate of gluconeogenesis from alanine in tumor-bearing animals compared to nontumor-bearing animals prior to the onset of cachexia. The latter study suggested that the increased rate of gluconeogenesis was not a function of weight loss, but possibly a specific tumor-related metabolic alteration.

Subsequent studies (Arbeit et al., 1982) were able to show differences in endogenous glucose production from alanine under the influence of exogenous glucose infusion, but with only minimal changes in alanine to glucose turnover when rats with and without a methyl cholanthrene-induced rhabdomyosarcoma were compared. Of more importance perhaps was that this study was in animals that had not lost significant quantities of weight, suggesting again that the abnormality might be related to the tumor-bearing state and not secondary to weight loss.

In man, a previous study (Waterhouse et al., 1979) demonstrated a significant increase in the rate of conversion of alanine to glucose in severely malnourished cancer patients with metastatic disease. These were compared to a previous group of patients studied by the same authors who did not have cancer. Again, it was difficult to differentiate the effect of weight loss in these two population groups.

MATERIALS AND METHODS

As part of an ongoing study of preoperative x-irradiation for localized esophageal carcinoma, we randomized patients to receive or not receive nutritional support, depending upon the degree of antecedent weight loss. All patients were then studied before and following two weeks of nutritional support. During the same period of time they received 1600 rads of mediastinal and esophageal irradiation in 400 rad fractions (Burt et al., 1982).

Following baseline studies for substrates and hormones, 50 μCi of D-[3-^{3}H]-glucose (17.54 mCi/mmol) and 50 μCi of L-[(U)^{14}C-] alanine (175 mCi/mmol) were rapidly injected into a peripheral vein, flushed with normal saline, and arterial blood sampled at 1, 3, 5, 10, 15, 30, 45, 60, 90, 120, and 190 minutes after tracer injection. For parallel glucose recycling studies, the protocol was identical except that 50 μCi D-[(U)^{14}C]-glucose (4.36 mCi/mmol) was injected instead of the alanine. All plasma samples were deproteinized by membrane filter centrifugation (Amicon-CF$_{50}$A, Amicon Corp., Lexington, MA). Alanine concentration was determined by a single column chromatographic method on a Beckman 121 MB Amino Acid Analyzer (Beckman Instruments Corp., Palo Alto, CA). Specific activity (DPM/mmol) of plasma ^{3}H and ^{14}C glucose was determined by sequentially passing deproteinized plasma through anion and cation resin exchange columns, evaporating the eluant to dryness, redissolving in water, scintillation counting, and then determining the glucose concentration. Specific activity of plasma ^{14}C alanine was determined by collecting the alanine fraction from a modified amino acid analyzer, scintillation counting an aliquot and determining the alanine concentration on the automated 121 MB.

The data was then analyzed using steady state assumptions (Kreisberg et al., 1970, Baker et al., 1959). Noncompartmental analysis of the specific activity versus time curves was then performed (Katz et al., 1974). Specific activity versus time curves were then best fitted to a curve expressed as a sum of three exponentials. With the integration from 0 time to infinity, the area under the specific activity versus time curve was calculated (Shipley and Clark, 1972). The turnover for the respective substrate was then obtained by dividing the dose of tracer injected by the area under the respective curve. The alanine pool was defined as the alanine mass of the body that dilutes the injected tracer (Baker et al., 1959). The percentage of glucose derived from alanine after injecting the uniformly labeled alanine was calculated from the area under the ^{14}C glucose specific activity versus time curve divided by the area under the ^{14}C alanine specific activity versus time curve multiplied by two (Kreisberg, 1970). The rate of glucose derived from alanine, the rate of alanine converted to glucose, and the percentage of alanine converted to glucose were then calculated according to Kreisberg et al. (1970) and Chochinov et al. (1978).

Total parenteral nutrition was provided in standard fashion utilizing a synthetic amino acid solution (4.25% Freamine II from American McGaw Laboratories, Glendale, CA). Vitamins, essential fatty acids, and trace elements were provided as outlined previously (Brennan, 1981). The energy source was glucose in a final concentration of 20%. The studies in which jejunal feedings provided the nutritional support were with Vivonex (Norwich-Eaton Pharmaceuticals, Norwich, NY) delivered at 106 ml/hr and provided isocaloric, but not isonitrogenous, equivalence to the TPN formula.

RESULTS

There were 17 males and one female with an age range of 48 to 75 years. These 18 patients were divided into four groups: a group of four that did not receive nutritional support and had lost less than 20% of their pre-illness body weight, a group (n = 6) that had lost less than 20% of their body weight and received total parenteral nutrition, a group (n = 3) that received jejunal feedings having lost greater than 20% body weight, and a group (n = 5) who had lost greater than 20% of their body weight and received total parenteral nutrition. All allocations to Groups I and II and between Groups III and IV were random. Values are mean ± s.d.

Substrate and Hormone Determinations

Statistical differences were noted in the arterial plasma glucose and blood lactates in patients receiving nutritional support, compared to their prefeeding control (Table 25-2). Patients receiving TPN demonstrated significant increases in serum insulin concentrations but no change in plasma glucagon, serum cortisol, serum growth hormone or serum T4 levels. Serum cholesterol fell in all groups receiving nutritional support. Although serum insulin concentrations tended to increase in the patients in Group III, this change was not significant and the plasma cortisol level decreased significantly in this group.

Alanine Kinetics

Two weeks of conventional in-hospital diet while receiving radiation therapy did not change alanine kinetics (Table 25-3). Patients receiving jejunal feeding and TPN had an increase in alanine pool size, but this was only significant in the patients who

Table 25-2
Arterial Substrate Levels

	n	Plasma Glucose mM Before*	Plasma Glucose mM During	Blood Lactatate mM Before*	Blood Lactatate mM During
< 20% Body Weight Loss					
Conventional nutritional support	4	5.06 ± 0.82	5.75 ± 0.77	0.4 ± 0.2	0.5 ± 0.1
TPN	5	4.98 ± 0.64	9.73 ± 5.47	0.6 ± 0.1	1.0 ± 0.4†
> 20% Body Weight Loss					
Jejunal Feeding	3	4.32 ± 0.34	7.98 ± 0.39†	0.6 ± 0.1	1.3 ± 0.1†
TPN	5	5.05 ± 0.36	8.23 ± 1.08‡	0.4 ± 0.1	1.0 ± 0.4†

*Before and During refer to nutritional support
†$p < 0.5$ (Before vs. During)
‡$p < 0.01$ (Before vs. During)

Table 25-3
Alanine Kinetics

	Ala Pool μmol kg^{-1} Before	Ala Pool μmol kg^{-1} During	Ala Turnover Rate μmol kg^{-1} min^{-1} Before	Ala Turnover Rate μmol kg^{-1} min^{-1} During	Ala Endogenous Production Rate μmol kg^{-1} min^{-1} During
< 20% BWL					
Conventional nutritional support	79.6 ± 17.7	104.4 ± 12.7	1.68 ± 0.5	2.21 ± 0.2	2.21 ± 0.2
TPN	76.0 ± 35.5	158.8 ± 55.7*	1.82 ± 0.5	4.13 ± 1.03*	3.15 ± 0.99*
> 20% BWL					
Jejunal feeding	84.7 ± 6.2	172.1 ± 43.3	2.09 ± 0.65	4.36 ± 1.26	4.01 ± 1.21
TPN	104.8 ± 39.0	197.2 ± 118.0	2.11 ± 0.66	4.93 ± 2.30	3.75 ± 2.30

Ala = Alanine
BWL = Body Weight Loss
*$p < 0.05$
Before and During refer to Nutritional Support

had lost less than 20% of body weight and received TPN (Group II). The endogenous alanine production rate rose significantly in this same group, increasing in the other groups but not to statistical significance. Alanine turnover rate increased in all fed groups, as did alanine clearance rate, but only in the TPN–no weight loss group was this significant. The alanine infusion rate in the TPN patients was approximately 0.34 mmol $kg^{-1}min^{-1}$. Alanine clearance rate was unchanged except in the weight loss group receiving TPN who had a significant increase from 18.0 to 22.3 mmol kg^{-1} min^{-1}.

Alanine conversion to glucose, a measure of gluconeogenesis, was not changed in the group that did not receive nutritional support (Table 25-4). Patients receiving total parenteral nutrition who had previously lost less than 20% of their pre-illness weight had a significantly decreased percentage of glucose derived from alanine, a decrease in the percentage of alanine converted to glucose and a decrease in the rate of alanine converted to glucose. Identical effects were noted in the weight loss group receiving nutritional support by either jejunal feedings or TPN. Changes between jejunally fed and the TPN group were identical, suggesting that such enteral feeding was equivalent to parenteral nutrition in decreasing the rate of gluconeogenesis in the cancer patient with weight loss.

DISCUSSION

As our intent was to provide isocaloric rather than isonitrogenous feeding, the TPN group received a higher quantity of alanine than the jejunally fed patients (TPN approx. 1.1 mmol•kg^{-1} min^{-1} compared to 0.34 for jejunal feeding). This is a function of the composition of the TPN solution and of the quantity of Vivonex needed to supply an isocaloric infusion.

The alanine rate and rate of alanine conversion to glucose is significantly different in our esophageal cancer patients (Table 25-5) when compared to rates in normal subjects determined by similar methods (Hall et al., 1979). A marked increase in the rate of alanine converted to glucose in esophageal patients with localized disease did not appear to be due to weight loss alone, for when the alanine turnover rate, percentage of glucose derived from alanine, and rate of alanine converted to glucose were independently plotted against the percentage of weight loss, no significant correlation was identified.

In another study, Sauerwein et al. (1981) used a similar single injection technique with U-^{14}C alanine kinetics of five patients with gastric carcinoma, but without weight loss, undergoing elective total gastrectomy. The patients in this study were examined in the basal state, after preoperative TPN and during TPN following the operative procedure. They demonstrated that alanine turnover rate increased 100% on TPN, a figure which compares well to the mean increase of 104% in the nutritionally supported patients in our study.

Conventionally, protein sparing with exogenous glucose alone has been accompanied by diminution in renal ammoniagenesis, decreased blood ketones concentration, and some decrease in urinary urea excretion. The degree of diminution of the latter appears dependent on the degree of antecedent starvation (Aoki et al., 1975) and amount of glucose infused or fed (O'Connell et al., 1974; Fitzpatrick et al., 1977). Regardless of the amount of glucose supplied, there appears to be a limit to

Table 25-4
Gluconeogenesis from Alanine: Response to Nutritional Support

	% Glucose from Alanine		% Ala to Glucose		Rate of Ala to Glucose (mmol/min/kg)	
	Before	*After*	*Before*	*After*	*Before*	*After*
< 20% BWL						
No nutritional support	7.3 ± 2.3	7.1 ± 2.2	71.8 ± 18.4	62.3 ± 23.4	1.2 ± 0.4	1.4 ± 0.6
TPN	7.8 ± 2.9	0.13 ± 0.11*	72.4 ± 18.0	0.47 ± 0.2	1.3 ± 0.4	0.02 ± 0.02*
> 20% BWL						
Jejunal feeding	6.6 ± 2.0	0.03 ± 0.02*	58.5 ± 10.6	0*	1.22 ± 0.38	0*
TPN	4.4 ± 2.3	0.14 ± 0.2†	44.8 ± 22.2	0.56 ± 0.98‡	0.92 ± 0.44	0.04 ± 0.07*

BWL = Body Weight Loss
*$p < .05$ (before vs. during)
†$p = 0.07$
‡$p = 0.054$

Table 25-5
Basal Alanine Kinetics

	Ala Turnover Rate $\mu mol\ kg^{-1}\ min^{-1}$	% Glucose from Alanine	Rate of Alanine to Glucose $\mu mol\ kg^{-1}\ min^{-1}$
Normal subjects[†]	7.54 ± 1.81	8.39 ± 4.50	0.66 ± 0.31
Esophageal cancer patients	1.91 ± 0.54*	6.72 ± 2.55	1.18 ± 0.40*

*$p < 0.02$ (normal vs. esophageal cancer)
[†]Data from Hall et al., 1979

the degree that ureagenesis and gluconeogenesis can be suppressed. Such changes are accompanied by changes in plasma alanine levels which increases with an infused glucose load. However, whether this is due to increased release from muscle or decreased splanchnic extraction cannot be determined.

Changes in plasma and red cell alanine levels in response to an exogenous protein meal in normal man are quite small. Under baseline, non-fed circumstances, alanine is released from muscle (Aoki et al., 1976). This decreases with the ingestion of the meal, although arterial levels rise only slightly.

When mixed amino acids are infused intravenously alone, despite large quantities of alanine in the infusate, levels of alanine will begin to fall as gluconeogenesis occurs (Tweedle et al., 1977).

Rates of alanine synthesis in young men vary according to the preceding dietary intake and fall with increasing dietary protein (Young, 1981). The change from zero protein intake to a high protein intake (1.5 g protein kg^{-1} day^{-1}) results in a decrease of approximately 50% in the alanine synthesis rate. In addition to the higher alanine synthesis rates at lower protein intakes, the ingestion of a meal (the fed state) increases alanine formation, an observation suggested by early glucose infusion studies (O'Connell et al., 1974). When glucose was infused to healthy young men at 4 mg kg^{-1} min^{-1}, alanine flux increased due to new alanine synthesis by an amount that could be obtained from 7% of the glucose disposal (Young, 1981). If this increase in alanine synthesis is an obligatory response to the disposal of the infused glucose, then it may be deleterious in situations where the aim is to prevent rather than promote nitrogen release from muscle. The hyperglycemia seen in injury may therefore increase the muscle wasting in such conditions.

Studies of protein turnover which suggest an increase in both synthesis and catabolism of tumor-bearing man might account for the mild increase in energy expenditure seen in some cancer patients. If the energy cost of protein synthesis and breakdown is 2.0 kcal/g (Young et al., 1977) and protein synthesis rates may increase by 50% to 100% (4 to 5 g protein $kg^{-1} \bullet day^{-1}$) (Norton et al., 1981), it is conceivable that an increase of energy expenditure by as much as 30% could occur due to the presence of tumor alone. Mild increases in energy expenditure over and above similar but not identical noncancer-bearing control patients have been identified (Warnold et al., 1978).

In our study insulin levels rose in patients receiving TPN. Normal men fasted for 48 hours and then infused with 1 to 5 mU Kg WB min of insulin will show a decrease in hepatic glucose production (Chiasson et al., 1980). At the low insulin infusion rate, this appears to be due to glycogen deposition, but at a higher rate of insulin administration it is more consistent with inhibition of gluconeogenesis. The concentrations of insulin obtained by the low dose infusion are similar or greater than the levels seen in our patients receiving nutritional support.

An earlier study by Chiasson and his colleagues (1980) demonstrated no increase in net splanchnic uptake of alanine, nor any alanine release from the gut. We have presumed that by two weeks of nutritional support, accompanied by weight gain, that the glycogen stores are adequately repleted. Perhaps in our own study the hyperglycemia induced was sufficient to diminish alanine extraction by the liver, as shown by Felig et al. (1974).

In our study, the suppression of gluconeogenesis from alanine by TPN appears complete and is associated with large increases in total glucose turnover and incomplete endogenous glucose suppression due to continued recycling (Burt et al., 1982). Although the turnover rate of alanine increases by a factor of two in these cancer patients when placed on standard enteral or total parenteral nutrition, the point must be emphasized that the rate of gluconeogenesis, as measured by the conversion of ^{14}C-alanine to ^{14}C-glucose, is suppressed to almost immeasurable levels. This, we feel, is a beneficial effect and hopefully reflects the ability of nutritional support to favorably impact on the protein economics of the cancer patient.

REFERENCES

Aoki, T.T., Muller, W.A., Brennan, M.F. and Cahill, G.F., Jr. (1975): Metabolic effects of glucose in brief and prolonged fasted man. *Am. J. Clin. Nutr.* 28:507–511.

Arbeit, J.MN., Burt, M.E., Rubinstein, L.V., Gorschboth, C.M. and Brennan, M.F. (1982): Glucose metabolism and gluconeogenesis from alanine. Response to exogenous glucose infusion in tumor bearing and non-tumor bearing rats. *Cancer Res.* (in press).

Baker, N., Shipley, R.A., Clark, R.E. and Incefy, G.E. (1959): C^{14} studies in carbohydrate metabolism: glucose pool size and rate of turnover in the normal rat. *Am. J. Physiol.* 196:245–252.

Brennan, M.F. (1981): Total parenteral nutrition in the cancer patients. *N. Engl. J. Med.* 305: 375–382.

Brennan, M.F. (1977): Uncomplicated starvation versus cancer cachexia. *Cancer Res.* 37: 2359–2364.

Burt, M.E., Gorschboth, C.M. and Brennan, M.F. (1982): A controlled prospective randomized trial evaluating the metabolic effects of enteral and parenteral nutrition in the cancer patient. *Cancer* 49:1092–1105.

Burt, M.E., Lowry, S.F., Gorschboth, C. and Brennan, M.F. (1981): Metabolic alteration in a non-cachectic animal tumor system. *Cancer* 47:2138–2146.

Carmichael, M.J., Claque, M.S., Keir, M.J. and Johnston, I.D.A. (1980): Whole body protein turnover, synthesis and breakdown in patients with colorectal carcinoma. *Br. J. Surg.* 67:736–739.

Chiasson, J.L., Atkinson, R.L., Cherrington, A.D., Keller, U., Sinclair-Smith, B.C., Lacy, W.W., Liljenquist, J.E. (1980): Effects of insulin at two dose levels on gluconeogenesis from alanine in fasting man. *Metabolism* 29:810–818.

Chochinov, R.H., Perlman, K. and Moorhouse, J.A. (1978): Circulating alanine production and disposal in healthy subjects. *Diabetes* 27:287–295.

Felig, P., Wahren, J. (1974): Influence of endogenous insulin in splanchnic glucose and amino acid metabolism in man. *J. Clin. Invest.* 50:1702–1711.

Fitzpatrick, G.F., Meguid, M.M., Gitlitz, P.H. and Brennan, M.F. (1977): Glucagon infusion in normal man: effects of 3-methylhistidine excretion and plasma amino acids. *Metabolism* 26:477–485.

Hall, S.E.H., Braaten, J.T., McKendry, J.B.R., Bolton, T., Foster, D. and Berman, M. (1979): Normal alanine-glucose relationships and their changes in diabetic patients before and after insulin treatment. *Diabetes* 28:737–745.

Hradec, J. (1958): Metabolism of serum albumin in tumor bearing rats. *Br. J. Cancer* 12: 290–304.

Katz, J., Rostami, H. and Dunn, A. (1974): Evaluation of glucose turnover, body mass and recycling with reversible and irreversible tracers. *Biochem J.* 142:161–170.

Kreisberg, R.A., Pennington, L.F. and Boshell, B.R. (1970): Lactate turn-over and glucogenesis in normal and obese humans. Effects of starvation. *Diabetes* 19:53–63.

Lukaski, H.C., Mendez, J., Buskirk, E.R., Cohn, S.H. (1981): A comparison of methods of assessment of body composition including neutron activation analysis of total body nitrogen. *Metabolism* 30:777–782.

Long, C.L., Kinney, J.M., and Geiger, J.W. (1976): Nonsuppressability of gluconeogenesis by glucose in septic patients. *Metabolism* 25:193–201.

Lowry, S.F., Norton, J.A. and Brennan, M.F. (1980): Glucose turnover and gluconeogenesis during hypocaloric glucose infusion in tumor bearing F344 male rats. *J. Natl. Cancer Inst.* 64:291–296.

Norton, J.A., Stein, T.P. and Brennan, M.F. (1981): Whole body protein synthesis and turnover in normal man and malnourished patients with and without known cancer. *Ann. Surg.* 194:123–128.

O'Connell, R.C., Morgan, A.P., Aoki, T.T., Ball, M.R. and Moore, F.D. (1974): Nitrogen conservation in starvation: graded responses to intravenous glucose. *J. Clin. Endocrin. Metab.* 39:555–563.

O'Keefe, S.J.D., Moldawer, L.L., Young, V.R. and Blackburn, G.L. (1981): The influence of intravenous nutrition on protein dynamics following surgery. *Metabolism* 30:1150–1158.

Sauerwein, H.P., Michels, R.P.J. and Ceijka, V. (1981): Alanine turnover in the post-absorptive state and during parenteral hyperalimentation before and after surgery. *Metabolism* 30:700–705.

Shipley, R.A. and Clark, R.E. (1972): *Tracer Methods for In Vivo Kinetics. Theory and Applications.* Academic Press, New York.

Tweedle, D.E.F., Fitzpatrick, G.F., Brennan, M.F., Culebras, J.M., Wolfe, B.M., Ball, M.R. and Moore, F.D. (1977): Intravenous amino acids as the sole nutritional substrate. *Ann. Surg.* 186:60–73.

Warnold, I., Falkheden, T., Hulten, B. and Isaksson, B. (1978): Energy intake and expenditure in selected groups of hospitalized patients. *Am. J. Clin. Nutr.* 31:722–729.

Waterhouse, C., Jeanpretre, N., and Keilson, J. (1979): Gluconeogenesis from alanine in patients with progressive malignant disease. *Cancer Res.* 39:1968–1972.

Young, V.R. (1977): Energy metabolism and requirements in the cancer patient. *Cancer Res.* 37:2336–2347.

Young, V.R. (1981): Dynamics of human whole body amino acid metabolism: use of stable isotope probes and relevance to nutritional requirements. *J. Nutr. Sci. Vitaminol.* 27:395–413.

26 Amino Acid Analogues: Metabolism and Use in Patients with Chronic Renal Failure

William E. Mitch

The major functions of the kidney are to excrete waste products resulting from catabolism of endogenous and exogenous protein and to regulate water and electrolyte balance. In patients with chronic renal failure (CRF), the capacity of the remaining kidney to fulfill these functions becomes progressively limited; consequently, these waste products accumulate in proportion to the loss of renal function. In addition, there can be abnormalities of water and electrolyte balance (Mitch and Wilcox, 1982). Usually, these can be controlled by changing the intake of electrolytes (sodium, potassium, etc.) and/or using diuretics, and thus, symptoms ascribable to abnormal water and electrolyte balance are absent until there is almost no remaining renal function. Unfortunately, there is no simple or effective means of increasing the excretion of the inorganic ions (phosphorus, sulphur, etc.) and organic waste products arising from protein catabolism. Therefore, a higher plasma level is required to excrete the quantity of waste products produced each day when renal function is impaired because the relationship between the plasma level and excretion of these waste products is determined by the reduced clearance capacity of the kidney. Since proteinaceous foods are the principal source of phosphate, sulphate, potassium, hydrogen ions, as well as organic waste products, it is clear that the only way to decrease their accumulation is to reduce the intake of protein. This has been recognized for decades and was the basis for manipulation of the diet with the aim of reducing uremic symptoms (Giordano, 1963; Giovannetti and Maggiore, 1964).

The use of dietary protein restriction to treat patients with CRF is limited, however, because the essential amino acids necessary for efficient protein synthesis must be provided in order to avoid protein malnutrition. For this reason, early therapeutic regimens restricted nitrogen intake to proteins that were relatively rich in essential amino acids, i.e., "high-quality" protein. This limitation made dietary therapy monotonous and consequently, long-term compliance with the regimen limited its effectiveness. Moreover, the degree of protein restriction was probably excessive since usually there was at least some degree of protein depletion before nitrogen balance became neutral (Giordano, 1963; Kopple and Coburn, 1973). Subsequently, it was suggested that dietary therapy of CRF could be improved further by adding a supplement of essential amino acids as such to a low-protein diet. This would ensure an adequate intake of essential amino acids and raise nitrogen intake closer to the level necessary for normal subjects. The supplements generally contained essential amino acids in the amounts and proportions required for normal adults (Rose and Wixom, 1955; Walser, 1981).

An interesting hypothesis arising from early studies was that patients with CRF had a lower nitrogen requirement than normal subjects because they could use nitrogen derived from urea degradation to synthesize amino acids and, hence, protein (Richards, 1972). This widely accepted hypothesis led to the suggestion that α-ketoacids of essential amino acids might be especially useful as a supplement in place of the essential amino acids because their amination would use nitrogen from urea and cause a further reduction in the pool of accumulated urea as well as an increase in the supply of essential amino acids. This should lead to an improvement in nitrogen balance (Schloerb, 1966). Use of α-ketoacids in this way seemed possible since it had been shown that they could be substituted for essential amino acids in the diet of experimental animals and that humans also could convert the α-ketoacids of branched-chain amino acids, phenylalanine, methionine, and tryptophan, to the respective amino acids (Walser, 1978). In 1973, Walser and associates reported that patients with CRF eating a 15 to 25 g/day protein diet could maintain a neutral or positive nitrogen balance when they were given a mixture of five α-ketoacids and four essential amino acids even though the dietary protein was not limited to "high-quality" type. In this same study, it was reported that when the supplement was withdrawn, urea nitrogen appearance (the sum of urea nitrogen excreted and the change in the urea nitrogen pool) increased by an average of 1.55 g N/day and nitrogen balance (corrected for changes in the urea nitrogen pool) decreased by an average of 1.73 g N/day. Since the amount of nitrogen that would be required to aminate the α-ketoacids contained in the mixture (0.57 g N/day) was two to three times lower than the amount of improvement in either urea nitrogen appearance or nitrogen balance, it was concluded that the α-ketoacids apparently have a beneficial effect on nitrogen metabolism beyond that derived from their conversion to essential amino acids.

The effects of α-ketoacids on nitrogen metabolism has been defined further. In a recent study of patients with normal renal function who were in negative nitrogen balance during voluntary starvation, we found that infusion of α-ketoisocaproate decreased their total nitrogen excretion and, therefore, improved their nitrogen balance compared to another period in which the same patients were starved, but received no infusions (Mitch et al., 1981). In a third period of starvation, infusion of an equimolar amount (as in the α-ketoisocaproate infusion) of leucine did not change nitrogen excretion, suggesting that α-ketoisocaproate promoted nitrogen retention and that the effect was specific for the analogue rather than the amino acid. Since α-ketoisocaproate and leucine are rapidly interconverted in many organs of the body, this finding was unexpected. Moreover, leucine itself should promote nitrogen retention through its ability to stimulate protein synthesis in incubated skeletal muscle of rats. Recently, Tischler et al. (1982) have reported that following conversion of leucine to α-ketoisocaproate that protein degradation in muscle was reduced. They incubated rat hemidiaphragms with leucine and showed that protein synthesis was increased while protein degradation was reduced, but when the incubation media also contained an inhibitor of transamination that prevented the conversion of leucine to α-ketoisocaproate, the rate of protein degradation was unchanged. Other studies showed that incubation with α-ketoisocaproate reduced protein degradation. Thus, it is possible that the nitrogen-sparing effect of α-ketoisocaproate in man occurs in part because α-ketoisocaproate decreases the rate of protein degradation in skeletal muscle.

The rationale, therefore, for using α-ketoacids in a dietary regimen for patients with CRF would be to reduce dietary nitrogen, to provide additional essential amino acids and to improve nitrogen retention. To study the effects of α-ketoacids in CRF, we gave patients with this illness a mixture of five α-ketoacids and the four remaining essential amino acids in proportions required for normal subjects as a supplement to a low-protein diet. Long-term results of this therapy were assessed. Another mixture with different proportions of amino acids and analogues was used also because evidence is accumulating that the amino acid requirements of patients with CRF are different from those of normal subjects.

In the first study, 27 patients with severe chronic renal insufficiency in whom the initial average creatinine clearance, serum creatinine and serum urea nitrogen were 8 ml/min, 10 mg/dl and 87 mg/dl, respectively, were treated for one or more months. Their diet consisted of 20 to 25 g/day of protein (protein quality unrestricted), 30 to 35 kcal/kg/day and a supplement of the calcium salts of nitrogen-free analogues of five essential amino acids (leucine, valine, isoleucine, methionine, phenylalanine) plus the four remaining essential amino acids as such (Table 26-1). The diseases causing CRF included glomerulonephritis, interstitial nephritis, inherited renal diseases and diabetes. Throughout the study, they were examined monthly or more frequently if required until completion of the study or until dialysis became necessary. The diet was designed according to the personal preferences of each patient and, at monthly intervals, the patient met with the research dietician (Mrs. Elizabeth Chandler) to review the diet and to continue dietary training. The patients were also treated with 1 mg/d folic acid, 50 mg/d pyridoxine and a B vitamin tablet each day plus antihypertensive medicines, phosphate binders, diuretics and other medicines as required.

At each visit, serum was obtained for measurement of urea nitrogen, creatinine, albumin, transferrin, calcium and phosphorus. These values were subsequently averaged for four periods: before beginning the therapy, after four to five weeks of therapy and at the end of the study. In addition, the average value for each patient throughout the study was calculated and from these values, the mean for each serum chemistry was calculated.

In the second study, the nitrogen-free analogue supplement included the branched-chain ketoacids given as salts of the basic amino acids, L-ornithine, L-lysine, and L-histidine. The mixture also contained L-tyrosine, L-threonine, and a small quantity of the hydroxyl-analogue of methionine (Table 26-1). Thus, the mixture

Table 26-1
Composition of Mixture D and EE of Nitrogen-free Analogues of Amino Acids and Essential Amino Acids

Mixture D		
Analogue (Calcium salt)	g	
α-Ketoisocaproate	4.00	
α-Keto-β-methylvalerate	2.92	
α-Ketoisovalerate	2.88	
D,L-α-hydroxy-γ-methylthiodutyrate	2.12	
L-Phenyllactate	2.00	
Amino Acid	g	
L-Threonine	0.67	
L-Tryptophan	0.33	
L-Lysine (HCl)	0.80	
L-Histidine	0.54	
Total Nitrogen	0.42	
Mixture EE		
Compound	mmol/day	mg N/day
L-Tyrosine	20	280
L-Threonine	15	210
L-Ornithine α-Ketoisovalerate	7	196
L-Ornithine α-Ketoisocaproate	7	196
L-Ornithine R, S-α-Keto-β-methylvalerate	7	196
L-Lysine α-Ketoisovalerate	7	196
L-Lysine α-Ketoisocaproate	7	196
L-Lysine R, S-α-Keto-β-methylvalerate	7	196
L-Histidine α-Ketoisocaproate	4	112
Calcium D, L-α-hydroxy-γ-methylthiodutyrate	2	0
Total	83	1178

was "unbalanced" since it did not contain tryptophan, phenylalanine or their analogues. The dietary regimen, vitamins and other medicine and dietary education were prescribed as before. For this group of nine patients with renal diseases that included glomerulonephritis, interstitial nephritis, diabetes and polycystic nephropathy, the initial average glomerular filtration rate was 4.8 ml/min and serum urea nitrogen and creatinine concentrations averaged 100 and 11.3 mg/dl, respectively.

RESULTS AND DISCUSSION

The patients receiving ketoacid-essential amino acid mixture D were treated for a total period of 207 patient-months. The average duration of therapy was 9.4 months per patient (range: 1 to 38 months). The serum chemistry data obtained is shown in Table 26-2. Throughout the study, there were no significant changes in weight or serum albumin and transferrin concentrations; since the latter values were within the normal range, it was concluded that protein nutrition was maintained. The values for serum urea nitrogen and urea nitrogen to creatinine ratio decreased

Table 26-2
Weight and Serum Chemistries of Patients Treated with α-Ketoacid-amino Acid Mixture D

	Initial	4–5 Weeks	Average	Final
Weight (kg)	70.3 ± 2.5	72.0 ± 2.9	72.0 ± 2.7	73.3 ± 3.1
Urea Nitrogen (mg/dl)	88 ± 5	70 ± 5†	81 ± 4	108 ± 6†
Creatinine (mg/dl)	10.0 ± 0.4	9.6 ± 0.4	11.8 ± 0.5*	15.5 ± 0.7†
Urea Nitrogen/Creatinine	8.8 ± 0.5	7.5 ± 0.6†	7.3 ± 1.7*	7.4 ± 0.5*
Calcium (mg/dl)	8.9 ± 0.3	9.0 ± 0.1	9.1 ± 0.2	9.0 ± 0.3
Phosphorus (mg/dl)	5.0 ± 0.3	4.3 ± 0.2*	4.5 ± 0.2	5.0 ± 0.4
Albumin (g/dl)	4.2 ± 0.1	4.1 ± 0.1	4.1 ± 0.1	4.1 ± 0.1
Transferrin (μg/dl)	266 ± 12	258 ± 16	274 ± 8	286 ± 17

Values expressed are mean ± SEM. Initial refers to values obtained before therapy was begun; four to five weeks' values are those obtained after this period of therapy; the average values are the mean of the average values for each patient throughout the period of therapy, and the final values are those obtained before dialysis was begun or at the end of the study. From Mitch, W.E., Collier, V.U. and Walser, M. (unpublished).
*†change from initial values significant at $p < 0.05$ and $p < 0.01$, respectively.

significantly after four to five weeks and the latter value remained lower throughout the study. Serum calcium concentration did not change significantly and was within the normal range during the study. Serum phosphorus concentration was initially high and decreased to normal levels after four to five weeks. The average value increased slightly above that obtained at four to five weeks and returned to the initial level by the end of the study. The increase in serum urea nitrogen concentration at the end of therapy could have been caused either by poor compliance with the diet or by progressively severe renal insufficiency. The lack of a change in the serum urea nitrogen to serum creatinine ratio suggests that the increase in the final value for serum urea nitrogen was related primarily to advancing renal insufficiency. Thus, the initial decrease in serum urea nitrogen was associated with a decrease in the SUN:serum creatinine ratio which was maintained throughout the study. Therefore, renal insufficiency, rather than a higher protein intake, presumably caused the rise in urea nitrogen. Because creatinine can be eliminated by degradation as well as by excretion in patients with CRF (Mitch et al., 1980), the ratio is not an accurate representation of renal function in severe CRF. However, elimination of creatinine by degradation could only raise the value of the SUN:creatinine ratio, especially if dietary compliance was poor.

The results obtained with mixture EE of basic amino acid salts of ketoacids indicated that nitrogen balance was neutral even though some essential amino acids or their nitrogen-free analogues were omitted and protein intake was inadequate (Mitch et al., 1982). Thus, nitrogen intake compared to the control period in which each patient was eating his/her customary diet was 1.36 g N less with mixture EE, but nitrogen balance corrected for changes in the urea nitrogen pool was neutral, as it was during the control period when nitrogen intake averaged 6.9 g N/day. The most marked change in the components of nitrogen balance that occurred on initiation of therapy with mixture EE was a sharp decrease in the urea nitrogen appearance rate (the sum of urine urea nitrogen and the rate of change of the urea nitrogen pool). Urea nitrogen appearance decreased by 1.1 g N/day ($p < 0.01$) from the control value of 4.5 g N/day when the low-protein diet EE supplement regimen was begun. There were no changes in the other components of nitrogen excretion which ranged from 1.63 to 3.11 g N/day, similar to those we have previously found in patients with severe chronic renal insufficiency (Mitch and Walser, 1977a,b).

Serum chemistry values obtained during long-term therapy with mixture EE and shown in Table 26-3 indicated that protein nutrition was well maintained during a treatment period of 63 patient-months (average: 7 months, range: 3 to 17 months). Serum urea nitrogen and creatinine concentrations fell significantly after four to six weeks of therapy with the analogue supplement, while serum albumin and transferrin concentrations increased significantly. Serum calcium changed only slightly, but serum phosphorus fell from a mean of 4.9 mg/dl to 3.9 mg/dl. This latter change was not statistically significant, but it is interesting that three of the patients who had hyperphosphatemia before therapy (average initial serum phosphate, 6.9 mg/dl) had a normal serum phosphorus concentration during therapy. There were no further statistically significant changes found during the ensuing months of therapy.

Plasma amino acid concentrations were measured during the fasting state in each subject before and again after four to five weeks of therapy with the amino acid analogue supplement. Compared to values obtained in normal subjects, plasma levels of taurine, citrulline, cystine, and 3-methyl-histidine were significantly increased in the patients before initiation of therapy. In addition, there were significant decreases in the values for threonine, serine, valine, isoleucine, leucine and tyrosine. These changes are similar to those reported by others during treatment of patients with CRF (Walser, 1981). During administration of the supplement, there were few statistically significant changes, although threonine increased by 38 ± 10 μM after four to five weeks. Tyrosine increased into the normal range from 45 ± 3 to 72 ± 9.5 μM by the second month and lysine increased slightly to 235 μM. Finally, alloisoleucine was increased in every sample taken after beginning therapy with EE because the mixture contains both R and S isomers of the α-ketoacids of isoleucine (Walser et al., 1981). There were no other significant changes in plasma amino acid concentrations including those of the branched-chain amino acids, ornithine or histidine.

These results show that nitrogen-free analogues of essential amino acids given as a supplement to a low-protein diet provides an effective and acceptable regimen that can be used in the long-term treatment of patients with CRF. Indices of protein nutrition were maintained for prolonged periods even though the diet contained an inadequate amount of protein. Moreover, there was a decrease in the quantity of accumulated urea nitrogen leading to a lower SUN. This, plus the constant finding of an increase in plasma alloisoleucine, indicates that there was good compliance with the regimen. Others also have reported that compliance is good with this type of regimen (Kampf et al., 1980).

The minimal daily protein requirement that can maintain nitrogen balance in patients with chronic renal failure is approximately 0.5 g/kg/day of "high-quality" protein (Kopple and Coburn, 1973). When dietary protein is restricted below this level, the accumulated pools of waste products will decrease at a rate proportional to the clearance of the molecules and symptoms will improve. However, protein depletion will develop leading to decreased values for plasma albumin, transferrin and other proteins. To avoid protein depletion, the patients in the present study were given a supplement of nitrogen-free analogues of essential amino acids plus amino acids. In both mixtures, branched-chain amino acid analogues were given as α-ketoacids and the methionine analogue was the α-hydroxy acid; in mixture D, the phenylalanine analogue was L-phenyllactate.

Branched-chain α-ketoacids are converted to the respective branched-chain amino acid by branched-chain amino acid transaminase. This enzyme is found in

Table 26-3
Serum Chemistry Values During Therapy with α-Ketoacid-amino Acid Mixture EE

	Initial	4–5 Weeks	8–11 Weeks
Creatinine (mg/dl)	11.3 ± 0.9	10.1 ± 0.8[†]	11.6 ± 1.1
Urea Nitrogen (mg/dl)	100 ± 5	85 ± 7*	88 ± 6*
Calcium (mg/dl)	9.0 ± 0.3	9.0 ± 0.3	9.1 ± 0.3
Phosphorus (mg/dl)	4.9 ± 0.6	3.9 ± 0.2	4.3 ± 0.3
Albumin (g/dl)	3.9 ± 1.3	4.1 ± 1.1*	4.1 ± 0.1*
Transferrin (μg/dl)	209 ± 22	267 ± 21[†]	250 ± 13[†]

Values are mean ± SE. Initial values refer to values obtained before therapy while four to five weeks and eight to 11 weeks refer to values obtained at those times.
*·$p < 0.01$,
†·$p < 0.05$ compared to initial value by paired "T" test. From Mitch et al., 1982, with permission.

many organs and accounts for the constant rate of release of a branched-chain amino acid when its α-ketoacids is perfused through kidney, liver, or muscle (Walser et al., 1973; Mitch and Chan, 1978). Besides being utilized in transamination reactions, branched-chain α-ketoacids also can be degraded by branched-chain ketoacid dehydrogenase. The liver contains a large amount of this enzyme, but a smaller amount of the transaminase so that branched-chain α-ketoacids are more readily degraded than the amino acids following gastrointestinal absorption (Khatra et al., 1977a). Hepatic dehydrogenase activity can increase with long-term feeding of branched-chain α-ketoacids (Khatra et al., 1977b) and some (Halliday et al., 1981), but not all (Epstein et al., 1980), reports suggest that conversion of α-ketoisovalerate to valine following oral administration may be subnormal in uremic patients. Moreover, plasma levels of branched-chain α-ketoacids are subnormal in uremic patients (Schauder et al., 1980). For these reasons, the quantities of branched-chain α-ketoacids used in mixtures D and EE were increased two- to threefold above the amounts of branched-chain amino acids that would be required by subjects with normal kidneys.

The α-hydroxy-analogues of methionine and phenylalanine were used because they are somewhat more palatable than the α-ketoacids analogue. These α-hydroxy-analogues are converted to the respective amino acid presumably by first being oxidized to the ketoacid derivative. Thus, perfusion of the kidney with L-phenyllactate results in the release of phenylpyruvate and phenylalanine (Collier et al., 1980). The release of phenylalanine can be increased by adding glutamine to the perfusate, and approximately 64% of the L-phenyllactate removed from the perfusate can be accounted for by the appearance of phenylpyruvate and L-phenylalanine.

Proof that this mixture of α-ketoacids, α-hydroxy-acids and amino acids were absorbed and utilized by uremic subjects was obtained by demonstrating that such patients were in neutral or positive nitrogen balance while they ate a virtually protein-free diet supplemented with glycine and ketoacid-amino acid mixture D (Mitch and Walser, 1977b). Since the nitrogen-free analogues were the only source of the respective essential amino acid in these experiments, maintenance of nitrogen balance indicates that the nitrogen-free analogues were absorbed and converted to the respective essential amino acids. It must be emphasized that α-ketoacids are useful only when dietary protein is restricted (Hecking et al., 1980). With a high-protein diet, they are rapidly degraded (Epstein et al., 1980).

Upon initiation of the low-protein diet–ketoacid regimen, the serum urea nitrogen concentration always decreases. This is important because the severity of uremic symptoms most closely parallels the degree of urea accumulation. The correlation of uremic symptoms with the SUN occurs because of the unique relationship of the metabolism of amino acids and, hence, protein to urea. Clearly, when urea production rises, the production of all putative uremic toxins arising during protein degradation increases. This relationship has recently been re-emphasized by Lowrie et al. (1981) in a report from the National Cooperative Study of factors affecting the adequacy of dialysis. One factor was urea. When the dialysis schedule or technique was altered so that the average SUN between dialyses was less than 80 mg/dl, morbidity and hospitalizations related to complications of uremia were significantly less compared to another group of patients eating similar amounts of protein, but being dialyzed less intensively so that their SUN between dialyses exceeded 100 mg/dl.

In addition to lowering nitrogen intake, the ketoacid of leucine, α-ketoisocaproate, may reduce the rate of endogenous protein catabolism and thus lower urea production (see above). Other explanations including the "urea nitrogen reutilization" hypothesis do not have a significant impact on the rate of urea accumulation. Evidence from several studies indicate that nitrogen derived from urea degradation is not nutritionally important in patients with CRF. For example, Varcoe et al. (1975) showed, in patients with CRF eating a mildly protein-restricted diet, that only 1.6% of the nitrogen in albumin could be derived from urea degradation, and Ell et al. (1978) confirmed this in patients being treated with a low-protein-ketoacid regimen. Using another approach, we suppressed urea degradation by giving nonabsorbable aminoglycoside antibiotics orally to subjects with CRF, some of whom were receiving the ketoacid regimen (Mitch et al., 1977; Mitch and Walser, 1977b). During the period of antibiotic administration, urea kinetics were measured using ^{14}C-urea. Significant suppression of urea degradation occurred in seven patients, but the amount of urea nitrogen appearing in urine and body fluids did not change compared to a control period in which the antibiotics had not been administered. Moreover, nitrogen balance improved significantly. These data indicate that urea degradation is not an important source of nitrogen for amino acid and, hence, protein synthesis. If urea nitrogen were being used for amination of ketoacids, then during suppression of urea degradation, more urea should appear in urine and body fluids and nitrogen balance should become more negative. Thus, it appears that the more likely nitrogen source for amination of α-ketoacids are amino acids (e.g., glutamate, glutamine) rather than urea nitrogen.

From the present results and those of others, it seems likely that the amino acid requirements of patients with CRF are different from those of normal subjects. Thus, concentrations of amino acids in plasma and in the intracellular compartment of muscle cells are abnormal and several defects in amino acid metabolism have been identified in patients with CRF. For example, the plasma concentrations of valine, isoleucine, and leucine are subnormal in almost all reports; in the intracellular compartment of muscle in uremic adults, isoleucine is normal in the absence of severe protein restriction, while leucine is somewhat reduced and valine more so (Alvestrand et al., 1981). Tyrosine is low, in part, because of reduced conversion of phenylalanine to tyrosine in patients with chronic renal insufficiency, while the concentration of serine is reduced because of diminished production of serine by the damaged kidney. Thus, it seems likely that amino acid requirements in CRF are different. In fact, many of these abnormalities can be corrected by supplementation of a low-protein diet with essential amino acids in different proportions than those recommended for normal subjects plus certain "nonessential" amino acids. Alvestrand et al. (1981) reported that using such a mixture in which there was more leucine than valine and more valine than isoleucine plus small amounts of threonine and phenylalanine and additional tyrosine, histidine and lysine fully corrected the concentrations of amino acids in plasma and muscle.

The unique feature of supplement EE used in the present study was that tryptophan and phenylalanine were absent in any form and the amount of the methionine analogue was quite low (about 1% of total). Regardless, the concentration of phenylalanine and methionine in plasma did not fall, also suggesting that their requirements are different from those of normal subjects. Tryptophan was not measured, but in studies of similar patients given a supplement which also did not contain tryptophan, its plasma concentration did not change (Abras et al., 1981). It appears that the amounts or proportions of branched-chain α-ketoacids were incorrect because plasma concentrations of branched-chain amino acids did not become normal even though nitrogen balance was neutral and there was a sustained improvement in serum albumin and transferrin during long-term (63 patient-months) administration. Inclusion of ornithine in supplement EE may have been useful since the ornithine concentration within muscle cells is subnormal in patients with CRF on moderate protein restriction. In addition, two reports indicate that patients with CRF have a small increase in blood ammonia concentration and ornithine would tend to lower blood ammonia.

In addition to the patients of this report, there are at least 120 other patients with moderate to severe renal impairment (75% had creatinine clearance of less than 10 ml/min) who have been treated with α-ketoacids. In virtually all studies, nitrogen balance improved or remained neutral, and there was a decrease in the SUN because of a lower rate of urea production (Mitch et al., 1981). An additional benefit of the α-ketoacid regimen is that it generally leads to a lower serum phosphorus concentration. This is important because a high-protein diet and a high serum phosphorus may be factors contributing to the progressive loss of residual renal function in patients with CRF. Indeed, Barsotti et al. (1981) measured the change in the rate of loss of creatinine clearance in 12 patients with CRF who were treated with a ketoacid regimen when creatinine clearance was between 3 and 9.6 ml/min. In eight of these patients, the rate of loss of renal function was halted or substantially slowed compared to the rate measured in the control period. Only one patient continued to lose renal function at the same rate. In the group as a whole, the mean change was significant ($p < 0.02$).

In summary, the data presented and those reported by others indicate that nitrogen-free analogues of essential amino acids can be used as a substitute for dietary essential amino acids in patients with CRF eating a low-protein diet. This regimen promotes neutral nitrogen balance and protein nutrition during long-term therapy. In addition, the accumulation of SUN and other waste products always decreases. Finally, the regimen might decrease the rate of loss of residual renal function, at least in some patients. It is likely that changes in the proportions and amounts of α-ketoacids, as well as addition of certain amino acids, might lead to further improvement, since amino acid requirements for patients with CRF are almost certainly different from those of normal subjects.

ACKNOWLEDGMENTS

Supported by RCDA AM 00750 and Program Project Grant AM 18020, Clinical Research Center Grant RR 00888 and RR 35. Ms. P. Dolan provided expert editorial assistance.

REFERENCES

Abras, E., Walser, M., and Mitch, W.E. (1981): Mixed salts of basic amino acids with branched chain ketoacids as the basis for new supplements designed to improve nutrition in chronic renal failure. In: *Metabolism and Clinical Implications of Branched Chain Amino and Ketoacids,* (eds: M. Walser and J.R. Williamson) p.593, Elsevier/North Holland, New York.

Alvestrand, A., Ahlberg, M., Bergstrom, J., and Furst, P. (1981): The effect of nutritional regimens on branched chain amino acid antagonism in uremia. In: *Metabolism and Clinical Implications of Branched Chain Amino and Ketoacids,* (eds: M. Walser and J.R. Williamson) pp.605–613, Elsevier/North Holland, New York.

Barsotti, G., Guiducci, A., Ciardella, F., and Giovannetti, S. (1981): Effects on renal function of a low-nitrogen diet supplemented with essential amino acids and ketoanalogues and of hemodialysis and free protein supply in patients with chronic renal failure. *Nephron* 27:113–117.

Collier, V.U., Butler, D.O., and Mitch, W.E. (1980): Metabolic effects of L-phenyllactate in perfused kidney, liver and muscle. *Am. J. Physiol.* 238:E450–E457.

Ell, S., Fynn, M., Richards, P., and Halliday, D. (1978): Metabolic studies with keto acid diets. *Am. J. Clin. Nutr.* 31:1776–1783.

Epstein, C.M., Chawla, R.K., Wadsworth, A., and Rudman, D. (1980): Decarboxylation of α-ketoisovaleric acid after oral administration in man. *Am. J. Clin. Nutr.* 33:1968–1974.

Giordano, C. (1963): Use of exogenous and endogenous urea for protein synthesis in normal and uremic subjects. *J. Lab. Clin. Med.* 62:231–246.

Giovannetti, S., and Maggiore, Q. (1964): A low-nitrogen diet with proteins of high biological value for severe chronic uremia. *Lancet* 1:1000–1003.

Halliday, D., Madigan, K., Chalmers, R.A., Purkiss, P., Ell, S., Berstrom, J., Furst, P., Neuhauser, M., and Richards, P. (1981): The degree of conversion of α-ketoacids to valine and phenylalanine in health and uremia. *Q. J. Med.* 50:53–62.

Hecking, E., Andrzejewski, L., Prellwitz, W., Opferkuch, W., and Muller, D. (1980): Double-blind cross-over study with oral α-ketoacids in patients with chronic renal failure. *Am. J. Clin. Nutr.* 33:1678–1681.

Kampf, O., Fischer, H.C., and Kessel, M. (1980): Efficacy of an unselected protein diet (25g) with minor oral supply of essential amino acids and keto analogues compared with a selective protein diet (40g) in chronic renal failure. *Am. J. Clin. Nutr.* 33:1673–1677.

Khatra, B.S., Chawla, R.K., Sewell, C.W., and Rudman, D. (1977a): Distribution of branched-chain alpha-keto acid dehydrogenases in primate tissues. *J. Clin. Invest.* 59:558.

Khatra, B.S., Chawla, R.K., Wadsworth, A.D., and Rudman, D. (1977b): Effect of dietary branched-chain alpha-keto acids on hepatic branched-chain, alpha-keto acid dehydrogenase in the rat. *J. Nutr.* 107:1528.

Kopple, J.D., and Coburn, J.W. (1973): Metabolic studies of low-protein diets in uremia. I. Nitrogen and potassium. *Medicine* 52:583–595.

Lowrie, E.G., Laird, N.M., Parker, T.F., and Sargent, J.A. (1981): The effect of hemodialysis prescription on patient morbidity: report from the National Cooperative Dialysis Study. *New Engl. J. Med.* 305:1176–1181.

Mitch, W.E., Abras, E., and Walser, M. (1982): Long-term effects of a new ketoacid-amino acid supplement in patients with chronic renal failure. *Kidney Int.* (In Press).

Mitch, W.E., and Chan, W. (1978): Transamination of branched-chain keto acids by isolated perfused rat kidney. *Am J. Physiol.* 235:E47–E52.

Mitch, W.E., Collier, V.U., and Walser, M. (1980): Creatinine metabolism in chronic renal failure. *Clin. Sci.* 58:327–335.

Mitch, W.E., Collier, V.U., and Walser, M. (1981): Treatment of chronic renal failure with branched-chain ketoacids plus the other essential amino acids or their nitrogen-free analogues. In: *Metabolism and Clinical Implications of Branched Chain Amino and Ketoacids,* (eds: M. Walser and J.R. Williamson) pp.587–592, Elsevier/North Holland, New York.

Mitch, W.E., Leitman, P.S., and Walser, M. (1977): Effects of oral neomycin and kanamycin in chronic renal failure: I. Urea metabolism. *Kidney Int.* 11:116–122.

Mitch, W.E., and Walser, M. (1977a): Effects of oral neomycin and kanamycin in chronic uremic patients. II. Nitrogen balance. *Kidney Int.* 11:123–127.

Mitch, W.E., and Walser, M. (1977b): Utilization of calcium L-phenyllactate as a substitute for phenylalanine by uremic subjects. *Metabolism* 26:1041–1044.

Mitch, W.E., Walser, M., and Sapir, D.G. (1981): Nitrogen-sparing induced by leucine compared with that induced by its keto-analogue, alpha-ketoisocaproate, in fasting obese man. *J. Clin. Invest.* 67:553–562.

Mitch, W.E., and Wilcox, C.S. (1982): Disorders of body fluids, sodium and potassium in chronic renal failure. *Am. J. Med.* 72:536–550.

Richards, P. (1972): Nutritional potential of nitrogen recycling in man. *Am. J. Clin. Nutr.* 25:615–625.

Rose, W.C., and Wixom, R.L. (1955): The amino acid requirements of man. XVI. The role of the nitrogen intake. *J. Biol. Chem.* 217:997–1004.

Schauder, P., Matthaei, D., Henning, H.V., Scheler, F., and Langenbeck, U. (1980): Blood levels of branched-chain amino acids and α-ketoacids in uremic patients given keto analogues of essential amino acids. *Am. J. Clin. Nutr.* 33:1660–1666.

Schloerb, P.R. (1966): Essential amino acid administration in uremia. *Am. J. Med. Sci.* 252:650–659.

Tischler, M.E., Desautels, M., and Goldberg, A.L. (1982): Does leucine, leucyl-tRNA, or some metabolite of leucine regulate protein synthesis and degradation in skeletal and cardiac muscle? *J. Biol. Chem.* 257:1613–1621.

Varcoe, R., Halliday, D., Carson, E.R., Richards, P., and Tavill, A.S. (1975): Efficiency of utilisation of urea nitrogen for albumin synthesis by chronically uremic and normal man. *Clin. Sci. Mol. Med.* 48:379–390.

Walser, M. (1978): Keto acid therapy in chronic renal failure. *Nephron* 21:57–74.

Walser, M. (1981): Conservative management of the uremic patient. In: *The Kidney,* (2nd edition) (eds: B. Brenner, F. Rector) pp.2383–2424, W.B. Saunders, Philadelphia.

Walser, M., Coulter, A.W., Dighe, S., and Crantz, F.R. (1973): The effect of keto-analogues of essential amino acids in severe chronic uremia. *J. Clin. Invest.* 52:678–690.

Walser, M., Lund, P., Ruderman, N.B., and Coulter, A.W. (1973): Synthesis of essential amino acids from their α-keto analogues by perfused rat liver and muscle. *J. Clin. Invest.* 52:2865–2877.

Walser, M., Sapir, D.G., Mitch, W.E., and Chan, W. (1981): Effects of branched chain ketoacids in normal subjects and patients. In: *Metabolism and Clinical Implications of Branched Chain Amino and Ketoacids,* (eds: M. Walser and J.R. Williamson) p.291, Elsevier/North Holland, New York.

27 Amino Acid Metabolism in Chronic Renal Failure

Joel D. Kopple

The plasma amino acid pattern in chronic renal failure is pathognomonic of this condition. This chapter will describe the alterations in plasma, red cell and muscle amino acid concentrations in uremia, the factors which may predispose to the abnormal patterns, and implications for treatment.

PLASMA AND TISSUE AMINO ACID CONCENTRATIONS

The postabsorptive plasma amino acid pattern of patients with chronic renal failure typically shows decreased concentrations of tryptophan, valine, and tyrosine, reduced ratios of essential/nonessential amino acids, tyrosine/phenylalanine, serine/glycine and valine/glycine, and increased concentrations of cystine, citrulline, N^{π}-methylhistidine (1-methylhistidine) and N^{τ}-methylhistidine (3-methylhistidine). Other amino acid concentrations are often normal but have been variably reported as being high or low. This amino acid pattern is present in clinically stable chronically uremic patients who are not dialyzed and in postabsorptive, predialysis specimens from patients who are undergoing maintenance hemodialysis. During hemodialysis treatment, plasma amino acids decrease transiently.

Red cell amino acid concentrations also are altered in nondialyzed chronically uremic patients and in those undergoing maintenance hemodialysis. In red cells from uremic patients and in predialysis specimens from hemodialysis patients, we found increased histidine, cystine, glutamate, glycine, ornithine, citrulline, taurine, N^{π}- and N^{τ}-methylhistidine concentrations and increased glycine-serine ratio (Flugel-Link et al., unpublished observations). Red cell valine, tyrosine and the tyrosine/phenylalanine and valine/glycine values were reduced. The altered amino acid pattern in red cells is similar to but not identical to that in plasma. During treatment with hemodialysis, red cell concentrations of many amino acids decreased, although not to the same magnitude as in plasma.

Muscle contains the largest pool of free amino acids and, hence, is of special interest for understanding amino acid metabolism in renal failure. Bergstrom and coworkers examined muscle intracellular amino acid concentrations in nondialyzed chronically uremic patients and patients undergoing maintenance intermittent peritoneal dialysis and hemodialysis (Bergstrom et al., 1978; Furst et al., 1980). In both groups of patients, there tended to be reduced muscle concentrations of threonine, valine, tyrosine and carnosine, and increased levels of phenylalanine, aspartate, ornithine, citrulline, arginine, and N^{π}-and N^{τ}-methylhistidine. Other amino acid concentrations were normal, increased or reduced depending on the type of diet ingested and the type of dialysis therapy, if any. The patients undergoing maintenance hemodialysis had increased muscle phenylalanine, lysine, histidine, alanine, glycine, aspartate, ornithine, citrulline and arginine concentrations. It is of interest that the altered patterns of plasma and muscle intracellular amino acid concentrations were not identical, suggesting that the transcellular movement of amino acids or the capacity to maintain intracellular gradients may be altered in renal failure. In the nondialyzed chronically uremic patients, supplementation of a low protein diet with specialized preparations of essential amino acids normalized concentrations of some amino acids in plasma and muscle (Furst et al., 1980).

CAUSES OF ALTERED AMINO ACID POOLS

General Causes

A number of investigators have examined the causes of altered amino acid levels in patients with chronic renal failure. These studies have been reviewed recently (Kopple and Jones, 1979), and it seems clear that there are many causes for the abnormal amino acid pattern.

The low protein intake or poor general nutrition of uremic patients is one cause of abnormal plasma amino acid concentrations. Kopple and Swendseid evaluated the effects of protein intake on plasma amino acid levels in patients with renal failure (Kopple and Swendseid, 1976; Kopple and Jones, 1979). Eleven normal and 18 chronically uremic subjects were fed high calorie diets providing 20, 40, or 60 g/day of protein primarily of high biological value. Seven patients undergoing maintenance hemodialysis were also fed diets varying in protein content. In most of the studies (79%), patients lived in a metabolic research ward for an average of 25 ± 12 (SD) days. The results indicated that plasma concentrations of some amino acids were altered in uremic patients *per se* and were not affected by protein intake. These included the elevated levels of cystine, citrulline and N^{π}- and N^{τ}-methylhistidine and low levels of tryptophan and the ratios of tyrosine/phenylalanine and serine/glycine. Other amino acid levels were primarily affected by low protein intakes. The low protein diets probably accounted for the decreased concentrations of histidine, isoleucine, leucine and lysine, the reduced ratios of essential/nonessential amino acids and the tendency for high glycine concentrations. Both renal failure and low protein diets contributed to the reduced concentrations of valine and tyrosine and the low valine/glycine ratio. If severe malnutrition supervenes, alterations of many other amino acids may occur. Indeed, the plasma amino acid pattern of chronically uremic patients has many similarities to that of patients with malnutrition. Plasma levels of some amino acids displayed a direct or inverse correlation with protein intake, and this relationship was often different in chronically uremic or hemodialysis patients as compared to normal subjects. Thus, the response of plasma concentrations of certain amino acids to protein restriction is also abnormal in uremia.

Another factor that can affect plasma amino acid pools is impaired renal metabolic activity. We studied this factor in a group of 11 normal and eight chronically uremic female mongrel dogs (Fukuda and Kopple, 1980a,b; Kopple and Fukuda, 1980). Renal failure was created in the uremic animals by repeated injections of uranyl nitrate. All dogs were fed one pound per day of horsemeat for four to seven days prior to the study. They were then fasted overnight and anesthetized with pentobarbital. A catheter was placed in the left renal vein, femoral artery, and left ureter. Renal blood flow was measured with para-aminohippurate; glomerular filtration rate was determined by the creatinine clearance. Dogs received an infusion of 0.45% sodium chloride, 5 ml/min, for 120 minutes and then an infusion for 120 minutes of 0.45% sodium chloride containing 22 different L-amino acids in quantities determined in previous studies to be sufficient to raise plasma amino acid concentrations to approximately postprandial levels. At the end of each of the two infusions, whole blood, plasma and urine were obtained for measurement of net production or utilization (Q_{met}) of amino acids and ammonia. The results of these studies are shown in Figure 27-1. During infusion of only salt solutions, which is considered to resemble the fasting state, there was net production of many amino acids from the kidney of the normal dogs. These included in greatest quantities alanine, serine and glutamate. Ammonia was also released, and there was net utilization, most prominently, of glutamine and glycine. After infusion of amino acids, the pattern changed dramatically. While there was a tendency toward net production of many amino acids during infusion of only electrolyte, in general, many amino acids were taken up during administration of amino acids. During this latter infusion, there was significant utilization of glutamine, alanine, lysine, glycine and the three branched-chain amino acids, valine, leucine and isoleucine, and aspartate and taurine.

The results for the uremic dogs are compared to the normal animals in Figure 27-2. It is clear that the pattern of response to infusion of 0.45% sodium chloride and amino acids in the two groups of animals was similar. However, there was a tendency for less net production of amino acids and ammonia during the infusion of only electrolytes and less net utilization of amino acids during the amino acid infusion. When these differences were factored by the creatinine clearance to normalize the results for the glomerular filtration rate, the ratio of the Q_{met}/creatinine clearance (fractional Q_{met}) for amino acids and ammonia in the uremic dogs tended

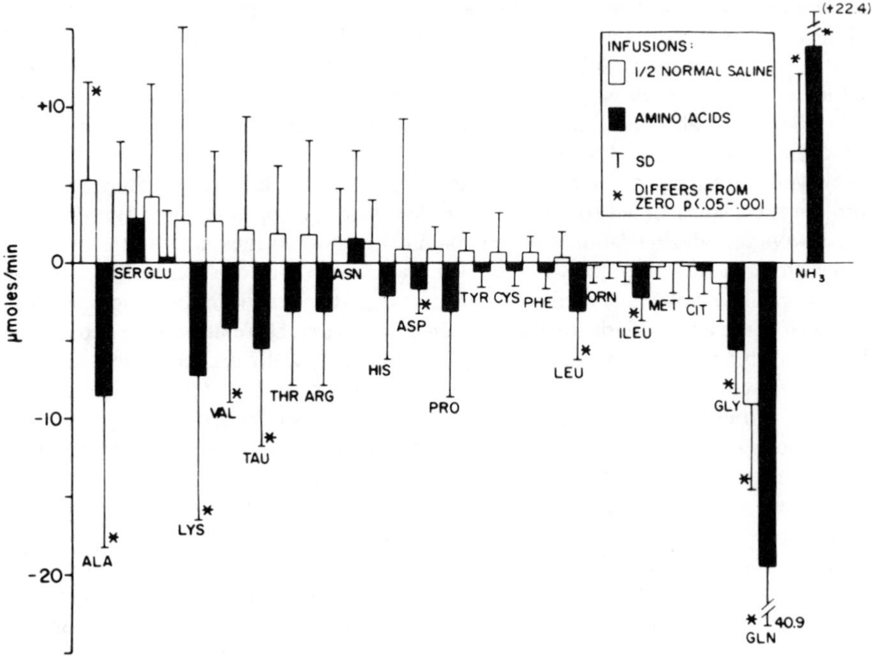

Figure 27-1 Net production (+) and utilization (−) of amino acids and ammonia (Q_{met}) by the left kidney in 11 adult female mongrel dogs with normal renal function who received infusions first with half-normal saline (white columns) and then with half-normal saline and amino acids (black columns). Bars represent the mean value; brackets indicate standard deviation. Asterisks depict values for Q_{met} which are significantly different from zero ($p < 0.05$ to $p < 0.001$). Reprinted from Kopple and Fukuda (1980) with permission.

to be equal to or greater than normal. These data suggest that during infusion of 0.45% sodium chloride in the chronically uremic dogs, the Q_{met} for many amino acids and ammonia were qualitatively similar to normal. After infusion of amino acids, the Q_{met} tended to change in the same direction as in the normal dogs. During infusion of 0.45% sodium chloride or amino acids, net production or utilization of amino acids by the kidneys of uremic dogs, when adjusted for the reduction in glomerular filtration rate, was usually equal to or greater than in the normal dogs.

Altered Metabolism of Specific Amino Acids

Serine and glycine The foregoing data also suggest that the impairment in renal metabolic activity may lead to altered plasma pools of some amino acids. An example of this is the plasma serine and glycine levels. As in humans, uremic dogs have a tendency toward lower plasma serine and higher plasma glycine levels, and the ratio of plasma serine to glycine is markedly reduced. There is a direct correlation between the serine/glycine ratio and the creatinine clearance in the normal and uremic dogs (Figure 27-3). Moreover, the Q_{met} for serine correlates directly with

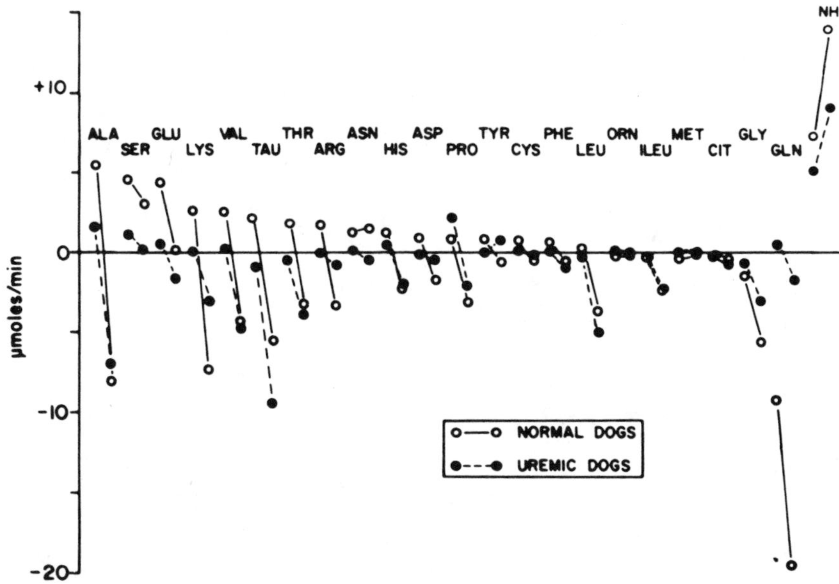

Figure 27-2 The mean renal Q_{met} for individual amino acids and ammonia in 11 normal (open circles) and eight chronically uremic (closed circles) adult female dogs. Dogs were infused first with 0.45% sodium chloride (half-normal saline) and then with 0.45% sodium chloride and amino acids. Lines connect the Q_{met} values for a single amino acid during the two infusions. Positive values indicate net production; negative values represent net utilization. Reprinted from Kopple and Fukuda (1980) with permission.

creatinine clearance ($r = 0.74$, $p < 0.001$). In addition, the Q_{met} for serine is inversely correlated with the Q_{met} for glycine ($r = -0.49$, $p < 0.01$). These data suggest that the altered ratio of serine/glycine in renal failure is due to the impaired conversion of glycine to serine by the kidney. Pitts and MacLeod (1972) demonstrated that the kidney converts glycine to serine and is a major source of serine in the body. Our studies also suggest that there is a relationship between renal function and plasma serine and glycine levels.

The data of Tizianello and co-workers are pertinent to this question (Tizianello et al., 1980a,b; De Ferrari et al., 1982). These investigators measured arterial-venous differences in whole blood across different organs in patients with normal renal function and in patients with moderate to advanced renal failure (glomerular filtration rates from about 6 to 33 ml/min•1.73m²). Patients were studied during diagnostic evaluation of various medical disorders. Catheters were placed in a peripheral artery and hepatic vein, the aorta and internal jugular vein, or the femoral artery and renal vein. The arterial-venous concentrations across the splanchnia measured the differences in amino acid concentrations across the liver and the nonhepatic splanchnia combined. For the renal studies, the renal blood flow was also measured, and therefore Q_{met} for the kidney could be determined. In contrast, only arterial-venous differences were measured for the splanchnia and brain; consequently, amino acid balances for these latter two organ systems could not be assessed, and only the net direction of uptake or release could be determined. The results are shown in Table 27-1.

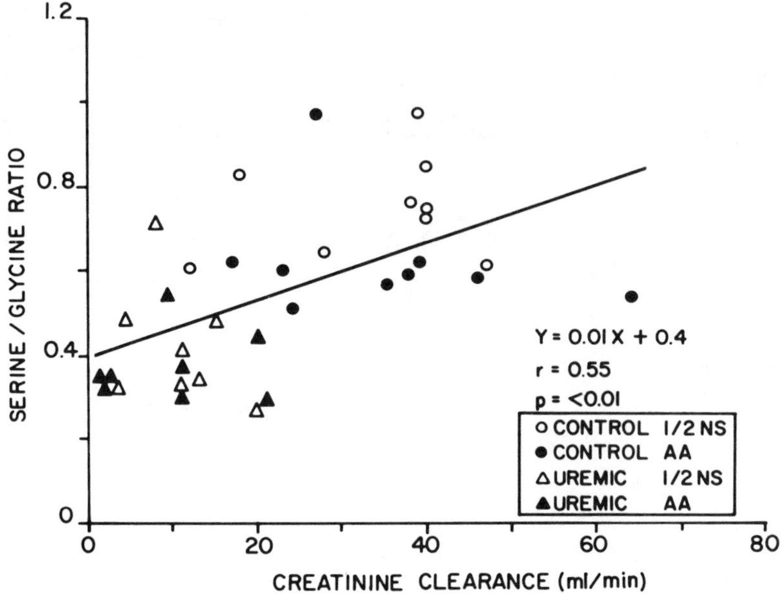

Figure 27-3 Direct correlation between the plasma ratio of serine/glycine and the creatinine clearance in female dogs with normal renal function (open symbols) and dogs with chronic renal failure (black symbols). Circles represent data obtained during infusion of half-normal saline. Triangles indicate values during administration of 0.45% sodium chloride (half-normal saline) and amino acids. Reprinted from Fukuda and Kopple (1980b) with permission.

These researchers found net uptake of glycine from the splanchnia and brain (1980b, 1982), but no net uptake or release from the kidney in the patients with either normal renal function or renal insufficiency (1980a). Serine was taken up from the splanchnia in the patients with normal renal function and from the brain in the patients with both normal and impaired renal function. In contrast, there was net production of serine by the kidney in patients with normal renal function and, to a lesser extent, in those with renal insufficiency. These data also suggest that a reduced serine output from the failing kidney may lead to a low plasma serine level and a low plasma ratio of serine to glycine. In advanced renal failure or in the anephric state, it is not known which organs provide serine to the extracellular pools.

Phenylalanine and tyrosine The following lines of evidence indicate that the conversion of phenylalanine to tyrosine is impaired in renal failure (Kopple et al., 1972; Pickford et al., 1973; Jones et al., 1978): 1) plasma tyrosine concentrations are often decreased; 2) the ratio of tyrosine to phenylalanine is impaired in plasma, muscle and red cells. Phenylalanine loading tests and studies of ^{14}C-phenylalanine kinetics indicate decreased metabolic clearance and impaired oxidation of phenylalanine. In contrast, load tests and analysis of ^{14}C-tyrosine kinetics indicate that tyrosine metabolism is normal in patients with renal failure.

Wang et al. (1975) assayed the *in vitro* activities of the enzyme phenylalanine hydroxylase, which catalyzes the hydroxylation of phenylalanine to tyrosine, and tyrosine aminotransferase, which catalyzes the first step along the main degradative pathway for tyrosine. Activities of these enzymes in liver homogenates were normal

Table 27-1
Splanchnic and Brain Arterial-Venous Differences and Net Renal Production or Utilization (Q_{met}) for Amino Acids in Subjects with Normal Renal Function or Chronic Renal Failure (CRF)*†‡

	Peripheral artery minus hepatic vein, μmol/L			Renal Q_{met} μmol/min/1.73m²			Peripheral artery minus internal jugular vein, μmol/L		
	Control	*CRF*	p§	*Control*	*CRF*	p§	*Control*	*CRF*	p§
Number of Subjects	6	6		8	5		8	6	
Essential									
Histidine	5.1 ± 1.5‖¶	4.9 ± 1.3¶		−3.5 ± 1.6	0.1 ± 0.5		1.3 ± 0.6	0.4 ± 1.4	
Isoleucine	1.6 ± 0.9	1.3 ± 1.6		1.4 ± 1.4	0.4 ± 0.3		3.1 ± 0.6#	1.5 ± 0.6¶	< 0.1
Leucine	4.8 ± 1.2¶	5.2 ± 2.3¶		−0.3 ± 2.3	−1.0 ± 0.6		6.1 ± 0.7**	4.8 ± 0.6**	
Lysine	10.7 ± 2.5#	7.3 ± 2.8¶		−3.3 ± 1.2¶	−0.9 ± 0.4¶		3.2 ± 1.0¶	3.6 ± 1.6¶	
Phenylalanine	9.0 ± 2.4¶	7.6 ± 1.9¶		1.3 ± 0.6¶	0.2 ± 0.5		1.3 ± 0.6	1.2 ± 0.6	
Threonine	12.8 ± 3.4¶	6.6 ± 2.0¶		−5.0 ± 1.7¶	−0.8 ± 0.4¶		2.0 ± 1.0	3.9 ± 1.8	
Valine	8.5 ± 0.8**	2.9 ± 1.3	< 0.005	−0.2 ± 3.2	−0.5 ± 0.8		9.0 ± 1.7#	4.0 ± 1.3¶	< 0.05
Semiessential									
Cystine							2.9 ± 0.3**	6.2 ± 1.5#	< 0.025
Tyrosine	8.1 ± 1.0**	5.3 ± 1.1#		−4.2 ± 1.4¶	−1.3 ± 0.4¶		0.7 ± 0.6	−0.1 ± 0.4	

Table 27-1 (continued)

	Peripheral artery minus hepatic vein, μmol/L		p§	Renal Q_{met} μmol/min/1.73m²		p§	Peripheral artery minus internal jugular vein, μmol/L		p§
	Control	*CRF*		*Control*	*CRF*		*Control*	*CRF*	
Nonessential									
Alanine	72.9 ± 5.0**	81.9 ± 9.8**		−10.6 ± 5.3	−4.1 ± 1.6¶		−0.1 ± 1.5	0.6 ± 3.6	
Arginine	9.7 ± 1.7#	6.7 ± 1.2#		−7.0 ± 1.2**	−2.7 ± 1.0¶	<0.05	1.9 ± 1.0	−1.3 ± 1.4	
Asparagine							0.9 ± 0.7	−0.1 ± 1.0	
Aspartate	−4.2 ± 2.1	−8.0 ± 4.6		1.2 ± 4.1	1.4 ± 1.1		2.1 ± 1.2	2.1 ± 2.4	
Citrulline	−6.0 ± 1.3#	−1.9 ± 1.5		6.9 ± 1.6#	2.9 ± 1.1**		1.6 ± 0.7	1.5 ± 0.7	
Glutamate	−64.1 ± 7.8**	−47.5 ± 12.9¶		−4.6 ± 3.2	−0.7 ± 0.6		2.3 ± 1.1	−0.5 ± 2.5	
Glutamine	73.2 ± 12.1**	39.7 ± 13.9¶		31.8 ± 6.4**	3.2 ± 1.5¶	<0.01	13.4 ± 4.5¶	−1.0 ± 4.0	<0.05
Glycine	19.1 ± 4.9#	20.8 ± 5.8#		2.7 ± 4.6	−0.3 ± 0.9		5.2 ± 1.1¶	11.7 ± 2.8¶	<0.05
Ornithine	2.5 ± 1.6	1.5 ± 1.6		−3.5 ± 1.7¶	0.03 ± 0.2		1.1 ± 0.5	3.0 ± 1.4	
Proline	7.1 ± 5.4	22.7 ± 7.4¶		14.6 ± 6.0¶	2.3 ± 0.6¶		6.1 ± 1.7#	5.6 ± 1.5¶	
Serine	14.3 ± 4.1#	2.0 ± 1.6	<0.02	−24.2 ± 4.0**	−5.3 ± 1.8#	<0.01	3.7 ± 1.1¶	3.4 ± 1.2¶	
Taurine	4.8 ± 6.0	10.4 ± 12.1		−6.8 ± 2.5¶	−1.9 ± 1.6		7.9 ± 4.7	0.6 ± 6.1	

*Measurements were made in whole blood.

†Adapted from Tizianello et al. (1980a, b) and De Ferrari et al. (1981).

‡Minus sign in front of number indicates net release or production of an amino acid; no sign indicates net uptake or utilization of an amino acid.

§Probability of no difference between control and chronically azotemic patients.

‖Mean ± standard error.

Probability that value is not significantly different from zero; ¶$p < 0.05$, #$p < 0.01$, **$p < 0.001$.

in chronically uremic rats as compared with pair-fed controls. However, phenylalanine hydroxylase activity in the kidney of uremic rats was reduced. The activity of this enzyme in the kidney is small and would seem to be insignificant relative to that of the liver (Ayling et al., 1975). However, Young and Parsons (1973) have reported that sera from uremic patients inhibit hepatic phenylalanine hydroxylase activity in normal rats by a mean of 15%. It is not clear whether this effect is sufficient to account for impaired conversion of phenylalanine to tyrosine in renal failure.

Fukuda and Kopple (1980a,b) found a small but significant net production of tyrosine by the kidney of normal dogs but not uremic dogs. Tizianello and coworkers (1980a) reported net uptake of phenylalanine and release of tyrosine by the kidney of the patients with normal renal function (Table 27-1). In the patients with renal failure, there was no uptake or release of phenylalanine, and tyrosine release was substantially reduced. There was net uptake of phenylalanine and tyrosine from the splanchnia in patients with normal and impaired renal function and no uptake or release from the brain of these patients (Tizianello et al., 1980b, De Ferrari et al., 1982). These observations suggest that the failure of renal metabolic activity may indeed play a role in the altered conversion of phenylalanine to tyrosine in uremic patients.

Citrulline and arginine Normally, the liver releases citrulline. The kidney has the enzymatic apparatus to convert citrulline to arginine. Featherston et al. (1973) reported that in rats, citrulline was taken up by the kidney which in turn released arginine. In previous studies in humans, the data concerning the uptake of citrulline and release of arginine by the normal kidney were not conclusive (Felig et al., 1969; Owen and Robinson, 1963). Chan et al. (1974) found in uremic rats that *in vitro* activity of ornithine transcarbamoylase in liver was increased and activity of arginine synthetase in kidney was decreased, whether calculated per milligram of protein or per total kidney mass. Liver arginase activity was decreased or increased in the uremic rats depending on the protein intake. In our normal and uremic dogs, we found a tendency for the kidney to produce arginine and utilize citrulline during infusion of 0.45% sodium chloride only when the Q_{met} was calculated from the plasma data (Fukuda and Kopple, 1980a,b). When calculated from the whole blood values, the Q_{met} was not significantly different from zero. Tizianello et al. (1980a) found that citrulline was taken up and arginine was released by the kidney of patients with normal renal function and in those with renal insufficiency; ornithine was also released from the normal kidney. The renal uptake of citrulline and release of arginine and ornithine were reduced in the patients with renal insufficiency. There was also net uptake of arginine and release of citrulline from the splanchnia of the patients with normal and impaired renal function and net splanchnic uptake of arginine from the patients with renal insufficiency (Tizianello et al., 1980b). There was no brain uptake or release of these amino acids (De Ferrari et al., 1982). These data support the thesis that in patients with renal failure, the elevated citrulline levels are due to impaired conversion of this amino acid to arginine in the failing kidney. The cause for the absent citrulline release from the splanchnia of the azotemic patients merits further investigation.

Hydroxyproline and proline Plasma total, free and peptide-bound hydroxyproline may be elevated in renal failure (Koevoet, 1965; Dubovsky et al., 1968). Impaired urinary excretion of these compounds may contribute to the elevated plasma concentrations. Collagen is a major reservoir for hydroxyproline and in conditions of enhanced bone reabsorption, such as during renal osteodystrophy, there may be increased release of hydroxyproline from bone. Hence, urine-free and peptide-bound hydroxyproline may also be elevated in renal failure (Koevoet, 1965, Kivirikko, 1970). A direct correlation has been observed between the severity of renal osteodystrophy and the degree of elevation of plasma-free and peptide hydroxyproline concentrations (Dubovsky et al., 1968; Koevoet, 1965). However, Avioli et al. (1969) have suggested that impaired activity of hepatic hydroxyproline oxidase contributes to increased plasma-free hydroxyproline. It has been suggested that osteodystrophy may be a cause of increased plasma proline concentrations in renal failure (Bishop et al., 1971).

Histidine Interest in histidine metabolism in uremia was stimulated by the observation that plasma histidine is sometimes low and the observation of Bergstrom et al. (1970) that addition of histidine to histidine-free diets improved nitrogen balance in uremic patients. Giordano et al. (1972) added histidine to histidine-free diets in two chronically uremic patients and observed increased incorporation of ^{14}C-leucine into the globin moiety of hemoglobin (1972).

Kopple and Swendseid (1975) reported evidence that histidine is an essential amino acid in both chronically uremic and normal men. When such subjects were fed histidine-devoid diets, there was an abrupt decrease in plasma histidine, nitrogen balance gradually became negative, and muscle-free histidine, serum albumin and hematocrit fell. In addition, a clinical syndrome developed which included malaise, anorexia, nausea, agitation, memory loss, confusion and a skin eruption that resembled asteatosis. Addition of histidine to the diet reversed this syndrome. Other investigators now have also provided evidence that histidine is an essential amino acid (Anderson et al., 1977; Cho et al., 1977; Wixom et al., 1977).

There is a question as to whether the metabolism of histidine is altered in renal failure. Furst et al. (1972) examined this question by giving ^{15}N-urea or ^{15}N-ammonium chloride to one normal subject, one catabolic patient, and two chronically uremic patients. They were able to identify the ^{15}N-label in histidine from plasma or muscle protein in the normal and catabolic subjects but not in the uremic patients. These data imply that synthesis of the ketoacid analogue of histidine, imidazolepyruvic acid, and/or transamination of this compound to form histidine does not occur normally in uremic patients. However, Giordano et al. (1968) gave ^{15}N-urea to normal and uremic individuals and found the ^{15}N-label in histidine obtained from plasma albumin in both groups of subjects.

Sheng et al. (1977) fed ^{15}N-ammonium chloride to a normal man receiving parenteral nutrition without histidine (1977). They detected the ^{15}N-label in both the alpha-amino nitrogen and in the imidazole ring from histidine and N^{τ}-methylhistidine isolated from globin or urine. These observations suggest that some histidine may be synthesized in normal humans at least during histidine deficiency, although it is possible that this synthesis occurs in intestinal bacteria.

Histidine is reported to be released from the kidney in dogs, pregnant sheep and rats in some, but not all, studies (Bergman et al., 1974; Fukuda and Kopple, 1980a,b; Squires et al., 1976). We found that less histidine was released into the renal venous plasma from dogs with chronic renal failure caused by administration of uranyl nitrate as compared to normal dogs (Fukuda and Kopple, 1980a,b). Curiously, there was no significant release of histidine from the kidney when values were measured in whole blood rather than in plasma. Plasma histidine concentrations were also decreased in renal venous plasma from the normal dogs. The kidney contains carnosinase, which catalyzes the hydrolysis of carnosine (beta-alanylhistidine). When dogs are infused with carnosine, there is a marked increase in the release of histidine from the kidney (Fukuda and Kopple, 1979). Tizianello et al. (1980a) described a slight, but not significant release of histidine from the kidney of normal individuals but not patients with chronic renal insufficiency (Table 27-1). Thus, it is possible, but not proven, that in patients with renal failure, loss of renal biochemical activity might also affect histidine metabolism by leading to a reduction in the release of histidine from the kidney.

There is also evidence from chronically uremic rats for altered histidine metabolism (Schmid et al., 1978). In comparison to sham-operated, pair-fed controls, these uremic rats had normal plasma histidine, reduced muscle histidine, and elevated brain histidine and its decarboxylation product, histamine. On the other hand, we observed no differences between normal and chronically uremic subjects in the metabolism of histidine, using tracer ^{14}C-histidine and, in preliminary studies, in the dietary requirements for histidine (Kopple et al., 1977; Kopple and Swendseid, 1981; Jones et al., 1982). Also, although plasma histidine concentrations are sometimes reduced in chronically uremic patients, when compared to normal individuals fed the same 20, 40 or 60 g protein diets, the fasting plasma histidine levels were similar to normals at each level of protein intake (Kopple and Swendseid, unpublished observations). There was a direct correlation between postabsorptive morning plasma histidine levels and the 24-hour urinary histidine excretion in normal and chronically uremic individuals (Kopple and Swendseid, 1981). However, for each level of plasma histidine, the amount of urinary histidine was lower in the uremic patients. The urinary clearance of histidine is reported to be directly correlated with inulin clearance (Whitehouse et al., 1975). However, the percent of tubular reabsorption of histidine falls and thus fractional excretion rises as the glomerular filtration rate decreases (Gulyassy et al., 1970; Whitehouse et al., 1975).

Although some investigators have reported improvement in hematocrit in uremic patients supplemented with histidine (Giordano et al., 1973, Jontofsohn et al., 1975), other workers have been unable to confirm these findings (Blumenkrantz et al., 1975).

N^{π}-methylhistidine and N^{τ}-methylhistidine N^{π}-methylhistidine (1-methylhistidine) and N^{τ}-methylhistidine (3-methylhistidine) are normally excreted in the urine and are increased in uremic plasma, red cells and muscle (Bergstrom et al., 1978; Kopple and Swendseid, 1981; Flugel-Link et al., unpublished observations). N^{τ}-methylhistidine is formed after histidine is incorporated into protein, primarily in muscle (Young et al., 1972). When protein is degraded, the released N^{τ}-methylhistidine is believed to be nonreutilizable and is excreted in the urine. Urinary excretion of this compound is considered to be an indicator of the absolute rate of muscle protein degradation. Although increased serum levels in clinically stable, chronically uremic patients reflect impaired urinary excretion, urinary N^{τ}-methylhistidine excretion is reduced in chronically uremic patients even when serum concentrations appear stable (Kopple and Swendseid, 1981). Decreased urinary N^{τ}-methylhistidine does not appear to be due to the lower protein intake of uremic patients because the excretion is reduced even when comparisons are made between normal and uremic subjects ingesting the same amino acid diets that contain no meat, which is a source of N^{τ}-methylhistidine. Decreased urinary excretion of N^{τ}-methylhistidine in uremia may be due to reduced muscle mass or turnover. Alternatively, elevated plasma N^{τ}-methylhistidine levels in uremic patients might predispose to degradation or incorporation into larger molecules.

Cystine Cystine is consistently elevated in the plasma of uremic patients. Cohen et al. (1977) reported elevated plasma and urinary levels of homocysteine, a metabolic intermediate between methionine and cystine. Vitamin B_6 is a co-factor for enzymes involved with the formation and metabolism of cystine, and vitamin B_6 deficiency has been described in renal failure (Kopple et al., 1981). Whether deficiency or altered metabolism or function of this vitamin contributes to elevated cystine levels is not known.

Tryptophan Plasma tryptophan levels are decreased in renal failure. Tryptophan differs from other amino acids in plasma in that a substantial fraction is bound to protein (De Torrente et al., 1974). In renal failure, low plasma total tryptophan appears to be due to decreased binding to albumin, and plasma concentrations of unbound tryptophan may be increased (Gulyassy et al., 1972). The quantity of tryptophan transported into brain is affected by the ratio of plasma total tryptophan to five other neutral amino acids, valine, leucine, isoleucine, phenylalanine and tyrosine, that compete for the same blood-brain transport system (Fernstrom and Wurtman, 1972). Whether in uremia the low ratio of tryptophan to these five competing amino acids may alter the transport of tryptophan across the blood-brain barrier, the synthesis of tryptophan metabolites and brain function is not known.

EFFECT OF DIETARY NUTRITION ON ALTERED AMINO ACID CONCENTRATIONS

Effect of Low Nitrogen Diets on Plasma and Muscle Amino Acid Concentrations

It has been suggested that altered amino acid pools might contribute to wasting, malnutrition, and abnormal metabolism in chronically uremic patients. We assessed the effect of different low protein and amino acid diets on plasma and muscle amino acid concentrations in uremic patients (Kopple, 1978; Kopple et al., 1981). Studies were conducted in nine normal men, in 11 men and two women with chronic renal failure who were not receiving dialysis therapy (serum creatinine 10 ± 2 mg/dl) and four men undergoing maintenance hemodialysis. The mean age of these three groups of subjects combined was 54 years, and the differences in age among the three groups were not significant. Five of the normal men ingested food *ad libitum;* the other normal men ate diets providing 0.55 to 0.60 g/kg•day of primarily high quality protein in a clinical study center. All of the nondialyzed chronically uremic patients were studied after they had ingested one or more of the following four high calorie diets while they lived in a clinical study center: a diet providing 0.55 to 0.60 g/kg of protein primarily of high biological value (HBV protein, nine patients); a diet providing 0.55 to 0.60 g/kg of amino acids proportioned as in the egg pattern (Egg pattern, seven patients); 21 g/day of a mixture of the nine essential amino acids and about 22 g/day of protein (EAA-protein, eight patients) as described by Bergstrom et al. (1975); or a diet providing 0.47 g/kg•day of essential amino acids (EAA, eight patients). Details of the study have been described previously (Kopple, 1978; Kopple et al., 1981). For some of the chronically uremic patients, amino acids were measured in plasma but not in muscle. Patients undergoing maintenance hemodialysis had received dialysis treatment for 26 months (range 12 to 45) at the time that plasma or muscle amino acids were obtained. The dialysis patients were prescribed a diet providing about 1.0 g protein/kg•day and about 35 cal/kg•day. Blood specimens and muscle biopsies were obtained between 8:00 AM and 10:30 AM in patients who had been fasting overnight. Plasma and muscle were prepared and analyzed for amino acids as described previously (Kopple et al., 1981). Diets were supplemented with vitamins, minerals and trace elements. Mean dietary nitrogen intake was 6.0 ± 0.7 g/day with the HBV protein diet, 5.4 ± 0.7 g/day with the Egg pattern diet, 5.8 ± 0.2 g/day with the EAA-protein diet and 4.2 ± 0.5 g/day with the 4.7 g/kg EAA diet. Energy intake was 35 kcal/kg•day in both the normal and uremic individuals.

In the chronically uremic patients, nitrogen balance was neutral or slightly positive with all four diets, although there were occasional patients who were in negative nitrogen balance. Urea nitrogen appearance tended to be lower with the EAA-protein diet and was lowest with the EAA diet. The plasma total essential and nonessential amino acids were often abnormal with all four diets in the chronically uremic patients (Figure 27-4). Total plasma essential amino acids were significantly low with the HBV protein and EAA-protein diets while the total nonessential amino acids were significantly increased with the Egg pattern diet. The ratio of essential to nonessential amino acids was also often decreased with all four diets, and the mean values were significantly reduced with the HBV protein, Egg pattern amino acid, and EAA-protein diets. There was no difference in the plasma total essential or total nonessential amino acids or the essential/nonessential ratio among the four diet groups.

Many individual amino acid concentrations were abnormal in the plasma or muscle of these patients with all four diets. With regard to the branched-chain amino acids, plasma isoleucine and valine were decreased in the chronically uremic patients fed the HBV protein diet. Plasma leucine was reduced in the chronically uremic patients with each of the four diets. No branched-chain amino acid was decreased in the plasma of the hemodialysis patients. There were no significant differences in branched-chain amino acid concentrations between any two groups of patients with chronic renal failure or between groups of chronically uremic patients and subjects undergoing maintenance hemodialysis. However, in the chronically uremic patients, the plasma concentrations of each of the branched-chain amino acids tended to be greater with the Egg pattern, EAA-protein and EAA diets, which had the highest concentrations of these three amino acids.

The intracellular muscle amino acid concentrations are shown as percent of normal in Figure 27-5, although statistical analyses were performed on the absolute values with the student's t test. Intracellular muscle isoleucine and leucine concentrations did not differ among the groups. However, mean muscle isoleucine levels tended to be normal or increased in the chronically uremic patients who received the EAA-protein and EAA diets, which had the highest branched-chain amino acid content (Kopple et al., 1981), and in the hemodialysis patients. In contrast, the mean values for leucine tended to be less than normal in each group of patients. In the chronically uremic patients ingesting the HBV protein diet, muscle intracellular valine concentrations were significantly lower than in the normal subjects or in the patients ingesting the EAA-protein or EAA diets. For each branched-chain amino acid, muscle levels tended to rise as dietary intake of that amino acid increased.

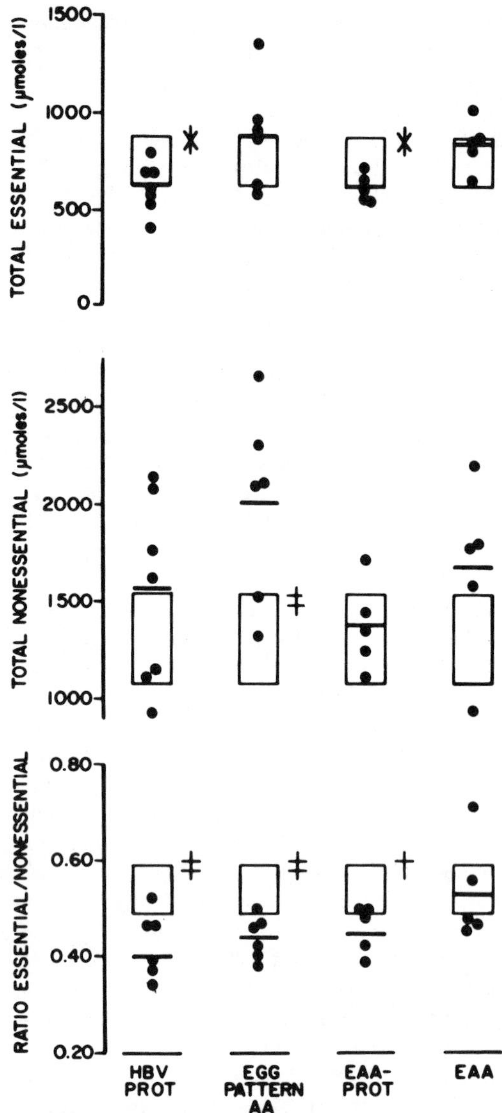

Figure 27-4 Postabsorptive plasma total essential amino acids, nonessential amino acids and ratio of essential/nonessential amino acids in chronically uremic patients fed low nitrogen diets. Diets provided 39 g/day of primarily high biological value protein (HBV protein), 44 g/day of essential and nonessential amino acids in the egg pattern (Egg pattern AA), 21 g/day of the nine essential amino acids and 22 g/day of protein (EAA-protein) or 30 g/day of the nine essential amino acids (EAA). Circles represent individual values obtained during the last one to three days of study with each diet. Horizontal bars indicate the mean values for the uremic patients with each diet. The vertical columns indicate the range of values within one standard deviation of the mean for normal subjects. The asterisk, single cross, and double cross next to the vertical columns indicate the probability that the values for the uremic patients are not different from normal subjects; $p < 0.05$, $p < 0.01$, and $p < 0.001$, respectively. Reprinted from Kopple (1978) with permission.

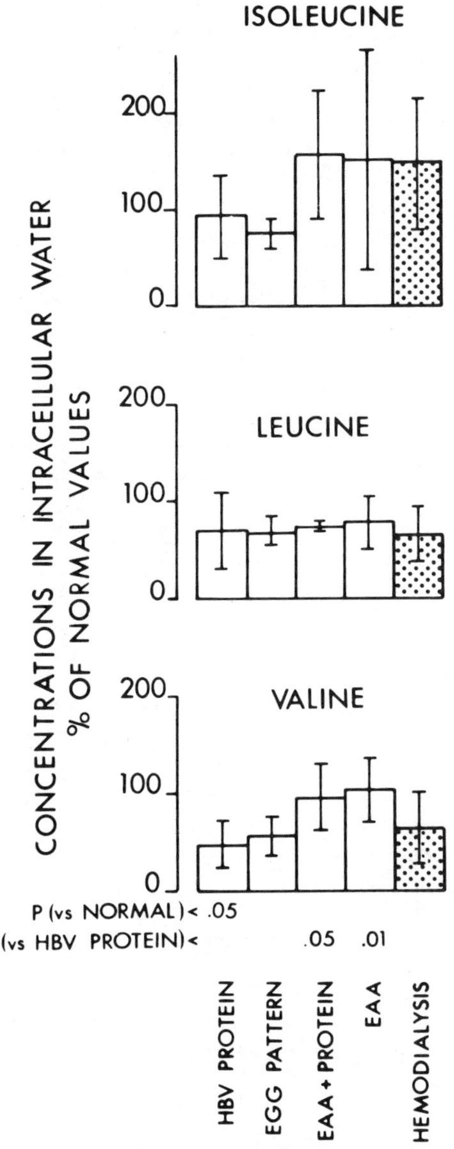

Figure 27-5 Mean postabsorptive muscle intracellular branched-chain amino acid concentrations in six chronically uremic patients fed 0.55 to 0.60 g/kg•day of primarily high quality protein, four patients fed 40 g/day of essential and nonessential amino acids in the egg pattern, four patients fed 21 g/day of essential amino acids and 22 g/day of protein, five patients fed 0.47 g/kg•day of essential amino acids, and four patients undergoing maintenance hemodialysis. Values are expressed as percent of normal intracellular concentrations determined in six normal men. Vertical columns indicate mean values; brackets represent one standard deviation. Reprinted from Kopple et al. (1981) with permission.

These studies indicate that in patients with renal failure, plasma and muscle concentrations of individual and total amino acids may be increased, normal or reduced depending upon the amino acid in question and the dietary intake of that amino acid. Although the diets providing greater quantities of the essential amino acids may raise some of the amino acid levels to normal values, no dietary formulation normalized all of the amino acid concentrations in plasma or muscle. Moreover, there was often a wide range of amino acid concentrations among the patients fed one diet. Thus, even when the mean value for an amino acid level was normal with a given diet formulation, there were some patients with excessively high or low values for that amino acid.

The studies of Bergstrom, Alvestrand and Furst are pertinent in this regard. These investigators describe an abnormal muscle intracellular amino acid pattern in uremia which differs from the alterations present in plasma (Alvestrand et al., 1978; Bergstrom et al., 1978; Furst et al., 1980).

The altered muscle amino acid pattern was not normalized by low protein diets, diets providing 18 g/day of miscellaneous protein supplemented with the nine essential amino acids proportioned in the Rose pattern, or with hemodialysis. It was of particular interest that despite a high intake of essential amino acids in the Rose pattern, muscle intracellular valine, phenylalanine, threonine, and tyrosine remained low while lysine and histidine concentrations were greater than normal. The muscle intracellular concentrations of the urea cycle amino acids citrulline, ornithine and arginine were each increased in each group of uremic patients studied. Plasma concentrations of certain amino acids were not uncommonly normal in the presence of altered muscle amino acid levels.

The authors then examined the use of a new pattern of amino acid supplementation with the 18-g protein diet. In the new formulation, there was a higher proportion of threonine and valine, and tyrosine was added. With tryptophan taken as the reference amino acid, the proportions of the other essential amino acids, histidine, leucine, isoleucine, lysine, methionine and phenylalanine, were reduced. The non-dialyzed chronically uremic patients fed this new formulation showed a normalization of muscle intracellular histidine, threonine, valine, and tyrosine concentrations, although lysine was still elevated in plasma and muscle, and histidine was increased in plasma.

These studies of Furst and co-workers indicate that the altered concentrations of some amino acids in uremic patients may be normalized with special amino acid formulations.

IMPLICATIONS FOR TREATMENT

Altering the Dietary Intake of Specific Amino Acids

The foregoing studies indicate that in chronically uremic patients, including those undergoing dialysis therapy, the amino acid pools in plasma, red cells, muscle and probably other tissues are altered. There are many causes for these alterations which include poor nutrition and alterations in synthesis, metabolism and possibly the ability to maintain transcellular concentration gradients for certain amino acids.

Preliminary studies suggest that the plasma and muscle concentrations of some amino acids can be normalized in chronically uremic patients by major changes in their dietary intake of amino acids. However, there is no evidence that altering dietary intake of these amino acids also corrects the underlying metabolic disorders. Also, it has not been demonstrated that uremic patients undergo clinical improvement when their plasma or muscle amino acid patterns are made more normal, although the possibility has been raised that their nitrogen balance becomes more positive (Furst et al., 1980). Moreover, the amino acid or ketoacid preparations used for uremic patients do not normalize the concentrations of every amino acid.

At the present time, almost all information concerning amino acid concentrations in clinically stable chronically uremic patients have been obtained during the postabsorptive state or before and after dialysis therapy. It would seem important to examine the effect of special amino acid formulations on the amino acid concentrations at other times of the day and during such conditions as the postprandial state, sleep or exercise.

Current evidence does suggest that histidine is an essential amino acid and should be included in amino acid preparations for uremic patients (Bergstrom et al., 1970; Giordano et al, 1972; Kopple and Swendseid, 1975). The beneficial effects of tyrosine in nonuremic individuals (see Wurtman, this publication) may indicate a role for this amino acid in the amino acid formulations for uremic patients, especially since there is impaired synthesis of tyrosine from phenylalanine in renal failure. Although the synthesis of arginine may be altered in renal failure (Chan et al., 1974), a dietary need for this amino acid has not yet been demonstrated in this condition, unless the patients receive large intakes of amino acids (e.g., greater than 50 to 60 g/day). The finding in uremic patients that plasma total tryptophan concentrations are decreased and free tryptophan is elevated may indicate that brain serotonin metabolism is abnormal. There may be a role for altering dietary intake of tryptophan and the five competing amino acids (valine, leucine, isoleucine, phenylalanine, and tyrosine) in order to normalize the transport of tryptophan into the brain (Fernstrom and Wurtman, 1972) and the metabolism of this amino acid and serotonin in the central nervous system.

Therapy with Diets Containing Amino Acids, Ketoacids or Hydroxyacids

Many researchers have reported beneficial effects in chronically uremic patients who have been fed semisynthetic low protein diets supplemented with the nine essential amino acids, or a mixture of calcium or sodium salts of ketoacid or hydroxyacid analogues of five essential amino acids (isoleucine, leucine, methionine, phenylalanine, and valine) and small quantities of the other essential amino acids (Furst et al., 1980; Walser, 1975; Walser et al., 1973). These diets generally contain 16 to 24 g of mixed quality protein and 10 to 21 g of the essential amino acids or approximately 12 g of ketoacid or hydroxyacid salts and about 2.4 g of essential amino acids. Diets containing essential amino acids or mixtures of essential and nonessential amino acids but virtually no protein have also been used (Kopple, 1978). In addition, newer formulations containing compounds of ketoacids or hydroxyacids bound to specific amino acids are currently under study for the treatment of uremic patients.

The potential advantages of these diets are related to the possibility that they may decrease uremic toxicity, improve nutritional status, and correct disorders in amino acid metabolism. In comparison to very low protein diets (i.e., 25 g protein/day or less), these semisynthetic diets seem to be utilized more efficiently for maintaining nitrogen balance and decreasing urea nitrogen appearance. This enhanced efficiency may be related to the greater proportions of protein given as essential amino acids or the ketoacid or hydroxyacid precursors, the lower quantities of nonamino acid nitrogen, the greater quantities of branched-chain amino acids or ketoacids in the diet, and the greater net absorption of nitrogen from the gut. Leucine and the ketoacid analogue of leucine may also have a specific nitrogen-sparing effect which may persist beyond the period of administration (Walser, 1975). As previously discussed, these diets may also normalize concentrations of some amino acids in plasma and other tissues. In patients with very low glomerular filtration rates (e.g., less than 4.0 to 5.0 ml/min) who are not undergoing regular dialysis therapy, these amino acid and ketoacid diets appear to be preferable to low protein intakes (Kopple, 1978; Walser, 1975). Ketoacids and hydroxyacids may also be utilized more efficiently than diets containing similar amounts of amino acids (Walser et al., 1973), although the differences in efficiency of utilization do not appear great.

The efficient utilization of essential amino acids, ketoacids and hydroxyacids diminishes as protein intake increases, and the potential advantages to these low nitrogen semisynthetic diets falls as the glomerular filtration rate rises. In patients with glomerular filtration rates greater than 4 to 5 ml/min, it has not been established that these amino acid and ketoacid diets have advantages over a diet providing 0.55 to 0.60 g/kg•day of primarily high biological value protein. Current data suggest that there are no major advantages (Kopple, 1978). However, the finding that low protein diets might retard the progression of renal failure and that this could be related to the low dietary content of protein, purines, phosphorus or some other constituent may indicate that there is a role for specialized amino acid or ketoacid formulations at higher levels of renal function (e.g., glomerular filtration rates of 4 to 15 ml/min). Also, if it can be established that normalizing plasma or muscle concentrations of specific amino acids is beneficial, then the indications for amino acid, ketoacid, or hydroxyacid diets may become clearer. Moreover, diets containing a small quantity of purified essential amino acids or ketoacids may enable the patient to eat a more varied intake that contains more low quality protein. Further studies are necessary to examine these questions.

Controlled prospective studies have not been carried out to examine whether these specialized amino acid and ketoacid formulations can maintain nutrition and minimize uremic toxicity as well as maintenance dialysis therapy with more liberal protein diets. Since the semisynthetic diets contain low quantities of total nitrogen and amino acids or ketoacids, they may not be as nutritious as higher protein intakes. Since maintenance dialysis therapy is currently available in most industrialized nations and uremic patients are often wasted, this question is of considerable importance. For underdeveloped societies where dialysis therapy is not readily available, these semisynthetic diets may have greater applicability for the patient with very low glomerular filtration rates (e.g., less than 5 ml/min).

SUMMARY

The amino acid concentrations in plasma, red cells, and muscle are altered in renal failure, and the pattern of amino acid concentrations in these tissues is unique to renal failure. There are many causes for the altered concentrations of amino acids, many of which have not been elucidated. Preliminary data suggest that specialized formulations of dietary amino acids can normalize many of the abnormal amino acid concentrations in plasma and muscle. Although normalizing the abnormal amino acid concentrations in plasma and intracellular sites would seem to be desirable, the benefits of such treatment have not yet been demonstrated.

REFERENCES

Alvestrand, A., Bergström, J., Fürst, P., Germanis, G., and Widstam, U. (1978): The effect of essential amino acid supplementation on muscle and plasma free amino acids in chronic uremia. *Kidney Int.* 14:323.

Anderson, H.L., Cho, E.S., Krause, P.A., Hanson, K.C., Krause, G.F., and Wixom, R.L. (1977): Effects of dietary histidine and arginine on nitrogen retention of men. *J. Nutr.* 107:2067.

Avioli, L.V., Scharp, C., and Birge, S.J. (1969): Catabolism of free hydroxyproline in chronic uremia. *Am. J. Physiol.* 217:536.

Ayling, J.E., Helfand, G.D., and Pirson, W.D. (1975): Phenylalanine hydroxylase from human kidney. *Enzyme* 20:6.

Bergman, E.N., Kaufman, C.F., Wolff, J.E., and Williams, H.H. (1974): Renal metabolism of amino acids and ammonia in fed and fasted pregnant sheep. *Am. J. Physiol.* 226:833.

Bergström, J., Fürst, P., Josephson, B., and Norée, L.O. (1970): Improvement of nitrogen balance in a uremic patient by the addition of histidine to essential amino acid solutions given intravenously. *Life Sci.* 9:787.

Bergström, J., Fürst, P., Norée, L.O., and Vinnars, E. (1978): Intracellular free amino acids in muscle tissue of patients with chronic uraemia: Effect of peritoneal dialysis and infusion of essential amino acids. *Clin. Sci. Mol. Med.* 54:51.

Bishop, M.C., Smith, R., Ledingham, J.G.G., and Oliver, D. (1971): Biochemical markers in renal bone disease. *Proc. Eur. Dial. Transplant Assoc.* 8:122.

Blumenkrantz, M.J., Shapiro, D.J., Swendseid, M.E., and Kopple, J.D. (1975): Histidine supplementation for treatment of anaemia of uraemia. *Br. Med. J.* 2:530.

Chan, W., Wang, M., Kopple, J.D., and Swendseid, M.E. (1974): Citrulline levels and urea cycle enzymes in uremic rats. *J. Nutr.* 104:678.

Cho, E.S., Krause, G.F., and Anderson, H.L. (1977): Effects of dietary histidine and arginine on plasma amino acid and urea concentrations of men fed a low nitrogen diet. *J. Nutr.* 107:2078.

Cohen, B.D., Patel, H., and Kornhauser, R.S. (1977): Proteins in atherogenesis. In: *Abstracts of First International Congress of Nutrition in Renal Disease.* Würzburg, Federal Republic of Germany.

De Ferrari, G., Garibotto, G., Robaudo, C., Ghiggeri, G.M., and Tizianello, A. (1981): Brain metabolism of amino acids and ammonia in patients with chronic renal insufficiency. *Kidney Int* 20:505.

DeTorrente, A., Glazer, B.G., and Gulyassy, P. (1974): Reduced in vitro binding of tryptophan by plasma in uremia. *Kidney Int.* 6:222.

Dubovský, J., Dubovská, E., Pacovský, V., and Hrba, J. (1968): Free and peptide hydroxyproline in chronic uremia. *Clin. Chim. Acta* 19:387.

Featherston, W.R., Rogers, Q.R., and Freedland, R.A. (1973): Relative importance of kidney and liver in synthesis of arginine by the rat. *Am. J. Physiol.* 224:127.

Felig, P., Owen, O.E., Warren, J., and Cahill, G.F., Jr. (1969): Amino acid metabolism during prolonged starvation. *J. Clin. Invest.* 48:584.

Fernstrom, J.D., and Wurtman, R.J. (1972): Brain serotonin content: Physiological regulation by plasma neutral amino acids. *Science* 178:414.

Fukuda, S., and Kopple, J.D. (1979): Evidence that dog kidney is an endogenous source of histidine. *Am. J. Physiol.* 237:E1.

Fukuda, S., and Kopple, J.D. (1980a): Uptake and release of amino acids by the normal dog kidney. *Min. Elect. Metab.* 3:237–247.

Fukuda, S., and Kopple, J.D. (1980b): Uptake and release of amino acids by the kidney of dogs made chronically uremic with uranyl nitrate. *Min. Elect. Metab.* 3:248–260.

Fürst, P. (1972): ^{15}N-studies in severe renal failure. II. Evidence for the essentiality of histidine. *Scand. J. Clin. Lab. Invest.* 30:307.

Fürst, P., Alvestrand, A., and Bergstrom, J. (1980): Effects of nutrition and catabolic stress on intracellular amino acid pools in uremia. *Am. J. Clin. Nutr.* 33:1387–1395.

Giordano, C., De Pascale, C., Balestrieri, C., Cittadini, D., and Crescenzi, A. (1968): Incorporation of urea ^{15}N in amino acids of patients with chronic renal failure on low nitrogen diet. *Am. J. Clin. Nutr.* 21:394.

Giordano, C., DeSanto, N.G., Rinaldi, S., De Pascale, C., and Pluvio, M. (1972): Histidine and glycine essential amino acids in uremia. In: *Uremia: An International Conference on Pathogenesis, Diagnosis and Therapy* (eds: R. Kluthe, G. Berlyne, and B. Burton), pp. 138–143. Georg Thieme Verlag, Stuttgart.

Giordano, C., De Santo, N.G., Rinaldi, S., Acone, D., Esposito, R., and Gallo, B. (1973): Histidine for treatment of uraemic anaemia. *Br. Med. J.* 4:714.

Gulyassy, P.F., Aviram, A., and Peters, J.H. (1970): Evaluation of amino acid and protein requirements in chronic uremia. *Arch Intern. Med.* 126:855.

Gulyassy, P.F., Peters, J.H., and Schoenfeld, P. (1972): Transport and protein binding of tryptophan in uremia. In: *Uremia: An International Conference on Pathogenesis, Diagnosis and Therapy,* (eds: R. Kluthe, G. Berlyne, and B. Burton), pp. 163–170, Georg Thieme Verlag, Stuttgart.

Jones, M.R., Kopple, J.D., and Swendseid, M.E. (1978): Phenylalanine metabolism in uremic and normal man. *Kidney Int.* 14:169–179.

Jones, M.R., Kopple, J.D., and Swendseid, M.D. (1982): $^{14}CO_2$ expiration after ^{14}C-histidine administration in normal and uremic men ingesting two levels of histidine. *Am. J. Clin. Nutr.* 35:15–23.

Jontofsohn, R., Heinze, V., Katz, N., Stuber, U., Wilke, H., and Kluthe, R. (1975): Histidine and iron supplementation in dialysis and pre-dialysis patients. *Proc. Eur. Dial. Transplant Assoc.* 2:391.

Kivirikko, K.I. (1970): Urinary excretion of hydroxyproline in health and disease. *Int. Rev. Connect. Tissue Res.* 5:93.

Koevoet, A.L. (1965): Plasma hydroxyproline in primary hyperparathyroidism and in chronic uremia. *Clin. Chim. Acta* 12:230.

Kopple, J.D., Wang, M., Vyhmeister, I., Baker, N., and Swendseid, M.E. (1972): Tyrosine metabolism in uremia. In: *Uremia: An International Conference on Pathogenesis, Diagnosis and Therapy* (eds: R. Kluthe, G. Berlyne and B. Burton), pp. 150–163, Georg Thieme Verlag, Stuttgart.

Kopple, J.D., and Swendseid, M.E. (1975): Evidence that histidine is an essential amino acid in normal and chronically uremic man. *J. Clin. Invest.* 55:881.

Kopple, J.D., and Swendseid, M.E. (1976): Effect of protein intake and uremia on plasma amino acid levels. *Kidney Int.* 10:560.

Kopple, J.D., Figueroa, W.G., and Swendseid, M.E. (1977): The dietary histidine requirement in normal and uremic man. *Fed. Proc.* 36:1092.

Kopple, J.D. (1978): Treatment with low protein and amino acid diets in chronic renal failure. In: *Proceedings VIIth International Congress of Nephrology,* pp. 497–507. S. Karger, Montreal, Canada.

Kopple, J.D., and Jones, M.R. (1979): Amino acid metabolism in patients with advanced uremia and in patients undergoing chronic dialysis. In: *Advances in Nephrology* (ed: M.H. Maxwell), Vol. 8, pp. 233–268. Year Book Medical Publishers, Chicago.

Kopple, J.D., and Fukuda, S. (1980): Effects of amino acid infusion and renal failure on the uptake and release of amino acids by the dog kidney. *Am. J. Clin. Nutr.* 33:1363–1372.

Kopple, J.D., Flugel, R., and Jones, M.R. (1981): Branched chain amino acids in chronic renal failure. In: *Metabolism and Clinical Implications of Branched Chain Amino and Ketoacids,* (eds: M. Walser and Williamson), pp. 555–567. Elsevier/North Holland, Amsterdam.

Kopple, J.D., Mercurio, K., Blumenkrantz, M.J., Jones, M.R., Tallos, J., Roberts, C., Card, B., Saltzman, R., Casciato, D.A., and Swendseid, M.E. (1981): Daily requirement for pyridoxine supplements in chronic renal failure. *Kidney Int.* 19:694–704.

Kopple, J.D., and Swendseid, M.E. (1981): Effect of histidine intake on plasma and urine histidine levels, nitrogen balance and N^{τ}-methylhistidine excretion in normal and chronically uremic men. *J. Nutr.* 111:931–942.

Owen, E.E., and Robinson, R.R. (1963): Amino acid extraction and ammonia metabolism by the human kidney during the prolonged administration of ammonium chloride. *J. Clin. Invest.* 42:263.

Pickford, J.C., McGale, E.H.F., and Aber, G.M. (1973): Studies on the metabolism of phenylalanine and tyrosine in patients with renal disease. *Clin. Chim. Acta* 48:77.

Pitts, R.F., and MacLeod, M.B. (1972): Synthesis of serine by the dog kidney in vivo. *Am. J. Physiol.* 222:394.

Schmid, G., Przuntek, H., Fricke, L., Heidland, A., and Hempel, K. (1978): Increased histidine and histamine content in the brain of chronic uremic rats. Cause of enhanced cerebral cAMP in uremia? *Am. J. Clin. Nutr.* 31:1665.

Sheng, Y.B., Badger, R.M., Asplund, J.M., and Wixom, R.L. (1977): Incorporation of $^{15}NH_4C1$ into histidine in adult men. *J. Nutr.* 107:621.

Squires, E.J., Hall, D.F., and Brosnan, J.T. (1976): Arteriovenous differences for amino acids and lactate across kidneys of normal and acidotic rats. *Biochem. J.* 160:125.

Tizianello, A., De Ferrari, G., Garibotto, G., Giovanna, G., and Robaudo, C. (1980a): Renal metabolism of amino acids and ammonia in subjects with normal renal function and in patients with chronic renal insufficiency. *J. Clin. Invest.* 65:1162–1173.

Tizianello, A., De Ferrari, G., Garibotto, G., and Robaudo, C. (1980b): Amino acid metabolism and the liver in renal failure. *Am. J. Clin. Nutr.* 33:1354–1362.

Walser, M. (1975): Ketoacids in the treatment of uremia. *Clin. Nephrol.* 3:180.

Walser, M., Coulter, A.W., Dighe, S., and Crantz, F.R. (1973): The effect of ketoanalogues of essential amino acids in severe chronic uremia. *J. Clin. Invest.* 52:678.

Wang, M., Vyhmeister, I., Swendseid, M.E., and Kopple, J.D. (1975): Phenylalanine hydroxylase and tyrosine aminotransferase activities in chronically uremic rats. *J. Nutr.* 105:122.

Whitehouse, S., Katz, N., Schaeffer, G., and Kluthe, R. (1975): Histidines and renal function. *Clin. Nephrol.* 3:24.

Wixom, R.L., Anderson, H.L., Terry, B.E., and Sheng, Y.B. (1977): Total parenteral nutrition with selective histidine depletion in man. I. Responses in nitrogen metabolism and related areas. *Am. J. Clin. Nutr.* 30:887.

Young, G.A., and Parsons, F.M. (1973): Impairment of phenylalanine hydroxylation in chronic renal insufficiency. *Clin. Sci. Mol. Med.* 45:89, 1973.

Young, V.R., Alexis, S.D., Baliga, B.S., and Munro, H.N. (1972): Metabolism of administered 3-methylhistidine, lack of muscle transfer ribonucleic acid charging and quantitative excretion as 3-methylhistidine and its N-acetyl derivative. *J. Biol. Chem.* 247:3592.

Communication

Purified Rat Kidney Branched-Chain Ketoacid Dehydrogenase Complex Contains Endogenous Kinase Activity

Richard Odessey

Branched-chain ketoacid dehydrogenase (BCKD)* catalyzes the rate-limiting step in the oxidation of the branched-chain amino acids in many tissues including heart, skeletal muscle, kidney and adipose tissue (Odessey and Goldberg, 1979; Goodman, 1978; Dawson and Hird, 1967). This enzyme is probably responsible for the changes in branched-chain amino acid oxidation which is observed during trauma and starvation (Odessey and Parr, 1982; Birkhahn et al., 1980). Recent work in this (Odessey, 1980a,b) and other laboratories (Parker and Randle, 1978, 1980; Hughes and Halestrap, 1981) have shown that in isolated mitochondria this enzyme can be inhibited by an ATP-dependent phosphorylation. Several factors that alter enzyme activity have reciprocal effects on ^{32}P-labeling of the enzyme. By analogy with the pyruvate dehydrogenase complex (PDH), it has been suggested that phosphorylation is mediated by an enzyme-associated protein kinase. However, previous purifications of this multienzyme complex have failed to detect phosphorylating activity (Pettit et al., 1978) or ATP-induced inhibition (Danner et al., 1979). Neither PDH kinase nor the catalytic subunit of cAMP-dependent protein kinase can stimulate ^{32}P incorporation into purified enzyme (Pettit et al., 1978). These results suggest that if a BCKD specific kinase exists, it must be lost or degraded during isolation. To test this hypothesis, co-purification of enzyme and kinase activity was attempted.

MATERIALS AND METHODS

Purification

Digitonin-washed mitochondria were prepared as described previously (Odessey, 1980b), suspended in potassium phosphate buffer (30 mg/ml) and frozen at −80°C. BCKD was purified by freeze-thawing, PEG precipitation, hydroxylapatite chromatography and ultracentrifugation (Odessey, 1982).

Assays

BCKD was assayed as described previously (Odessey, 1980b). To measure ATP inhibition, 2.5 nmol ATP was added to kinase assay buffer and the reaction was

* Abbreviations: BCKD—branched-chain ketoacid dehydrogenase (EC 1.2.4.4), PDH—pyruvate dehydrogenase complex (EC 1.2.4.1 + EC 2.3.1.12 + EC 1.6.4.3).

started by addition of enzyme (final vol. – 25 μl). After five minutes, the reaction was terminated by transfer of the mixture to ice cold tubes containing 20 nmol of adenylyl 5′ – [b,γ-imido] diphosphate (Odessey, 1980a). BCKD activity was assayed immediately.

To measure phosphorylation, the incubation mixture described above also contained [γ – ^{32}P] ATP (2500 cpm/pmol). The reaction was terminated by spotting an aliquot of the mixture on ITLC strips (Fisher Scientific) and separating unbound radioactivity by chromatography (Odessey, 1982). Blanks of the incubation mixture without enzyme were run in triplicate and subtracted from the experimental values. Blanks were less than 5% of the maximum amount of labeled enzyme.

To measure dephosphorylation, an aliquot of ^{32}P-labeled enzyme was incubated with various phosphatase preparations (Odessey, 1982; Parker and Randle, 1980). Phosphatase activity was measured as an increase in BCKD activity and/or a decrease in acid-precipitable radioactivity.

Protein was assayed using a dye-binding reagent (Biorad Lab.) with bovine serum albumin as a standard. This method gave values equivalent to the Lowry procedure on purified BCKD. Phosphoamino acids were analyzed by high-voltage electrophoresis (Odessey, 1982).

RESULTS AND DISCUSSION

The introduction of washing the digitonin-treated mitochondria with hypotonic solutions resulted in the solubilization of 100% of the BCKD activity after a single freezing and thawing. Furthermore, the BCKD activity in the freeze-thaw extract was inhibited 95% by ATP (Table 1). However, further purification by precipitation with 50% ammonium sulfate or by 3% PEG in the presence of 10 mM $MgCl_2$ and 0.05M NaCl caused the loss of ATP-inhibiting activity. These results suggest that previous failures to demonstrate BCKD kinase activity (Pettit et al., 1978; Danner et

Table 1
Purification and BCKD and Associated Kinase Activity*

Fraction	Protein (mg)	Total Activity† (U)	Specific Activity (U/mg)	+/– ATP‡
Freeze-thaw extract	580	45.1	0.078	0.05
PEG precipitate	65.5	38.8	0.59	0.06
Total hydroxyl-apatite peak	22.1	33.6	1.46	–
Low kinase (0.21–0.24M)	9.9	13.6	1.23	0.53
High kinase (0.24–0.28M)	12.2	20.0	1.64	0.11
Ultracentrifuge pellet	6.1	19.3	3.19	0.12

*From about 340 g of rat kidney.
†Unit = micromoles NADH formed/min at 37°C in the presence of excess dihydrolipoyl dehydrogenase and with (3-methyl)-2-ketobutyrate as substrate.
‡Ratio of activity before and after incubation with ATP (0.1 mM) for five minutes (see methods).

al., 1979) were probably due to the omission of the digitonin washing step during mitochondrial isolation and/or the use of ammonium sulfate or PEG (in the presence of high salt) as precipitants. The loss of kinase activity may be due to enzyme inactivation since remixing the supernatant (with or without the removal of the precipitant) failed to restore the ability to inhibit BCKD by ATP. If however, the freeze-thaw extract was adjusted to pH 6.6 (in the absence of $MgCl_2$), slow addition of PEG to a final concentration of 3.2% precipitated 85% of the BCKD activity and resulted in a 7.5-fold purification (Table 1). BCKD could still be inhibited 94% by ATP (Table 1). Further purification yielded a preparation, which when subjected to SDS-PAG electrophoresis contained only three bands (Figure 1). These bands correspond to the decarboxylase dimer (37K and 46K daltons) and the transacylase (52K daltons) (Pettit et al., 1978). Furthermore, incubation of the purified enzyme with [$\gamma - {}^{32}P$] ATP for five minutes caused intense labeling of the 46K band exclusively. This is also the subunit phosphorylated when the labeling is performed with intact mitochondria (Odessey, 1980b). The failure to observe a band corresponding to the endogenous kinase suggests that this component may be a small fraction of the total protein.

To demonstrate the relationship between phosphorylation and activity, 20 mU of purified enzyme was incubated with [^{32}P] ATP (0.1 mM) in kinase assay buffer. Inhibition occurred rapidly with a halftime of approximately 1.5 minutes. Concomitantly, ^{32}P was incorporated in the enzyme protein with a $t_{1/2}$ of 1.5 minutes (Figure 2). Thus ^{32}P incorporation into BCKD mirrored enzyme inhibition. Maximum incorporation corresponded to 0.72 nmol/U. The Km of the kinase for ATP is approximately 14μM. Acid hydrolysis and high voltage electrophoresis of the labeled enzyme (see methods) showed that ^{32}P is incorporated exclusively into serine

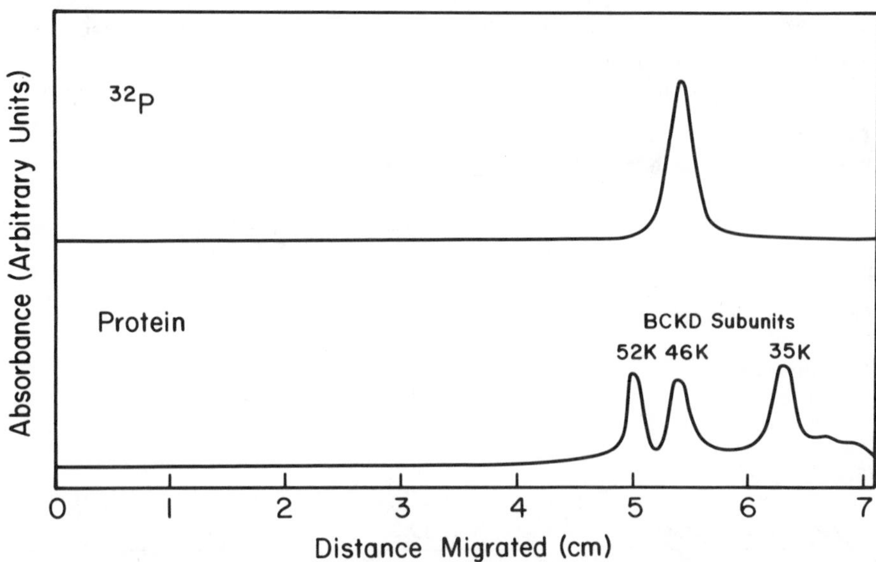

Figure 1 SDS polyacrylamide gel electrophoresis of [^{32}P] BCKD. SDS slab gels (8%) were run for four hours as described previously (Odessey, 1980b). In the bottom scan (at 520 nm) the gel is stained for protein with Coomassie brilliant blue. The top scan is an autoradiograph of the same gel.

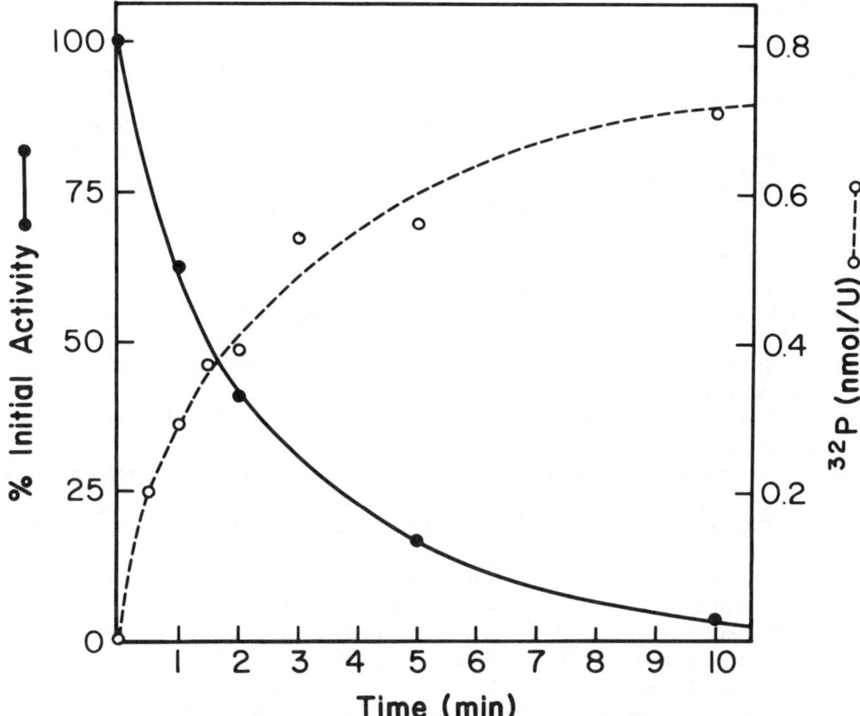

Figure 2 Time course of ATP inhibition and enzyme phosphorylation of BCKD. Purified BCKD was incubated with [$\gamma - {}^{32}P$] ATP (0.1 mM, 2400 cpm/pmol) in kinase assay buffer. At various intervals aliquots were taken for measurement of enzyme activity and ^{32}P incorporation (see methods).

residues. Calculation of the degree of 46K subunit phosphorylation must await precise knowledge of the molecular weight and subunit stoichiometry of the complex.

Although the BCKD complex, purified as described, retains endogenous kinase activity, phosphatase activity (in the presence or absence of Ca^{++}) is not observed. Further, purified pig heart or beef liver PDH phosphate phosphatase (gift of T. E. Roche) failed to activate the enzyme or liberate ^{32}P when incubated as described previously (Parker and Randle, 1980; Pettit et al., 1978). In addition, Pettit et al. (1978) have reported that PDH kinase does not phosphorylate the BCKD complex. It is, therefore, likely that the enzymes controlling the phosphorylation of BCKD are distinct from those regulating PDH.

ACKNOWLEDGMENTS

I would like to thank Dr. J. Larner for his advice and discussions. This project was aided by an institutional Biomedical Research Support Grant from LSU Medical Center (BRSG-SORR5376) with funds provided by the Division of Research, NIH.

REFERENCES

Birkhahn, R.H., Long, C.L., Fitkin, D. et al (1980): Effects of major skeletal trauma on whole body protein turnover in man measured by L – [1 – ^{14}C] leucine. *Surgery* 88:294–300.

Danner, D.J., Lemmon, S.K., Besharse, J.C. and Elsas, L.J. (1979): Purification and characterization of branched chain α-ketoacid dehydrogenase from bovine liver mitochondria. *J. Biol. Chem.* 254:5522–5526.

Dawson, A.J. and Hird, F.J.R. (1967): Oxidation of L-valine by rat kidney preparations. *Arch. Biochem. Biophys.* 122:426–433.

Goodman, H.M. (1977): Site of action of insulin in promoting leucine utilization in adipose tissue. *Am. J. Physiol.* 233:E97–E103.

Hughes, W.A. and Halestrap, A.P. (1981): The regulation of branched-chain 2-oxo acid dehydrogenase of liver, kidney and heart by phosphorylation. *Biochem. J.* 196:459–469.

Odessey, R. and Goldberg, A.L. (1979): Leucine degradation in cell-free extracts of skeletal muscle. *Biochem. J.* 178:475–489.

Odessey, R. (1980a): Reversible ATP-induced inactivation of branched chain 2-oxo acid dehydrogenase. *Biochem. J.* 192:155–163.

Odessey, R. (1980b): Direct evidence for the inactivation of branched-chain oxo-acid dehydrogenase by enzyme phosphorylation. *FEBS Lett.* 121:306–308.

Odessey, R. and Parr, B. (1982): Effect of insulin and leucine on protein turnover in rat soleus muscle after burn injury. *Metabolism* 31:82–87.

Odessey, R. (1982): Purification of rat kidney branched chain oxoacid dehydrogenase complex with endogenous kinase activity. *Biochem. J.* 204:353–356.

Parker, P.J. and Randle, P.J. (1978): Inactivation of rat heart branched chain 2-oxoacid dehydrogenase complex by ATP. *FEBS Lett.* 95:153–156.

Parker, P.J. and Randle, P.J. (1980): Active and inactive forms of branched chain 2-oxoacid dehydrogenase complex in rat heart and skeletal muscle. *FEBS Lett.* 112:186–190.

Pettit, F.H., Yeaman, S.J. and Reed, L.J. (1978): Purification and characterization of branched-chain α-keto acid dehydrogenase complex of bovine kidney. *Proc. Natl. Acad. Sci. USA* 75:4881–4885.

LIVER FAILURE

28 Branched-Chain Amino Acids in Hepatic Encephalopathy

H. Franklin Herlong
Anna Mae Diehl

Hepatic encephalopathy is a complex neuropsychiatric syndrome which can complicate both acute and chronic liver disease (Schenker et al., 1974). It is characterized by mental status alterations, such as personality disturbances, impairment of cognitive ability and depression of the level of consciousness. Neuromuscular function is also disordered, with tremors and asterixis commonly seen. Although the electroencephalogram is abnormal in patients with hepatic encephalopathy, the pattern of abnormality is nonspecific and can be seen in a variety of toxic or metabolic disorders (Conn and Lieberthal, 1978).

The exact cause of hepatic encephalopathy remains obscure. A number of biochemical alterations typically appear in patients with hepatic encephalopathy, but which ones of these are important in the pathogenesis is unknown. The most commonly incriminated toxin is ammonia, but several other substances are abnormally elevated in the blood of patients with hepatic encephalopathy. These candidate "toxins" include short-chain free fatty acids and sulfur-containing compounds such as methionine and mercaptans (Zieve et al., 1974). An abnormal plasma amino acid profile characterized by a decrease in the ratio of branched-chain amino acids (BCAA) to aromatic amino acids is found, and may influence the development of hepatic encephalopathy (Fischer et al., 1974; Munro et al., 1975).

ETIOLOGY OF PLASMA AMINO ACID ABNORMALITIES IN CIRRHOSIS

A number of factors may contribute to the abnormal amino acid pattern seen in patients with chronic liver disease and portal systemic shunting. Elevation in plasma concentrations of the aromatic amino acids is a consistent finding and may develop for several reasons (Iber et al., 1957). Increased muscle catabolism is present in cirrhosis, probably from an effect of disturbances in carbohydrate metabolism and the level of the pancreatic glucoregulatory hormones, insulin and glucagon. This increased muscle degradation leads to release of amino acids into the blood. Aromatic amino acids derived from muscle and dietary sources are preferentially metabolized by the liver. With impairment in liver function, a reduction in the metabolism of the aromatic amino acids results in elevation of their plasma levels. In addition, patients with cirrhosis have portal systemic shunting. When portal blood bypasses the liver, dietary aromatic amino acids and their bacterial degradation products escape into the systemic circulation. Thus, aromatic amino acids are elevated due to a combination of muscle catabolism, hepatic dysfunction, and portal-systemic shunting.

The plasma concentrations of BCAA are low in patients with cirrhosis and portal systemic shunting. Unlike the aromatic amino acids, the BCAA are metabolized primarily by extrahepatic tissues such as muscle and fat. Increased plasma levels of insulin seen in cirrhosis may favor transport of these amino acids into muscle and fat where they are oxidized as energy sources. It is also possible that reduced liver cell mass may contribute to a decrease in hepatic sources of BCAA and lead to a further reduction in their plasma levels. For these reasons, the characteristic amino acid pattern of chronic liver disease is a reduction in the molar ratio of BCAA to the aromatic amino acids. This value, which is normally 3.0 to 3.5, is reduced to below 1.0 in patients with cirrhosis (Munro et al., 1975, Morgan et al., 1978).

Certain individual amino acids may be particularly important in the pathogenesis of hepatic encephalopathy. Tryptophan, for example, has been reported to induce encephalopathy in dogs with Eck fistulae in the absence of hyperammonemia (Ogihara et al., 1966). Most tryptophan circulates in the plasma bound to albumin. In patients with cirrhosis, free (unbound) tryptophan is elevated despite normal or decreased levels of conjugated tryptophan. This increased free tryptophan may result from a complex interaction of several factors which are operative in patients with chronic liver disease. For example, cirrhotic patients with encephalopathy have elevated levels of circulating free fatty acids which may displace tryptophan from albumin. In addition cirrhotic patients are often hypoalbuminemic and, hence, have fewer binding sites for tryptophan. Finally, decreased degradation of tryptophan in the liver may also be important in elevating plasma tryptophan levels in these patients (Knell et al., 1974; Ono et al., 1978).

ETIOLOGY OF AMINO ACID ABNORMALITIES IN ACUTE LIVER FAILURE

Hepatic encephalopathy which develops as a result of fulminant liver failure is clinically indistinguishable from that which occurs in chronic liver disease. The plasma amino acid abnormalities are qualitatively similar to those seen in chronic liver disease, with a decrease in the ratio of BCAA to aromatic amino acids. However, some important quantitative differences exist. Fulminant liver disease is characterized by striking elevations of all amino acids except the BCAA which are usually present in normal concentrations. This generalized increase in amino acid concentrations may occur because of amino acid release from damaged liver cells. The liberated BCAA are metabolized in muscle and fat, but the aromatic amino acids which would ordinarily be metabolized in the liver escape degradation because of liver dysfunction. Hence, in this situation the ratio of BCAA to aromatic amino acids is decreased despite generalized elevation of circulating amino acids (Rosen et al., 1977).

AMINO ACIDS AND THE PATHOGENESIS OF HEPATIC ENCEPHALOPATHY

While characteristic plasma amino acid patterns have been noted in patients with hepatic encephalopathy in both acute and chronic liver disease, the importance of these abnormalities in the pathogenesis of the central nervous system dysfunction is speculative. One theory attempts to link the abnormalities in plasma amino acids to disordered neurotransmitter synthesis (Fischer, 1982). Phenylalanine and tyrosine (precursors of the neurotransmitters norepinephrine and dopamine) and tryptophan (the precursor of serotonin), compete with other neutral amino acids for transport across the blood brain barrier. In cirrhotic patients the relatively high plasma concentration of these aromatic amino acids would favor their transport into the CNS. Some investigators have suggested that other factors operative in patients with encephalopathy, i.e., hyperammonemia and elevated levels of CNS glutamine, may further facilitate accumulation of aromatic amino acids in the CNS. Disproportionately elevated CNS concentrations of the monamine precursors is thought to "overwhelm" normal synthetic pathways and favor the formation of false neurotransmitters such as octopamine and phenylethanolamine (James, 1979). These theories are appealing because they link documented plasma abnormalities with plausible chemical changes within the nervous system and, hence, with the clinically observed neuropsychiatric syndrome of encephalopathy. However, going from biochemical abnormalities to behavioral changes requires a significant leap of faith. Some important inconsistencies must be considered. Most notably, the plasma amino acid pattern of a decreased ratio of BCAA to aromatic amino acids is typical of most cirrhotic patients with portal-systemic shunting in general, not only those who are encephalopathic (Conn and Lieberthal, 1978). The fact that some patients with abnormal plasma amino acid patterns develop clinical encephalopathy while others do not suggest that surely other factors, such as alterations in the blood brain barrier, modulate in the pathogenesis of this syndrome (Fischer, 1982).

Despite this controversy, the detection of altered plasma amino acid patterns in hepatic encephalopathy and the hypothesis that they are causally related has led to a number of clinical trials of amino acid therapy. All of these trials have attempted to normalize the abnormalities in amino acid concentrations in the blood by administering BCAA themselves or BCAA-enriched amino acid mixtures.

TRIALS OF AMINO ACID THERAPY FOR HEPATIC ENCEPHALOPATHY

Rakette et al. (1981) studied 37 patients with cirrhosis and varying degrees of hepatic encephalopathy. The patients were divided into three groups. One group received parenterally 50 g per day of a BCAA-enriched mixture. Another group received a similar concentration of BCAA but without methionine, tryptophan and phenylalanine. A third group received glucose alone. In both groups of patients receiving the BCAA-enriched mixtures, plasma levels of BCAA increased. The aromatic amino acids, phenylalanine and tyrosine, fell with therapy, but the changes were only significant for phenylalanine. Administration of glucose alone normalized plasma tyrosine and decreased phenylalanine slightly. Glucose infusion caused a further reduction in the low pretreatment concentrations of leucine, isoleucine and valine. The degree of hepatic encephalopathy improved in both groups receiving the BCAA-enriched solutions but not in those who received the glucose infusion.

Fischer et al. (1976) administered a BCAA-enriched mixture to eight patients with cirrhosis and three patients with severe viral hepatitis. In the patients with chronic liver disease, infusion of the BCAA-enriched mixture led to a fall in plasma phenylalanine and tyrosine and a rise in the BCAA concentrations. These changes in plasma amino acid concentrations were accompanied by improvement in mental status and electroencephalographic abnormalities. One of three patients with severe viral hepatitis had some clinical improvement but no significant changes occurred in the amino acid profile.

Okada et al. (1981) studied 21 patients with liver disease treated with a BCAA mixture at a dose of 50 to 70 g per day. All of these patients had grade three to four encephalopathy. Sixteen patients had chronic liver disease while five patients had fulminant hepatitis. The amino acid infusion improved the grade of coma in both groups of patients. Ammonia concentration was not affected by therapy in either group. The only significant change in serum amino acid abnormalities was a reduction in the plasma phenylalanine concentration in the patients with chronic liver disease. No significant change occurred in the amino acid pattern in patients with fulminant hepatitis.

Eriksson and Wahren (1981) compared oral BCAA supplementation with a placebo in a double-blinded, randomized cross-over study in seven patients with chronic encephalopathy. Thirty grams of a mixture of the three BCAA were given daily in four divided doses. The results of six psychometric tests did not indicate a difference in response to BCAA and placebo administration. Moreover, the clinical status did not suggest a more beneficial effect of BCAA than for placebo. Three hours after a 7.5-g dose of BCAAs, there was a rise in the plasma BCAA concentrations and a fall in the plasma concentration of phenylalanine and tyrosine. In the postabsorptive state, 12 hours after the last dose of BCAA, there was no significant difference in the plasma amino acid levels compared to basal levels.

Holm et al. (1981) compared a BCAA-enriched mixture containing small amounts of methionine, phenylalanine and tryptophan with a BCAA-enriched mixture which lacked these amino acids. The amino acid mixtures were infused at a dose of 50 or 80 g per day. One hundred-twenty patients were studied, of whom 66 had clinical encephalopathy prior to the study. An improvement in the clinical grade of encephalopathy was noted in 41 of these 66 patients. Amino acid data for the group as a whole were reported but not specifically for the encephalopathic patients. Therefore, correlations between the effect of improvement in the plasma amino acid pattern and subsequent effect on the clinical grade of encephalopathy could not be determined.

Michel et al. (1980) performed a controlled study comparing intravenous infusion of a conventional amino acid preparation containing a low ratio of BCAA to aromatic amino acids with an amino acid solution modified to contain a high proportion of BCAA to aromatic amino acids. The degree of clinical improvement in the two groups was not significantly different. The patients receiving the BCAA-enriched mixture had a significant improvement in their plasma ratio of BCAA to aromatic amino acids. Those receiving the conventional mixture did not. Thus, in this study, the infusion of a BCAA-enriched solution did not improve hepatic encephalopathy despite correction of the abnormal plasma amino acid ratio. However, the acute mortality in this controlled study was greater than 25%, suggesting that the patient population studied had severe liver disease or that there were significant complicating factors.

Rossi-Fanelli et al. (1981) reported an uncontrolled trial in 19 patients with grade three to four hepatic encephalopathy who were treated with parenteral infusion of approximately 4.2 g of BCAA daily. After 24 hours of infusion, all patients had clinical improvement. There was also a statistically significant rise in BCAA concentrations and a fall in aromatic amino acid concentrations. The infusion was then continued for another 48 hours after mental recovery. Surprisingly, despite continued BCAA infusion, plasma levels of both aromatic and BCAAs returned toward pre-infusion levels. Free tryptophan concentration decreased with recovery and remained low throughout the infusion.

In summary, a number of studies report that BCAA therapy improves clinical hepatic encephalopathy. In some of these trials clinical improvement was accompanied by favorable alteration in plasma amino acid abnormalities. However, consistent changes in plasma amino acid patterns have not always paralleled clinical improvement.

How might these discrepancies be explained? It is possible that factors other than amino acid abnormalities are more important in the pathogenesis of hepatic encephalopathy. However, it is more likely that the differences among the studies reflect uncontrolled study designs with small numbers of patients, differences in patient populations, lack of objective measures of hepatic encephalopathy, and differences in dose and route of administration of the amino acids.

KETO ANALOGUES OF THE BRANCHED-CHAIN AMINO ACIDS IN THE THERAPY OF HEPATIC ENCEPHALOPATHY

It appears that measures directed toward increasing the BCAA concentrations and lowering the aromatic amino acid concentrations are beneficial in the treatment of hepatic encephalopathy. We have compared the BCAA with their nitrogen-free analogues (ketoacids) in patients with chronic hepatic encephalopathy. We performed a double blind cross-over comparison of the BCAAs (68 mmol/d) versus ornithine salts of ketoacids (34 mmol/d) in eight patients with chronic hepatic encephalopathy who were symptomatic despite protein restriction and lactulose therapy. Both treatments improved the clinical grade of encephalopathy and electroencephalographic abnormalities, but the degree of improvement in both of these parameters was greater with the ornithine salts of ketoacids. With both therapies, the BCAA concentrations in the plasma improved, and both led to a significant fall in plasma tyrosine concentration. However, ornithine salts of branched-chain ketoacids significantly reduced plasma concentrations of tryptophan while BCAA themselves did not (Herlong et al., 1980). A recent study by Rossle et al. (1981) has shown that when BCAAs are supplemented with ornithine and arginine and administered parenterally to patients with hepatic encephalopathy significant clinical improvement ensued. During this treatment, plasma concentrations of the BCAA increased by 32% over the original values. The aromatic amino acids, tyrosine, phenylalanine and tryptophan, decreased by 50%. In addition, the CSF concentrations of tyrosine and phenylalanine declined by 55%, while the concentration of tryptophan fell by 67%.

Thus, it appears that the ornithine salts of branched-chain ketoacids and ornithine-supplemented BCAA infusions are both efficacious in the treatment of hepatic encephalopathy. Perhaps these beneficial effects are due to a synergism between stimulation of the urea cycle by ornithine and a peripheral anticatabolic action of the branched-chain compounds.

Because of the variable course of hepatic encephalopathy, more controlled trials with large numbers of patients are necessary before the optimal formulation and dose of branched-chain amino acid or ketoacid supplementation can be determined.

REFERENCES

Conn, H.O., Lieberthal, M.M. (1978): *the Hepatic Coma Syndromes and Lactulose,* pp. 1–122. Baltimore, William and Wilkins Co.

Ericksson, S. and Wahren, T. (1981): Failure of branched chain amino acid administration to improve chronic hepatic encephalopathy. In *Metabolism and Clinical Implications of Branched-Chain Amino Acids and Ketoacids* (eds: M. Walser and J.R. Williamson), pp. 481–485. New York, Elsevier/North Holland.

Fischer, J.E., Yoshimura, N., Aguirre, et al. (1974): Plasma amino acids in patients with hepatic encephalopathy: Effects of amino acid infusions. *Am. J. Surg.* 127:40–70.

Fischer, J.E. (1982): Amino acids in hepatic coma. *Dig. Dis. Sci.* 27:97–102.

Fischer, J.E., Rosen, H.M., Ebeid, A.M., James, J.H., Keane, J.M., Soeters, P.B. (1976): The effect of normalization of plasma amino acids on hepatic encephalopathy in man. *Surgery* 80:77–91.

Herlong, H.F., Maddrey, W.C., Walser, M. (1980): The use of ornithine salts of branched-chain keto acids in portal systemic encephalopathy. *Ann. Intern. Med.* 93:545–550.

Holm, E., Streibel, J.P., Moller, P., Hartmen, M. (1981): Amino acid solutions for parenteral nutrition and for adjuvant treatment of encephalopathy in liver cirrhosis. Studies concerning 120 patients. In *Metabolism and Clinical Implications of Branched-Chain Amino and Ketoacids* (eds: M. Walser, J.R. Williamson), pp. 513–530. New York, Elsevier/North Holland.

Iber, F.L., Rosen, H., Levenson, S.M., Chalmers, T.C. (1957): The plasma amino acids in patients with liver failure. *J. Lab. Med.* 50:417–425.

James, J.H., Jeppsson, B., Ziparo, V., Fischer, J.E. (1979): Hyperammonemia, plasma amino acid imbalance, and blood-brain amino acid transport: A unified theory of portal-systemic encephalopathy. *Lancet* 2:772–775.

Knell, A.J., Davidson, A.R., Williams, R., Kantamaneni, B.D., Curzon, G. (1974): Dopamine and serotonin metabolism in hepatic encephalopathy. *Br. Med. J.* 1:549–551.

Michel, H., Pomier-Layrargues, G., Duhamel, O., Lacombe, B., Cuilleret, G., Bellit, H. (1980): Intravenous infusion of ordinary and modified amino acid solutions in the management of hepatic encephalopathy (controlled study, 30 patients). *Gastroenterology* 79:1038.

Morgan, M., Milson, J.P., Sherlock, S. (1978): Plasma ratio of valine, leucine and isoleucine to phenylalanine and tyrosine in liver disease. *Gut* 19:1068–1073.

Munro, N.M., Fernstrom, J.D., Wurtman, R.J. (1975): Insulin, plasma amino acid imbalance and hepatic coma. *Lancet* 1:722–724.

Ogihara, K., Mozai, T., Hirai, S. (1966): Tryptophan as cause of hepatic coma. *N. Engl. J. Med.* 275:1255–1256.

Okada, A., Kamata, S., Kim, C.W., Kawashima, Y. (1981): Treatment of hepatic encephalopathy with BCAA-rich amino acid mixture. In *Metabolism and Clinical Implications of Branched-Chain Amino and Ketoacids* (eds: M. Walser, J.R. Williamson), pp. 447–452. New York, Elsevier/North Holland.

Ono, J., Hutson, D.G., Dombro, R.S., Levi, J.U., Livingstone, A., Zeppa, R. (1978): Tryptophan and hepatic coma. *Gastroenterology* 74:196–200.

Rakette, S., Fischer, M., Reimann, H.J., Sommoggy, S.V. (1981): Effects of special amino acid solutions in patients with liver cirrhosis and hepatic encephalopathy. In *Metabolism and Clinical Implications of Branched-Chain Amino and Ketoacids* (eds: M. Walser, J.R. Williamson), pp. 419–427. New York, Elsevier/North Holland.

Rosen, H.M., Yoshimura, N., Hodgman, J.M., Fischer, J.E. (1977): Plasma amino acid patterns in hepatic encephalopathy of differing etiology. *Gastroenterology* 72:483–487.

Rossi-Fanelli, F., Cangiano, C., Cuscino, A., et al. (1979): The therapeutic effect of branched chain amino acids in hepatic encephalopathy. *Clin. Res.* 27:579.

Rossle, M., Herz, R., Gerok, W. (1981): Treatment of hepatic encephalopathy with an adapted amino acid solution: Influence on amino acid and ammonia concentration in plasma and CSF. *Hepatology* 1:541.

Schenker, S., Breen, K.A., Hoyumpa, A.M., Jr. (1974): Hepatic encephalopathy: current status. *Gastroenterology* 66:121–151.

Zieve, L., Doizaki, W.M., Zieve, F.J. (1974): Synergism between mercaptans and ammonia or fatty acids in the pathogenesis of hepatic coma. *J. Lab. Clin. Med.* 83:16–28.

Cystine and Tyrosine Requirements During the Nutritional Repletion of Cirrhotic Patients

Daniel Rudman, Rajender K. Chawla, and Julie C. Bleier

When a patient is unable to meet nutritional needs because of inability to eat, gastrointestinal malabsorption, or hypermetabolism, parenteral nutrition is often the therapy of choice. Until 1960 it was impossible to provide even maintenance nutritional needs by the parenteral route, to say nothing of the two to four times greater requirements of repletion. Use of the parenteral route was limited because of the 600 mosm/L tolerance of peripheral veins. However, when Dudrick et al. (1969) showed that central veins would tolerate up to 1800 mosm/L, the door was opened to central hyperalimentation or total parenteral nutrition (TPN). Another recent advance in parenteral nutrition has been reduction of the osmolar content of the solution without reducing its energy content, by shifting the energy source from carbohydrate to triglyceride (Jeejeebhoy et al., 1976).

Regardless of the carbohydrate to triglyceride ratio, current parenteral nutrition supplies 40 to 120 g a day of free amino acids. Originally, the amino acids were furnished in the form of a chemical or enzymatic hydrolysate of fibrin or casein; such hydrolysates contained all 20 natural amino acids, although the utilization of peptides was questionable. Once it became economically feasible to use synthetic amino acids, the hydrolysates were phased out. Currently, the most commonly used solutions are mixtures of synthetic amino acids, including the eight essentials, and arginine and histidine, with most of the nonessential nitrogen being supplied as glycine. Cystine and tyrosine are omitted on the assumption that the patient will synthesize these materials from methionine and phenylalanine, respectively.

To assess whether the patient's nutritional needs are being met by the TPN solution, the nitrogen balance, anthropometric measures of adipose and muscle mass, creatinine/height ratio, hematocrit and serum albumin concentration are determined. In successful maintenance regimens nitrogen balance is zero, and there is no deterioration of anthropometric and chemical nutritional indicators. Effective repletion of nutrients produces a nitrogen balance of +5 to +10 g/day/70 kg body weight (BW), expansion of both lean body mass and adipose mass, and a rise in albumin and hematocrit.

Central hyperalimentation was first clinically applied in cachectic individuals whose undernutrition was caused by anorexia or gastrointestinal malabsorption. Central hyperalimentation was highly successful in such individuals (Keating and Ternberg, 1971; Scribner et al., 1970). Protein-energy malnutrition (PEM) now affects about 30% of hospitalized patients (Bistrian, 1976). In only a small proportion of such individuals, however, is the PEM caused by hypophagia or gastrointestinal malabsorption. Instead, malnutrition in the hospital is usually caused by underlying organic diseases outside the GI tract: cirrhosis, renal insufficiency, cancer, congestive heart failure, pulmonary disease, chronic infection or recurrent surgical trauma.

Investigators are now striving to apply TPN to each of these diverse categories to learn whether the undernutrition can be corrected. This report concerns our at-

Table 1
Nutritional Assessment of Cirrhotics in Three Hospitals

A. Boston City Hospital (52 patients) (Bistrian, 1976)

	<60% of Standard	60–90% of Standard	>90% of Standard
Triceps skinfold	56%	19%	25%
Arm muscle circumference	0	44%	56%
Weight/Height	2%	31%	67%

B. Grady Memorial Hospital (100 patients), Atlanta, 1979

	<70% of Standard	70–90% of Standard	>91% of Standard
Triceps skinfold	15%	35%	50%
Creatinine/height	23%	69%	8%

C. Veterans Administration Hospital (140 patients), East Orange, N.J. (Leery, et al, 1970)

	% of Cirrhotics with Subnormal Vitamin Blood Level
Thiamin	58%
Niacin	33%
B_6	60%
B_{12}	25%
Folic acid	78%

tempt to apply TPN to undernourished cirrhotic patients, most of whom have some degree of PEM (Table 1).

During 1970–1973, our colleagues, Ansley, Slovis, and Rypins used TPN to treat 10 emaciated patients with cirrhosis. In half of these patients nutritional status failed to improve, and indeed clinical status deteriorated. Therefore, we undertook a study to compare the nutritional responses of 12 patients with cirrhosis and six patients with short gut syndrome with comparable degrees of PEM. A complete report has been published (Rudman et al., 1981) and the findings are summarized below.

The subjects are described in Table 2. As shown in this table, the degrees of reduction in adipose mass and lean body mass were similar in the two groups. Each patient had a four- or five-week course of TPN. The composition of the TPN solution is shown in Table 3. The clinical and nutritional indicators before and at one- to three-day intervals during TPN are shown in Table 4.

The results of the study are shown in Figures 1 through 4. First consider the nitrogen balance (Figure 1). Patients with malabsorption showed uniformly positive nitrogen balance averaging +6 g/70 kg BW/day. Eight cirrhotic patients showed positive nitrogen balance, as did the patients with short gut syndrome, while four patients with cirrhosis failed to show significant nitrogen retention. The cirrhotic patients were therefore subdivided on the basis of nitrogen balance, into subgroup 1, those with nitrogen retention of 4 to 8 g/day, and subgroup 2, with nitrogen balance of −2 to 2 g/day.

Table 2
Clinical Features of the Patients Who Were Observed During Four to Five Weeks of TPN

	Malabsorption	Cirrhosis	Cirrhotic Subgroup 1	Cirrhotic Subgroup 2
Age: Average (SD)	48.3 (5.6)	46.9 (7.1)	44.8 (6.8)	51.3 (6.3)
Sex: M/F	4/2	8/4	5/3	3/1
Duration since diagnosis (yrs)	1–24	3–16	4–15	3–16
Diagnosis				
Massive resection of small intestine	3			
Regional ileitis	3			
Alcoholic cirrhosis		12	8	4
Ascites				
0	6	2	1	1
1		6	4	2
2		4	3	1
Child's score				
A			1	0
B			7	4
C			0	0

Table 3
Contents of One Liter of the TPN Solution

dextrose	250 g	*Per day:*	
amino acids	39 g	Zn	2 mg
isoleucine	2.9 g	Mn	0.4 mg
leucine	3.8 g	Cu	1 mg
lysine	3.1 g	Cr	10 mcg
phenylalanine	2.4 g	ascorbic acid	500 mg
methionine	2.2 g	vitamin A	10,000 IU
cysteine	<0.02 g	vitamin D	1,000 IU
threonine	1.7 g	thiamine	50 mg
tryptophan	0.65 g	riboflavin	10 mg
valine	2.8 g	pyridoxine	15 mg
alanine	3.0 g	niacinamide	100 mg
arginine	1.55 g	pantothenic acid	15 mg
glycine	8.5 g	vitamin E	5 IU
histidine	1.2 g		
proline	4.7 g	*Per week: intramuscular*	
serine	2.5 g	folic acid	10 mg
Na	50 meq	vitamin K	10 mg
K	40 meq	*Per month: intramuscular*	
Cl	50 meq	vitamin B_{12}	1 mg
P	465 mg		
Ca	5 meq		
Mg	5 meq		

Table 4
Clinical and Nutritional Indicators Measured at Baseline and at One- to Three-Day Intervals during TPN

Clinical:	Hematocrit, prothrombin time, serum albumin, serum cholesterol, serum bilirubin, serum LDH, serum SGOT, serum creatinine, venous plasma NH_3, EEG, neurological grade.
Nutritional:	MAMA, TSF, 24-hr urine creatinine/ht ratio, daily N balance.
Plasma Amino Acids:	Glycine, alanine, citrulline, α-aminobutyric acid, valine, cystine, methionine, isoleucine, leucine, tyrosine, phenylalanine, ornithine, lysine, histidine, tryptophan, arginine.

The two subgroups differed in most measurements. Creatinine/height ratio and mid-arm muscle area, albumin, hematocrit, and liver function tests all improved in subgroup 1 but not in subgroup 2. Ascites tended to improve in subgroup 1 and to worsen in subgroup 2. Only in terms of enlargement of adipose mass, as reflected in the triceps skinfold, were the two subgroups similar.

The plasma aminograms offered some explanation of the diverse behavior of cirrhotic subgroup 1 and 2. Before hyperalimentation, the patients with short gut syndrome showed generalized hypoaminoacidemia. During hyperalimentation, these patients showed progressive weight gain and positive nitrogen balance and their plasma amino acids rose into or above the normal fasting range. Cirrhotic patients in subgroup 1 before hyperalimentation, showed a plasma aminogram typical of cirrhosis with reduced branched-chain amino acids, and elevated methionine, tyrosine and phenylalanine. During hyperalimentation, all plasma amino acid levels rose into or above the normal fasting ranges. In subgroup 2, the pre-TPN plasma aminogram was similar to that of subgroup 1. During hyperalimentation, however, subgroup 2 differed from subgroup 1 with respect to four amino acids: cystine, tyrosine, taurine and α-aminobutyric acid. These four amino acids declined below the normal fasting range during TPN in all four members of subgroup 2 and in some individuals virtually disappeared. The relationship between the depression of plasma cystine and tyrosine levels and the degree of nitrogen retention during TPN is shown in Figure 4.

In subgroup 1, the lowest amino acid level in the amino acid profile during TPN was at least 80% of the normal fasting mean. On the other hand, in subgroup 2, either the cystine or tyrosine level declined to below 20% of the normal fasting mean during hyperalimentation. These findings led us to postulate that the factor which prevented nutritional repletion during TPN in subgroup 2 was either the inability to synthesize tyrosine from the phenylalanine in the nutrient solution, or the inability to synthesize cystine from the methionine. In two members of subgroup 2 we were able to add a fifth week of TPN, during which the patient received an oral supplement of 0.9 g/day each of cystine and tyrosine. The supplements promptly normalized the depressed cystine and tyrosine levels. Simultaneously, nitrogen balance rose from zero to about plus 5 g per day (Table 5). In addition, there were improvements in albumin, hematocrit and prothrombin time. These findings led us to postulate that in some patients with cirrhosis the biosynthetic pathways leading from phenylalanine to tyrosine (Figure 5), and from methionine to cystine (Figure 6) were impaired.

Therefore, these patients were unable to synthesize cystine and tyrosine at rates sufficient to maintain the repletion process. The simultaneous declines in α-aminobutyric acid and taurine levels are consistent with the metabolic relationships of these two compounds to methionine and cystine.

Our data suggest that during TPN, the cirrhotic patients of subgroup 2 lacked the ability to synthesize tyrosine and cystine at an adequate rate during repletion.

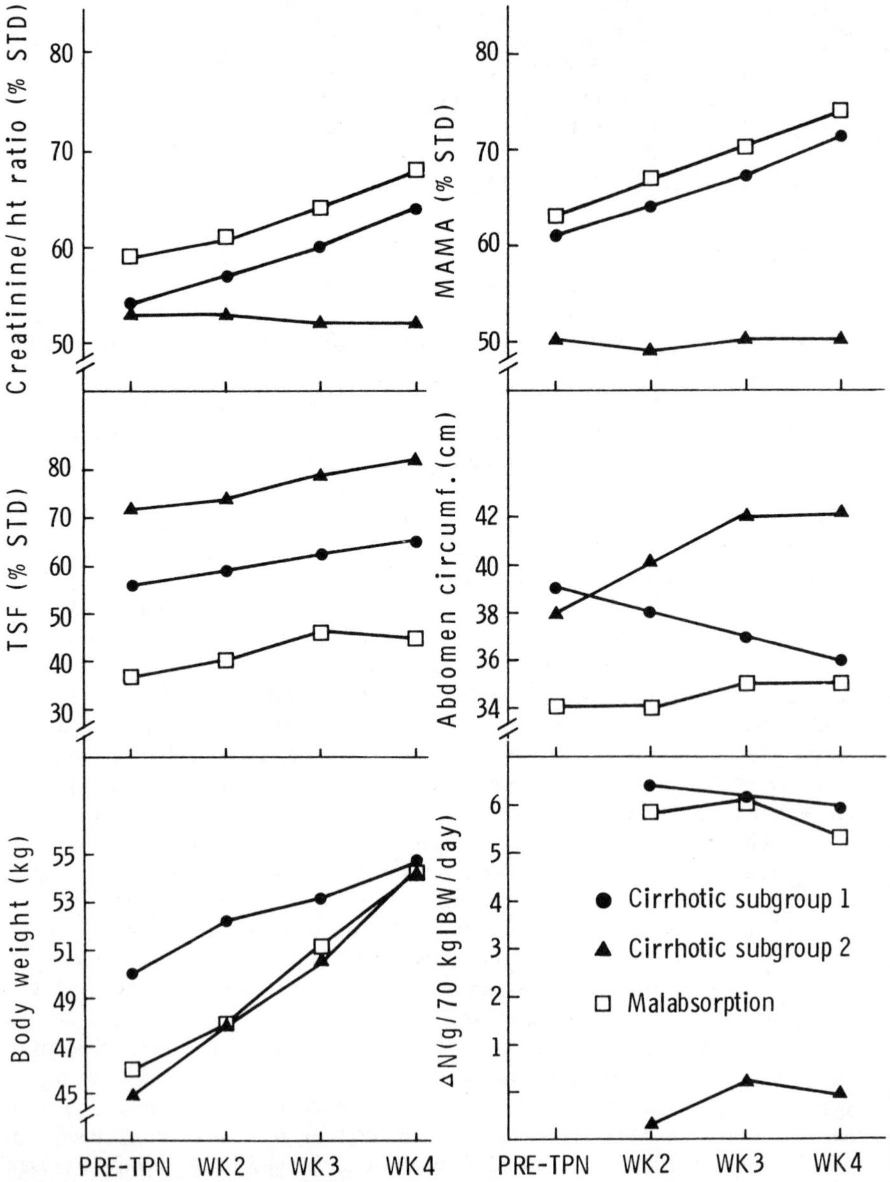

Figure 1 Nutritional and clinical indicators during four weeks of TPN. Average values are shown for each group or subgroup of patients.

However, the nutritional requirements during repletion are known to be two to four times greater than during maintenance. Therefore, while the biosynthetic capacities in these patients may be insufficient for repletion, they could be adequate for maintenance.

The proposed biosynthetic deficiencies in subgroup 2 are analogous to certain inborn errors in metabolism. The postulated block in the biosynthesis of tyrosine is

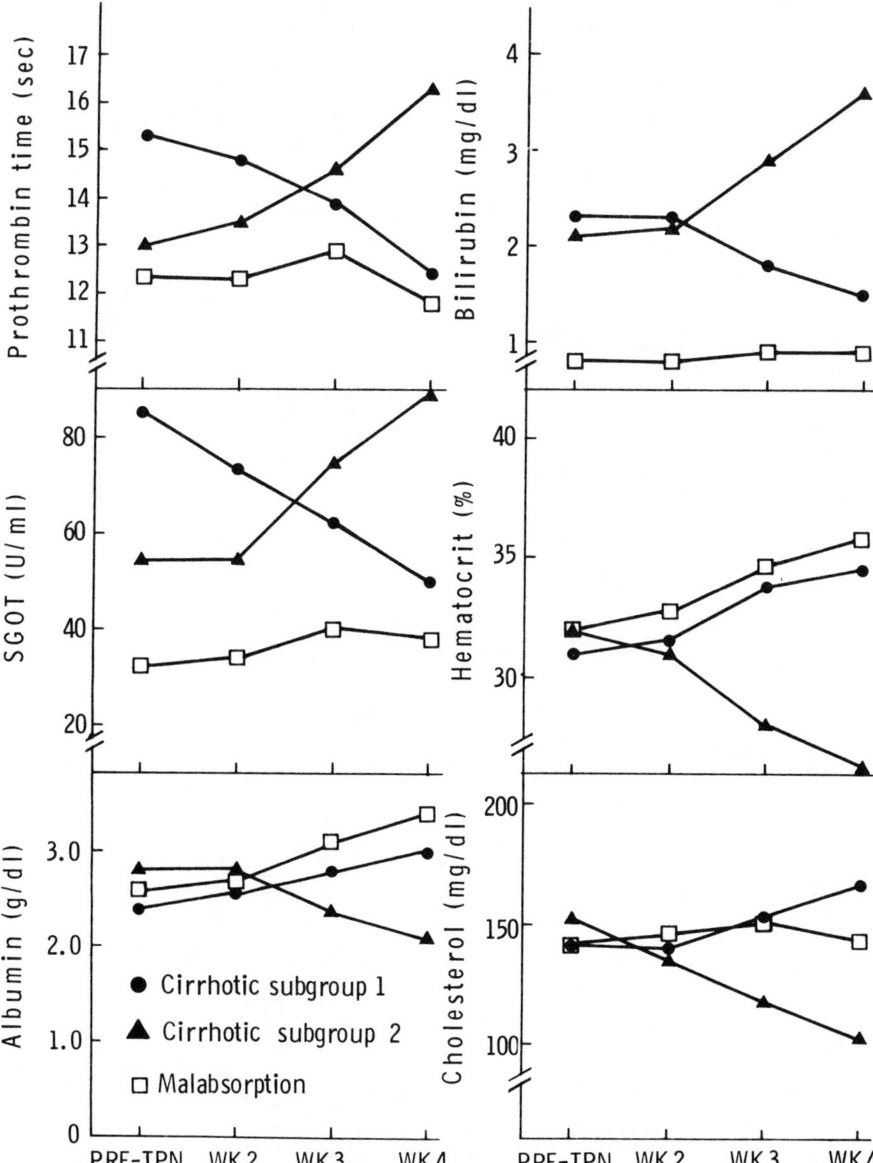

Figure 2 Nutritional and clinical indicators during four weeks of TPN. Average values are shown for each group or subgroup of patients.

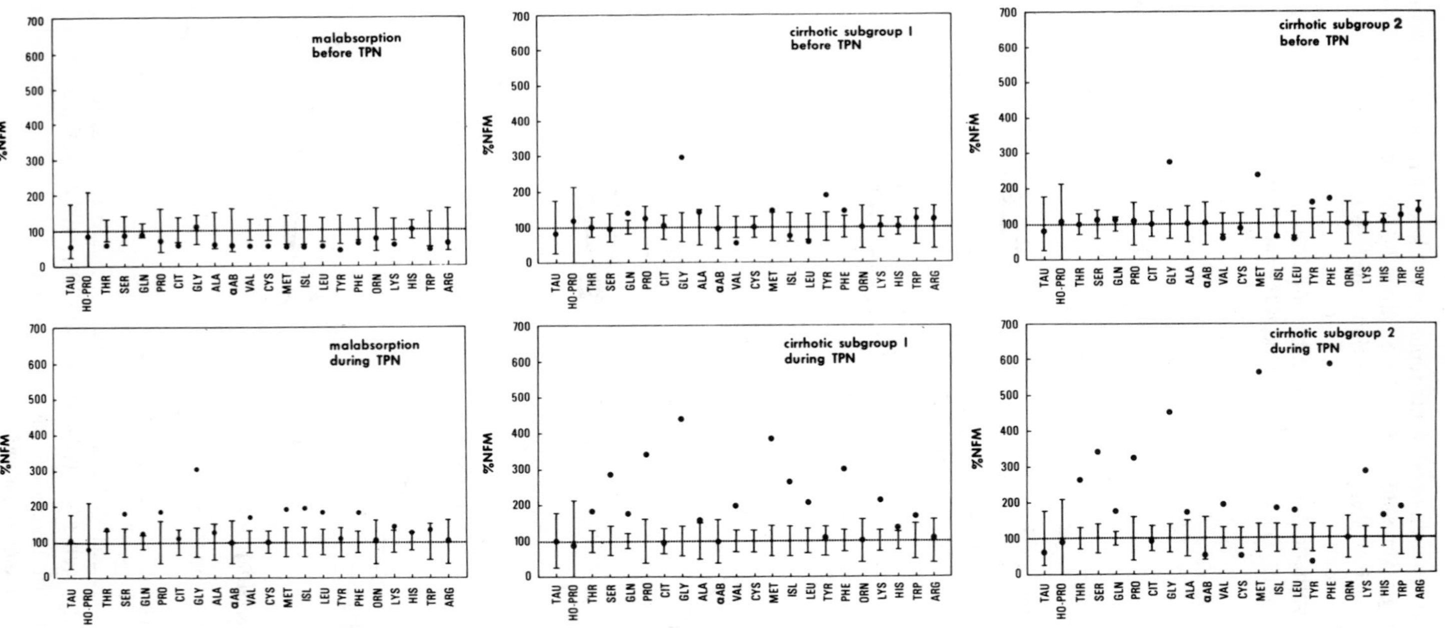

Figure 3 Plasma aminograms before and during weeks of TPN. Average values are shown for each group or subgroup of patients. NFM = Normal fasting range. See Rudman et al. (1981) for complete data.

similar to that in phenylketonuria (Knox, 1972), and the block in cystine synthesis may be comparable to the block between methionine and cystine in homocystinuria and in cystathioninuria (Brenton et al., 1966; Frimpter, 1972).

How can we reconcile the postulated requirement for tyrosine with the pre-TPN fasting hypertyrosinemia in the subgroup 2 cirrhotic patients? The explanation may have to do with blocks of tyrosine metabolism distal to tyrosine in cirrhosis. In patients with advanced liver disease after an oral load of tyrosine, clearance of plasma

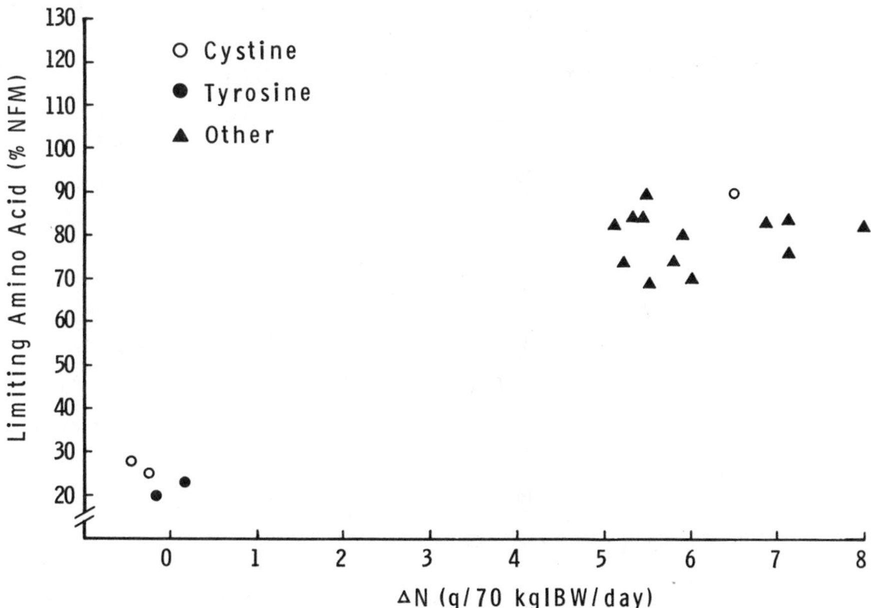

Figure 4 Relation during TPN of average nitrogen balance to average plasma level of the limiting amino acid, i.e., the amino acid with lowest % of normal fasting mean. Patients of cirrhotic subgroup 2 are clustered in the lower left of the graph; cirrhotic subgroup 1 and malabsorbers are clustered in the upper right.

Table 5
Metabolic Course of the Two Cases in Subgroup 2 Who Received an Oral Cystine and Tyrosine Supplement in the Fifth Week

	Case #1				Case #2			
	Wk2	Wk3	Wk4	Wk5	Wk2	Wk3	Wk4	Wk5
Hematocrit	30.0	28.0	25.5	28.0	31.5	28.0	26.5	30.0
Serum albumin	2.7	2.4	2.0	2.4	2.8	2.3	2.0	2.4
Plasma taurine	47	39	42	127*	58	45	48	126*
Plasma α-amino-butyric acid	37	30	26	135*	39	30	28	143*
Plasma cystine	34	28	14	157*	51	38	38	154*
Plasma tyrosine	77	36	34	160*	29	15	17	142*
Δ N	−0.9	−0.5	−0.4	+6.5*	−0.8	0.2	0.1	+5.1*

*$p<.05$ for comparison with weeks 2–4.

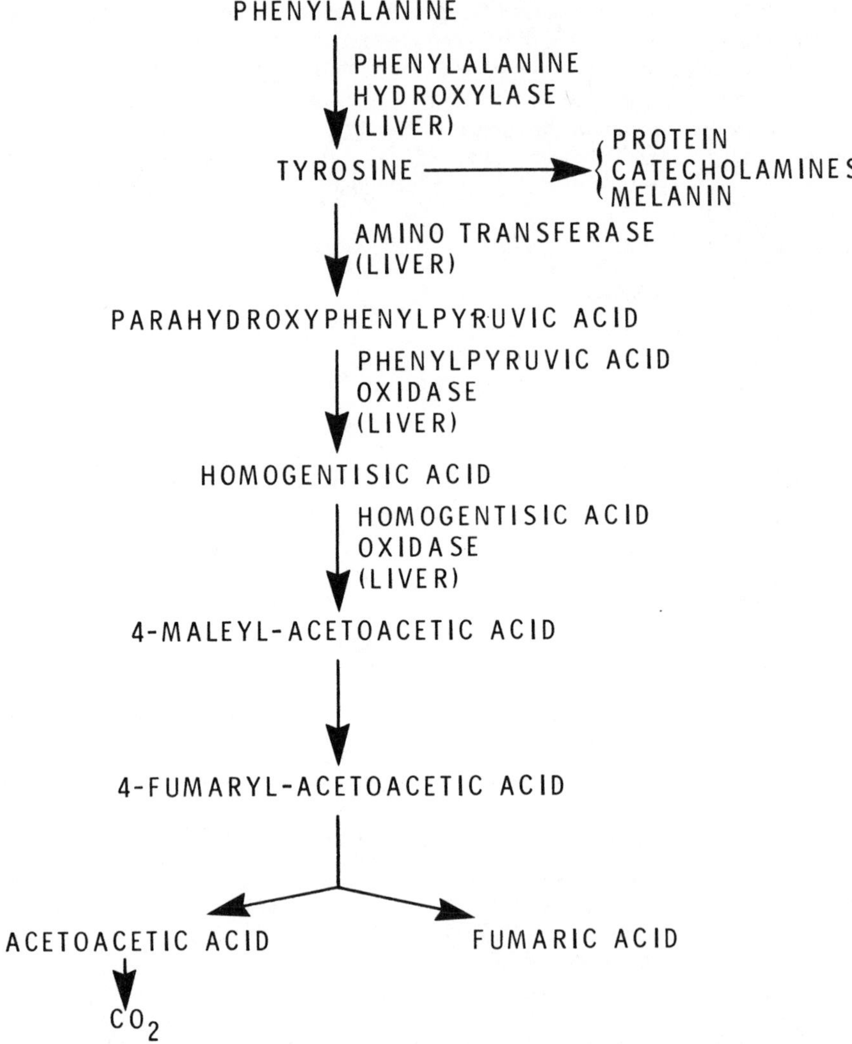

Figure 5 Pathway for the metabolism of phenylalanine via tyrosine, parahydroxyphenylpyruvic acid, and homogentisic acid. Those enzymes which are primarily confined to the liver in mammals are identified.

tyrosine is delayed and parahydroxyphenylpyruvic and homogentistic acids are excreted in abnormally large amounts (Fulenwider et al., 1978).

These findings show an impairment in the main pathway of tyrosine degradation. Therefore, we propose that in some cirrhotic patients there is a disturbance in the homeostasis of tyrosine with blocks both proximal and distal to the amino acid. When such an individual is on a tyrosine-free diet, he may become rapidly hypotyrosinemic. On the other hand, a tyrosine-rich diet will cause hypertyrosinemia.

Why should the cirrhotic patients of subgroup 2 have blocks in one or the other

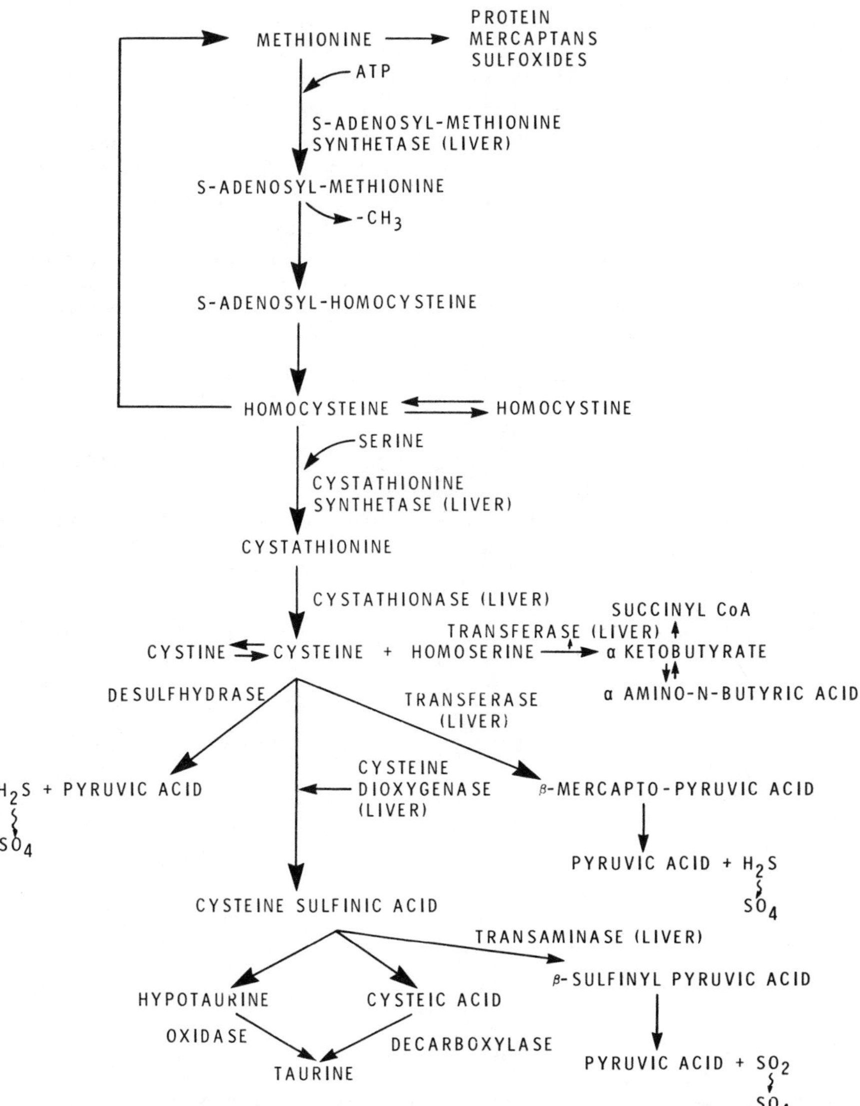

Figure 6 Transsulfuration pathway for the metabolism of methionine. Those enzymes which are primarily confined to the liver in mammals are identified.

of these pathways, while those in subgroup 1 do not? One of the responsible factors could be the degree of portal perfusion. As Stegink and Den Besten showed in 1972, when a methionine-containing, cystine-free amino acid solution is given orally to a normal individual, the plasma cystine level tends to be maintained. But when the same solution is given intravenously, the subject becomes hypocystinemic. Therefore, the delivery of dietary methionine to the liver via the portal vein is important in promoting the conversion of methionine to cystine. In many cirrhotic patients portal perfusion is lost either spontaneously or because of shunt surgery (Galambos,

1979). The difference between the two subgroups could also be attributed to differences in the metabolism of B_6 and folate, both of which are involved in the two pathways under discussion (Finkelstein, 1970). Pyridoxal phosphate and folate are frequently depleted in cirrhosis (Labadarios et al., 1977; Leery et al., 1970).

Similarly, the phenylalanine to tyrosine conversion, depressed in subgroup 2, may be due not only to inadequate portal perfusion but also to the impaired hepatic metabolism of tetrahydropteridine, a co-factor required for this enzymatic reaction.

The transsulfuration pathway generates not only cystine from methionine, but also other physiologically essential compounds: taurine, choline, carnitine, and glutathione (Figure 7). The former three substances are plentiful in a mixed diet. But a cystine-free, nothing by mouth, TPN regimen in a cirrhotic patient with a block in the transsulfuration pathway could theoretically cause depletion of all four substances. Supporting this notion we have already seen that in the cirrhotic patients that are on synthetic TPN, as plasma cystine declined, taurine declined simultaneously.

Table 6 shows the amino acid composition of all the intravenous solutions in current use. Because nearly all are deficient in cystine and tyrosine, the problem of cystine and tyrosine depletion during TPN in cirrhotic patients could have a wide prevalence.

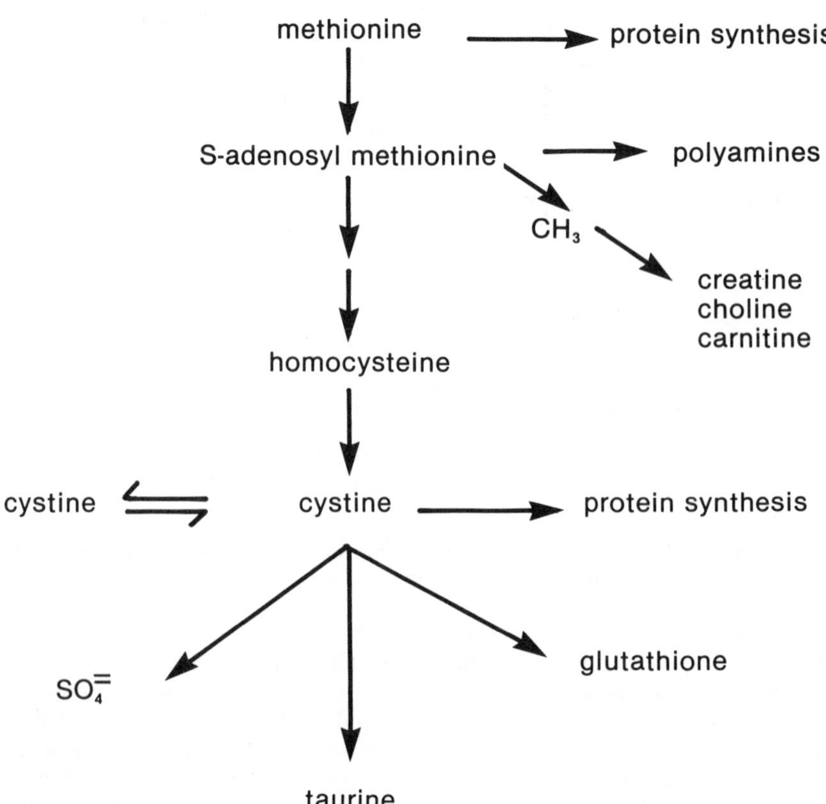

Figure 7 Products of the transsulfuration pathway which serve vital physiologic functions.

Table 6
Cystine, Cysteine and Tyrosine Contents (g/100 g) of Various Parenteral and Enteral Amino Acid Solutions in Current Use

	g/100 g Amino Acids		
	Cystine	*Cysteine*	*Tyrosine*
Egg protein§	2.4	0	4.2
Casec*	0.2	0	5.5
Isocal*	0.5	0	4.6
Vivonex*	0	0	0.9
Hepatic-aid*	0	0	0
Freamine*	0	<0.2	0
Freamine III*	0	<0.2	0
Freamine II*	0	<0.2	0
Travasol*	0	0	0.4
Amigen*	0	0	1.2
F080*	0	0	0
Aminosol°	0	0.8	2.9
Intramin°	0	0	0
Vamin°	0	2.0	0.7
Aminoplasmal⁺	0	0.5	1.3
Aminofusin⁺	0	0	0
Aminomel⁺	0	0	0
Aminonorm⁺	0.1	0	0.3
Aminosteril⁺	0	0	0
Sohamin ⊕	0	0	0

*U.S.A. ⁺Germany °Sweden ⊕ Japan
§For comparison, the contents of egg protein, a standard reference protein of high biologic value, are also given.

During January–March in 1981, plasma amino acid levels were analyzed in 48 patients who were being nourished primarily by TPN at Emory University Hospital. Blood was drawn while TPN was being infused at a rate of about 125 ml/hr and analyzed for plasma amino acids. The source of the TPN amino acids was Freamine III, which contains neither cystine nor tyrosine. Table 7 shows the nature of the subject population. Twenty-five percent of the patients had low plasma cystine, 13% had low plasma taurine, and 21% had low plasma tyrosine. Taurine concentration was directly proportional to cystine concentration ($r = 0.68$, $p < .01$). There were occasional (3% to 7% of cases) subnormal values for serine or histidine. When hypocystinemia, hypotaurinemia and hypotyrosinemia were analyzed according to disease category (Table 7), we found that the frequency of one or more such depletion was about 50% in cirrhosis, and 5% to 15% in individuals without diffuse hepatic disease. These data bear out our previous conclusion that patients with cirrhosis nourished solely by cystine- and tyrosine-free TPN are prone to hypocystinemia, hypotaurinemia and hypotyrosinemia. In addition, they show that the problem is not restricted to cirrhosis, but affects noncirrhotic individuals as well.

Table 7
Number of Patients Whose Plasma Level of Cystine, Taurine or Tyrosine Was Below the Normal Fasting Range*

	Cirrhosis n = 12	Cancer n = 18	GI Obstruction n = 8	Other n = 10
Cystine	6	3	1	2
Taurine	4	1	0	1
Tyrosine	5	2	1	2

*Range defined as ± 2 SD about normal fasting mean.

The latter deduction is consistent with the work of Stegink and Den Besten (1972) showing that even normal individuals, when given a cystine-free amino acid solution intravenously, may become hypocystinemic.

REFERENCES

Bistrian, B.R. (1976): Prevalence of malnutrition in general medical patients. *J. Am. Med. Assoc.* 235:1567–1570.

Brenton, D.P., Cusworth, D.C., Dent, C.E., and Jones, E.E. (1966): Homocystinuria, clinical and dietary studies. *Q. J. Med.* 35:325–346.

Dudrick, S.J., Wilmore, D.W., Vars, H.M., and Rhoads, J.E. (1969): Can intravenous feeding as the sole means of nutrition support growth in the child and restore weight loss in an adult? *Ann. Surg.* 169:974–984.

Finkelstein, J.D. (1970): Control of sulfur metabolism in mammals. In: *Symposium: Sulfur in Nutrition* (ed: O.H. Myth) pp. 36–40, Avi Publishing Co., Westport, Conn.

Frimpter, G.W. (1972): Cystathioninuria, sulfite oxidase deficiency, and "β-mercaptolactate-cysteine disulfiduria". In: *The Metabolic Basis of Inherited Disease* (eds: J. Stanbury, J. Wynggarden, and D. Frederickson), Chapter 20, pp. 413–425. McGraw-Hill, New York.

Fulenwider, J.T., Nordlinger, B.M., Faraj, B.A., Ivey, G.I., and Rudman, D. (1978): Deranged tyrosine metabolism in cirrhosis. *Yale J. Biol. Med.* 51:625–633.

Galambos, J. (1979): Cirrhosis. Vol. VII, In: *Major Problems in Internal Medicine.* W.B. Saunders Co., Philadelphia, Pa.

Jeejeebhoy, K.N., Anderson, G.H., Nakhooda, A.F., et al (1976): Metabolic studies in total parenteral nutrition with lipid in man. Comparison with glucose. *J. Clin. Invest.* 57:125–136.

Keating, J.P., and Ternberg, J.L. (1971): Amino acid-hypertonic glucose treatment for intractable diarrhea in infants. *Am. J. Dis. Child.* 122:226.

Knox, W.E. (1972): Phenylketonuria. In: *The Metabolic Basis of Inherited Disease* (eds: J. Stanbury, J. Wynggarden, and D. Frederickson) Chapter 11, p. 266–295. McGraw-Hill, New York.

Rudman, D., Kutner, M., Ansley, J., Jansen, R., Chipponi, J., and Bain, R.P. (1981): Hypotyrosinemia, hypocystinemia, and failure to retain nitrogen during total parenteral nutrition of cirrhotic patients. *Gastroenterology* 81:1025–1035.

Scribner, B.H., Cole, J.J., Christopher, T.G., et al (1970): Long-term total parenteral nutrition. *J. Am. Med. Assoc.* 212:457.

Stegink, L.D., and Den Besten, L. (1972): Synthesis of cysteine from methionine in normal adult subjects: Effect of route of alimentation. *Science* 178:514–516.

Intravenous Administration of Branched-Chain Amino Acids in the Treatment of Hepatic Encephalopathy

John Wahren, Jaque Denis, Philippe Desurmont, Ljusk-Siw Eriksson, Jean-Marc Escoffier, A.P. Gauthier, Lars Hagenfeldt, Henri Michel, Pierre Opolon, J.C. Paris, and M. Veyrac

In recent years it has been repeatedly suggested that intravenous or oral administration of branched-chain amino acids (BCAA) may be beneficial in patients with liver cirrhosis and encephalopathy (Fischer, et al., 1976; Freund et al., 1979; de Aguilar et al., 1979; Pellegrino et al., 1980). However, these reports are primarily concerned with case reports or uncontrolled trials. So far, results from properly controlled clinical trials have not been presented. The present study was designed as a double blind, randomized multicenter trial to evaluate the possible influence of BCAA administration on brain function in patients with liver coma.

PATIENTS AND METHODS

The study included 52 patients with acute hepatic encephalopathy (29 male, 23 female) from five medical centers (Paris, Marseille, Montpellier, Lille and Stockholm). All patients showed clinical and laboratory signs of liver cirrhosis; histological verification was available in 36 patients. Before admission to the study each patient was examined twice with a minimum interval of six hours and found to have encephalopathy grade II (n = 2), III (n = 19) or IVa–IVd (n = 31) (Denis et al., 1978).

A double blind, randomized study design was employed. BCAAs were given intravenously (20 g/L, 70% leucine, 20% valine, 10% isoleucine) in 5% glucose. Glucose (5%) alone was given as placebo. Two liters of BCAA (40 g) or placebo were given daily. The BCAA and placebo solutions were generously supplied by KabiVitrum, Sweden. The intravenous infusions were given for 20 hours per day and therapy was continued for one day after the encephalopathy had improved to grade 0 or I or for a maximum of five days. Nutritional support (30 kcal/kg body weight) was provided with equal proportions of calories from carbohydrate (50% glucose) and fat (20% Intralipid, KabiVitrum, Sweden). In addition, eight patients (four BCAA and four placebo) received conventional therapy involving lactulose and/or neomycin administration.

Daily neurological examinations were carried out. Daily venous blood samples for analyses of amino acids, enzymes and ammonia were collected in the morning four hours after the end of the intravenous infusions of BCAA or placebo. Amino acid concentrations in plasma were analyzed using ion exchange chromatography. Biochemical determinations were carried out in the routine chemical laboratory at each centre. Data in the text are given as mean ± SE. Cumulative mortality data for the two groups were compared as described by Cramér (1946), otherwise standard statistical methods were employed (Snedecor and Cochran, 1967).

RESULTS

At the end of the study 27 patients had been given BCAA and 25 had received placebo. In the BCAA group 14 patients woke up (grade 0-II), while 13 were unchanged or deteriorated. Among those who received placebo, 12 woke up and 13 were unchanged or deteriorated. There was no statistically significant difference between the two groups in this regard.

Plasma amino and analysis before the start of the study demonstrated elevated venous levels of tyrosine (165 ± 21 μmol/L) phenylalanine (141 ± 18 μmol/L) and methionine (63 ± 7 μmol/L) as well as low concentrations of all three BCAA. After one day of BCAA infusion, significant reductions in the venous concentrations of tyrosine (−65%, $p < 0.01$), phenylalanine (−30% $p < 0.05$) and methionine (−25%, $p < 0.05$) could be detected. The concentrations of the three BCAA all tended to rise but the increments did not reach statistical signficance. No changes in the concentrations of liver enzymes, creatinine or potassium were seen in either group during the treatment. However, the urea level increased in the BCAA group while it decreased in the placebo group; on the third day of treatment the urea level was 12.1 ± 1.9 mmol/L in the BCAA group and 7.0 ± 1.3 mmol/L in the placebo group ($p < 0.05$).

The cumulative survival during the five days of study is illustrated in Figure 1. Survival tended to be consistently lower in the BCAA group. Thus, after five days, 13 of the 27 patients in the BCAA group had died, as compared to five out of 25 in the placebo group ($p < 0.05$). After the study, this difference tended to even out, so that 25 days after end of the trial the survival was approximately 30% in both groups. Examination of the causes of death for those who died during the first five days revealed no difference between the two treatment groups.

The BCAA-treated patients and the placebo group were quite similar with regard to the severity of the encephalopathy as reflected by the clinical grading. Moreover, the laboratory data did not differ between the two groups, with the exception that plasma ammonia levels were 50% greater in the placebo group. The incidence of precipitating factors (gastrointestinal bleeding, infection, hepatitis, etc.) was no different in the two groups. However, the patients in the placebo group were somewhat younger (52 ± 2 yr) than those in the BCAA group (62 ± 2 yr, $p < 0.05$).

DISCUSSION

Previous studies involving BCAA administration to patients with liver cirrhosis and hepatic encephalopathy have reported a positive therapeutic effect, which in part has been attributed to a decrease in the concentrations of the aromatic amino acids (Fischer et al., 1976; Watanabe et al., 1979; Holm et al., 1978; Higashi et al., 1981). However, it should be noted that none of these studies is an adequately controlled clinical trial. In the present study, the patients treated with BCAA but not those receiving placebo showed a marked diminution in the plasma levels of the aromatic amino acids and methionine. Despite this, there was no greater improvement in encephalopathy compared with patients receiving placebo. Thus, these observations do not support the notion that BCAA administration is beneficial in patients with hepatic encephalopathy. In agreement with this conclusion,

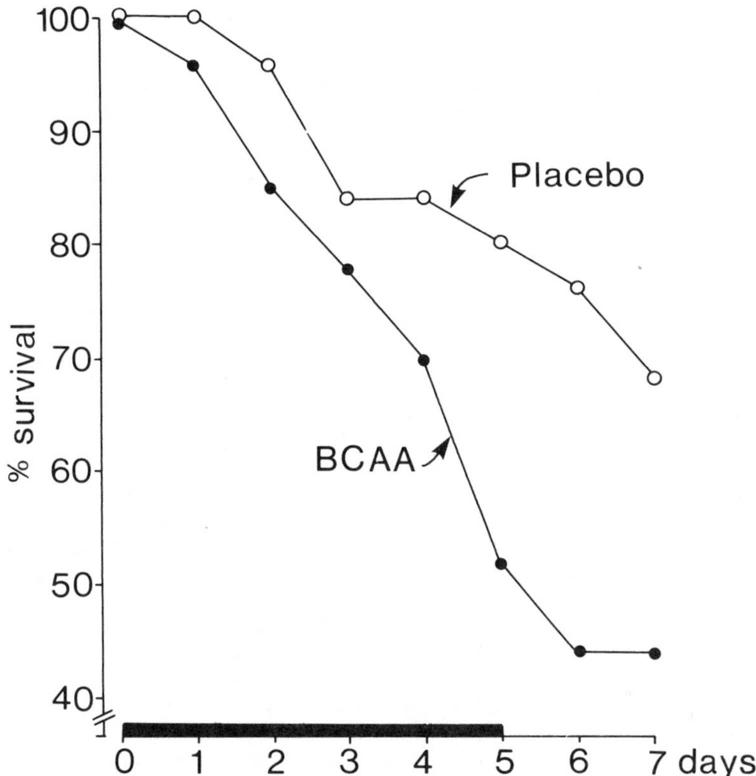

Figure 1 Cumulative survival in the BCAA and placebo groups, respectively, during (solid box) and after the study. The difference between the two groups on day five is statistically significant, $p < 0.05$.

preliminary findings from another controlled clinical study (Michel et al., 1980) suggest that a BCAA solution with a different composition to that used in the present study also fails to improve patients with acute liver coma. Similarly, a randomized double-blind cross-over study on the influence of oral BCAA ingestion in patients with chronic as opposed to acute hepatic encephalopathy demonstrated no improvement in the altered brain function in this condition (Eriksson et al., 1982). These findings emphasize the importance of controlled, randomized trials, especially in a situation where the spontaneous clinical course or conventional therapy results in clinical improvement in about 50% of the patients.

It is surprising that the mortality during the first five days in the present study was significantly higher among the patients who received BCAA. Careful examination of possible differences in clinical course or laboratory data between the BCAA and placebo groups did not offer an explanation for the increased mortality after BCAA administration. Although the BCAA-treated patients were somewhat older, the conclusion cannot be avoided that BCAA infusion in patients with acute hepatic coma not only fails to improve cerebral function but also may have deleterious effects as reflected by an increased early mortality.

ACKNOWLEDGMENTS

This study was supported by grants from KabiVitrum, Stockholm, Sweden and Paris, France, the Swedish Medical Research Council (No. 3108, 722) and the Petrus and Augusta Hedlund Foundation.

REFERENCES

Cramer, H. (1946): *Mathematical Methods of Statistics.* Princeton University Press, Princeton, N.J.

de Aguilar, T.C.F., Martines, J.L. and Perez Picouto, F. (1979): Nutricioon parenteral en 29 enfermos afectos de encefalopatia hepatica tratados con F.080. *Rev. Clin. Esp.* 355–361.

Denis, J., Opolon, P., Nusinovici, V., Granger, A. and Darnis, F. (1978): Treatment of encephalopathy during fulminant hepatic failure by hemodialysis with high permeability membrane. *Gut* 19:787–793.

Eriksson, L.S., Persson, A. and Wahren, J. (1982): Branched-chain amino acids in the treatment of chronic hepatic encephalopathy. *Gut* (In Press).

Fischer, J.E., Rosen, H.M., Ebeid, A.M., Howard James, J., Keane, J.M. and Soeters, P.B. (1976): The effect of normalization of plasma amino acids on hepatic encephalopathy in man. *Surgery* 80:77–91.

Freund, H., Yoshimura, N. and Fischer, J.E. (1979): Chronic hepatic encephalopathy. Long-term therapy with a BCAA-enriched diet. *J.A.M.A.* 242:347–349.

Higashi, T., Watanabe, A., Hayashi, S., Obata, T., Takei, N. and Nagashima, H. (1981): Effect of branched-chain amino acid infusion on alterations in CSF neutral amino acids and their transport across the blood-brain barrier in hepatic encephalopathy. In: *Metabolism and Clinical Implications of Branched Chain Amino and Ketoacids.* (eds: M. Walser and J.R. Williamson), pp. 465–470. Elsevier/North Holland, Amsterdam.

Holm, E., Striebel, J.P., Meisinger, E., Haux, P., Langhans, W. and Becker, H.D. (1978): Aminosäurengemische zur parenteralen Ernährung bei Leberinsuffizienz. *Infusionstherapie* 5:274–292.

Michel, H., Pomier-Layrargues, G., Duhamel, O., Lacombe, B., Cuilleret, G. and Bellet, H. (1980): Intravenous infusion of ordinary and modified amino acid solutions in the management of hepatic encephalopathy. *Gastroenterology* 79:1038.

Pellegrino, F., Zola, C. and Ghinelli, F. (1980): L'impiego delle soluzioni selettive di aminoacidi nel trattamento pre- e post- operatorio dei cirrotici. *Minerva Chir.* 35:439–444.

Snedecor G.W. and Cochran, W.G. (1967): *Statistical Methods,* 6th ed. Iowa State University Press, Ames, Iowa.

Watanabe, A., Takesue, A., Higashi, T. and Nagashima, N. (1979): Serum amino acids in hepatic encephalopathy—Effects of branched-chain amino acid infusion on serum aminogram. *Acta Hepato-Gastroenterol.* 26:346–357.

INDEX

Acetate salts, in parenteral nutrition, 330, 331
Acetoacetate, 90
Acetoacetic acid, 91
Acetylcholine
  brain function and, 220
  food consumption and synthesis of, 220–222
Acetylglutamate (AGA), 81–82, 83
Acid-base balance
  parenteral nutrition and, 328–329
  ureagenesis and, 77–78
Acidosis, renal, 5
Acid phosphotase, 38, 39, 40
Acylcarnitine, 342
Adenosine, 220
S-adenoxylmethionine, 32
Adipose tissue
  amino acid metabolism in, 5–6
  arteriovenous measurements of amino acids in, 3–4
  valine oxidation in, 147, 153
Adrenocorticotrophic hormone, 344–345
Aging
  albumin synthesis and, 40, 44
  amino acid requirements and, 24
  amino acid and protein metabolism and, 37–45
  organ function and alterations associated with, 39–43
  protein intake and, 43–44
  protein turnover and, 44
Alanine
  arteriovenous measurement in muscle of, 3–5
  cancer and, 10, 212, 429–437
  epinephrine and, 70
  fasting and, 90, 292
  glucagon and, 68–70, 72–75
  gluconeogenesis and, 66, 68–70
  glutamate and, 132
  hepatic utilization of amino acids and, 212
  hyperammonemia and, 84
  hyperglucagonemia and, 97
  hyperketonemia and, 91
  indispensable amino acids and, 110, 114–115
  insulin and, 7, 70, 72
  insulin-glucagon interaction and, 72–75
  ketone bodies and, 89–93
  nitrogen in urea biosynthesis and, 80
  nitrogen transport with, 2, 114, 115
  norepinephrine and, 72
  nutritional state of hepatocyte and, 185, 186, 187
  peripheral tissue release of, 5
  portacaval shunt and transport of, 243
  protein balance in skeletal muscle and, 201
  protein intake and synthesis of, 436
  protein synthesis and, 184, 185
  renal failure and, 452, 453
  sepsis and, 9, 417–420
  skeletal muscle metabolism of, 275
  sodium β-hydroxybutyrate and, 92
  stressed nutritional states and, 296, 304
  threonine brain uptake and, 116–117
  total parenteral nutrition (TPN) with, 429–437
  transamination reaction with, 2–3, 112
  traumatic injury and, 391
L-alanine
  hospitalized patient metabolism of, 273
  sepsis and, 417
Albumin
  aging and synthesis of, 40, 44
  amino acids and synthesis of, 168, 172
  cancer and, 430
  cirrhosis and, 478, 484, 487
  intravenous hyperalimentation (IVH) and, 406, 407, 408, 411
  isotopic measurements of, 276
  liver protein synthesis and, 176–177
  malnutrition and, 348, 353–354
  nitrogen balance technique with, 268
  renal failure and, 441, 442, 445, 448
Alkaline phosphatase, 406–407
Amino acid catabolism
  nutrient flow in liver and, 183
  protein turnover and, 49
Amino acid metabolism, 63–104
  aging and, 37–45
  amino acid requirements and, 18–24
  cancer and, 10
  diabetes and, 7
  disease states and, 5–10
  dispensable amino acids in, 24–27
  factors influencing, 13
  fasting and, 5–6
  fever and sepsis and, 8–9
  gluconeogenesis and, 63–75
  indispensable amino acids in, 14–16
  in isolated hepatocyte, 183–187
  liver failure and, 8
  in muscle, 159
  protein and energy intakes in, 13–26
  renal failure and, 7–8
  sulfur amino acids and developmental aspects of, 29–34
  whole body, 1–62
Amino acid requirement estimates, 23, 265–285, 291–292
  aging and, 24

amino acid concentrations and, 269–270
arteriovenous differences technique in, 274–275
Catabolic Index in, 284–285
degree of metabolic stress and, 283–285
identification of parameters to use in, 266
interpretation of amino acid changes and, 269–270
isotopically labeled amino acids in, 275–282
in Japanese young men, 55–62
limitations of model in, 279–282
nitrogen balance in, 268–282
pool sizes and significance in, 270–271
whole body protein turnover and, 282–283
Amino acids
health and, 1–5
interrelationships among, 105–164
organ relationships with, 167–261
overview and synthesis in, 1–10
D-amino acids, in intestine, 256, 258
L-amino acids
crystalling, in enteral solutions, 309
intestinal absorption of, 256, 258
Amino acid solutions
Catabolic Index and, 284–285
crystalline, in parenteral nutrition, 328–331
goals of use of, 266–268
stressed nutritional states and, 304–305
see also Enteral nutrition; Nutritional support solutions; Parenteral nutrition
α-aminobutyric acid, 487, 488
Aminopeptidase A, 259
Aminoplex 5, 295
Aminosol, 298
Aminosyn, 124, 125, 328, 329
Ammonia
glutamine and, 4
hemodialysis reactions and, 80
hepatic encephalopathy and, 480, 497
hyperammonemia and, 328
protein synthesis and, 79
protein turnover in severely ill patients and, 401–405
renal failure and, 448, 453–454
threonine transamination release of, 113
ureagenesis and, 77–78, 80, 81
Amphetamine, 233
Amygdala, 244
Amylase
intravenous hyperalimentation (IVH) and, 407
malnutrition and, 351
Arachidonate, and protein breakdown, 206–207, 208
Arachidonic acid, 206–207
Arginase, 78
Arginine
blood-brain barrier transport of, 239, 250
brain uptake of, 118
creatine synthesis and, 2
dispensable and indispensable amino acids in synthesis of, 115–116
hepatic encephalopathy and, 482
hepatic failure and, 318, 319, 320
hepatic utilization of amino acids in cancer and, 213
hyperammonemia and, 83, 84
parenteral nutrition and, 328, 484
renal failure and, 452, 459, 466, 467
starvation and, 293
ureagenesis with, 78, 83
Arginine synthetase, 459
Arginyl, 213
Aromatic amino acids
amino acid infusion with, 304
hepatic encephalopathy and, 477, 478, 479, 480, 481, 482
hepatic failure and, 318
starvation and, 295, 296
Arrhythmias, 352
Aryl sulphatase, 38
Asparagine
portacaval shunt and transport of, 243
protein catabolism and, 184
protein composition with, 123, 124
ureagenesis and, 84
Aspartate
enteral nutrition with, 126–130
factors influencing utilization of, 123–141
indispensable amino acids and concentrations of, 110
liver failure and, 317
neurotoxicity of, 124, 136
nutritional state of hepatocyte and, 185, 186
parenteral solutions with, 124–127, 135–141, 329
protein composition with, 123, 124
renal failure and, 452, 453
transport of, 239
traumatic injury and, 390
ureagenesis with, 78, 80, 83, 84
Aspartate-oxaloacetate aminotransferase, 80
Aspartic acid, 25
Aspirin, 207
ATP
kidney branched-chain ketoacid dehydrogenase and, 473–474
protein breakdown and, 208

Bacteria, gastrointestinal, 351
Basal metabolic rate, in malnutrition, 369

BCAA, *see* Branched-chain amino acids (BCAA)
BCKA, *see* Branched-chain ketoacids (BCKA)
Beef fibrin protein hydrolysate, 298
Bicarbonate
  gluconeogenesis measurement with, 66
  ureagenesis and, 77–78
Bile acids, 351
Bilirubin, in intravenous hyperalimentation (IVH), 407
Blastogenesis, lymphocyte, 414, 415
Blood-brain barrier
  brain metabolism and, 250
  cirrhosis and, 479
  neurotransmitter synthesis and, 231
  portacaval shunting and, 239–251
  transport system in, 219–220
  tryptophan and, 462
Blue Cross, 336
Body mass
  elderly and, 337, 338
  nutritional therapy for depletion of, 360
  starvation and, 348–349
Body weight
  elderly and, 338
  intravenous hyperalimentation (IVH) and, 406, 407, 408, 411
  muscle decrease in starvation and, 349
Bombesin, 234
Bradycardia, 352
Brain, 219–251
  blood-brain barrier transport system and, 219–220
  dispensable and indispensable amino acid interactions in, 116–118
  dispensable and indispensable amino acid pools in, 108–110
  food consumption and neurotransmitter synthesis in, 220–222
  ketone bodies utilized by, 91
  metabolism of, and blood-brain barrier, 250
  muscle factor and BCKA dehydrogenase in, 192, 194, 197
  parenteral and enteral amino acid mixtures and, 219–223, 330
  portacaval shunting and amino acid transport in, 239–251
  starvation and changes in, 348, 349, 355
Branched-chain amino acids (BCAA)
  albumin synthesis in liver and, 184
  amino acid solutions with, 304, 305
  branched-chain α-ketoacid metabolism and, 101
  endocrine system control of, 96
  fever and sepsis and, 9
  free fatty acids (FFA) and, 90–91
  hepatic encephalopathy and, 477–482, 497–499
  high performance liquid chromatography (HPLC) for quantiation of, 101–104
  hospitalized patient metabolism of, 272–274
  hypercatabolic patients and, 382
  indispensable amino acids and transamination of, 112–113
  injury and, 269, 300, 304, 389, 393
  insulin in diabetes and, 7
  in vivo and *in vitro* interactions of, 147–153
  liver failure and, 8, 318, 319
  low birth-weight infants and, 321
  nitrogen in cancer patients and, 421–427
  nitrogen in urea biosynthesis and, 80, 83
  nutritional state of hepatocyte and, 185, 186, 187
  peripheral tissues with, 5
  protein synthesis and, 89
  renal failure and, 440, 453, 468
  starvation and, 6, 291, 292, 295, 296
  transfer of, 3
  uremia and, 8
Branched-chain amino acid transaminase, in renal failure, 445–446
Branched-chain ketoacid dehydrogenase (BCKD)
  kinase activity and, 472–475
  renal failure and, 446
Branched-chain ketoacids (BCKA)
  hepatic encephalopathy and, 482
  indispensable amino acids and transamination of, 112–113
Branched-chain α-ketoacid (BCKA) dehydrogenase
  muscle in regulation of, 191–198
  plasma factor in, 192–193, 198
Branched-chain α-ketoacids
  branched-chain amino acid metabolism and, 101
  high performance liquid chromatography (HPLC) in quantitation of, 101–104
  renal failure and, 446, 447
Bronchitis, 354
Burn patients
  amino acid flux in, 390
  amino acid requirements of, 266, 274, 282, 300
  nitrogen balance in, 209
  nitrogen intake in, 380
  protein dynamics in, 396–400

Cachexia
  cancer and, 430, 431
  cardiac mass and, 352

elderly and, 339
gastrointestinal mass in, 350
nitrogen balance and, 206
Cadmium, 83
Calcium, in renal failure, 441, 444
Calorie malnutrition, *see* Malnutrition
Cancer, 348, 429–437
alanine kinetics in, 429–437
amino acid metabolism and, 7, 10
branched-chain amino acid solutions and nitrogen accretion in, 421–427
cachexia and, 430, 431
elemental diet for, 325
hepatic utilization of amino acids in, 212–217
intravenous hyperalimentation (IVH) and, 407, 409
malnutrition in, 424–425, 484
marasmus in, 425
protein and amino acid metabolism in, 429–437
protein turnover in, 403–405
Carbamoyl phosphate synthetase (CPS), and ureagenesis, 81–84
Carbohydrates
branched-chain amino acids and, 3
dispensable amino acid synthesis and, 115
as energy source in malnutrition, 370–371
food intake regulation and, 232
glutamate metabolism and, 132–134
hepatic encephalopathy and, 478, 497
intravenous hyperalimentation (IVH) and, 413
liver and muscle in metabolism of, 5–6
neurotransmitter synthesis and, 221, 222, 223
protein intake regulation and, 227
serotonin and, 232–233
thermic effect of protein intake and, 383
Carbon dioxide
amino acid measurements with, 293
respiratory function in malnutrition and, 354–355, 373
stress in burn patients and, 397
thermic effect of protein intake and, 383
Carboxyglutamate, 107
Cardiac muscle
branched-chain amino acid oxidation in, 201
leucine and protein synthesis in, 188–190
malnutrition and, 351–352
protein balance in, 202
Cardiopulmonary support techniques, 348
Carnitine
BCKA dehydrogenase and, 197
cirrhosis and, 494
lysine as precursor of, 113
partial parenteral nutrition and, 342–345
Carnityl fatty acid esters, 90
Carnosinase, 461
Carnosine, 452, 461
Casein
enteral nutrition with, 312, 484
protein intake and, 228, 233
Casein hydrolysate, 328
Catabolic Index, 284–285
Catecholamines
brain function and, 220
feeding behavior and, 232–234, 235
food consumption and synthesis of, 220–222, 225–226, 231
gluconeogenesis and, 63, 70–72
parenteral mixtures and, 223
postoperative patients and, 426
protein breakdown and, 208
synthesis of, 239
tyrosine and, 231
Cathepsin B, H, and L, 208
Cathepsin D, 38, 39, 40
Central nervous system
food intake regulation and, 228
hepatic encephalopathy and, 479
Chemotherapy, 348
p-Chlorophenylanine, 223
Cholecystokinin (CCK)
amino acid uptake and, 226
food intake and, 226, 228, 234–235
malnutrition and, 351
Cholesterol, in total parenteral nutrition (PTN), 432
Choline
brain function and, 220
cirrhosis and, 494
neurotransmitter synthesis and, 220, 221 222
parenteral mixtures with, 220, 223
Choline acetyltransferase, 221
Chromatography, high performance liquid (HPLC), 101–104
Chymotrypsin, 351
Cirrhosis
amino acid concentrations in, 269
amino acid metabolism and, 6, 7, 8
amino acid requirements in, 300
branched-chain amino acids and, 497, 498
cystine and tyrosine reuirements in, 484–496
enteral nutrition and, 318–320
plasma amino acid abnormalities in, 478
Citrulline
indispensable amino acids in synthesis of, 115
nitrogen in urea biosynthesis and, 80
renal failure and, 444, 451, 452, 453, 459, 466
Clonidine, 233
Collagen, 284, 459
Coma, liver, 497, 499

Complement system, 284
Concanavalin A (Con A), 414
Congestive heart failure, 352, 484
Copper, 83
Coronary insufficiency, 325
Corticosteroids, 284
Cortisol, 345
Costs, health care, 334, 335
Creatine
  postoperative patients and, 425
  synthesis of, 2
Creatinine
  cirrhosis and, 484, 487
  hepatic encephalopathy and, 498
  postoperative patients and, 425
  protein turnover rates and, 53
  renal failure and, 441, 442, 444, 448, 453, 454, 455
Cycloheximide, 202
Cyclooxygenase inhibitors, 209
Cycloserine, 205
Cystathionase, and liver activity, 30, 31
Cystathionine
  function of, 33
  transulfuration and, 30, 31, 32–33
Cystathioninuria, 491
Cysteine
  low birth-weight infants and, 317, 321
  methionine as precursor of, 113
  parenteral nutrition and, 329
  ureagenesis and, 84
Cyst(e)ine
  infant requirement for, 31–34
  methionine and, 29–31
  milk as source of, 31–32
Cystine
  cirrhosis and, 487–488, 491, 493, 494, 495, 496
  as indispensable amino acid, 106
  nutritional state of hepatocyte and, 186
  parenteral nutrition with, 329, 484
  portacaval shunt and transport of, 243
  renal failure and, 444, 451, 452, 453, 462
Cystinuria, 256
Cystoscopy, 389
Cytochrome oxidase, 353
Cytochrome P-450, 351

Diabetes
  amino acid metabolism and, 6, 7, 8
  amino acid requirements in, 274
  amino acid transport in, 257, 258
  leucine concentrations in, 270
  parenteral mixtures and neurotransmission in, 220
Dialysis, 348
Diarrhea, and starvation, 351
Dibutyryl cyclic AMP, 208
Dicarboxylic amino acids, 126, 136–140
Diet
  brain neurotransmitter synthesis and, 225–226
  dispensable and indispensable amino acid concentrations and, 116–118
  nutritional classification of amino acids in, 106–107
  weight reduction with, 48–53
  see also Food intake; Nutritional support solutions
Digestive tract, *see* Gastrointestinal tract
5,7-Dihydroxytryptamine, 233
Dipeptidase I and II, 259
Dipeptides
  enteral nutrition and, 260–261
  transport system for, 257–258
Dipeptidyl aminopeptidase (IV), 259
Dispensable amino acids
  amino acid degradation and, 113–115
  brain transport interactions with, 116–118
  classification of amino acids as, 106–107
  interrelationship of indispensable amino acids with, 105–119
  metabolism of, 24–27
  nitrogen and, 24–25, 111–112, 123
  protein intake and, 109–110
  protein synthesis and, 107, 110–112
  protein turnover and, 282
  see also Nonessential amino acids
DNA, brain, 330
Dopamine
  brain function and, 220
  feeding behavior and, 231
  hepatic encephalopathy and, 479
  tyrosine and synthesis of, 222
Duodenal ulcer disease, 389

EDTA, 249
Egg protein, 344
  enteral solutions with, 310
  indispensable amino acids and, 111
  leucine infusion studies with 160–161
  nitrogen requirements and, 55–62
Elderly, 335–341
  age distribution of, 334, 336
  cost-effectiveness considerations in, 340–341
  cost of health care and, 334, 335
  increases in number of, 334
  nutrient requirements of, 339–340
  nutritional status assessment in, 337–339
  nutritional support services for, 336–337, 340
Elemental diet, *see* Enteral nutrition
Elental, 310–313, 314–317
  administration of, 311–312
  clinical applications of, 317

contraindications of, 316, 317
efficacy of, 311
schedules in, 314, 315
Emphysema, 354
Endocrine system, 96
Endogenous pyrogens, 284, 392
Endotoxin, and alanine, 417, 418
Energy expenditures
body mass changes with, 360
nitrogen balance estimates of, 362
Energy homeostasis
food intake and control of, 225
protein balance in skeletal muscle and, 201
Energy intakes
amino acid metabolism and, 13–26
fat and carbohydrates as, 370–371
intravenous hyperalimentation (IVH) and, 411–413
nitrogen balance and, 363–370
Enteral nutrition, 126–134, 309–325
administration of, 311–312
amino acid and peptide absorption in intestine and, 260–261
amino acid concentration changes in, 269
aminogram in, 317, 318
brain function and, 219–223
as chemically defined diet, 310
crystalline L-amino acids in, 309
efficacy of, 311
elderly and, 339, 340
healing rate with, 312, 313
hepatic failure and, 317–320
for infants, 320–324
nutritional therapy with, 317–324
schedules for, 314, 315
Ep-475, 208
Epinephrine
brain function and, 220
gluconeogenesis and, 70
Erythrocyte amino acids, 139–140
Esophageal cancer, 403, 431
Essential amino acids
human requirements for, 55–62
postoperative patients and, 389
protein synthesis and, 89
renal failure and, 441, 442, 445, 448, 453, 463, 466, 467, 468
semi-essential amino acids and, 106
traumatic injury and muscle pool of, 392–393
ureagenesis and, 79
see also Indispensable amino acids
Essential fatty acids (EFA)
low birth-weight infants and, 321
malnutrition and, 371
parenteral nutrition with, 331
Fasting
leucine and protein turnover in, 204
metabolic changes associated with, 89–90
muscle protein in, 201
protein synthesis and, 185
protein turnover in, 51
see also Starvation
Fat
in injury and infection, 380
liver and muscle in metabolism of, 5–6
malnutrition and absorption of, 363, 367
nitrogen balance in malnutrition and, 363, 367
protein intake regulation and, 227
Fatty acids, 90
Feeding behavior, and serotonin, 231–233
Fenfluramine, 222
Fever
amino acid metabolism and, 8–9
amino acid requirements and, 284
nitrogen balance and, 206, 209
Fibrin, 484
Fibrin hydrolysates, 138, 328
Fibrinogen, 184
Food intake
age and, 43
amino acid fluctuations and, 16–18, 20
amino acids in regulation of, 228–234
gut peptides and, 234–235
neurotransmitter synthesis and, 220–222
plasma amino acids and, 228–231
protein intake regulation in, 227–228
protein levels and amount in, 226–227
FreAmine II, 124, 125, 432
FreAmine III, 124, 125, 328, 329
Free amino acids
cancer and hepatic utilization of, 214, 217
food intake control mechanisms and, 225
hypercatabolic patients and, 381–382
hyperornithinemia and, 77
protein synthesis in hepatocyte and, 186
Free fatty acids (FFA)
branched-chain amino acid oxidation and, 90–91
hepatic encephalopathy and, 478
insulin in diabetes and, 7
protein balance in skeletal muscle and, 203
stressed nutritional states and, 296
Fructose diphosphatase, 353
Fumarate, 78

Gamma-amino-butyric acid, 233
Gas liquid chromatography, 101
Gastric carcinoma, 434–436
Gastrin, 234
Gastrocnemius muscle
branched-chain α-ketoacids (BCKA) dehydrogenase and, 192, 194, 196–197
leucine and protein synthesis in, 188–190

Gastrointestinal malignancies, 404, 407
Gastrointestinal surgery, 324
Gastrointestinal tract, 255–261
  amino acid and peptide absorption in, 255–261
  feeding behavior regulation and, 234
Glomerular filtration rate
  malnutrition and, 352
  renal failure and, 453, 454, 455, 461, 468
Glomerulonephritis, 441
Glucagon
  alanine uptake in liver and, 68–70
  fever and sepsis and, 8
  food intake and, 234
  gluconeogenesis and, 63, 66, 67–70, 72–75
  hepatic encephalopathy and, 478
  insulin interaction with, 72–75
  leucine or valine consumption and, 148
  liver amino acid homeostasis with, 391
  nitrogen balance in stress and, 421
  postoperative patients and, 426
  protein turnover and, 97, 99
  total parenteral nutrition (TPN) in cancer and, 432
  ureagenesis and, 84
Glucagonomas, 84
Glucocorticoids
  fever and sepsis and, 8
  leucine and, 96, 97–99
Gluconeogenesis
  alanine in, 417, 419
  amino acids and, 63–75
  arteriovenous (AV) difference techniques in measurement of, 64–65
  biochemical steps in, 63–64, 65
  cancer and, 10, 212, 213, 217
  catecholamines and, 70–72
  components of regulation of, 63, 64
  diabetes and, 7
  dispensable and indispensable amino acids and, 108
  epinephrine and, 70
  glucagon and, 67–70
  glucose trace technique in, 65–66
  hormonal actions and, 67–75
  hyperglucagonemia and, 97
  insulin and, 63, 67, 68, 70, 72–75
  insulin-glucagon interaction in, 72–75
  in vivo measurement of, 64–67
  ketone bodies in brain and, 91
  liver in starvation and, 353
  norepinephrine and, 70–72
  protein in skeletal muscle and, 201
  sepsis and, 9
  skeletal muscle after surgery and, 425
  starvation and, 292
  stressed nutritional state and, 304
  total parenteral nutrition (TPN) in cancer and, 430, 431, 434, 436
Glucose
  alanine and, 417, 419
  blood-brain barrier transport of, 249, 250
  brain function and, 223
  cancer and, 10
  carnitine and, 345
  fasting and, 90
  gluconeogenesis and, 63
  glutamate absorption in intestine and, 132–133
  hepatic encephalopathy and, 497
  leucine consumption and, 148
  leukocyte endogenous mediator (LEM) and, 284
  nitrogen balance and, 381
  potassium in malnutrition and, 372
  protein balance in skeletal muscle and, 203
  protein in malnutrition and, 371
  protein turnover in weight reduction diets and, 48
  respiratory problems in malnutrition and, 373
  sepsis and, 8–9
  stressed nutritional states and, 298
  total parenteral nutrition (TPN) in cancer and, 430, 431, 432, 434, 436, 437
  valine consumption and, 148
L-glucose, and blood-brain barrier, 249
Glucose-6-phosphatase, 353
Glucose-6-phosphate dehydrogenase, 43
B-glucuronidase, 38, 39, 40
Glutamate
  alanine in intestine and, 132
  blood-brain barrier transport and, 219
  carbohydrate and metabolism of, 132–134
  enteral nutrition with 126–134
  factors influencing utilization of, 123–141
  hyperketonemia and, 91
  liver failure and, 317
  neurotoxicity of, 124, 136
  nitrogen transfer and, 114
  nutritional state of hepatocyte and, 186
  parenteral nutrition and, 124–127, 135–141, 329
  protein composition with, 123, 124
  protein synthesis and, 111
  renal failure and, 452, 453
  transamination of, 112, 114
  transport of, 239
  traumatic injury and, 390
  ureagenesis with, 83, 84
Glutamate dehydrogenase, 79, 80
Glutamic acid, 2–3, 113
Glutaminase, 393

Glutamine
acidosis in kidney and, 5
alanine transamination with, 2–3
arteriovenous measurement in muscle and, 3–5
cancer and, 10
hyperammonemia and, 84, 328
hypercatabolic patients and, 381, 382
indispensable amino acids and, 110, 114–115
injury and infection and, 269, 300
nitrogen in urea biosynthesis and, 80
nitrogen metabolism and, 25
nitrogen transport with, 2, 114
peripheral tissue release of, 5
portacaval shunt and transport of, 243
protein balance in skeletal muscle and, 201
protein composition with, 123, 124
protein synthesis and, 172
renal failure and, 446, 453
sepsis and, 9
Glutamine aminotransferase, 113
Glutamine synthetase, 393
Glutathione, 494
Glutathione 5-transferases, 351
Glycerol
gluconeogenesis with, 63
hepatic utilization of amino acids in cancer and, 212, 213
starvation and, 84
Glycine
ammonia and, 84
creatine synthesis and, 2
enteral nutrition with, 126, 130
factors influencing utilization of, 123–141
gluconeogenesis with, 66
hyperammonemia with, 135
injury and infection and, 269, 300
metabolism of, 185
neurotransmitter precursors and, 233
nutritional state of hepatocyte and, 185, 186
parenteral nutrition with, 124–127, 135–141, 329, 330, 484
portacaval shunt and transport of, 243
protein intake and concentrations of, 110
protein synthesis and, 111, 185
protein turnover and, 48–53, 283, 401–405
renal failure and, 446, 451, 452, 453, 454–456
starvation and, 293
threonine as precursor of, 113
threonine brain uptake and, 117
Glycogen
aging and, 42
amino acid metabolism and, 5–6
gluconeogenesis with, 66
potassium in malnutrition and, 372
total parenteral nutrition (TPN) in cancer with, 436, 437
Glycolysis, and aging, 42
Growth hormone, 432
Guanidoacetic acid, 2
Gut
food intake regulation and, 234–235
leucine and protein synthesis in, 188–190

Hartnup disease, 256
Healing rate, with enteral solutions, 312, 313
Health care costs, 334, 335
Heart
malnutrition and mass and function of, 351–352
muscle factor and BCKA dehydrogenase in, 192, 194, 197
starvation and changes in, 348, 349
see also Cardiac muscle
Hematoma, 378
Hemodialysis, 80, 451
Hepatic Aid, 319, 320
Hepatic failure, *see* Liver failure
Hepatitis, 480
Hepatocyte
amino acid metabolism in, 183–187
glucagon in protein turnover and, 97
malnutrition and, 353
High performance liquid chromatography (HPLC), 101–104
Hippocampus, 244
Histamine
neurotransmitter precursors with, 233
renal failure and, 461
Histidine
food intake regulation and, 229, 233–234
liver regulation of, 3
nutritional state of hepatocyte and, 185
parenteral nutrition with, 328, 484
portacaval shunt and transport of, 243
protein catabolism and, 184
protein intake and, 111
renal failure and, 447, 452, 453, 460–461, 466, 467
starvation and, 293
transport of, 239
ureagenesis and, 84
L-histidine, and renal failure, 441
Homocysteine
infant development and, 32
methionine as precursor of, 113
renal failure and, 462
Homocystinuria, 491
Homogentistic acid, 492

Homoserine, 113
Hospitalized patients
  amino acid profiles and nutritional considerations in, 291–305
  amino acid requirement estimates for, 265–285
  branched-chain amino acid metabolism in, 272–274
  metabolic stress in, 283–285
  stressed state amino acid patterns in, 296–305
  whole body protein turnover in, 282–283
Host defense, 166, 168
Hydrochloride salts, 330
Hydrogen, 439
Hydrolases, peptide, 259–261
Hydroxyacids, and renal failure, 467–468
β-Hydroxybutyrate, 90, 91, 92, 93
p-Hydroxy-phenylpyruvate oxidase, 320
Hydroxyproline, 107
  absorption of, 126
  renal failure and, 459–460
  traumatic injury and, 390
Hydroxyproline oxidase, 460
Hyperaminoacidemia, 84
Hyperammonemia, 78, 80
  amino acids in, 83, 84
  arginine and, 83
  glycine metabolism defects and, 135
  hepatic encephalopathy and, 478, 479
  parenteral nutrition with, 328, 330
Hypercapnia, 413
Hypercatabolic patient, 377–384
  balance between amino acids and nonprotein calories in, 377–378
  free amino acids of plasma and muscle in, 381–382
  nitrogen balance in, 378
  nitrogen intake in, 379–380
  nitrogen loss in, 378–379
  peripheral amino acids in, 380–381
  thermic effect of protein intake in, 382–383
  traumatic injury and, 388
  use of term, 378
Hypercatabolism
  amino acid patterns in, 296
  malnutrition and, 366, 369, 371
Hyperglucagonemia, 67, 97
Hyperglycemia, 8, 419, 426, 436, 437
Hyperglycinemia, 329
Hyperketonemia, 91, 93
Hyperlactacidemia, 419
Hypermetabolism, 388
Hyperornithinemia, 77
Hyperphosphatemia, 444
Hypertriglyceridemia, 426
Hypertyrosinemia, 491, 492
Hypoalaninemia, 70
Hypoalbuminemia, 478
Hypoaminoacidemia, 391, 487
  low birth-weight infants and, 320
  ureagenesis and, 84
Hypoammonemia, 77
Hypocystinemia, 495, 496
Hypoglycemia, 419
Hypotaurinemia, 495
Hypotension, 352
Hypothalamus
  amino acid transport and, 244
  food intake regulation and, 228, 234, 235
  glutamate and neuronal necrosis in, 136
Hypothyroidism, 343
Hypotyrosinemia, 495

Imidazolepyruvic acid, 460
Immune response
  amino acids and, 166
  elderly and, 339
  nutrient support and, 414
  stressed nutritional states and, 303
Indispensable amino acids
  amino acid degradation and, 113–115
  brain transport interactions with, 116–118
  classification of amino acids as, 106–107
  interrelationships among dispensable amino acids and, 105–119
  nitrogen equilibrium and, 111–112
  protein intake and, 14–16
  protein synthesis and, 107, 110–112
  protein turnover and, 282
  semi-indispensable amino acids and, 106
  see also Essential amino acids
Indomethacin, 207
Infancy
  cyst(e)ine requirements in, 31–34
  elemental diet for, 320–324
  parental amino acid solutions in, 135–141, 327–332
Infection
  adrenocorticotrophic hormone in, 344–345
  amino acid requirements in, 266, 283
  fat stores as energy source in, 380
  malnutrition and, 484
  protein dynamics of blood lymphocytes and, 414–416
  protein loss in, 379
  protein synthesis and, 266–268
  traumatic injury and, 388
Inflammation
  amino acid requirements and, 284
  prostaglandins in, 206
Injury
  adrenocorticotrophic hormone in, 344–345

amino acid requirements in, 266, 279–280, 283, 284, 296
fat stores as energy source in, 380
free amino acids in plasma and muscle in, 382
hyperglycemia in, 436
leucine concentrations in, 270
protein loss in, 379
protein synthesis and, 266–268
Insulin
alanine levels and, 70, 72
amino acid metabolism and, 5–6
amino acid uptake and, 226
blood-brain barrier transport of, 249
branched-chain amino acid metabolism and, 6, 7
disease states and levels of, 5–10
fever and sepsis and, 8–9
food intake and, 234
glucagon interaction with, 72–75
gluconeogenesis and, 63, 67, 68, 70, 72–75
hepatic encephalopathy and, 478
hypoaminoacidemia and, 84
leucine and, 96, 148, 149
leukocyte endogenous mediator (LEM) and, 284
muscle protein in malnutrition and, 371
nitrogen balance and, 268, 421
nutritional state of hepatocyte and, 185, 186–187
postoperative patients and, 426
protein balance in skeletal muscle and, 203
protein in fasts and, 91
protein synthesis and, 39, 41, 172, 183, 185, 186
protein turnover and, 99
renal failure and, 7–8, 461
stressed nutritional states and, 298
total parenteral nutrition (TPN) in cancer and, 432, 435–436
valine consumption and, 148
Insulin resistance, in sepsis, 419
Interleukin I, 284
Interstitial nephritis, 441
Intestine
amino acid and peptide absorption in, 130, 255–261
leucine and protein synthesis in, 188–190
Intravenous hyperalimentation (IVH)
alanine tolerance in, 417–420
nutritional and metabolic response to, 406–413
Isoleucine
branched-chain α-ketoacids (BCKA) and catabolism of, 191
hepatic encephalopathy and, 480, 497
high performance liquid chromatography (HPLC) and, 102, 104
hospitalized patient metabolism of, 273, 274
hypercatabolic patients and, 381
leucine ingestion and, 147, 153
muscle amino acid metabolism and, 159
neurotransmitter synthesis and, 231
portacaval shunt and transport of, 242
protein intake regulation and, 229
protein synthesis and, 89
renal failure and, 441, 445, 447, 453, 462, 463, 467
stressed nutritional states and, 299, 301
transport of, 239
ureagenesis and, 84
Isoproterenol, 284
Isotope techniques
amino acid studies with, 275–282
body mass changes with, 360
protein turnover in severely ill patients with, 401

Japanese young men, and amino acid requirements, 55–62
Jejunum
amino acid absorption in, 130, 133, 257, 258
leucine and protein synthesis in, 188–190

Kanamycin, 80
α-Ketoacid dehydrogenase, 153
Ketoacids, and renal failure, 467–468
α-Ketoacids
branched-chain amino acid metabolism and, 89
high performance liquid chromatography (HPLC) for quantitation of, 101–104
indispensable amino acids and, 107, 112
renal failure and, 440, 441, 442, 445, 447, 448
Keto analogues, 481–482
α-Ketocaproate, 101–102, 103
Ketogenesis, 108
α-ketoglutarate, 113
branched-chain amino acid metabolism and, 89
glutamate and intestinal, 132
muscle protein breakdown with leucine and, 151, 153
L-ketoisocaproate, 280
α-Ketoisocaproate
BCKA dehydrogenase and, 197
branched-chain α-ketoacid analysis with, 102

leucine formation and, 113
leucine infusion and, 159–164
renal failure and, 440–441, 446
α-ketoisocaproic acid, 205
leucine in protein breakdown and, 205
stress in burn patients and, 396–400
Ketoisovalerate, in muscle protein breakdown with leucine, 151, 153
α-Ketoisovalerate
branched-chain α-ketoacid analysis with, 102
renal failure and, 446
α-Ketomethiolbutyrate, 102
α-Ketomethylvalerate, 102, 103
Ketone bodies
blood-brain barrier and, 250
carnitine and, 345
insulin in diabetes and, 7
leucine and alanine metabolism and, 89–93
parenteral nutrition and, 371
protein balance in skeletal muscle and, 203
starvation and, 296
total parenteral nutrition (TPN) in cancer and, 436
Ketonuria, 50
Kidney
acidosis and glutamine in, 5
arteriovenous techniques for amino acids in, 274
branched-chain ketoacid dehydrogenase (BCKD) and kinase activity in, 472–475
gluconeogenesis in, 63
glutamine as source of ammonia in, 4
muscle factor and BCKA dehydrogenase in, 192, 194, 197, 198
starvation and changes in, 348, 349, 352–353
Kinase, and kidney branched-chain ketoacid dehydrogenase (BCKD) complex, 472–475

Labile protein, 363
Lactalbumin, 109
Lactate
alanine and, 417, 419
cancer and, 10
gluconeogenesis and, 7, 63
hepatic utilization of amino acids in cancer and, 212, 213
hyperketonemia and, 91
total parenteral nutrition (TPN) in cancer and, 430, 432
Lactulose, 481, 497
Laparotomy, 280
LDH phosphoglucomutase, 353
Lecithin, 221, 222
Leucine
albumin and fibrinogen synthesis in liver and, 184
adipose tissue valine oxidation and, 147
aging and protein synthesis and, 38–39, 40
alanine nitrogen transport and, 115
amino acid requirements and, 19–23, 277–279, 280–282
branched-chain amino acid synthesis and, 272
branched-chain α-ketoacid (BCKA) dehydrogenase and, 197
branched-chain α-ketoacids (BCKA) and catabolism of, 191
cancer and, 10
glucocorticoids and, 97–99
hepatic encephalopathy and, 480, 497
high performance liquid chromatography (HPLC) quantitation for, 102, 104
hormonal regulation of metabolism of, 96–99
hospitalized patient metabolism of, 273, 274
hypercatabolic patient and, 381
hyperglucagonemia and, 97
injury or burns and, 266, 270
insulin and, 96, 148, 149
in vitro branched-chain amino acid interactions with, 151–152
α-ketoisocaproate and formation of, 113, 159–164
ketone bodies and, 89–93
liver protein synthesis and, 169–171
meal intake and metabolism of, 17–18
muscle proteins with, 39, 41, 147, 151–153
neurotransmitter synthesis and, 231
peripheral tissue glutamine and, 5
pool sizes and significance in, 270–271
portacaval shunt and transport of, 240, 242, 244, 245–248, 250
postoperative patients and, 426
protein balance in skeletal muscle and, 203–204
protein catabolism and, 184
protein dynamics in infection and, 414, 415
protein intake and, 3, 14–16, 161–163, 229
protein synthesis and, 169–171, 188–190, 205–206, 421
renal failure and, 440–441, 445, 446, 447, 453, 462, 467, 468
requirements for, 23, 55, 58
similarities between plasma concentrations and appearance in, 270–271

sodium β-hydroxybutyrate and, 92
stressed nutritional states and, 296, 299, 301
stress in burn patients and, 396–400
transport of, 239
traumatic injury and, 392, 394
ureagenesis and, 83, 84
valine interactions with, 147–151
whole body protein turnover and, 282–283
L-leucine
amino acid reqirements estimates with, 278–279
insulin and, 149
similarities between plasma concentrations and appearance of, 270–271
whole body protein turnover and, 282–283
Leucyl tRNA synthetase, 206
Leukocyte endogenous mediator (LEM), 284
Leukocyte pyrogen, 284
Leupeptin, 208
Lipase, 351
Lipogenesis, 108
Lipase, 351
Lipogenesis, 108
Liver, 167–198, 477–499
aging and protein synthesis in, 37–45
albumin mRNA and protein synthesis in, 176–177
albumin synthesis in, 184
amino acid metabolism in, 5–6
amino acid metabolism in isolated hepatocyte in, 183–187
amino acid regulation in, 3
arteriovenous techniques for amino acids in, 274
branched-chain amino acids in encephalopathy in, 477–482, 497–499
cancer-induced malnutrition and, 212–217
cystathionase activity in, 30, 31
dispensable and indispensable amino acid pools in, 108, 110
glucagon and alanine uptake in, 68–70
glucagon and amino acid homeostasis in, 391
glucagon and protein breakdown in, 97
gluconeogenesis in, 63–75
hyperglycemia and alanine in, 437
indispensable amino acid oxidation in, 159
insulin-glucagon interactions in, 72–75
intravenous hyperalimentation (IVH) and, 407
leucine and protein synthesis in, 169–171, 188–190
methionine and protein synthesis in, 179–180
muscle factor and BCKA dehydrogenase in, 192–198
peripheral plasma amino acid concentrations and, 381
protein synthesis in, 37, 167–180
protein turnover in, 402–403
ribosomal cycle subunits and protein synthesis in, 168, 174–178
starvation and changes in, 348, 349, 353–354
thermic effect of amino acids and, 383
tRNA aminoacylation and protein synthesis in, 172–174
tryptophan deficiency and, 172
Liver failure
amino acid changes in, 317, 478–479
amino acid metabolism and, 7, 8
aminogram in, 317, 319, 321
depletion in malnutrition and, 372
elemental diet for, 317–320, 325, 331
parenteral mixtures and neurotransmission in, 220
protein in, 283
Low birth-weight infants
amino acid changes in, 317
elemental diet for, 320–324
Lymphocyte activating factor, 284
Lymphocytes, and protein dynamics in infection, 414–416
Lymphoma, 430
Lysine, 79
alanine nitrogen transport with, 115
blood-brain barrier transport of, 118, 239, 249
carnitine and, 113, 342, 344, 345
estimated requirement of, 19–20, 23
as indispensable amino acid, 107
indispensable amino acids and concentrations of, 108, 110, 112
liver regulation of, 3
methionine binding and, 180
nutritional state of hepatocyte and, 186
parenteral nutrition with, 328
portacaval shunt and transport of, 240, 242, 244, 245–248, 250–251
protein intake regulation and, 228
protein synthesis and, 250–251
renal failure and, 447, 453, 466
starvation and, 293, 294
stressed nutritional states and, 299, 303, 304
transamination reactions and, 112
traumatic injury and, 393
ureagenesis and, 84
whole body protein turnover and, 283
L-lysine, in renal failure, 441

MacEight, 312
Macrophages, in injury, 284
Malabsorption, 351
Malignant diseases, 348, 429; *see also* Cancer
Malnutrition, 317, 347–373
  brain mass and function in, 355
  cancer and, 424–425
  carnitine and, 343
  cirrhosis and, 484, 485
  elderly and, 337, 340
  fat and carbohydrate as energy sources in, 370–371
  hepatic utilization of amino acids in, 212–217
  incidence of, 347–348
  organ mass and function and, 347–353
  postoperative patients and, 389
  protein intake and protein synthesis in, 268, 400, 404
  renal failure and, 440
  repletion in, 359–373
  respiratory mass and function in, 354–355
  see also Starvation
Marasmus, in cancer, 425
Meals, *see* Food intake
Meclofenamate, 207
Medicare, 336
Melatonin, 219
Mental retardation, 330
Mercaptans, 477
Metabolic acidosis, in starvation, 352
Metabolic alkalosis, in parenteral nutrition, 329
Methionine
  cancer and, 430
  carnitine and, 342, 344
  cirrhosis and, 487, 488, 491, 493
  cyst(e)ine and, 29–34
  food intake and levels of, 227
  glutamine aminotransferase and, 113
  hepatic encephalopathy and, 477, 480, 498
  high performance liquid chromatography (HPLC) for quantitation of, 102, 104
  hospitalized patient metabolism of, 273
  human requirements for, 55
  hypercatabolic patients and, 382
  indispensable amino acids and, 106
  injury or trauma and, 269, 390
  liver failure and, 317, 320
  liver protein synthesis and, 179–180
  liver regulation of, 3
  low birth-weight infants and, 317, 320, 321
  metabolic pathways of, 29, 30
  milk as source for, 31–32
  nutritional state of hepatocyte and, 186
  parenteral nutrition with, 330, 484
  portacaval shunt and transport of, 243
  as precursor in amino acid degradation, 113
  protein catabolism and, 184
  renal failure and, 440, 441, 445, 446, 462, 466, 467
  starvation and, 292, 296
  stressed nutritional states and, 298, 300
  ureagenesis with, 84
Methyl cholanthrene, 431
3-methylhistidine, 107
  myofibrillar protein degradation with, 44
  renal failure and, 444, 451, 461–462
  stressed nutritional states and, 296, 298, 299
  traumatic injury and, 387
Milk, and cyst(e)ine, 31–32
Mitochondria
  malnutrition and, 353
  muscle factor and BCKA dehydrogenase and, 191–192
  protein breakdown and, 208
  ureagenesis and, 81–82
Monoamines
  feeding behavior and, 231–234
  metabolism of, 250
mRNA, and liver protein synthesis, 168, 176–177
Muscle, 201–217
  alanines and, 436
  amino acid metabolism and, 5–6
  arteriovenous measurement of amino acids in, 3–5, 274
  branched-chain amino acid interactions in, 113, 151, 159
  branched-chain α-ketoacids (BCKA) dehydrogenase activity in, 191–198
  contractile activity of, and protein breakdown, 205
  dispensable and indispensable amino acid pools in, 108–110
  elderly and measurements of, 338–339
  indispensable amino acid metabolism in, 114
  leucine and protein activity in, 147, 151–153, 188–190
  leucine incorporated into, 39, 41
  protein balance in, 201–209
  protein synthesis in, 37
  traumatic injury and breakdown of, 390
  see also specific muscles
Muscular dystrophy, 208
Myofibrillar protein, 44, 204

Neomycin, 80, 497
Neopham, 124, 125
Nephrotic syndrome, 339

Nervous system development, 330
Neurotensin, 234
Neurotransmission
  amino acid levels and, 250
  food consumption and, 220–222
  parenteral mixtures and, 220
  precursor control of, 231
Neutron activation analysis, 360
Neutrophils, in injury, 284
Nitrogen
  alanine metabolism and, 25
  amino acid requirement estimates with, 277, 278
  branched-chain amino acid solution in cancer and, 421–427
  Catabolic Index with, 284–285
  dispensable and indispensable amino acids and, 24–25, 106, 107, 108
  fasting and, 89
  enteral nutrition and, 260, 261
  fat and carbohydrate as energy sources in malnutrition and, 370–371
  glycine as source of, 124
  hypercatabolic patients and, 377, 378–379
  indispensable amino acid metabolism and, 14, 15, 114–115
  injury or infection and, 283
  leucine and, 188, 189
  malnutrition and, 363–370
  precursors of, in ureagenesis, 80
  protein intake and requirements for, 55–62
  protein synthesis and, 1–2
  protein turnover in liver and, 402
  renal failure and, 441, 442–444, 445, 446, 447
  reutilization of, in ureagenesis, 79–80
  starvation and losses of, 349
  total parenteral nutrition (TPN) with, 359–360
  traumatic injury and, 387, 388, 389, 390, 391
  ureagenesis and, 78–79
  urea metabolism and, 77–84
Nitrogen balance
  amino acid requirement estimates and, 55, 60, 266, 268–269, 285, 291–292
  amino acid solutions and, 305
  basal metabolic rate in, 369
  cirrhosis and, 484, 485, 487
  cyclooxygenase inhibitors and, 209
  dispensable amino acid concentrations and, 111–112
  energy expenditure estimates in, 362
  enteral nutrition and, 312, 316
  factors affecting, 206
  glucose infusions and, 381
  hypercatabolic patient and, 378, 379–380, 381
  intravenous hyperalimentation (IVH) and, 406
  leucine and, 205
  nitrogen and energy intake and, 363–370
  nitrogen intake and, 379–380
  nutritional state of hepatocyte and, 185
  ornithine aminotransferase deficiency and, 77
  parenteral nutrition and, 329
  protein dynamics in infection and, 414, 415
  renal failure and, 440, 444, 445, 446, 447, 448, 460, 463, 467, 468
  stress and, 421
  technical problems with, 360–362
  traumatic injury and, 394
  tumor growth and, 212, 213
  weight reduction diets and, 48, 52–53
Nonessential amino acids
  postoperative patients and, 389
  renal failure and, 447, 453, 463
  ureagenesis and, 79
  see also Dispensable amino acids
Norepinephrine
  brain function and, 220
  feeding behavior and, 231, 235
  gluconeogenesis and, 70–72
  hepatic encephalopathy and, 479
Norleucine, 101
Nutritional classification of amino acids, 106–107
Nutritional support solutions
  alanine tolerance in, 417–420
  cost-effectiveness considerations in, 340–341
  elderly and, 336–337, 340
  intravenous hyperalimentation (IVH) in, 406–413
  nitrogen accretion in cancer patients and, 421–427
  see also Amino acid solutions; Elenal; Enteral nutrition; Parenteral nutrition; Total parenteral nutrition (TPN)

Octanoate, 90
Octopamine, 479
Oligopeptides, 255, 256
Ornithine
  brain uptake and transport systems for, 118
  dispensable and indispensable amino acid interrelationships with, 115
  hepatic encephalopathy and, 482
  nutritional state of hepatocyte and, 186
  renal failure and, 448, 452, 466

transport of, 239
ureagenesis and, 83, 84
L-orinithine, and renal failure, 441
Ornithine aminotransferase deficiency, 77, 84
Ornithine carbamoyltransferase deficiency, 78
Ornithine salts, 481, 482
Ornithine transcarbamoylase, 459
Orotic aciduria, 328, 330
Ovarian tumor, 404
Oxygen
body mass changes and, 360
stress in burn patients and, 396
traumatic injury and, 390

Pain, and nutritional status, 284
Palmitate, 90
Pancreas
food intake and, 234
proteolytic enzymes of, 255
starvation and exocrine function of, 351
Pancreatitis, 280
Para-aminohippurate, 453
Parahydroxyphenylpyruvic acid, 492
Parenteral nutrition, 309
amino acid changes during, 269, 295
amino acid composition of, 124–126
brain function and, 219–223
carnitine excretion in, 342–345
choline in, 220
crystalline amino acid solutions in, 328–331
elderly and, 339, 340
erythrocyte amino acids in, 139–140
glycine, glutamate, and aspartate in, 135–141
hyperammonemia and, 328, 330
in infants, 327–332
metabolic alkalosis in, 329
metabolic effects of second-generation, 329–330
protein hydrolysates in, 327–328
ranking order of amino acids in, 295
third generation of, 331–332
traumatic injury with, 393
see also Total parenteral nutrition (TPN)
Pentobarbitol, 351
Peptides
enteral nutrition and, 260–261
food regulation and, 234–235
hydrolases of, 259
intestinal absorption of, 255–261
parenteral nutrition with, 328
Peripheral tissues
hepatic utilization of amino acids in cancer and, 212–217
hypercatabolic patients and amino acids in, 380–381
Phagocytosis, in injury, 284
Phenylalanine
amino acid solutions and, 305
cholecystokinin stimulation with, 234
cirrhosis and, 487, 494
food intake and levels of, 227, 229, 234
glutamine aminotransferase and, 113
hepatic encephalopathy and, 479, 480, 482
hypercatabolic patients and, 382
as indispensable amino acid, 106
injury or trauma and, 269, 390, 393
liver failure and, 317, 318, 320
liver metabolism of, 3
low birth-weight infants and, 317, 320, 321
neurotransmitter synthesis and, 231
nutritional state of hepatocyte and, 185, 186
parenteral nutrition with, 484
portacaval shunt and transport of, 240, 243, 244, 245–248, 250
protein catabolism and, 184
protein synthesis and, 188, 189, 206
protein turnover in skeletal muscle and, 202
renal failure and, 440, 441, 442, 445, 446, 447, 451, 452, 453, 456–459, 462, 466, 467
skeletal muscle catabolism with, 392
starvation and, 292, 293, 294, 295, 296
stressed nutritional states and, 298, 300
transport of, 239, 249
tyrosine metabolism and, 113, 155–158
whole body protein turnover and, 283
L-phenylalanine
renal failure and, 446
tyrosine metabolism and, 155
Phenylalanine hydroxylase
low birth-weight infants and, 320
renal failure and, 456, 459
Phenylalanine tRNA, 206
Phenylethanolamine, 479, 498
β-phenylethylamine, 189
Phenylketonuria, 491
L-phenyllactate, 445, 446
Phenylpyruvate, 446
Phosphatase, 197
Phosphate
renal failure and, 439
total parenteral nutrition (TPN) with, 359–360
Phosphatidylcholine, 221
6-Phosphoglucodehydrogenase, 353
Phosphohexose isomerase, 353
Phosphorus
injury or infection and, 284

malnutrition and, 352
renal failure and, 439, 441, 444, 468
Phytohemagglutin (PHA), 414
Pituitary, 344
Pneumococcal infection, 414–416
Pokeweed mitogen (PWM), 414
Portacaval shunting, and amino acid transport, 239–251
Potassium
hepatic encephalopathy and, 498
nitrogen balance techniques and, 268, 370
repletion in malnutrition and, 371–372
total parenteral nutrition (TPN) and, 359–360
Prealbumin, 350, 354
Premature infants
cystathionase activity in, 30
nutritional solutions for, 137
Progesterone, 219
Proline
absorption of, 126
nitrogen in urea biosynthesis and, 80
renal failure and, 459–460
ureagenesis and, 84
Proline dipeptidase, 259
Prostacyclins, 206, 207
Prostaglandin E_2 (PGE_2), 206–208
Prostaglandins, and protein breakdown, 206–208
Protein
amino acid composition of typical, 123, 124
amino acids in intake regulation in, 228–234
arteriovenous studies of effects of, 274
enteral nutrition with, 126–134
factors affecting balance of, 202–205
fasting and, 90
fat and carbohydrate as energy sources in malnutrition and, 371
food intake and levels of, 226–227
glucose and insulin and skeletal muscle balance of, 203
intestinal absorption of, 255–261
labile, 363
leucine and skeletal muscle balance of, 203–204
parenteral nutrition with, 124–127, 327–328
pneumococcal infection and, 414–416
regulation of intake of, 227–234
renal failure and, 461
skeletal muscle and balance of, 201–209
stress and, 396–400
weight loss and, 380
Protein anabolism, and trauma patients, 393–394
Protein breakdown
amino acid requirement estimates with, 274, 276, 279
arteriovenous techniques in, 274
branched-chain amino acid solutions and, 424
contractile activity of muscle and, 205
hypercatabolic patient and, 378
leucine and, 151–153, 205–206
prostaglandins and, 206–208
starvation and, 270, 292, 296
traumatic injury and, 387–388
tyrosine metabolism and, 155, 156–157
Protein-calorie malnutrition, *see* Malnutrition
Protein catabolism, 317
amino acids and, 184
enteral nutrition and, 312
hospitalized patient and, 272
insulin and, 185, 186
measurement of, in muscle, 202
stress in burn patients and, 396–400
traumatic injury and, 393
Protein depletion
cardiac mass and function and, 351–352
gastrointestinal tract mass and function and, 350–351
injury or infection and, 379
liver mass and function in, 353–354
renal mass and function with, 352–354
skeletal muscle mass and function and, 349–350
starvation and, 349–355
Protein hydrolysate, 294
Protein intake
aging and, 43–44
alanine and, 25, 436
amino acid metabolism and, 13–26
amino acid requirements by age and, 24
carnitine and, 343–344
dispensable and indispensable amino acids and, 109–110
indispensable amino acid metabolism and, 14–16
leucine catabolism and, 3
leucine infusion studies with, 161–163
liver regulation of amino acids and, 3
nitrogen requirements and, 55–62
renal failure and, 439–440, 452
thermic effect of, 382–383
valine plasma concentration and, 127
Protein loads, in urea production, 81, 83
Protein metabolism
aging and, 37–45
leucine and, 147
meal intake and, 16–18
nutritional state and, 185–186
skeletal muscle and aging and, 44
total parenteral nutrition (TPN) in

cancer and, 429–437
Protein synthesis
albumin mRNA in liver and, 176–177
amino acid concentrations and, 183, 184, 271
amino acid metabolism and, 1–2
amino acid requirements and, 274, 276, 179, 291–292
amino acid solutions and, 304, 305
arteriovenous technique in, 274
blood-brain barrier synthesis and, 250–251
burn patients and, 400
cancer and, 10
dispensable and indispensable amino acids and, 107, 110–112
elderly and, 339
essential amino acids and, 89
glucocorticoids and, 98–99
glutamine and, 172
hepatic utilization of amino acids in cancer and, 212–213, 217
hospitalized patients and, 272
injury or infection and, 266–268, 415
insulin and, 39, 41, 172, 185, 186
leucine and, 159–160, 169–171, 188–190, 205–206
liver amino acid availability and, 167–180
low birth-weight infants and, 321
lysine and, 250–251
measurements of, 167–168
methionine and, 179–180
ribosome cycle subunits and, 168, 174–178
severely ill patients and, 401–405
stressed nutritional states and, 298, 303
trauma and, 393–394
tRNA aminoacylation in liver and, 172–174
tryptophan deficiency and, 172
tyrosine and, 157
ureagenesis and, 78–79
Protein turnover
aging and, 44
amino acid requirement estimates and, 282–283
cancer and, 403–405
compartmentation hypothesis in, 402–403
elderly and, 339
glucagon and, 97
hormonal regulation of leucine metabolism and, 96–97
insulin and, 99
leucine and, 204
muscle and, 215
severely ill patients and, 401–405
skeletal muscle and, 202
weight reduction diets and, 48–53
Proteolytic enzymes, 208, 255
Psychosis, 355
Pulmonary disease, 484
Pulmonary function, and malnutrition, 354, 373
Purines, 468
Pyrmidine, 328
Pyruvate
gluconeogenesis and, 7, 63, 66
glutamate absorption in intestine and, 133
protein synthesis and, 184
Pyruvate dehydrogenase (PDH), 472

Renal disease, 441
Renal failure, 372, 439–448
altered amino acid pools in, 452–462
amino acid analogues in, 439–448
amino acid metabolism in, 7–8, 451–469
amino acid solutions for, 325, 331
chronic, 439–469
citrulline and arginine in, 459
histidine in, 460–461
hydroxyproline and proline in, 459–460
ketoacids and hydroxyacids in, 467–468
leucine and nitrogen balance in, 205
low nitrogen diets in, 462–466
methylhistidine in, 461–462
nutrition support and, 462–468
phenylalanine and tyrosine in, 456–459
protein intake and, 439–440
serine and glycine in, 454–456
Renal insufficiency, 484
Respiration
amino acids and, 383
thermic effect of protein intake and, 383
starvation and, 354–355
Reticular formation, 244
Rhabdomyosarcoma, 431
Ribosomal cycle subunits, in protein synthesis, 168, 174–178

Secretin
food intake and, 234
malnutrition and, 351
Semi-essential amino acids, 106
Semi-indispensable amino acids, 106
Sepsis
alanine tolerance in, 417–420
amino acid metabolism and, 8–9
amino acid requirements and, 284, 296
amino acid solutions and, 298, 299, 300, 301–304
intravenous hyperalimentation (IVH) and, 407
nitrogen balance in, 206, 209

nitrogen losses in, 379
nutritional state of hepatocyte and, 186
protein wasting in, 414
Serine
amino acid degradation and, 113
gluconeogenesis with, 66
protein intake and concentrations of, 110
protein metabolism and, 185
protein synthesis and, 111
renal failure and, 445, 451, 452, 453, 454–456
threonine brain uptake and, 116–117
ureagenesis and, 84
Serotonin
brain function and, 220
carbohydrates and, 232–233
feeding behavior and, 231–233, 235
food consumption and synthesis of, 220–222, 225–226, 231
parenteral nutrition and, 223
synthesis of, 239
uremia and, 467
SGOT, 407
SGPT, 407
Short gut syndrome, 485
Skeletal muscle
aging and amino acid metabolism in, 37, 39, 42, 44
amino acid patterns in, 296–305
amino acid requirement estimates in, 274–275, 279–280
arteriovenous techniques for amino acids in, 274–275
BCKA dehydrogenase and, 191–198
branched-chain amino acid solutions and, 424, 426
leucine and nitrogen balance in, 394
leucine and protein synthesis in, 188–190, 205–206
nitrogen balance and, 381, 394
phenylalanine as marker of catabolism in, 392
prostaglandins in protein breakdown in, 206–208
protein balance in, 201–209
protein depletion in starvation and, 349–350
protein turnover measurement in, 202
repletion of nutrients in, 372
traumatic injury to, 206, 390, 394
tyrosine oxidation in, 279–280
work capacity and, 350
Skin tests, for immune response, 339
Small intestine
amino acid absorption in, 257
glutamine as precursor of alanine in, 4
Sodium bicarbonate, 92
Sodium β-hydroxybutyrate, 91, 92
Somatostatin
food intake and, 234
gluconeogenesis measurement and, 67, 70
leucine metabolism and, 96
protein turnover and, 99
Starvation
amino acid patterns in, 292–295
amino acid solutions in, 304–305
body composition changes with, 348–349
brain mass and function in, 355
cardiac mass and function in, 351–352
effects of, 291, 296
gastrointestinal tract mass and function in, 350–351
hypercatabolic patients and, 378
leucine concentrations in, 270
liver mass and function in, 353–354
organ function and, 347
protein depletion in, 349–353
renal mass and function in, 352–353
respiratory mass and function in, 354–355
skeletal muscle mass and function in, 349–350
work capacity in, 350
see also Fasting; Malnutrition
Steroids, 393
Stomach cancer, 434–436
Stress
amino acid patterns in, 296–305
elderly and, 337
intravenous hyperalimentation (IVH) in, 406–413
operative procedures and, 388
protein dynamics in, 396–400
Substance P, 234
Sucrose, 249
Sulphate, 439
Sulfur
injury or infection and, 283
renal failure and, 439
Sulfur amino acids, 29–34
Sustagen, 312

T4, 432
Taurine
cirrhosis and, 487, 488
methionine as prescursor of, 113
renal failure and, 444, 452, 453
Tetrahydropteridine, 494
Tetrapeptides, 259
Thermal injury, 269, 284
Thermogenesis, with protein intake, 382–383
Threonine, 79, 105
amino acid solutions with, 304
brain uptake and transport systems for,

116–117
estimated requirement of, 23, 55
gluconeogenesis and, 66
as glycine precursor, 113
as indispensable amino acid, 105, 107
indispensable amino acids and concentrations of, 108, 110, 112
injury and infection and, 300
liver regulation of, 3
neurotransmitter precursors and, 233
nutritional state of hepatocyte and, 186
portacaval shunt and transport of, 242
renal failure and, 445, 447, 452, 466
transamination reactions and, 112, 113
transport of, 239
ureagenesis and, 84
L-threonine, and renal failure, 441
Thromboxanes, 206
Total parenteral nutrition (TPN), 359–373
alanine kinetics in cancer patients and, 429–437
cystine and tyrosine requirements for cirrhosis and, 484–496
elderly and, 340
hypercatabolic patients and, 377
insulin levels and, 435–436
nitrogen accretion in cancer patients with, 422–427
nitrogen balance and, 360–362
protein turnover in severely ill patients with, 403–404
thermogenic effects of, 383
see also Parenteral nutrition
Transamination
alanine, 92–93
amino acids in protein synthesis and, 184
branched-chain amino acids and, 89, 112–113, 159
branched-chain ketoacids (BCKA) in, 112–113
insulin in, 186
nitrogen and ammonia and, 79
nutritional state of hepatocyte and, 186, 187
renal failure and, 441, 460
Transferrin
malnutrition and, 350, 354
renal failure and, 441, 442, 445, 448
Transulfuration
cystathionine and, 30, 31, 32–33
methionine-cyst(e)ine relationships in, 29–31
Traumatic injury, 387–394
amino acid flux in, 390–391
amino acid requirements and, 284, 296–305
definition and scope of, 388–389
exogenous amino acids on protein anabolism in, 393–394
liver amino acid homeostasis in, 391
malnutrition and, 484
muscle intracellular free amino acid concentrations in, 392–393
muscle proteolysis regulation in, 392
nitrogen balance in, 206
plasma amino acid concentrations in, 389–390
protein breakdown in, 387–388
skeletal muscle catabolism in, 392
Travasol, 124, 125, 328, 329
Triglycerides, in intravenous hyperalimentation (IVH), 413
Trimethyllysine, 107
Tripeptides
enteral nutrition with, 260–261
transport system for, 257–258
tRNA, in liver protein synthesis, 172–174
Trypsin, 195, 351
Tryptophan
brain function and, 220
cholecystokinin stimulation with, 234, 235
food intake regulation and, 227, 228, 229, 232–234, 235
hepatic encephalopathy in, 478, 479, 480, 481, 482
human requirements for, 55
liver failure and, 318
liver protein synthesis and, 172
liver regulation of, 3
neurotransmitter synthesis and, 225, 231
parenteral nutrition with, 223
portacaval shunt and transport of, 240, 242, 243, 244, 245–248, 250
protein catabolism and, 184
protein intake regulation and, 228
renal failure and, 440, 442, 447, 451, 453, 462, 466, 467
starvation and, 293
transport of, 239, 240
ureagenesis and, 84
Tryptophan hydroxylase, 221
Tryptophan oxygenase, 3
Tryptophan pyrollase, 353
Tumors, *see* Cancer
Tyramine, 239, 240
Tyrosine
alanine nitrogen transport with, 115
amino acid requirement estimates with, 279–280
brain function and, 220
cirrhosis and, 487–488, 489–492, 494, 495
food intake and regulation with, 229, 232
glutamine aminotransferase and, 113
hepatic encephalopathy and, 479, 480, 481, 482, 498

hospitalized patient metabolism of, 272–273
hypercatabolic patients and, 382
as indispensable amino acid, 106
injury and, 266
liver failure and, 317, 318
low birth-weight infants and, 317, 320–321
neurotransmitter synthesis and, 222, 223, 225, 231
parenteral nutrition with, 220, 223, 329, 484
phenylalanine and, 113, 155–158, 392
portacaval shunt and transport of, 240, 243, 244, 245–248, 250
protein breakdown and, 155, 156–157
protein catabolism and, 184
protein turnover in skeletal muscle and, 202
renal failure and, 445, 447, 451, 452, 453, 456–459, 462, 466, 467
starvation and, 292, 293
ureagenesis and, 84
whole body protein turnover and, 282–283
L-tyrosine
phenylalanine and, 155
renal failure and, 441
Tyrosine aminotransferase, 456
Tryosine hydroxylase, 221, 222
Tyrosine transaminase, 353

Ulcers, 351, 389
Uranyl nitrate, 453
Urea
alanine-N formation with, 25–26
amino acid requirement estimates with, 277, 278
dispensable and indispensable amino acids and, 108, 115
hemodialysis and, 80
hepatic utilization of amino acids in cancer and, 212, 214
malnutrition and, 352
nitrogen sources and regulation of, 77–84
starvation and, 378
Ureagenesis, 77–84
acid-base balance in, 77–78
carbamoyl phosphate synthetase (CPS) and, 81–84
impairment of, 84
nitrogen and, 78–80
ornithine and, 83
protein synthesis and, 78–79
precursors of nitrogen in, 80
regulation of, 81–84
total parenteral nutrition (TPN) with, 436
Uremia, *see* Renal failure

Vagotomy, 389
Valine
adipose tissue oxidation of, 147, 153
amino acid requirements and, 20–23
amino acid solutions with, 304
branched-chain α-ketoacids (BCKA) and catabolism of, 191
estimated requirements of, 23, 55
food intake and levels of, 227, 229
glycine, aspartate, and glutamate plasma concentrations and, 130
hepatic encephalopathy and, 480, 497
hepatocyte protein with, 184
high performance liquid chromatography (HPLC) for quantitation of, 102, 104
hospitalized patient metabolism of, 273, 274
in vitro branched-chain amino acid interaction in, 151–152
leucine interactions with, 147–151
muscle amino acid metabolism and, 159
neurotransmitter synthesis and, 231
nutritional state of hepatocyte and, 184, 185, 186, 187
portacaval shunt and transport of, 242
protein and plasma concentrations of, 127
protein synthesis and, 89, 185
renal failure and, 441, 445, 446, 447, 451, 452, 453, 462, 463, 466, 467
starvation and, 293, 294
stressed nutritional state and, 298, 304
transport of, 239
ureagenesis and, 84
valine turnover and oxidation and intake of, 149, 150
Viral hepatitis, 480
Vitamin B_6, 462
Vitamin B_{12}, 351
Vivonex, 260, 261, 310, 432

Weight loss
malignancy and, 429
protein and, 380
see also Body weight
Weight reduction diets, 48–53
Work capacity, and starvation, 350

Xanthine oxidase, 353
D-xylose, 351

Zinc, 83

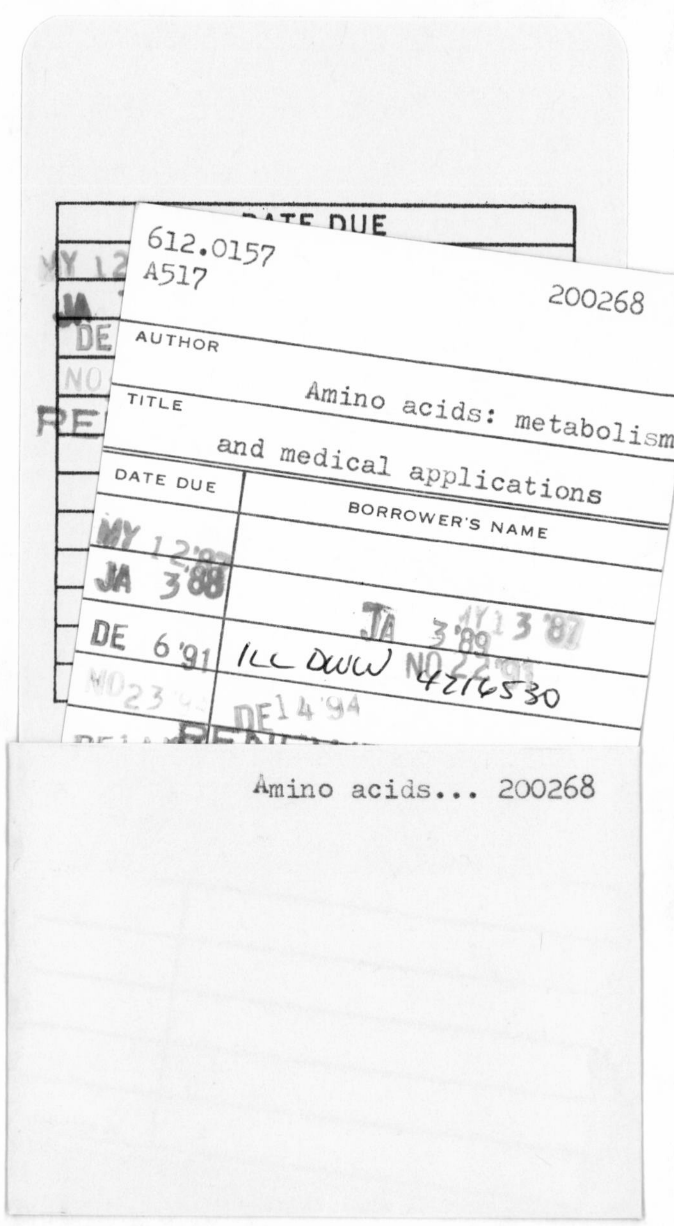
DATE DUE
612.0157
A517
200268
AUTHOR
TITLE
Amino acids: metabolism
and medical applications
DATE DUE
BORROWER'S NAME
MY 12 '87
JA 3 '88
DE 6 '91
ILL DWW
4216530
Amino acids... 200268